Don't Forget Your Online Access to ExpertConsult.com

Mobile. Searchable. Expandable.

ACCESS it on any Internet-ready device

SEARCH all Expert Consult titles you own

LINK to PubMed abstracts

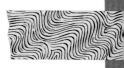
ExpertConsult.com

Davidson's
Essentials of
Medicine

Davidson's Essentials of

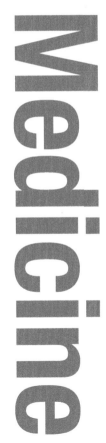

3rd Edition

Edited by

J. Alastair Innes
PhD FRCP (Ed)
Consultant Physician and Honorary Reader
in Respiratory Medicine
Western General Hospital
Edinburgh, United Kingdom

**For additional online content
visit** StudentConsult.com

ELSEVIER   Edinburgh London New York Oxford Philadelphia St Louis Sydney 2021

First edition 2009
Second edition 2016
Third edition 2020

Notices

Practitioners and researchers must always rely on their own experience and knowledge in evaluating and using any information, methods, compounds or experiments described herein. Because of rapid advances in the medical sciences, in particular, independent verification of diagnoses and drug dosages should be made. To the fullest extent of the law, no responsibility is assumed by Elsevier, authors, editors or contributors for any injury and/or damage to persons or property as a matter of products liability, negligence or otherwise, or from any use or operation of any methods, products, instructions, or ideas contained in the material herein.

ISBN: 978-0-7020-7875-0
978-0-7020-7876-7

Executive Content Strategist: Laurence Hunter
Content Development Specialist: Carole McMurray
Content Coordinator: Susan Jansons
Project Manager: Louisa Talbott/Anne Collett
Design: Brian Salisbury
Illustration Manager: Paula Catalano
Illustrator: TNQ
Marketing Manager: Deborah Watkins

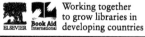

Working together
to grow libraries in
developing countries

www.elsevier.com • www.bookaid.org

Contents

Sir Stanley Davidson (1894–1981)

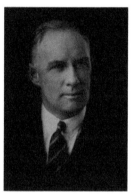

Davidson's Principles and Practice of Medicine was the brainchild of one of the great Professors of Medicine of the 20th century. Stanley Davidson was born in Sri Lanka and began his medical undergraduate training at Trinity College, Cambridge; this was interrupted by World War I and later resumed in Edinburgh. He was seriously wounded in battle, and the carnage and shocking waste of young life that he encountered at that time had a profound effect on his subsequent attitudes and values.

In 1930 Stanley Davidson was appointed Professor of Medicine at the University of Aberdeen, one of the first full-time Chairs of Medicine anywhere and the first in Scotland. In 1938 he took up the Chair of Medicine at Edinburgh and was to remain in this post until retirement in 1959. He was a renowned educator and a particularly gifted teacher at the bedside, where he taught that everything had to be questioned and explained. He himself gave most of the systematic lectures in Medicine, which were made available as typewritten notes that emphasised the essentials and far surpassed any textbook available at the time.

Principles and Practice of Medicine was conceived in the late 1940s with its origins in those lecture notes. The first edition, published in 1952, was a masterpiece of clarity and uniformity of style. It was of modest size and price, but sufficiently comprehensive and up to date to provide students with the main elements of sound medical practice. Although the format and presentation have seen many changes in 21 subsequent editions, Sir Stanley's original vision and objectives remain. More than half a century after its first publication, his book continues to inform and educate students, doctors and health professionals all over the world.

Preface

In the 67 years since *Davidson's Principles and Practice of Medicine* was first published, the profusion of molecular and genetic knowledge about disease, and of the number of diagnostic tests and possible treatments, has posed an increasing challenge to those seeking to summarise clinical medicine in a single textbook. An inevitable consequence has been a parallel growth in the physical size of all the major textbooks, including *Davidson*.

Davidson's Essentials of Medicine seeks to complement the parent volume by helping those who also need portable information to study on the move – whether commuting, travelling between training sites or during remote attachments and electives. In this third edition, the entire content of *Essentials* has been comprehensively revised and updated in line with the core content from *Davidson*, while retaining a size which can easily accompany readers on their travels. Although the text is concise, every effort has been made to maximise readability and to avoid dry and unmemorable lists; the intention has been to produce a genuine miniature textbook. The text draws directly on the enormous depth and breadth of experience of the parent *Davidson* writing team and presents the essential elements in a format to suit hand luggage. Key *Davidson* illustrations have been adapted and retained, and new sections include chapters on Clinical therapeutics and prescribing, Acute medicine and critical care, Medical ophthalmology and Oncology.

In an age when on-line information is ever more accessible to doctors in training, most still agree that there is no substitute for the physical page when systematic study is needed. With this book, we hope that the proven value of the parent *Davidson* can be augmented by making the essential elements accessible while on the move.

J.A.I.
Edinburgh 2020

Acknowledgements

I am very grateful to the chapter authors of *Davidson's Principles and Practice of Medicine*, without whom this project would have been impossible. I would also like to acknowledge the invaluable contribution of the team of assistant editors who helped to sift and select the relevant information during preparation of the first edition: Kenneth Baillie, Sunil Adwani, Donald Noble, Sarah Walsh, Nazir Lone, Jehangir Din, Neeraj Dhaun and Alan Japp.

I remain indebted to Nicki Colledge and Brian Walker for inviting me to help create *Essentials* and for their support and guidance in the early stages. Thanks also to Laurence Hunter, Carole McMurray, Louisa Talbott and Anne Collett at Elsevier for their support and meticulous attention to detail.

Finally, I would like to thank Hester and all my family for their encouragement and support during the preparation of this book, and to dedicate it to the memory of my father, James Innes, who worked with Stanley Davidson on the early editions of *Davidson's Principles and Practice of Medicine*.

J.A.I.
Edinburgh 2020

Contributors to *Davidson's Principles and Practice of Medicine*, 23rd Edition

The core of this book is based on the contents of *Davidson's Principles and Practice of Medicine*, with material extracted and re-edited to make a uniform presentation to suit the format of this book. Although some chapters and topics have, by necessity, been cut or substantially edited, contributors of all chapters drawn upon have been acknowledged here in recognition of their input into the totality of the parent textbook.

Brian J Angus BSc, DTM&H, FRCP, MD, FFTM(Glas)
Associate Professor, Nuffield Department of Medicine, University of Oxford, UK

Quentin M Anstee BSc(Hons), PhD, MRCP
Senior Lecturer, Institute of Cellular Medicine, Newcastle University, Newcastle upon Tyne; Honorary Consultant Hepatologist, Freeman Hospital, Newcastle upon Tyne, UK

Leslie Burnett MBBS, PhD, FRCPA, FHGSA
Medical Director, Garvan Institute of Medical Research, Sydney; Conjoint Professor, St Vincent's Clinical School, Faculty of Medicine, University of New South Wales; Honorary Professor in Pathology and Genetic Medicine, Faculty of Medicine, Sydney Medical School; Honorary Associate of the School of Information Technologies, University of Sydney, Australia

Mark Byers *OBE,* MRCGP, MCEM, MFSEM, DA(UK)
General Practitioner, Ministry of Defence, Royal Centre for Defence Medicine, University Hospitals Birmingham, UK

Harry Campbell MD, FRCPE, FFPH, FRSE
Professor of Genetic Epidemiology and Public Health, Centre for Global Health Research, Usher Institute of Population Health Sciences and Informatics, University of Edinburgh, UK

Gavin PR Clunie BSc, MD, FRCP
Consultant Rheumatologist and Metabolic Bone Physician, Cambridge University Hospitals NHS Foundation Trust, Addenbrooke's Hospital, Cambridge, UK

Lesley A Colvin BSc, FRCA, PhD, FRCPE, FFPMRCA
Consultant, Department of Anaesthesia, Critical Care and Pain Medicine, Western General Hospital, Edinburgh; Honorary Professor in Anaesthesia and Pain Medicine, University of Edinburgh, UK

Bryan Conway MB, MRCP, PhD
Senior Lecturer, Centre for Cardiovascular Science, University of Edinburgh; Honorary Consultant Nephrologist, Royal Infirmary of Edinburgh, UK

Nicola Cooper FAcadMEd, FRCPE, FRACP
Consultant Physician, Derby Teaching Hospitals NHS Foundation Trust, Derby; Honorary Clinical Associate Professor, Division of Medical Sciences and Graduate Entry Medicine, University of Nottingham, UK

Alison L Cracknell FRCP
Consultant, Medicine for Older People, Leeds Teaching Hospitals NHS Trust, Leeds; Honorary Clinical Associate Professor, University of Leeds, UK

Dominic J Culligan BSc, MD, FRCP, FRCPath
Consultant Haematologist, Aberdeen Royal Infirmary, Aberdeen; Honorary Senior Lecturer, University of Aberdeen, UK

Graham G Dark FRCP, FHEA
Senior Lecturer in Medical Oncology and Cancer Education, Newcastle University, Newcastle upon Tyne, UK

Richard J Davenport DM, FRCPE, BMedSci
Consultant Neurologist, Royal Infirmary of Edinburgh and Western General Hospital, Edinburgh; Honorary Senior Lecturer, University of Edinburgh, UK

David H Dockrell MD, FRCPI, FRCPG, FACP
Professor of Infection Medicine, Medical Research Council/University of Edinburgh Centre for Inflammation Research, University of Edinburgh, UK

Emad El-Omar BSc(Hons), MD(Hons), FRCPE, FRSE
Professor of Medicine, St George and Sutherland Clinical School, University of New South Wales, Sydney, Australia

Marie Fallon MD, FRCP
St Columba's Hospice Chair of Palliative Medicine, University of Edinburgh, UK

David R FitzPatrick MD, FRCPE
Professor, Medical Research Council Human Genetics Unit, Institute of Genetics and Molecular Medicine, University of Edinburgh, UK

Neil R Grubb MD, FRCP
Consultant in Cardiology, Royal Infirmary of Edinburgh; Honorary Senior Lecturer in Cardiovascular Sciences, University of Edinburgh, UK

Sally H Ibbotson BSc(Hons), MD(with commendation), FRCPE
Professor of Dermatology, University of Dundee, UK

J Alastair Innes BSc, PhD, FRCPE
Consultant, Respiratory Unit, Western General Hospital, Edinburgh; Honorary Reader in Respiratory Medicine, University of Edinburgh, UK

Sara J Jenks BSc(Hons), MRCP, FRCPath
Consultant in Metabolic Medicine, Department of Clinical Biochemistry, Royal Infirmary of Edinburgh, UK

Sarah L Johnston FCRP, FRCPath
Consultant Immunologist, Department of Immunology and Immunogenetics, North Bristol NHS Trust, Bristol, UK

David EJ Jones MA, BM, PhD, FRCP
Professor of Liver Immunology, Institute of Cellular Medicine, Newcastle University, Newcastle upon Tyne; Consultant Hepatologist, Freeman Hospital, Newcastle upon Tyne, UK

Peter Langhorne PhD, FRCPG
Professor of Stroke Care, Institute of Cardiovascular and Medical Sciences, University of Glasgow, UK

Stephen M Lawrie MD(Hons), FRCPsych, FRCPE(Hon)
Professor of Psychiatry, University of Edinburgh, UK

John Paul Leach MD, FRCPG, FRCPE
Consultant Neurologist, Institute of Neuroscience, Southern General Hospital, Glasgow; Head of Undergraduate Medicine and Honorary Associate Clinical Professor, University of Glasgow, UK

Gary Maartens MBChB, FCP(SA), MMed
Professor of Medicine, University of Cape Town, South Africa

Lucy Mackillop BM, MA(Oxon), FRCP
Consultant Obstetric Physician, Oxford University Hospitals NHS Foundation Trust, Oxford; Honorary Senior Clinical Lecturer, Nuffield Department of Obstetrics and Gynaecology, University of Oxford, UK

Michael J MacMahon FRCA, FICM, EDIC
Consultant in Anaesthesia and Intensive Care, Victoria Hospital, Kirkcaldy, UK

Rebecca Mann BMedSci MRCP, FRCPCh
Consultant Paediatrician, Taunton and Somerset NHS Foundation Trust, Taunton, UK

Lynn M Manson MD, FRCP, FRCPath
Consultant Haematologist, Scottish National Blood Transfusion Service, Edinburgh; Honorary Clinical Senior Lecturer, Department of Transfusion Medicine, Royal Infirmary of Edinburgh, UK

Sara E Marshall FRCP, FRCPath, PhD
Professor of Clinical Immunology, Medical Research Institute, University of Dundee, UK

Amanda Mather MBBS, FRACP, PhD
Renal Staff Specialist, Department of Renal Medicine, Royal North Shore Hospital, Sydney; Conjoint Senior Lecturer, Faculty of Medicine, University of Sydney, Australia

Simon R Maxwell BSc, MD, PhD, FRCP, FRCPE, FHEA
Professor of Pharmacology, Clinical Pharmacology Unit, University of Edinburgh, UK

David A McAllister MSc, MD, MRCP, MFPH
Wellcome Trust Intermediate Clinical Fellow and Beit Fellow, Senior Clinical Lecturer in Epidemiology, and Honorary Consultant in Public Health Medicine, University of Glasgow, UK

Rory J McCrimmon MD, FRCPE
Reader, Medical Research Institute, University of Dundee, UK

Mairi McLean MRCP, PhD
Senior Clinical Lecturer in Gastroenterology, School of Medicine, Medical Sciences and Nutrition, University of Aberdeen; Honorary Consultant Gastroenterologist, Aberdeen Royal Infirmary, UK

Francesca EM Neuberger MRCP(UK)
Consultant Physician in Acute Medicine and Obstetric Medicine, Southmead Hospital, Bristol, UK

David E Newby BA, BSc(Hons), PhD, BM DM DSc, FMedSci, FRSE, FESC, FACC
British Heart Foundation John Wheatley Professor of Cardiology, British Heart Foundation Centre for Cardiovascular Science, University of Edinburgh, UK

John DC Newell-Price MA, PhD, FRCP
Reader in Endocrinology, Department of Human Metabolism, University of Sheffield, UK

John Olson MD, FRPCE, FRCOphth
Consultant Ophthalmic Physician, Aberdeen Royal Infirmary; Honorary Reader, University of Aberdeen, UK

Ewan R Pearson PhD, FRCPE
Clinical Reader, Medical Research Institute, University of Dundee, UK

Paul J Phelan BAO, MD, FRCPE
Consultant Nephrologist and Renal Transplant Physician, Royal Infirmary of Edinburgh; Honorary Senior Lecturer, University of Edinburgh, UK

Stuart H Ralston MRCP, FMedSci, FRSE
Arthritis Research UK Professor of Rheumatology, University of Edinburgh; Honorary Consultant Rheumatologist, Western General Hospital, Edinburgh, UK

Peter T Reid MD, FRCPE
Consultant Physician, Respiratory Medicine, Lothian University Hospitals, Edinburgh, UK

Jonathan AT Sandoe PhD, FRCPath
Associate Clinical Professor, University of Leeds, UK

Gordon R Scott BSc, FRCP
Consultant in Genitourinary Medicine, Chalmers Sexual Health Centre, Edinburgh, UK

Alan G Shand MD, FRCPE
Consultant Gastroenterologist, Western General Hospital, Edinburgh, UK

Robby M Steel MA, MD, FRCPsych
Consultant Liaison Psychiatrist, Department of Psychological Medicine, Royal Infirmary of Edinburgh; Honorary (Clinical) Senior Lecturer, Department of Psychiatry, University of Edinburgh, UK

Grant D Stewart BSc(Hons), FRCSE(Urol), PhD
University Lecturer in Urological Surgery, Academic Urology Group, University of Cambridge; Honorary Consultant Urological Surgeon, Department of Urology, Addenbrooke's Hospital, Cambridge; Honorary Senior Clinical Lecturer, University of Edinburgh, UK

Peter Stewart MBBS, FRACP, FRCPA, MBA
Associate Professor in Chemical Pathology, University of Sydney; Area Director of Clinical Biochemistry and Head of the Biochemistry Department, Royal Prince Alfred and Liverpool Hospitals, Sydney, Australia

Mark WJ Strachan BSc(Hons), MD, FRCPE
Consultant Endocrinologist, Metabolic Unit, Western General Hospital, Edinburgh; Honorary Professor, University of Edinburgh, UK

David R Sullivan MBBS, FRACP, FRCPA, FCSANZ
Clinical Associate Professor, Faculty of Medicine, University of Sydney; Physician and Chemical Pathologist, Department of Clinical Biochemistry Royal Prince Alfred Hospital, Sydney, Australia

Shyam Sundar MD, FRCP(London), FAMS, FNASc, FASc, FNA
Professor of Medicine, Institute of Medical Sciences, Banaras Hindu University, Varanasi, India

Victoria R Tallentire BSc(Hons), DipMedEd, MRCP, MD
Consultant Physician, Western General Hospital, Edinburgh; Honorary Senior Lecturer, University of Edinburgh, UK

Katrina Tatton-Brown BA, MD, FRCP(Paeds)
Consultant and Reader in Clinical Genetics and Genomic Education, South West Thames Regional Genetics Service, St George's Universities Hospital NHS Foundation Trust, London, UK

Simon HL Thomas MD, FRCP, FRCPE
Professor of Cellular Medicine, Institute of Cellular Medicine, Newcastle University, Newcastle upon Tyne, UK

Henry G Watson MD, FRCPE, FRCPath
Consultant Haematologist, Aberdeen Royal Infirmary, UK

Julian White MB, BS, MD, FACTM
Head of Toxinology, Women's and Children's Hospital, North Adelaide; Professor, University of Adelaide, Australia

John PH Wilding DM, FRCP
Professor of Medicine, Obesity and Endocrinology, University of Liverpool, UK

Miles D Witham PhD, FRCPE
Clinical Senior Lecturer in Ageing and Health, University of Dundee, UK

List of abbreviations

ABGs	arterial blood gases	**CRP**	C-reactive protein
ACE	angiotensin-converting enzyme	**CSF**	cerebrospinal fluid
ACTH	adrenocorticotrophic hormone	**CT**	computed tomography/tomogram
ADH	antidiuretic hormone	**CVP**	central venous pressure
AIDS	acquired immuno-deficiency syndrome	**CXR**	chest X-ray
ANA	antinuclear antibody	**DEXA**	dual-energy X-ray absorptiometry
ANCA	antineutrophil cytoplasmic autoantibody	**DIC**	disseminated intra-vascular coagulation
ANF	antinuclear factor	**DIDMOAD**	diabetes insipidus, diabetes mellitus, optic atrophy, deafness
ANP	atrial natriuretic peptide		
APECED	Autoimmune polyendocrinopathy-candidiasis-ectodermal dystrophy	**dsDNA**	double-stranded deoxyribonucleic acid
		DVT	deep venous thrombosis
APS	Antiphospholipid syndrome	**ECG**	electrocardiography/electrocardiogram
APTT	activated partial thromboplastin time	**ELISA**	enzyme-linked immunosorbent assay
ARDS	acute respiratory distress syndrome	**ERCP**	endoscopic retrograde cholangiopancreat-ography
ASO	antistreptolysin O		
AST	aspartate aminotransferase	**ESR**	erythrocyte sedimenta-tion rate
AXR	abdominal X-ray	**FBC**	full blood count
BCG	Calmette–Guérin bacillus	**FDA**	Food and Drug Admin-istration
BMI	body mass index	**FEV$_1$/FVC**	forced expiratory volume in 1 sec/forced vital capacity
BP	blood pressure		
CK	creatine kinase		
CNS	central nervous system	**FFP**	fresh frozen plasma
CPAP	continuous positive airways pressure	**5-HT**	5-hydroxytryptamine; serotonin
CRH	corticotrophin-releasing hormone	**FOB**	faecal occult blood
		GI	gastrointestinal

GMC	General Medical Council	**MSU**	mid-stream sample of urine
GU	genitourinary	**NG**	nasogastric
HDL	high-density lipoprotein	**NICE**	National Institute for Health and Care Excellence
HDU	high-dependency unit		
HIV	human immuno-deficiency virus	**NIV**	non-invasive ventilation
HLA	human leucocyte antigen	**NSAID**	non-steroidal anti-inflammatory drug
HRT	hormone replacement therapy	**PA**	postero-anterior
ICU	intensive care unit	**PCR**	polymerase chain reaction
IL	interleukin		
IM	intramuscular	**PE**	pulmonary embolism
INR	International Normalised Ratio	**PET**	positron emission tomography
IV	intravenous	**PTH**	parathyroid hormone
IVU	intravenous urogram/ urography	**RBC**	red blood count
		RCT	randomised controlled clinical trial
JVP	jugular venous pressure	**SPECT**	single-photon emission computed tomography
LDH	lactate dehydrogenase		
LDL	low-density lipoprotein		
LFTs	liver function tests	**STI**	sexually transmitted infection
MRA	magnetic resonance angiography	**TB**	tuberculosis
MRC	Medical Research Council	**TFTs**	thyroid function tests
		TNF	tumour necrosis factor
MRCP	magnetic resonance cholangiopancreat-ography	**U&Es**	urea and electrolytes
		USS	ultrasound scan
		VTE	venous thromboembolism
MRI	magnetic resonance imaging	**WBC/WCC**	white blood/cell count
MRSA	meticillin-resistant *Staphylococcus aureus*	**WHO**	World Health Organization

Picture credits

We are grateful to the following individuals and organisations for permission to reproduce the figures and boxes listed below.

Chapter 5
Clinical examination of patients with infectious disease (p. 99)
Splinter haemorrhages inset: Dr Nick Beeching, Royal Liverpool University; Roth's spots inset: Prof. Ian Rennie, Royal Hallamshire Hospital, Sheffield. **Fig. 5.11** Malaria retinopathy inset: Dr Nicholas Beare, Royal Liverpool University Hospital; blood films insets, *P. vivax* and *P. falciparum*: Dr Kamolrat Silamut, Mahidol Oxford Research Unit, Bangkok, Thailand. **Box 5.20** WHO. Severe falciparum malaria. In: Severe and complicated malaria. 3rd edn. Trans Roy Soc Trop Med Hyg 2000; 94 (suppl. 1): S1–41

Chapter 6
Fig. 6.3 Adapted from Flenley D. Lancet 1971; 1: 1921

Chapter 7
Clinical examination of the kidney and urinary tract (p. 207)

Chapter 8
Clinical examination of the cardiovascular system (p. 249) Splinter haemorrhage, jugular venous pulse, malar flush and tendon xanthomas insets: Newby D, Grubb N. Cardiology: An Illustrated Colour Text. Edinburgh: Churchill Livingstone; 2005. **Fig. 8.4** Resuscitation Council (UK). **Fig. 8.18** NICE Clinical Guideline 127, Hypertension; August 2011) **Box 8.7** European Society of Cardiology Clinical Practice Guidelines: Atrial Fibrillation (Management of) 2010 and Focused Update (2012). Eur Heart J 2012; 33: 2719–2747

Chapter 9
Clinical examination of the respiratory system (p. 311) Idiopathic kyphoscoliosis inset: Dr I. Smith, Papworth Hospital, Cambridge. **Fig. 9.8** Adapted from Detterbeck FC, Boffa DJ, Tanoue LT. The new lung cancer staging system. Chest 2009; 136:260–271). **Fig. 9.9** Johnson N McL. Respiratory Medicine. Oxford: Blackwell Science; 1986

Chapter 10
Fig. 10.3 Toxic multinodular goitre inset: Dr P.L. Padfield, Western General Hospital, Edinburgh

Chapter 12
Fig. 12.3 Hayes P, Simpson K. Gastroenterology and Liver Disease. Edinburgh: Churchill Livingstone; 1995

Chapter 13
Clinical examination of the abdomen for liver and biliary disease (p. 509) Spider naevi inset: Hayes P, Simpson K. Gastroenterology and liver disease. Edinburgh: Churchill Livingstone; 1995. Aspiration inset: Strachan M. Davidson's clinical cases. Edinburgh: Churchill Livingstone; 2008 (Fig. 65.1). Palmar erythema inset: Martin P. Approach to the patient with liver disease. In: Gold L and Schafter AI. Goldman's Cecil Medicine. 24th edn. Philadelphia: WB Saunders; 2012 (Fig. 1148-2, p. 954)

Chapter 14
Blood disease Box 14.6 From Wells PS. New Engl J Med 2003; 349: 1227; copyright © 2003 Massachusetts Medical Society

Chapter 16
Fig. 16.7 Courtesy of Dr B Cullen. **Fig. 16.10** Courtesy of Dr A. Farrell and Professor J. Wardlaw

Chapter 18
Skin disease Fig. 18.13 White GM, Cox NH. Diseases of the skin. London: Mosby; 2000; copyright Elsevier

Chapter 19
Comprehensive geriatric assessment (p. 775) Wasted hand and kyphosis insets: Afzal Mir M. Atlas of Clinical Diagnosis. 2nd edn. Edinburgh: Saunders; 2003. **Box 19.5** Hodkinson HM, Evaluation of a mental test score for assessment of mental impairment in the elderly Age and Ageing 1972; 1(4): 233–238

Chapter 20
Clinical examination of the cancer patient (p. 785)

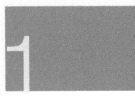

Clinical decision making

How doctors think, reason and make decisions is arguably their most critical skill. Knowledge is necessary, but not sufficient, for good safe care.

The problem of diagnostic error

It is estimated that the diagnosis is wrong in 10% to 15% of cases in many specialties, causing much preventable morbidity.

Diagnostic error has been defined as 'a situation in which the clinician has all the information necessary to make the diagnosis but then makes the wrong diagnosis'. Root causes include:

- No fault—for example, rare or atypical presentation.
- System error—for example, results not available, poorly trained staff.
- Human cognitive error—for example, inadequate data gathering, errors in reasoning.

Clinical reasoning

'Clinical reasoning' describes the thinking and decision-making processes associated with clinical practice. Errors may occur because of lack of knowledge, misinterpretation of diagnostic tests and cognitive bias (e.g. accepting another's diagnosis unquestioningly). Other key elements include patient-centred evidence-based medicine and shared decision making with patients and/or carers.

Clinical skills and decision making

Despite diagnostic technology, the history remains crucial; studies show that physicians make a diagnosis in 70% to 90% of cases from the history alone.

Additional knowledge is needed for correct interpretation of the history and examination. For example, students learn that meningitis presents with headache, fever and meningism (photophobia, nuchal rigidity). However, the frequency with which patients present with particular features and the diagnostic weight of each feature are important in clinical reasoning.

The likelihood ratio (LR) is the probability of a finding in someone with a disease (judged by a diagnostic standard, e.g. lumbar puncture in meningism) divided by the probability of that finding in someone without disease.

An LR greater than 1 increases the probability of disease; an LR of less than 1 reduces that probability. For example, in a person presenting with headache and fever, the clinical finding of nuchal rigidity (neck stiffness) may carry little diagnostic weight, because many patients with meningitis do not have classical signs of meningism (LR of around 1).

LRs do not determine the prior probability of disease, only how a single clinical finding changes it. Clinicians have to take all available information from the history and physical examination into account. If the prior probability is high, a clinical finding with an LR of 1 does not change this.

'Evidence-based history and examination' is a term used to describe how clinicians incorporate knowledge about the prevalence and diagnostic weight of clinical findings into the history and physical examination.

Use and interpretation of diagnostic tests

No diagnostic test is perfect. To correctly interpret test results requires understanding of the following factors:

Normal values

Many quantitative measurements in populations have a Gaussian or 'normal' distribution, in which the normal range is defined as that which includes 95% of the population (± 2 SD around the mean). Because 2.5% of the normal population will be above, and 2.5% below the range, it is better described as the 'reference range' rather than the 'normal range'.

Results in abnormal populations also have a Gaussian distribution, with a different mean and standard deviation, although sometimes there is overlap with the reference range. The greater the difference between the result and the limits of the reference range, the higher the chance of disease.

Clinical context can affect interpretation. For example, a normal $PaCO_2$ in the context of a severe asthma attack indicates life-threatening asthma. A low ferritin level in a young menstruating woman is not considered to be pathological.

Factors other than disease that influence results

These include:
• age • ethnicity • pregnancy • sex • technical factors (e.g., high K^+ in haemolysed sample).

Operating characteristics

Tests may be affected or rendered nondiagnostic by: • Patient motivation and technique (e.g. spirometry) • Operator skill • Patient's body habitus and clinical state (e.g. echocardiography) • Paroxysmal illness (e.g. normal EEG between fits in epilepsy) • The incidental discovery of a benign abnormality

Test results should always be interpreted in the light of the patient's history and examination.

i 1.1 Sensitivity and specificity		
	Disease	**No disease**
Positive test	A (True positive)	B (False positive)
Negative test	C (False negative)	D (True negative)

Sensitivity = A/(A+C) × 100
Specificity = D/(D+B) × 100

Sensitivity and specificity

Sensitivity is the ability to detect true positives; specificity is the ability to detect true negatives. Even a very good test with 95% sensitivity will miss 1 in 20 people with the disease. Every test therefore has 'false positives' and 'false negatives' (Box 1.1).

A very sensitive test detects most cases of disease but generates abnormal findings in healthy people. A negative result reliably excludes disease, but a positive result does not mean disease is present. Conversely, a very specific test may miss significant pathology, but can firmly establish the diagnosis if positive. Clinicians need to know the sensitivity and specificity of the tests they use.

In choosing how a test is used, there is a trade-off between sensitivity and specificity. This is illustrated by the receiver operating characteristic curve of the test (Fig. 1.1).

An extremely important concept is this: the probability that a person has a disease depends on both the pretest probability and the sensitivity and specificity of the test. In a patient whose history suggests a high pretest probability of disease, a normal test result does not exclude the condition, but in a low-probability patient, it makes it very unlikely. This principle is illustrated in Fig. 1.2.

Prevalence of disease

The prevalence of disease in the patient's population subgroup should inform the doctor's estimate of pretest probability. Prevalence also influences the chance that a positive test result indicates disease. Consider a test with a false-positive rate of 5% for a disease whose prevalence is 1:1000. If 1000 people are tested, there will be 51 positive results: 50 false positives and one true positive. The chance that a person found to have a positive result actually has the disease is only 1/51, or 2%.

Predictive values combine sensitivity, specificity and prevalence, allowing doctors to address the question: 'What is the probability that a person with a positive test actually has the disease?'. This is illustrated in Box 1.2.

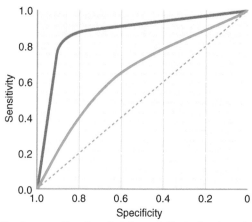

Fig. 1.1 Receiver operating characteristic graph illustrating the trade-off between sensitivity and specificity for a given test. The curve is generated by 'adjusting' the cut-off values defining normal and abnormal results, calculating the effect on sensitivity and specificity and then plotting these against each other. The closer the curve lies to the top left-hand corner, the more useful the test. The red line illustrates a test with useful discriminant value, and the green line illustrates a less useful, poorly discriminant test.

Dealing with uncertainty

Clinicians must frequently deal with uncertainty. By expressing uncertainty as probability, new information from diagnostic tests can be incorporated more accurately. However, intuition and subjective estimates of probability can be unreliable.

Knowing the patient's true state is often unnecessary in clinical decision making. The requirement for diagnostic certainty depends on the penalty for being wrong. Different situations require different levels of certainty before starting treatment. How we communicate uncertainty to patients will be discussed later in this chapter (p. 8).

The treatment threshold combines factors such as the risks of the test and the risks versus benefits of treatment. A less effective or high risk test increases the treatment threshold.

Cognitive biases

Human thinking and decision making are prone to error. Cognitive biases are subconscious errors that lead to inaccurate judgement and illogical interpretation of information.

Humans have two distinct types of processes when it comes to thinking and decision making: type 1 and type 2 thinking.

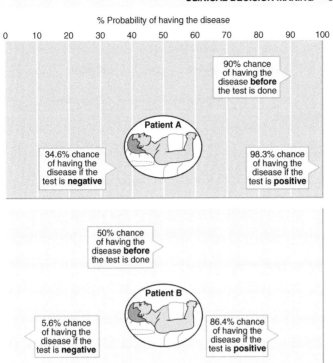

% Probability of having the disease

90% chance of having the disease **before** the test is done

Patient A

34.6% chance of having the disease if the test is **negative**

98.3% chance of having the disease if the test is **positive**

50% chance of having the disease **before** the test is done

Patient B

5.6% chance of having the disease if the test is **negative**

86.4% chance of having the disease if the test is **positive**

Fig. 1.2 The interpretation of a test result depends on the probability of the disease before the test is carried out. In the example shown, the test being carried out has a sensitivity of 95% and a specificity of 85%. Patient A has very characteristic clinical findings, which make the pretest probability of the condition for which the test is being used very high—estimated as 90%. Patient B has more equivocal findings, such that the pretest probability is estimated as only 50%. If the result in Patient A is negative, there is still a significant chance that he has the condition for which he is being tested; in Patient B, however, a negative result makes the diagnosis very unlikely.

Type 1 and type 2 thinking

Cognitive psychology identifies two distinct processes when it comes to decision making: intuitive (type 1) and analytical (type 2). This has been termed 'dual process theory'. Box 1.3 explains this in more detail.

Psychologists estimate that we spend 95% of our daily lives engaged in type 1 thinking—the intuitive, fast, subconscious mode of decision making. Learning to drive involves moving from the deliberate, conscious, slow and effortful first lesson to the automatic, fast and effortless process of an experienced driver. The same applies to medical practice, and intuitive thinking is highly efficient in many circumstances; however, in others it is prone to error.

1.2 Predictive values: 'What is the probability that a person with a positive test actually has the disease?'

	Disease	No disease
Positive test	A (True positive)	B (False positive)
Negative test	C (False negative)	D (True negative)

Positive predictive value = A/(A+B) × 100
Negative predictive value = D/(D+C) × 100

1.3 Type 1 and type 2 thinking

Type 1	Type 2
Intuitive, heuristic (pattern recognition)	Analytical, systematic
Automatic, subconscious	Deliberate, conscious
Fast, effortless	Slow, effortful
Low/variable reliability	High/consistent reliability
Vulnerable to error	Less prone to error
Highly affected by context	Less affected by context
High emotional involvement	Low emotional involvement
Low scientific rigour	High scientific rigour

Clinicians use both type 1 and type 2 thinking. When encountering a familiar problem, clinicians employ pattern recognition and reach a differential diagnosis quickly (type 1 thinking). When encountering a problem that is more complicated, they use a slower, systematic approach (type 2 thinking). Both types of thinking interplay—they are not mutually exclusive in the diagnostic process. Errors can occur in both type 1 and type 2 thinking; for example, people can apply the wrong rules or make errors in their application while using type 2 thinking. However, it has been argued that the common cognitive biases encountered in medicine tend to occur when clinicians are engaged in type 1 thinking.

Common cognitive biases in medicine

These include:
• Overconfidence bias—the tendency to believe we know more than we actually do • Availability bias—the likelihood of diagnosing recently seen conditions • Ascertainment bias—seeing what we expect to see • Confirmation bias—only looking for evidence to support a theory, not to refute it

• Commission bias—the assumption that doing something is better than waiting • Omission bias—the belief that doing nothing is better rather than causing harm.

The mark of a well-calibrated thinker is the ability to recognise what mode of thinking is being employed and to anticipate and recognise situations in which cognitive biases and errors are more likely to occur.

Human factors

The science of 'human factors' is the study of the limitations of human performance, and how technology, the work environment and team communication can adapt for this to reduce diagnostic and other types of error.

For example, performance is adversely affected by factors such as poorly designed processes and equipment, frequent interruptions and fatigue. The areas of the brain required for type 2 processing are most affected by things like fatigue and cognitive overload, and the brain reverts to type 1 processing to conserve cognitive energy.

In focusing on what we are trying to see to filter out distractions, we may not notice the unexpected. In a team context, what is obvious to one person may be completely missed by someone else. Safe and effective team communication therefore requires us to never assume and to verbalise things, even though they may seem obvious.

Reducing errors in clinical decision making

Knowledge and experience do not eliminate errors. Instead, there are a number of ways in which we can act to reduce errors in clinical decision making. Examples are:

- Adopting 'cognitive debiasing strategies'.
- Using clinical prediction rules and other decision aids.
- Engaging in effective team communication.

Cognitive debiasing strategies

There are some simple and established techniques that can be used to avoid cognitive biases and errors in clinical decision making.

History and physical examination

A thorough history and physical examination are essential, and bias and error will result if these are carried out inadequately.

Problem lists and differential diagnosis

The ability to identify key clinical data and create a problem list is a key step in clinical reasoning. Some problems (e.g. low serum potassium) require action, but not necessarily a differential diagnosis. Other problems (e.g. vomiting) require a differential diagnosis. The process of generating a problem list ensures nothing is missed and helps avoid anchoring on a particular diagnosis too early.

Mnemonics and checklists

These are used frequently in medicine to reduce reliance on fallible human memory. ABCDE (airway, breathing, circulation, disability, exposure/examination; sometimes prefixed with 'C' for 'control of any obvious problem') is probably the most successful checklist in medicine, and is commonly used during stressful assessment of critically ill patients.

Red flags and ROWS (rule out worst case scenario)

These are strategies that force doctors to consider serious diseases that can present with common symptoms. Red flags in back pain are listed in (Box 15.3, p. 597). Considering and investigating for possible pulmonary embolism in patients who present with pleuritic chest pain and breathlessness is a common example of ruling out a worst-case scenario, as pulmonary embolism can be fatal if missed.

Using clinical prediction rules and other decision aids

Clinical prediction rules use the patient's symptoms, signs and other data to determine the numerical probability of a disease or an outcome. They only work for the population used to create the rule.

Commonly used examples include the Wells score in suspected deep vein thrombosis (see Box 4.7, p. 71), the GRACE score in acute coronary syndromes (see Box 8.12, p. 284) and the CURB-65 score in community-acquired pneumonia (see Fig 9.6, p. 335).

Patient-centred evidence-based medicine and shared decision making

This requires the application of best-available research evidence while taking individual patient factors into account, including both clinical and non-clinical factors (e.g. the patient's social circumstances, values and wishes).

As this chapter has described, clinicians frequently deal with uncertainty/probability. Clinicians need to be able to explain the risks and benefits of treatment accurately and understandably. Providing the relevant statistics is seldom sufficient, because a patient's perception of risk may be influenced by irrational factors and individual values.

Avoid nebulous terms such as 'common' and 'rare'. Whenever possible, clinicians should quote numerical information using consistent denominators (e.g. '90 out of 100 patients who have this operation feel much better, one will die during the operation and two will suffer a stroke'). Visual aids can be used to present complex statistical information (Fig. 1.3).

Studies demonstrate a correlation between effective clinician–patient communication and improved health outcomes. If patients feel they have been listened to and understand the problem and proposed treatment plan, they are more likely to follow the plan and less likely to re-attend.

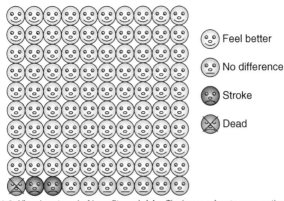

Fig. 1.3 Visual portrayal of benefits and risks. The image refers to an operation that is expected to relieve symptoms in 90% of patients, but cause stroke in 2% and death in 1%. *(From Edwards A, Elwyn G, Mulley A. Explaining risks: turning numerical data into meaningful pictures. BMJ 2002; 324:827–830. With permission from the BMJ Publishing Group.)*

Clinical therapeutics and prescribing

Prescribing medicines is the major tool used by doctors to restore or preserve the health of patients. Therapeutic benefits must be weighed against cost, adverse effects and interactions. Harm can also result from injudicious prescribing decisions and prescribing errors. The increasing number of available drugs and treatment indications, together with the complexity of individual treatment regimens ('polypharmacy'), are challenging for the modern prescriber. This chapter outlines the principles and practice of good prescribing (Box 2.1).

Principles of clinical pharmacology

Prescribers need to understand what the drug does to the body (pharmacodynamics) and what the body does to the drug (pharmacokinetics, Fig. 2.1). Most drugs are synthetic small molecules, but the same principles apply to 'biological' therapies, including peptides, proteins and monoclonal antibodies.

2.1 Steps in good prescribing

- Make a diagnosis
- Consider factors that might influence the patient's response to therapy (age, concomitant drug therapy, renal and liver function etc.)
- Establish the therapeutic goal[a]
- Choose the therapeutic approach[a]
- Choose the drug and its formulation (the 'medicine')
- Choose the dose, route and frequency
- Choose the duration of therapy
- Write an unambiguous prescription (or 'medication order')
- Inform the patient about the treatment and its likely effects
- Monitor treatment effects, both beneficial and harmful
- Review/alter the prescription

[a]These steps in particular take the patient's views into consideration, thereby establishing a therapeutic partnership (shared decision making to achieve 'concordance').

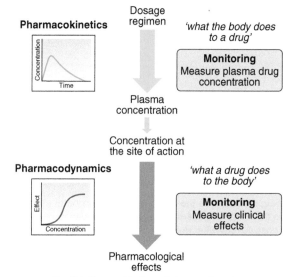

Fig. 2.1 Pharmacokinetics and pharmacodynamics.

Pharmacodynamics

Drug targets and mechanisms of action

Drugs usually either stimulate or block the function of a specific molecular target relevant to a particular disease (Box 2.2). Other drugs have less selective chemical properties, such as chelators (e.g. for iron overload), osmotic agents (for cerebral oedema) or general anaesthetics (which alter the biophysical properties of membranes). The interaction of drugs with receptors depends on:

- *Affinity:* how well the drug binds to a receptor, reflecting the 'molecular fit' and the strength of the bond. Some such interactions are irreversible, attributed to a strong affinity or because the drug modifies its target.
- *Selectivity:* how well the drug binds to one target relative to another. Drugs that target one receptor subtype commonly also affect other subtypes. For example, 'cardioselective' β-blockers have antianginal effects ($β_1$), but may also cause bronchospasm ($β_2$).
- *Agonists* bind to receptors, producing a response proportional to the agonist concentration and the proportion of receptors occupied. *Partial agonists* cannot produce a maximal response, even when all receptors are occupied.
- *Antagonists* bind to a receptor without initiating a response. *Competitive antagonists* compete with endogenous ligands to occupy receptors, and their potency depends on the relative affinities and concentrations of drug and ligand. *Noncompetitive antagonists* inhibit agonist effects by affecting other mechanisms (e.g. postreceptor signalling).

	2.2 Examples of target molecules for drugs	
Drug target	**Description**	**Examples**
Receptors		
Channel-linked receptors	Ligand binding controls a 'ligand-gated' ion channel	Nicotinic acetylcholine receptor
GPCRs	Ligand binding affects a 'G-protein' that mediates signal transduction	β-adrenoceptors Opioid receptors
Kinase-linked receptors	Ligand binding activates intracellular protein kinase, triggering phosphorylation	Insulin receptor Cytokine receptors
Transcription factor receptors	Intracellular; ligand binding promotes or inhibits gene transcription	Steroid receptors Retinoid receptors
Other targets		
Voltage-gated ion channels	Mediate electrical signalling in muscle and nervous system	Na^+ and Ca^{2+} channels
Enzymes	Catalyse biochemical reactions; drugs interfere with binding of substrate	ACE Xanthine oxidase
Transporter proteins	Carry ions or molecules across cell membranes	Na^+/K^+ ATPase
Cytokines/other signalling molecules	Small proteins that are important in cell signalling, especially immune responses	Tumour necrosis factors Interleukins
Cell surface antigens	Block recognition of cell surface molecules	CD20, CD80

ACE, Angiotensin-converting enzyme; GPCR, G-protein-coupled receptor.

Dose–response relationships

Plotting the logarithm of drug dose against drug response typically produces a sigmoidal dose–response curve (Fig. 2.2). Increases in dose produce increasing responses, but only within a particular range; further increases produce little extra effect. Drug responses are characterised by:

- *Efficacy:* the extent to which a drug produces a specific response when all available receptors are occupied. Efficacy is maximal for a full agonist; a partial agonist at the same receptor shows lower efficacy.
- *Therapeutic efficacy:* the effect of the drug on a desired biological endpoint. Used to compare drugs acting via different mechanisms (e.g. diuresis following loop diuretics versus thiazides).
- *Potency:* the amount of drug required for a given response. More potent drugs act at lower doses.

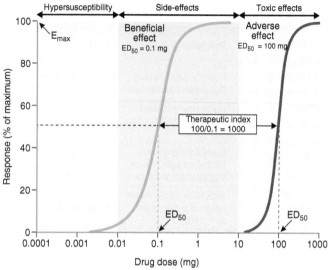

Fig. 2.2 Dose–response curve. The green curve represents the beneficial effect of the drug. The dose or concentration producing half the maximum response ($E_{max}/2$) is the ED_{50} (or EC_{50}). The red curve is the dose–response relationship for the key adverse effect, which occurs at higher doses. Adverse effects occurring above the therapeutic range are called 'toxic effects', whereas those occurring within the therapeutic range are 'side effects'.

The dose–response relationship varies between patients because of variations in pharmacokinetics and pharmacodynamics. The prescriber cannot know the dose–response curve for individuals, so most drugs are licensed within a dose range predicted to reach close to the top of the dose–response curve in most patients.

Therapeutic index

Adverse effects of drugs, like beneficial effects, are often dose-related, although the dose–response curve for adverse effects is shifted to the right (Fig. 2.2). The ratio of the dose effective in 50% of patients to the dose causing adverse effects in 50% is called the 'therapeutic index'. Many drugs have multiple adverse effects, so the therapeutic index is usually based on those that require dose reduction or discontinuation. For most drugs, the therapeutic index is greater than 100, but some have therapeutic indices of less than 10 (e.g. digoxin, warfarin, insulin, phenytoin, opioids). These must be titrated to maximise benefits while avoiding toxicity.

Desensitisation and withdrawal effects

Desensitisation means that the response to a drug diminishes with repeated dosing. Sometimes the response can be restored by increasing the dose; however, the tissues may ultimately become completely refractory to the drug.

i 2.3 Examples of drugs with withdrawal effects

Drug	Symptoms	Signs	Treatment
Alcohol	Anxiety, panic, paranoid delusions, visual and auditory hallucinations	Agitation, delirium, tremor, tachycardia, ataxia, disorientation, seizures	Treat immediate withdrawal syndrome with benzodiazepines
Barbiturates, benzodiazepines	Similar to alcohol	Similar to alcohol	Substitute long-acting benzodiazepine, then gradually wean off
Glucocorticoids	Weakness, fatigue, anorexia, weight loss, nausea, vomiting, diarrhoea, abdominal pain	Hypotension, hypoglycaemia	Prolonged therapy suppresses the HPA axis, causing adrenal insufficiency; gradual withdrawal required
Opioids	Rhinorrhoea, sneezing, yawning, lacrimation, abdominal and leg cramps, nausea, vomiting, diarrhoea	Dilated pupils	Transfer addicts to long-acting agonist methadone
SSRIs	Dizziness, sweating, nausea, insomnia, tremor, delirium, nightmares	Tremor	Reduce slowly to avoid withdrawal effects

HPA, Hypothalamic pituitary adrenal; SSRI, selective serotonin reuptake inhibitor.

- *Tachyphylaxis* describes very rapid desensitisation, sometimes with the initial dose. This implies depletion of chemicals necessary for the drug to act (e.g. a stored neurotransmitter) or receptor phosphorylation.
- *Tolerance* describes a gradual loss of response over days to weeks. This implies changes in receptor numbers or counter-regulatory physiological changes offsetting the drug's effect.
- *Drug resistance* means the loss of effectiveness of an antimicrobial or chemotherapy drug.
- A reduced response may also be caused by lower drug concentrations as a result of altered *pharmacokinetics* (see later).

When drugs induce chemical, hormonal and physiological changes that offset their actions, discontinuation may cause 'rebound' withdrawal effects (Box 2.3).

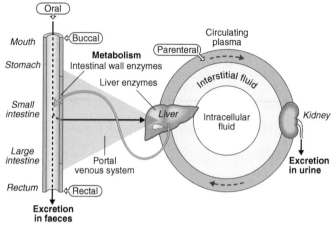

Fig. 2.3 Pharmacokinetics summary. Most drugs are taken orally, absorbed from the intestine and conveyed to the liver by the portal system, where they may undergo first-pass metabolism and/or excretion in bile. The active drug then enters the systemic circulation, from which it may diffuse (or sometimes be actively transported) into the interstitial and intracellular fluid compartments. Drug in the plasma undergoes liver metabolism and renal excretion. Drugs excreted in bile may be reabsorbed, creating an enterohepatic circulation. First-pass metabolism in the liver is avoided if drugs are administered via the buccal or rectal mucosa, or by injection.

Pharmacokinetics

Understanding 'what the body does to the drug' allows the optimal administration route and dose regimen to be chosen, and explains the majority of inter-individual variation in drug responses.

Drug absorption and routes of administration

How drug molecules access the blood stream depends on the route of administration (Fig. 2.3). 'Bioavailability' describes the proportion of the dose that reaches the systemic circulation.

Enteral (gastrointestinal) administration

- *Oral:* this is simple and convenient for patients, but the effect of an oral dose may be altered by ineffective swallowing, gastric acid, food binding, disease affecting intestinal absorption and by enteric or liver metabolism ('first-pass metabolism').
- *Buccal, intranasal and sublingual:* these routes allow rapid absorption into the systemic circulation, bypassing the complexities of oral administration. Commonly used for nitrates in angina.
- *Rectal:* occasionally used when the oral route is compromised by nausea, vomiting or unconsciousness (e.g. diazepam in status epilepticus).

Parenteral administration

- *Intravenous:* this route enables the entire dose to enter the systemic circulation reliably, unaffected by absorption or first-pass metabolism. It is ideal when a high plasma concentration is needed quickly (e.g. benzylpenicillin for meningococcal meningitis).
- *Intramuscular:* easier than the IV route (e.g. adrenaline (epinephrine) for anaphylaxis), but absorption is less predictable.
- *Subcutaneous:* this is ideal for self-administered parenteral drugs (e.g. insulin, heparin).
- *Transdermal patches:* these enable a drug to be absorbed through the skin into the circulation (e.g. oestrogens, nicotine, nitrates).

Other routes of administration

- *Topical:* direct administration to the site of action (e.g. skin, eye, ear). Achieves sufficient concentration at this site while minimising systemic exposure and adverse effects.
- *Inhaled:* administration allows direct delivery to the airways (e.g. salbutamol, beclometasone). However, a significant proportion of the dose may be absorbed from the lung or swallowed and can reach the systemic circulation. Correct use of a metered-dose inhaler is difficult for many patients. A 'spacer' device or a breath-powered dry powder inhaler can improve drug delivery. Nebulisers use pressurised oxygen or air to generate an aerosol from liquid drug that can be inhaled directly with a mouthpiece or mask.

Drug distribution

Distribution is the process by which drug molecules move into and out of the blood. It is influenced by molecular size, lipid solubility, plasma protein binding, affinity for surface-bound drug transporters and binding to molecular targets and other cellular proteins. Most drugs diffuse passively from the plasma to the interstitial fluid until the concentrations equalise. As the plasma concentration falls through metabolism or excretion, the drug diffuses back from the interstitium into the blood and is eliminated, unless additional doses enter the plasma.

Volume of distribution, V_d

This is the volume into which a drug appears to have distributed following intravenous injection. It is calculated as follows:

$$V_d = \text{Dose given} / \text{Intial plasma concentration}$$

Drugs that bind to plasma proteins (e.g. warfarin) have a V_d below 10 L; those that enter the interstitial fluid but not the cells (e.g. gentamicin) have a V_d of 10 to 30 L. Lipid-soluble and tissue-bound drugs (e.g. digoxin) may have a V_d of greater than 100 L. Drugs with a larger V_d have longer half-lives than those with a smaller V_d, and take longer to reach steady state on repeated administration.

Drug elimination

Drug metabolism

Metabolism is the process by which drugs are altered from a lipid-soluble form suitable for absorption and distribution to a more water-soluble form that is necessary for excretion. Some drugs, known as 'prodrugs', are inactive when administered but are converted to an active metabolite in vivo.

Phase I metabolism most commonly involves oxidation by the cytochrome P450 family of enzymes in the endoplasmic reticulum of hepatocytes.

Phase II metabolism involves combining phase I metabolites with an endogenous substrate to form an inactive conjugate that is much more water-soluble, thereby enabling renal excretion.

Drug excretion

Renal excretion is the usual route of elimination for drug metabolites of low molecular weight that have sufficient water-solubility to avoid tubular reabsorption. Drugs bound to plasma proteins are not filtered by the glomeruli. Urine is more acidic than plasma, so some drugs (e.g. salicylates) become un-ionised in the kidneys and tend to be reabsorbed. Alkalination of the urine can hasten excretion (e.g. after a salicylate overdose). For other drugs (e.g. methotrexate, penicillin), active secretion into the proximal tubule lumen is the main mechanism of excretion.

Faecal excretion is the predominant route for drugs with high molecular weight, those that are excreted in the bile after hepatic glucuronide conjugation and those that are not absorbed after enteral administration. After biliary excretion, some lipid-soluble drugs are reabsorbed in the small intestine, returning to the liver via the portal vein ('enterohepatic circulation'), thus prolonging the residence of the drug in the body.

Elimination kinetics

The net removal of drug from the circulation by metabolism and excretion is described as 'clearance', that is, the volume of plasma that is completely cleared of drug per unit time.

For most drugs, elimination is a high capacity process that does not become saturated, so elimination is proportional to drug concentration. This results in 'first-order' kinetics, in which the time that it takes for the plasma drug concentration to halve (half-life, $t_{1/2}$) is constant, causing an exponential decline in concentration (Fig. 2.4A). In this situation, a doubled dose leads to a doubled concentration at all time points.

For a few common drugs (e.g. phenytoin, alcohol), the elimination capacity is saturated within the usual dose range ('zero-order' kinetics). In this situation, if the rate of administration exceeds the maximum rate of elimination, the drug accumulates progressively, with serious toxicity.

▌ Repeated dose regimens

The goal of therapy is usually to maintain drug concentrations within the therapeutic range (see Fig. 2.2) over several days (e.g. antibiotics), or even for months or years (e.g. antihypertensives, lipid-lowering drugs). This requires the correct dose and frequency of administration.

As illustrated in Fig 2.4B, the time taken to reach therapeutic concentrations depends on the half-life of the drug. Typically, it takes approximately five half-lives to reach a steady state in which drug elimination equals drug administration, and drug concentrations stay within the therapeutic range. This means the effects of a new dose of a drug with a long half-life (e.g. digoxin, which has a half-life of 36 hours) may not be known for several days. In contrast, drugs with a short half-life (e.g. dobutamine) have to be given continuously by infusion but reach a steady state within minutes.

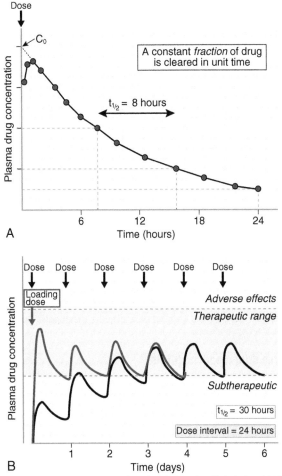

Fig. 2.4 Drug concentrations in plasma following single and multiple dosing. **A** Following a single IV dose, the time required for the plasma drug concentration to halve (half-life, $t_{1/2}$) is constant throughout the elimination process. **B** With multiple dosing, the peak, average and trough concentrations rise progressively if each dose is administered before the previous dose is entirely cleared (*black line*). For most of the first 3 days, drug concentrations are below the therapeutic range. This can be overcome by using a larger loading dose (*red line*) to achieve a steady state more rapidly.

For drugs with a long half-life, a large initial 'loading dose' can be given to achieve a therapeutic concentration rapidly, which is then maintained by subsequent doses. A steady state actually involves fluctuations in drug concentrations, with peaks after administration and troughs before the next dose. Manufacturers recommend dosing regimens that create, for most patients, troughs inside the therapeutic range and peaks low enough to avoid adverse effects. The optimal dose interval is a compromise between patient convenience and a constant level of drug exposure. Frequent administration (e.g. four times daily) achieves a smoother plasma concentration than once daily, but is much less convenient for patients. 'Modified-release' formulations allow drugs with short half-lives to be absorbed more slowly, reducing the oscillations in blood levels. This is especially useful for drugs with a low therapeutic index.

Inter-individual variation in drug responses

Generic prescribing advice is based on average dose–response data derived from many patients. Inter-individual pharmacodynamic and pharmacokinetic variability (Box 2.4) may require prescribers to adjust their prescriptions. Some of this variability can be explained by differences in individual genes ('pharmacogenetics') or the effects of multiple gene variants ('pharmacogenomics'). These concepts aim to identify patients most likely to benefit from specific treatments and those most susceptible to adverse effects, opening the way for 'personalised medicine'.

Adverse outcomes of drug therapy

Prescribing a drug always involves balancing the therapeutic benefits and the risk of adverse effects.

Adverse drug reactions (ADRs)

Important definitions include:

- *Adverse event.* A harmful event that occurs while a patient is taking a drug, irrespective of whether the drug is the cause.
- *Adverse drug reaction (ADR).* An unwanted or harmful reaction following normal use of a drug and suspected to be related to the drug.
- *Side effect.* Any effect of a drug other than the intended therapeutic effect. The term is often used interchangeably with ADR, although 'side effect' usually implies an ADR occurring at therapeutic drug concentrations (e.g. vasodilator-induced ankle oedema).
- *Hypersensitivity reaction.* An immunological ADR that often occurs at subtherapeutic drug concentrations. Some are immediate, when drug antigens interact with IgE on mast cells and basophils, releasing mediators (e.g. penicillin-related anaphylaxis). 'Anaphylactoid' reactions occur through a direct non-immune-mediated release of the same mediators or through direct complement activation. Hypersensitivity reactions also occur via other antibody-dependent, immune-complex or cell-mediated pathways.

2.4 Patient-specific factors that influence pharmacokinetics

Age
- Drug metabolism is low in the fetus and newborn, may be enhanced in young children and becomes less effective with age
- Drug excretion falls with the age-related decline in renal function

Sex
- Women have a greater proportion of body fat than men, increasing the volume of distribution and half-life of lipid-soluble drugs

Body weight
- Obesity increases volume of distribution and half-life of lipid-soluble drugs
- Patients with higher lean body mass have larger body compartments into which drugs are distributed, and may require higher doses

Liver function
- Metabolism of most drugs depends on cytochrome P450 enzymes that are impaired in advanced liver disease
- Hypoalbuminaemia influences the distribution of drugs that are highly protein-bound

Kidney function
- Renal disease and the decline in renal function with ageing may lead to drug accumulation

Gastrointestinal function
- Small intestinal absorption of oral drugs may be delayed by reduced gastric motility
- Absorptive capacity of the intestinal mucosa may be reduced in disease (e.g. Crohn or coeliac disease) or after surgical resection

Food
- Food in the stomach delays gastric emptying and reduces the rate (but not usually the extent) of drug absorption
- Some food constituents bind to certain drugs and prevent their absorption

Smoking
- Tar in tobacco smoke stimulates the oxidation of certain drugs

Alcohol
- Regular alcohol consumption stimulates liver enzyme synthesis, whereas binge drinking may temporarily inhibit drug metabolism

Drugs
- Drug–drug interactions cause marked variation in pharmacokinetics (see Box 2.8)

- *Drug toxicity.* Adverse effects caused by the drug concentrations exceeding the therapeutic range, either unintentionally or intentionally (overdose).
- *Drug abuse.* The misuse of recreational or therapeutic drugs that may lead to addiction, dependence, physiological derangement (e.g. hepatotoxicity), psychological harm or death.

2.5 How to take a drug history

Information from the patient (or carer)

Use clear language (e.g. 'medicines' not 'drugs', which may be misunderstood as drugs of abuse) while gathering the following information:

- Current prescribed drugs, including formulations, doses, routes of administration, frequency and timing, duration of treatment
- Commonly forgotten medications (e.g. contraceptives, over-the-counter drugs, herbal remedies, vitamins)
- Drugs recently stopped and reasons for stopping
- Previous drug hypersensitivity reactions; nature and time course (e.g. rash, anaphylaxis)
- Previous ADRs; nature and time course
- Adherence to therapy

Information from GP and/or pharmacist

- Up-to-date list of medications
- Previous ADRs
- Last order dates for each medication

Inspection of medicines

- Drugs and their containers should be inspected for name, dosage and the number of doses taken since dispensed

Prevalence of ADRs

ADRs are a common cause of illness, emphasising the importance of taking a careful drug history (Box 2.5). The prevalence of ADRs is rising with the ageing population; polypharmacy; increasing availability of over-the-counter medicines, herbal and traditional medicines; and the availability of medicines online without prescription. Additional risk factors for ADRs include comorbidity altering pharmacokinetics (e.g. renal impairment), low therapeutic index and poor prescribing practice.

ADRs reduce quality of life for patients, reduce adherence to beneficial treatments, cause diagnostic confusion, undermine the confidence of patients in their doctors and consume resources. Analysis shows that over half of ADRs that occur could be avoided if the prescriber took more care in anticipating the hazards of drug therapy. Drugs that commonly cause ADRs are listed in Box 2.6.

Prescribers and patients commonly want to know the frequency of particular ADRs. The words used to describe frequency can be easily misinterpreted, but widely accepted definitions include: very common (≥10%), common (1%–10%), uncommon (0.1%–1%), rare (0.01%–0.1%) and very rare (≤0.01%).

Classification of ADRs

ADRs may be classified into groups:

- *Type A ('augmented') ADRs.* Predictable, dose-dependent, common and usually mild.
- *Type B ('bizarre') ADRs.* Not predictable, not obviously dose-dependent in the therapeutic range, rare and often severe.

i	**2.6 Drugs that are common causes of adverse drug reactions**

Drug or drug class	Common adverse drug reactions
ACE inhibitors (e.g. lisinopril)	Renal impairment Hyperkalaemia
Antibiotics (e.g. amoxicillin)	Nausea Diarrhoea
Anticoagulants (e.g. warfarin, heparin)	Bleeding
Antipsychotics (e.g. haloperidol)	Falls Sedation Delirium
Aspirin	Gastrotoxicity (dyspepsia, gastrointestinal bleeding)
Benzodiazepines (e.g. diazepam)	Drowsiness Falls
β-blockers (e.g. atenolol)	Cold peripheries Bradycardia
Calcium channel blockers (e.g. amlodipine)	Ankle oedema
Digoxin	Nausea and anorexia Bradycardia
Diuretics (e.g. furosemide, bendroflumethiazide)	Dehydration Electrolyte disturbance (hypokalaemia, hyponatraemia) Hypotension Renal impairment
Insulin	Hypoglycaemia
NSAIDs (e.g. ibuprofen)	Gastrotoxicity (dyspepsia, gastrointestinal bleeding) Renal impairment
Opioid analgesics (e.g. morphine)	Nausea and vomiting Delirium Constipation

SPC, Summary of Product Characteristics.

- *Type C ('chronic/continuous') ADRs.* Occur only after prolonged continuous drug exposure.
- *Type D ('delayed') ADRs.* Occur long after drug exposure; diagnosis difficult.
- *Type E ('end-of-treatment') ADRs.* Occur after abrupt drug withdrawal.

A teratogen is a drug with the potential to affect the development of the fetus in the first 10 weeks of intrauterine life (e.g. phenytoin, warfarin). The thalidomide disaster in the early 1960s highlighted the risk of teratogenicity, and led to mandatory testing of new drugs.

i	**2.7 TREND analysis of suspected adverse drug reactions**	
Factor	Key question	Comment
Temporal relationship	What is the time interval between the start of drug therapy and the reaction?	Most ADRs occur soon after starting treatment, and within hours in the case of anaphylactic reactions
Re-challenge	What happens when the patient is re-challenged with the drug?	Re-challenge is rarely possible because of the need to avoid exposing patients to unnecessary risk
Exclusion	Have concomitant drugs and other nondrug causes been excluded?	ADR is a diagnosis of exclusion following clinical assessment and relevant investigations for nondrug causes
Novelty	Has the reaction been reported before?	The suspected ADR may already be recognised and mentioned in the SPC approved by the regulatory authorities
De-challenge	Does the reaction improve when the drug is withdrawn or the dose is reduced?	Most, but not all, ADRs improve on drug withdrawal, although recovery may be slow

SPC, Summary of Product Characteristics.

Detecting ADRs—pharmacovigilance

Type A ADRs become apparent early in drug development. By the time a new drug is licensed, however, a relatively small number of patients may have been exposed to it, so rarer type B ADRs may remain undiscovered. Pharmacovigilance is the process of detecting and evaluating ADRs to help drug regulatory agencies advise prescribers and patients, restrict the licensed indications or withdraw the drug.

Voluntary reporting is an early-warning system for previously unrecognised rare ADRs, but its weaknesses include low reporting rates (only 10% of serious ADRs are reported), an inability to quantify risk (because the ratio of ADRs to prescriptions is unknown) and the influence of prescriber awareness on the likelihood of reporting.

Many health care systems routinely collect patient-identifiable data on prescriptions (a surrogate marker of exposure to a drug), health care events (e.g. hospitalisation, operations, new diagnoses) and other clinical data (e.g. haematology, biochemistry). Using record linkage, with appropriate data protection safeguards, the harms and benefits of drugs may be assessed.

Prescribers who see patients experiencing possible ADRs should consider the features in Box 2.7. Other features suggesting an ADR include:

- Concern expressed by a patient that a drug has harmed them.
- Abnormal clinical measurements or laboratory results while on a drug.

- New therapy started that could be in response to an ADR (e.g. omeprazole, allopurinol).
- The presence of risk factors for ADRs (see previously).

Drug interactions

These occur when administration of one drug changes the beneficial or adverse responses to another drug. Although the potential number of drug interactions is large, only a few are common in practice. Interactions are most likely when the affected drug has a low therapeutic index, a steep dose–response curve, high first-pass or saturable metabolism or a single mechanism of elimination.

Mechanisms of drug interactions

Pharmacodynamic interactions occur when two drugs have additive, synergistic or antagonistic effects on the same target or physiological system (Box 2.8).

Pharmacokinetic interactions occur when one drug alters the concentration of another at its site of action. Mechanisms include:

- *Absorption interactions.* Drugs affecting gastric emptying alter the rate of absorption of other drugs. Drugs that bind to others (e.g. antacids to ciprofloxacin) can reduce absorption.
- *Distribution interactions.* Co-administration of drugs that compete for plasma protein binding (e.g. phenytoin and diazepam) can increase unbound drug concentration.
- *Metabolism interactions.* Hepatic cytochrome P450 (CYP) inducers (e.g. rifampicin) reduce plasma concentrations of other drugs, but may enhance activation of prodrugs. CYP inhibitors (e.g. clarithromycin) have the opposite effect.
- *Excretion interactions.* Drug-induced reductions in the glomerular filtration rate can reduce the clearance of drugs such as digoxin, lithium and aminoglycoside antibiotics, causing toxicity.

Avoiding drug interactions

Prescribers can avoid drug interactions by taking a careful drug history, only prescribing for clear indications and taking care when prescribing drugs with a narrow therapeutic index (e.g. warfarin). Good prescribers inform their patients of the risks and arrange for monitoring of the clinical effects (e.g. coagulation tests for warfarin) or of plasma concentration (e.g. digoxin).

Medication errors

A medication error is any preventable event that may lead to inappropriate medication use or patient harm while the medication is in the control of the health care professional or patient. This includes errors in prescribing, dispensing, preparing solutions, administration or monitoring. Many adverse events considered by one prescriber to be an unfortunate ADR might be considered by another to be a prescribing error.

i 2.8 Common drug interactions

Mechanism	Object drug	Precipitant drug	Result
Pharmaceutical			
Chemical reaction	Sodium bicarbonate	Calcium gluconate	Precipitation of insoluble calcium carbonate
Pharmacokinetic			
↓absorption	Tetracyclines	Ca^{++}, Al^{+++}, Mg^{++} salts	↓tetracycline absorption
↓protein binding	Phenytoin	Aspirin	↑unbound and ↓total phenytoin plasma concentration
↓metabolism:			
CYP3A4	Warfarin	Clarithromycin	↑anticoagulation
CYP2C19	Phenytoin	Omeprazole	Phenytoin toxicity
CYP2D6	Clozapine	Paroxetine	Clozapine toxicity
Xanthine oxidase	Azathioprine	Allopurinol	Azathioprine toxicity
Monoamine oxidase (MAO)	Catecholamines	MAO inhibitors	Hypertensive crisis attributed to monoamine toxicity
↑metabolism	Ciclosporin	St John's wort	Loss of immunosuppression
↓renal elimination	Methotrexate	NSAIDs	Methotrexate toxicity
Pharmacodynamic			
Direct antagonism at same receptor	Salbutamol	Atenolol	↓bronchodilator effect
Direct potentiation in same system	ACE inhibitors	NSAIDs	↑risk of renal impairment
Indirect potentiation by actions in different systems	Warfarin	Aspirin, NSAIDs	↑risk of bleeding because of gastrotoxicity + antiplatelet effects

Recent UK studies suggest that 7% to 9% of hospital prescriptions contain an error, and most are written by junior doctors. Common errors in hospitals include omission of regular medicines on admission or discharge ('medicines reconciliation' errors, 30% of errors), dosing errors, unintentional prescribing and poor documentation.

Most prescription errors result from a combination of failures by the individual prescriber and the health-service systems in which they work (Box 2.9). Health care organisations increasingly encourage 'no-blame'

2.9 Causes of prescribing errors

Systems factors

- Working hours and caseload of prescribers (and others)
- Professional support and supervision by colleagues
- Availability of information (medical records)
- Design of prescription forms
- Distractions
- Checks (e.g. pharmacist review)
- Reporting and reviewing of incidents

Prescriber factors

Knowledge

- Clinical pharmacology principles
- Common drugs and therapeutic problems with them
- Knowledge of workplace systems

Skills

- Taking a good drug history
- Obtaining supporting prescribing information
- Communicating with patients
- Numeracy/calculations
- Prescription writing

Attitudes

- Coping with risk and uncertainty
- Monitoring of prescribing
- Checking routines

reporting of errors and 'root cause analysis' of incidents using human error theory (Fig. 2.5). Prevention is targeted at the causes in Box 2.9, can be supported by electronic prescribing, which avoids errors caused by illegibility or dosing mistakes, and can incorporate clinical decision algorithms and warnings of contraindications and interactions.

Responding to an error

All prescribers make errors. When they do, the patient's safety should be protected by clinical review, remedial treatment, monitoring, documenting events in the patient record and informing colleagues. Patients who have been exposed to potential harm should be informed. The prescriber must also report errors that do not reach the patient, so that others can learn from and avoid similar incidents.

Drug regulation and management

The production and use of drugs are strictly regulated by government agencies. Regulators are responsible for licensing, safety monitoring, approving clinical trials and setting standards for drug development and manufacture. In addition, because of costs and adverse effects, health services must prioritise drug use by considering evidence of benefit and harm, through 'medicines management'.

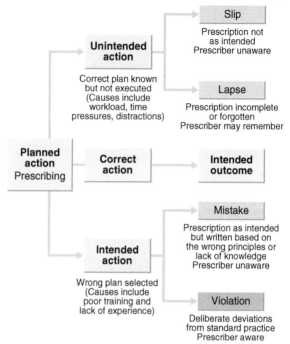

Fig. 2.5 Human error theory. To prevent unintended errors, the system must provide appropriate checking routines. Intended errors occur when the prescriber acts incorrectly as a result of lack of knowledge (a mistake); prevention must focus on training the prescriber.

Drug development and marketing

Naturally occurring drugs include morphine from the opium poppy, digitalis from the foxglove plant and quinine from the bark of the *Cinchona* tree. Although plant and animal sources remain important, most new drugs come from the identification or synthesis of small molecules with specific interactions with a molecular target.

Drug development involves screening numerous compounds for those that interact in vitro with a specific molecular target, optimising the formulation of lead compounds, testing efficacy and toxicity in vitro and in animals , and then undertaking a clinical trial programme:

- Phase 1: Healthy volunteers, single then repeated-dose studies to establish pharmacokinetics, pharmacodynamics and short-term safety.
- Phase II: Investigate clinical effectiveness, safety and dose–response relationship in target patients; identify optimal dosing regimen for larger studies.

- Phase III: Large, expensive trials to confirm safety and efficacy relative to placebo or alternative treatments in the target patients, using relevant clinical endpoints.
- Phase IV: Postmarketing for first indication—to evaluate new indications, doses or formulations, long-term safety or cost-effectiveness.

This process typically takes longer than 10 years and may cost up to US$1 billion. Manufacturers then have a defined patent period (10–15 years) in which to recoup the development costs. After the patent has expired, 'generic' manufacturers may produce cheaper formulations of the drug.

Newer 'biological' products (e.g. recombinant antibodies) require complex manufacturing involving specific cell lines, molecular cloning and purification. After patent expiry, other manufacturers may develop similar products ('biosimilars') with similar pharmacological actions.

The number of new drugs produced by the pharmaceutical industry has declined in recent years. Novel therapeutic agents increasingly target complex second-messenger systems, cytokines, nucleic acids and cellular networks. Examples include monoclonal antibodies, small interfering RNA, gene therapy and stem cell therapy.

Licensing new medicines

New drugs are given 'market authorisation' based on the evidence presented by the manufacturer. The regulator also ensures that the accompanying information (summary of product characteristics) reflects the evidence that has been presented.

Categories of approval include:

- *Controlled drug.* Subject to legal control of supply and possession, to prevent abuse (e.g. opioids).
- *Prescription-only medicine.* Available only from a pharmacist following prescription by an appropriate practitioner.
- *Pharmacy.* Available from a pharmacist without a prescription.
- *General sales list.* May be bought 'over the counter' without a prescription.

Prescribers may sometimes direct use of a drug outside the usual indication ('off-label' prescribing), for example, prescribing outside the approved age group. They may also be prescribing for an indication with no approved medicines, or where all approved medicines have caused adverse effects. When prescribing is 'off-label' or 'unlicensed', there is an increased requirement for prescribers to be able to justify their actions and to inform and agree on the decision with the patient.

Drug marketing

The pharmaceutical industry markets drugs actively to prescribers and, in some countries, to patients. Prescribers are targeted indirectly through sponsored educational meetings and journal advertisements, and directly by company representatives. Such largesse can potentially create conflicts of interest and bias towards one drug over another, despite conflicting evidence.

Managing the use of medicines

Although prescribers can legally prescribe any approved medicine, it is desirable to limit their choice to focus on the most effective and cost-effective options. In this way, prescribers (and patients) become familiar with a smaller number of medicines, and pharmacies can maintain their stocks efficiently.

The process of ensuring optimal use of available medicines usually involves both national (e.g. NICE in the United Kingdom) and local (e.g. drug and therapeutics committees) organisations.

Evaluating evidence

Drugs are often evaluated in high-quality randomised controlled trials (RCTs), the results of which can be considered by systematic review (Fig. 2.6). Ideally, data include comparison with placebo and also 'head-to-head' comparison with alternative therapies. Trials conducted in selected populations, however, may not be applicable to individual patients. Subtle bias may be introduced because of industry funding and investigators favouring research with a 'positive' impact. A common example of bias is the difference between relative and absolute risk of clinical events reported in prevention trials. If a clinical event is encountered in 1 of 50 patients (2%) receiving placebo, but only 1 of 100 patients (1%) receiving active treatment, the impact of treatment can be described as either a 50% relative risk reduction or a 1% absolute risk reduction. Although the former sounds impressive, the latter is of more importance to the patient. It means that 100 patients must be treated for one to benefit (vs placebo). This illustrates how large clinical trials can produce highly statistically significant reductions in relative risk but only have a very modest clinical impact.

Evaluating cost effectiveness

New drugs are often better but more expensive than standard care. Budgets are limited, so it is impossible to fund all new medicines, and difficult ethical and financial decisions are needed. Cost-effectiveness analysis expresses the relative costs and outcomes of different treatments by dividing the cost of a health gain by the size of the gain. It is particularly difficult to compare the value of interventions for different clinical outcomes. One method is to calculate the cost per quality-adjusted life year gained if a new drug is used rather than standard treatment (Box 2.10). Problems with this approach include the need to extrapolate outcomes beyond the duration of trial data, the assumption that QALYs gained at all ages are equally valuable and the fact that different standard treatments often exist. These assessments are complex and are normally undertaken at national level, for example, by NICE in the United Kingdom.

Implementing recommendations

Many recommendations about drug therapy feature in clinical guidelines written by an expert group after systematic review of the evidence. Guidelines provide recommendations rather than obligations for prescribers and are helpful in promoting more consistent and higher-quality prescribing.

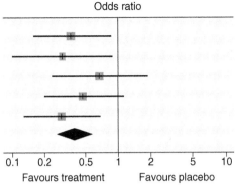

Odds ratio

0.1   0.2   0.5   1   2   5   10
Favours treatment   Favours placebo

Fig. 2.6 Systematic review of the evidence from RCTs. This forest plot shows the effect of warfarin compared with placebo on the likelihood of stroke in patients with atrial fibrillation in the five RCTs included in a meta-analysis. For each trial, the purple box is proportionate to the number of participants. The tick marks show the mean odds ratio, and the black lines indicate its 95% confidence intervals. Not all the trials showed statistically significant effects (the confidence intervals cross 1.0). However, the metaanalysis (*black diamond*) confirms a highly significant benefit. The overall odds ratio is 0.4, indicating a mean 60% risk reduction with warfarin treatment in patients matching the participants in these trials.

 2.10 Cost-effectiveness analysis

A clinical trial lasting 2 years compares two interventions for the treatment of colon cancer:
- Treatment A: standard treatment, cost = £1000/year, oral therapy
- Treatment B: new treatment, cost = £6000/year, monthly intravenous infusions, often followed by a week of nausea

The new treatment (B) significantly increases the average time to progression (18 months vs 12 months) and reduces overall mortality (40% vs 60%). The health economist models the survival curves from the trial to undertake a cost–utility analysis and concludes that:
- Intervention A: allows an average patient to live for 2 extra years at a utility 0.7 = 1.4 QALYs (cost £2000)
- Intervention B: allows an average patient to live for 3 extra years at a utility 0.6 = 1.8 QALYs (cost £18 000)

The health economists conclude that treatment B provides an extra 0.4 QALYs at an extra cost of £16 000, meaning that the ICER = £40 000/QALY. They recommend that the new treatment should not be funded on the basis that their threshold for cost acceptability is £30 000/QALY.

ICER, Incremental cost-effectiveness ratio; QALY, quality-adjusted life year.

They are often written without concern for cost-effectiveness, however, and may be limited by the quality of available evidence. Guidelines cannot anticipate the extent of the variation between individual patients who may have unexpected contraindications or choose different treatment priorities. When deviating from national guidance, prescribers should be able to justify their practice.

Additional prescribing recommendations are often implemented locally or imposed by bodies who fund health care. Most health care units have a drug and therapeutics committee comprised of medical staff, pharmacists, nurses and managers. This group develops local prescribing guidelines, maintains a local formulary and evaluates requests to use new drugs. The local formulary contains a more limited list than the national formulary, because the latter lists all available licensed medicines, not only those approved for local use.

Prescribing in practice

Decision making in prescribing

Prescribing should be based on a rational approach to a series of challenges (see Box 2.1).

Making a diagnosis

Ideally, this should be a confirmed diagnosis but in reality many prescriptions are based on the most likely of several possible diagnoses.

Establishing the therapeutic goal

This is clear when relieving symptoms (e.g. pain, nausea, constipation), but other goals are less obvious to patients, such as in the case of preventive treatments (e.g. ACE inhibitors to prevent hospitalisation and extend life in patients with chronic heart failure). Prescribers should agree on goals and measures of success with patients (concordance).

Choosing the therapeutic approach

Drug therapy is often only one of several available approaches. Prescribers should consider if it is better than no treatment or than an alternative treatment (e.g. physiotherapy, psychotherapy, surgery). Factors that should be considered when assessing the balance of benefit and harm are summarised in Box 2.11.

Choosing a drug

For most indications, more than one drug or class of drugs is available. Prescribers need to consider the optimal choice for the individual patient, considering:

Absorption: Patients may find some oral formulations intolerable or may be vomiting and require parenteral administration.

Distribution: Distribution to a particular tissue sometimes dictates choice (e.g. lincomycin and clindamycin concentrate in bones).

Metabolism: Drugs that are extensively metabolised should be avoided in patients with severe liver disease.

2.11 Factors to consider when balancing benefits and harms of drug therapy

- Seriousness of the disease or symptom
- Efficacy of the drug
- Seriousness of potential adverse effects
- Likelihood of adverse effects
- Efficacy of alternative drugs or nondrug therapies
- Safety of alternative drugs or nondrug therapies

Excretion: Drugs that depend on renal excretion should be avoided in patients with impaired renal function.

Efficacy: Drugs with the greatest efficacy are preferred unless alternatives are more convenient, safer or less expensive.

Avoiding adverse effects: Prescribers should avoid drugs that are likely to cause adverse effects or worsen coexisting conditions (e.g. β-blockers for angina in patients with asthma).

Features of the disease: Antibiotic therapy should be based on the known or suspected sensitivity of the organism.

Severity of disease: The choice of drug (e.g. analgesic) should be appropriate to disease severity.

Coexisting disease: This may either be improved by a planned treatment or may rule that treatment out.

Avoiding adverse drug interactions: Prescribers should avoid giving combinations of drugs that might interact (Box 2.8).

Patient adherence: Prescribers should choose drugs with a simple dosing schedule or easy administration.

Cost: Prescribers should choose the cheaper drug (e.g. a generic or biosimilar) if two drugs are of equal efficacy and safety.

Genetic factors: Rarely, genotype may influence the choice of drug (pharmacogenomics).

Choosing a dosage regimen

Prescribers have to choose a dose, route and frequency of administration to achieve an effective steady-state drug concentration in the target tissue without toxicity. Manufacturers' dosage recommendations are based on average patients, but the optimal regimen for an individual patient is never certain. Rational prescribing involves some general principles:

Dose titration: It is usual to start with a low dose and titrate slowly upwards as necessary. This is particularly important if the patient is prone to adverse pharmacodynamic effects or altered pharmacokinetic handling (e.g. renal or hepatic impairment), and when using drugs with a low therapeutic index. In contrast, when early effect is important but the drug has a long half-life (e.g. digoxin, warfarin, amiodarone), an initial loading dose is given before the appropriate maintenance dose (Fig. 2.4).

If adverse effects occur, the dose should be reduced, or an alternative drug prescribed. A lower dose may suffice if combined with another

| **i** | **2.12 Factors influencing the route of drug administration** |

Reason	Example
Only one route possible	Gliclazide (oral)
Patient adherence	Phenothiazines (two weekly IM depot injections, not daily tablets, in schizophrenia)
Poor absorption	Furosemide (IV, not oral, in severe heart failure)
Rapid action	Haloperidol (IM, not oral, in acute behavioural disturbance)
Vomiting	Phenothiazines (PR or buccal, not oral, in nausea)
Avoidance of first-pass metabolism	Glyceryl trinitrate (SL, in angina)
Topical, avoiding systemic exposure	Inhaled steroids in asthma
Ease of access	Diazepam (PR, if IV access is difficult in status epilepticus)
Comfort	Morphine (SC, not IV, in terminal care)

synergistic drug (e.g. azathioprine reduces glucocorticoid requirements in inflammatory disease). The shape of the dose–response curve means that higher doses may not increase therapeutic effect but may increase toxicity.

Route: Factors influencing route of administration are shown in Box 2.12.

Frequency: Less frequent doses are more convenient but result in greater fluctuation between peaks and troughs in drug concentration (Fig 2.4). Peaks can cause adverse effects (e.g. dizziness with antihypertensives), and troughs may be associated with loss of effect (e.g. antiparkinsonian drugs). Modified-release formulations or split dosing are possible solutions.

Timing: For many drugs the time of administration is unimportant; however, for others the timing of effect makes a difference (e.g. morning diuretics to avoid nocturnal diuresis).

Formulation: For some drugs there is a choice of formulation, which may influence palatability, absorption and bioavailability. Where these effects are important, drugs should occasionally be prescribed by brand name rather than 'generic' international name.

Duration: This ranges from a single dose (e.g. thrombolysis for myocardial infarction) to a course of treatment (e.g. antibiotics) to long-term treatment (e.g. insulin, antihypertensives, levothyroxine).

Involving the patient

Patients should, whenever possible, be involved in choices about drug therapy. It is important for them to be provided with sufficient information to understand the choice, know what to expect from the treatment and be aware of any monitoring required.

Evidence shows that up to half of drug doses for chronic preventative therapy are not taken. This is termed 'nonadherence' and may or may not be intentional. Nonadherence reduces the likelihood of benefits to the patient and is costly in terms of wasted medicines and unnecessary health care episodes. An important reason may be lack of concordance with the prescriber about the goals of treatment. A more open and shared decision-making process might resolve any misunderstandings at the outset and foster improved adherence, as well as improved satisfaction with health care services and confidence in prescribers. Fully engaging patients in shared decision making is sometimes constrained by various factors, such as limited consultation time and challenges in communicating complex numerical data.

Stopping drug therapy

It is important to review long-term treatment regularly to assess whether continuation is required. Elderly patients are keen to reduce their medication burden and are often prepared to compromise on long-term preventative therapy to achieve this.

Prescribing in special circumstances

Prescribing for patients with renal disease

Patients with renal impairment (eGFR <60 mL/min) require reduced maintenance doses of drugs eliminated predominantly by the kidneys, to avoid accumulation and toxicity. Examples of drugs that require extra caution in patients with renal disease are listed in Box 2.13.

Prescribing for patients with hepatic disease

The liver has a large reserve capacity for drug metabolism, so dosages only need modified in patients with advanced liver disease, for example, when jaundice, ascites, hypoalbuminaemia, malnutrition or encephalopathy are present. Hepatic drug clearance may also be reduced in patients with acute hepatitis, hepatic congestion or intrahepatic arteriovenous shunting (e.g. cirrhosis). There are no good tests of hepatic drug-metabolising capacity, so dosage should be guided by response and adverse effects. Some drugs that require extra caution in patients with hepatic disease are listed in Box 2.13.

Prescribing for elderly patients

Elderly patients require particular care when prescribing because of: • impaired excretion/renal function • increased sensitivity to drugs, notably in the brain (sedation or delirium) • multiple comorbidities • drug interactions caused by polypharmacy • poor drug adherence attributed to cognitive impairment, difficulty swallowing and complex regimens (dosette boxes can help).

Prescribing for women who are pregnant or breastfeeding

Prescribing in pregnancy should be avoided where possible to minimise risk to the fetus; however, it may be necessary for a preexisting problem

2.13 Some drugs that require extra caution in patients with renal or hepatic disease

Kidney disease	Liver disease
Pharmacodynamic effects enhanced	
ACE inhibitors and ARBs (renal impairment, hyperkalaemia) Metformin (lactic acidosis) Spironolactone (hyperkalaemia) NSAIDs (impaired renal function) Sulphonylureas (hypoglycaemia) Insulin (hypoglycaemia)	Warfarin (increased anticoagulation because of reduced clotting factor synthesis) Metformin (lactic acidosis) Chloramphenicol (bone marrow suppression) NSAIDs (gastrointestinal bleeding, fluid retention) Sulphonylureas (hypoglycaemia) Benzodiazepines (coma)
Pharmacokinetic handling altered (reduced clearance)	
Aminoglycosides (e.g. gentamicin) Vancomycin Digoxin Lithium Other antibiotics (e.g. ciprofloxacin) Atenolol Allopurinol Cephalosporins Methotrexate Opioids (e.g. morphine)	Phenytoin Rifampicin Propranolol Warfarin Diazepam Lidocaine Opioids (e.g. morphine)

(e.g. epilepsy, asthma) or a pregnancy-related problem (e.g. morning sickness, gestational diabetes). About 35% of women take medication at least once during pregnancy, and 6% take medication during the first trimester (excluding iron, folic acid and vitamins). Particular prescribing issues in pregnancy are:

- *Teratogenesis:* particularly relevant for drugs taken between 2 and 8 weeks of gestation. Common teratogens include retinoids, cytotoxics, ACE inhibitors, antiepileptics and warfarin.
- *Adverse fetal effects in late gestation:* for example, tetracyclines may stain growing teeth and bones.
- *Altered maternal pharmacokinetics:* extracellular fluid volume and V_d increase. Some binding globulins increase. Placental metabolism and increased glomerular filtration enhance drug clearance. The overall effect is a fall in plasma levels of many drugs.

Drugs that are excreted in breast milk may cause adverse effects in the baby. Prescribers should always consult datasheets for each drug or a reliable formulary when treating a pregnant woman or breastfeeding mother.

Writing prescriptions

A prescription should be precise, accurate, clear and legible. The information supplied must include:

- date
- identification details of the patient
- name, formulation and dose of the drug
- frequency, route and method of administration
- amount to be supplied and instructions for labelling (primary care only)
- prescriber's signature

Prescribing in hospital

Although GP prescribing is increasingly electronic, most hospital prescribing continues to be based around the prescription and administration record (the 'drug chart', Fig. 2.7). A variety of charts are in use, and prescribers must familiarise themselves with the local version. Most contain the following sections:

- *Basic patient information*: (often on an addressograph label) including name, age, date of birth, hospital number and address.
- *Previous adverse reactions/allergies*: based on a drug history and/or the medical record.
- *Other medicines charts*: these note any other hospital prescriptions (e.g. anticoagulants, insulin, oxygen, fluids).
- *Once-only medications*: for prescribing medicines to be used infrequently, such as single-dose prophylactic antibiotics.
- *Regular medications*: medicines to be taken for days or continuously, for example, a course of antibiotics, antihypertensive drugs.
- *'As required' medications*: those prescribed for symptomatic relief, usually administered at the discretion of nursing staff (e.g. antiemetics, analgesics).

Prescribers should be aware of the risks of prescription error (Boxes 2.14 and 2.9), consider the rational basis for their prescribing, then follow the guidance illustrated in Fig. 2.7 to write the prescription.

Hospital discharge ('to take out') medicines

The prescription provided on hospital discharge is crucial, because it defines therapy at the point of transfer of prescribing responsibility to primary care. Accuracy is vital, in particular when ensuring that any hospital medicines that should be stopped are not included, and that those intended to be administered short-term are clearly identified. Record any significant ADRs experienced in hospital and any specific monitoring or review required.

Prescribing in primary care

In many health care systems, community prescribing is electronic, making issues of legibility irrelevant, limiting the range of doses that can be written and highlighting potential interactions. Important additional issues more relevant to GP prescribing are:

- *Formulation.* The prescription needs to specify the formulation for the dispensing pharmacist (e.g. tablets or oral suspension).
- *Amount to be supplied.* In the hospital the pharmacist organises this. Elsewhere it must be specified either as the number of tablets

PRESCRIPTION AND ADMINISTRATION RECORD

A

Standard Chart		

Hospital/Ward: **W26**	Consultant: **Maxwell**	Name of patient: **John Smith**
Weight: **78 Kg**	Height: **1.84 m**	Hospital number: **WGH5522589**
If rewritten, date: **14. 2.18**		D.O.B.: **16/10/64**
DISCHARGE PRESCRIPTION Date completed:–	Completed by:–	(Attach printed label here)

OTHER MEDICINES CHARTS		PREVIOUS ADVERSE REACTIONS (This must be completed before prescribing on this chart)			
Date	Type of chart	Medicine	Description of reaction	Completed by	Date
14. 2.18	Oxygen	Penicillin	Serious reaction (hospitalised) age 15	S. Jones	14. 2.18
14. 2.18	Warfarin	Cefalexin	Rash (discontinued) 2006	S. Jones	14. 2.18

B

ONCE-ONLY MEDICINES							
Date	Time	Medicine (approved name)	Dose	Route	Prescriber – sign and print	Time given	Given by
14. 2.18	16.00	MORPHINE SULFATE	5 mg	IV	⟶ S. JONES	16.20	ST
14. 2.18	16.00	GLYCERYL TRINITRATE	2 mg	Buccal	⟶ S. JONES	16.10	DK
14. 2.18	16.00	METOCLOPRAMIDE	10 mg	IV	⟶ S. JONES	16.20	ST

C

REGULAR MEDICINES		Date → Time ↓	February 2018							
			14	15	16	17	18	19	20	21
Drug (approved name) **AMOXICILLIN**		6								
Dose **500 mg**	Route **ORAL**	(8)	X	DK	RB	RB	DK	X	X	X	X
		12								
Prescriber–sign and print S. JONES	Start date **14. 02.18**	(14)	X	DK	2	RB		X	X	X	X
		18								
Notes **For chest infection**	Pharmacy	(22)	X	DK	RB	RB		X	X	X	X
Drug (approved name) **AMLODIPINE**		6								
Dose **5 mg**	Route **ORAL**	(8)	X	DK	RB	Discontinued due to persistent ankle oedema S. Maxwell 16.02.18				
		12								
Prescriber–sign and print S. JONES	Start date **14. 02.18**	14								
		18								
Notes **For hypertension**	Pharmacy	22								

D

AS-REQUIRED THERAPY						
Drug (approved name) **PARACETAMOL**		Date	16.2			
		Time	11.15			
Dose and frequency **1g 4-hrly**	Route **ORAL**	Dose	1g			
		Initials	DK			
Prescriber–sign and print S. JONES	Start date **16. 02.18**	Date				
		Time				
Indication/notes **For pain** **Maximum 4g/24 hr**	Pharmacy	Dose				
		Initials				

Fig. 2.7 Example of a hospital prescription and administration record. **A** *Front page.* Includes identification of the patient, weight and height, responsible consultant, other prescription charts in use and previous adverse reactions. **B** *'Once-only medicines'.* Used for medicines that are unlikely to be repeated regularly. Generic, international, nonproprietary drug names are written legibly in block capitals. The only exceptions are alternative branded formulations that differ importantly (e.g. modified-release preparations) and combination products with no generic name. Dose units: 'g' and 'mg' are acceptable, but 'units' and 'micrograms' must be written in full. For liquids, write the dose in mg; use 'mL' only for a combination product or if the strength is not expressed in weight (e.g. adrenaline 1 in 1000). Always include the dose for inhaled drugs, in addition to numbers of 'puffs', as strengths vary. Widely accepted abbreviations for the route of administration are: IV, IM, SC, SL, PR, PV, NG, INH and TOP. 'ORAL' is preferred to 'PO'. Specify 'RIGHT' or 'LEFT' for eye and ear drops. The prescriber should sign and print his or her name clearly, and the prescription should be dated and show an administration time. **C** *'Regular medicines'.* The name, dose, route and frequency of administration is required for each medicine. Latin abbreviations for dose frequency are: once daily—'OD'; twice daily—'BD'; three times daily—'TDS'; four times daily—'QDS'; as required—'PRN'; in the morning—'OM'; at night—'ON'; and immediately—'stat'. The times specified for regular medicines should coincide with drug rounds, and these are circled. If treatment is for a finite time, cross off subsequent days. The 'notes' box is used to communicate additional information (e.g. inhaler device, times for drug level sampling etc.). Prescriptions are discontinued by drawing a vertical line at the time of discontinuation and diagonal lines through the drug details and administration boxes. This notation should be signed and dated, and a note should be written to explain it. **D** *'As-required medicines'.* The administration of these prescribed drugs is at the discretion of the nursing staff. The prescription must describe clearly the indication, frequency, minimal time interval between doses and maximum dose in a day.

---

or the duration of treatment. Creams and ointments are specified in grams, and lotions in mL.

- *Controlled drugs.* These prescriptions (e.g. opioids) are subject to additional laws. In the United Kingdom, they must contain the address of the patient and prescriber, the form and strength of the preparation and the total quantity/number of dose units in both words and figures.
- *'Repeat prescriptions'.* Much of GP prescribing involves 'repeat prescriptions' for chronic medication. These are often generated automatically, but the prescriber remains responsible for regular review.

Monitoring drug therapy

Prescribers should measure the beneficial and harmful effects of drugs, to inform decisions about dose titration, discontinuation or substitution of treatment. Monitoring can be subjective, through symptoms, or objective, by measuring effect. Alternatively, the plasma drug concentration may be measured, on the basis that it will be closely related to the effect of the drug.

2.14 High-risk prescribing moments

- Trying to amend an active prescription (e.g. altering the dose/timing)—*always avoid and start again*
- Writing up drugs in the immediate presence of more than one prescription chart or set of notes—*avoid*
- Allowing one's attention to be diverted in the middle of completing a prescription—*avoid*
- Prescribing 'high-risk' drugs (e.g. anticoagulants, opioids, insulin, sedatives)—*ask for help if necessary*
- Prescribing parenteral drugs—*take care*
- Rushing prescribing (e.g. in the midst of a busy ward round)—*avoid*
- Prescribing unfamiliar drugs—*consult the formulary and ask for help if necessary*
- Transcribing multiple prescriptions from an expired chart to a new one—*review the rationale for each*
- Writing prescriptions based on information from another source, such as a referral letter (the list may contain errors and some of the medicines may be the cause of the patient's illness)—*review the justification for each as if it is a new prescription*
- Writing up 'to take out' drugs (because these will become the patient's regular medication for the immediate future)—*take care and seek advice if necessary*
- Calculating drug doses—*ask a colleague to perform an independent calculation, or use approved electronic dose calculators*
- Prescribing sound-alike or look-alike drugs (e.g. chlorphenamine and chlorpromazine)—*take care*

Clinical and surrogate endpoints

Ideally, clinical endpoints are measured directly, and the drug dosage is titrated to achieve effective therapy and avoid toxicity. Sometimes this is impractical because the clinical endpoint is a future event (e.g. prevention of myocardial infarction by statins); in these cases, a 'surrogate' endpoint may be chosen to predict success or failure. Examples include serum cholesterol as a surrogate for risk of myocardial infarction, or serum C-reactive protein as a measure of inflammation in chest infection.

Plasma drug concentration measurement

This can be justified if:

- Clinical endpoints and surrogate effects are difficult to monitor.
- The relationship between plasma concentration and clinical effects is predictable.
- The therapeutic index is low.
  Common examples are listed in Box 2.15.

2.15 Drugs commonly monitored by plasma drug concentration		
Drug	Half-life (hours)[a]	Comment
Digoxin	36	Steady state takes several days to achieve. Sample 6 hours postdose. Levels useful to confirm toxicity or nonadherence, but clinical effectiveness is better assessed by ventricular heart rate.
Gentamicin	2	Predose trough concentration should be <1 µg/mL to ensure that accumulation (causing nephrotoxicity and ototoxicity) is avoided.
Levothyroxine	>120	Steady state may take up to 6 weeks to achieve.
Lithium	24	Steady state takes several days to achieve. Sample 12 hours postdose.
Phenytoin	24	Predose trough concentration should be 10–20 mg/L to avoid accumulation.
Theophylline (oral)	6	Steady state takes 2–3 days to achieve. Sample 6 hours postdose. Low therapeutic index.
Vancomycin	6	Predose trough concentration should be 10–15 mg/L to ensure efficacy and avoid accumulation and nephrotoxicity.

[a]Half-lives vary considerably with different formulations and between patients.

Timing of samples in relation to doses

Measurements made during the initial absorption and distribution phases are unpredictable, so samples are usually taken at the end of the dosage interval ('trough' or 'predose'). A steady state takes five half-lives to achieve after the drug is introduced or the dose is changed (unless a loading dose is given).

Interpreting the results

A target range is provided for many drugs, based on average thresholds for therapeutic benefit and toxicity, but individuals may develop toxic side effects within the therapeutic range. For heavily protein-bound drugs (e.g. phenytoin), only the unbound drug is pharmacologically active. Patients with hypoalbuminaemia may therefore have a therapeutic or even toxic concentration of unbound drug, despite a low 'total' concentration.

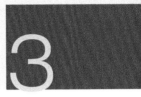

3

Poisoning

Acute poisoning accounts for around 1% of hospital admissions in the UK. In developed countries, intentional self-harm using prescribed or 'over-the-counter' medicines is most common, with paracetamol, antidepressants and drugs of misuse being the most frequently used. Accidental poisoning is also common in children and the elderly. Poisoning is a major cause of death in young adults, and death usually occurs before hospital admission. In developing countries, self-harm with OP pesticides and herbicides is endemic, and frequently fatal.

General approach to the poisoned patient

Triage

• Assess vital signs immediately. • Identify poison(s) involved and obtain information about them. • Identify patients at risk of further self-harm and remove remaining hazards from them.

Critically ill patients must be resuscitated.

History

Try to establish:
• What toxin(s) have been taken and how much • When and how were they taken • Whether alcohol or other drugs have been taken too • Whether any witness can corroborate the information • What drugs the GP has prescribed • What the risk of suicide is • Whether the patient is capable of making rational decisions • Whether there are any other significant medical conditions.

Be aware that, occasionally, patients may conceal information, exaggerate or deliberately mislead staff.

In envenomed patients, establish:
• When the patient was exposed to the bite/sting • What the causal organism looked like • How it happened • Whether there were multiple bites/stings • What first aid was given • What the patient's symptoms are • Whether the patient has other medical conditions, regular treatments, has had previous similar episodes or has known allergies.

Clinical examination of the poisoned patient

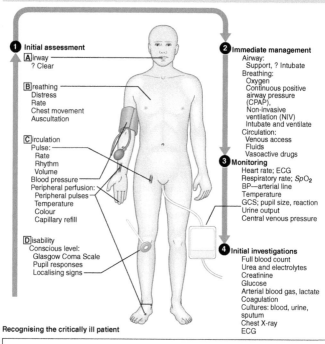

1 Initial assessment

Airway
? Clear

Breathing
Distress
Rate
Chest movement
Auscultation

Circulation
Pulse:
Rate
Rhythm
Volume
Blood pressure
Peripheral perfusion:
Peripheral pulses
Temperature
Colour
Capillary refill

Disability
Conscious level:
Glasgow Coma Scale
Pupil responses
Localising signs

2 Immediate management
Airway:
Support, ? Intubate
Breathing:
Oxygen
Continuous positive
airway pressure
(CPAP),
Non-invasive
ventilation (NIV)
Intubate and ventilate
Circulation:
Venous access
Fluids
Vasoactive drugs

3 Monitoring
Heart rate; ECG
Respiratory rate; SpO_2
BP—arterial line
Temperature
GCS; pupil size, reaction
Urine output
Central venous pressure

4 Initial investigations
Full blood count
Urea and electrolytes
Creatinine
Glucose
Arterial blood gas, lactate
Coagulation
Cultures: blood, urine,
sputum
Chest X-ray
ECG

Recognising the critically ill patient

Cardiovascular signs	Respiratory signs	Neurological signs

• Cardiac arrest
• Pulse rate <40 or >140 bpm
• Systolic blood pressure (BP) <100 mmHg
• Tissue hypoxia:
  Poor peripheral perfusion
  Metabolic acidosis
  Hyperlactataemia
• Poor response to volume resuscitation
• Oliguria: <0.5 mL/kg/hr (check urea, creatinine, K⁺)
	• Threatened or obstructed airway
	• Stridor, intercostal recession
	• Respiratory arrest
	• Respiratory rate <8 or >35/min
	• Respiratory 'distress': use of accessory muscles; unable to speak in complete sentences
	• SpO_2 <90% on high-flow O_2
	• Rising $PaCO_2$ >8 kPa (>60 mmHg), or >2 kPa (>15 mmHg) above 'normal' with acidosis
		• Threatened or obstructed airway
		• Absent gag or cough reflex
		• Failure to maintain normal PaO_2 and $PaCO_2$
		• Failure to obey commands
		• Glasgow Coma Scale (GCS) <10
		• Sudden fall in level of consciousness (GCS fall >2 points)
		• Repeated or prolonged seizures

Clinical examination

This is summarised on the previous page. There may be needle marks or evidence of previous self-harm, for example, razor marks on forearms. Pupil size, respiratory rate and heart rate may help to narrow down the potential list of toxins. The GCS (p. 69) is most frequently used to assess the degree of impaired consciousness. The patient's weight helps to determine whether toxicity is likely to occur, given the dose ingested. When patients are unconscious and no history is available, other causes of coma must be excluded (especially meningitis, intracerebral bleeds, hypoglycaemia, diabetic ketoacidosis, uraemia and encephalopathy). Certain classes of drug cause clusters of typical signs, for example, cholinergic, anticholinergic, sedative or opioid effects, which can aid diagnosis.

Investigations

U&Es and creatinine should be measured in all patients, and ABGs in those with circulatory or respiratory compromise. Drug levels are a useful guide to treatment for some specific toxins, for example, paracetamol, salicylate, iron, digoxin, carboxyhaemoglobin, lithium and theophylline. Urinary drug screens have a limited clinical role.

Psychiatric assessment

Patients presenting with drug overdose in the context of self-harm should undergo professional psychiatric evaluation before discharge, but ideally after recovering from poisoning. The purpose is to establish the short-term risk of suicide and to identify potentially treatable problems, either medical, psychiatric or social. Risk factors for suicide are shown in Box 3.1.

Management of the poisoned patient

Eye or skin contamination should be treated with appropriate washing or irrigation. Patients who have recently ingested significant overdoses need further measures to prevent absorption or increase elimination:

 3.1 Risk factors for suicide

- Psychiatric illness (depression, schizophrenia)
- Older age
- Male sex
- Living alone
- Unemployment
- Recent bereavement, divorce or separation
- Chronic physical ill health
- Drug or alcohol misuse
- Suicide note written
- Previous attempts (especially if violent method)

• Oral activated charcoal slurry (50 g orally) can be given if a potentially toxic amount of poison has been ingested less than 1 hour before presentation. Agents that do not bind to activated charcoal include ethylene glycol, iron, lithium, mercury and methanol. • Gastric aspiration is no more effective than charcoal and is rarely indicated. • Whole-bowel irrigation with polyethylene glycol can be used for iron or lithium overdose, or to flush out packets of illicit drugs. • Urinary alkalinisation using IV sodium bicarbonate enhances elimination of salicylates and methotrexate. • Haemodialysis is occasionally used for serious poisoning with salicylates, ethylene glycol, methanol, lithium or sodium valproate. • Haemoperfusion can help to eliminate theophylline, phenytoin, carbamazepine and barbiturates. • Infusions of lipid emulsion can be used to reduce tissue concentrations of lipid-soluble drugs such as TCAs.

Antidotes are available for some poisons and work by a variety of mechanisms (Box 3.2).

For most poisons, antidotes and methods to accelerate elimination are inappropriate, unavailable or ineffective. Outcome depends on supportive care and treatment of complications.

3.2 Antidotes for poisoning and their mechanisms of action		
Mechanism of action	**Examples of antidote**	**Poisoning treated**
Glutathione repleters	Acetylcysteine Methionine	Paracetamol
Receptor antagonists	Naloxone	Opioids
	Flumazenil	Benzodiazepines
	Atropine	Organophosphorus compounds Carbamates
Alcohol dehydrogenase inhibitors	Fomepizole Ethanol	Ethylene glycol Methanol
Chelating agents	Desferrioxamine	Iron
	Hydroxocobalamin Dicobalt edetate	Cyanide
	DMSA Sodium calcium edetate	Lead
Reducing agents	Methylthioninium chloride	Organic nitrites
Cholinesterase reactivators	Pralidoxime	Organophosphorus compounds
Antibody fragments	Digoxin Fab fragments	Digoxin

Poisoning by specific pharmaceutical agents

Paracetamol

In overdose, paracetamol causes hepatic damage and occasionally renal failure. The antidote of choice is NAC given IV (orally in some countries), which protects against toxicity if given less than 8 hours after overdose. Threshold blood levels for treatment are shown in Fig. 3.1. A patient presenting more than 8 hours after ingestion should receive NAC immediately; the infusion can later be stopped if the paracetamol level is below the treatment line.

Liver and renal function, prothrombin ratio (or INR) and venous bicarbonate should be measured. ABGs and lactate are indicated in patients with reduced bicarbonate or severe liver function abnormalities.

Liver transplantation should be considered for paracetamol poisoning with life-threatening liver failure. If multiple paracetamol ingestions have taken place over time (a staggered overdose), plasma paracetamol concentration will be uninterpretable. NAC may still be indicated, although treatment thresholds vary between countries.

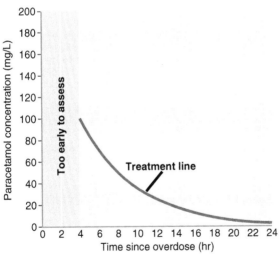

Fig. 3.1 Paracetamol treatment nomogram (United Kingdom). Above the treatment line, benefits of treatment outweigh risk. Below it, risks of treatment outweigh benefits.

Salicylates (aspirin)

Symptoms of salicylate overdose include nausea, vomiting, tinnitus and deafness. Direct stimulation of the respiratory centre produces hyperventilation. Signs of serious poisoning include vasodilation with sweating, hyperpyrexia, metabolic acidosis, pulmonary oedema, renal failure, agitation, delirium, coma and fits.

Activated charcoal is useful within 1 hour of ingestion. Plasma salicylate concentration is measured 2 hours after ingestion in symptomatic patients, then repeated because of continued drug absorption. Clinical status is more important than salicylate concentration when assessing severity. Dehydration should be corrected by careful fluid replacement, and metabolic acidosis treated with IV sodium bicarbonate (8.4%) after plasma potassium has been corrected. Urinary alkalinisation is indicated for adults with salicylate concentrations greater than 500 mg/L. Haemodialysis should be considered if serum salicylate is greater than 700 mg/L, if there is resistant metabolic acidosis or if severe CNS effects (coma, convulsions) are present.

Nonsteroidal antiinflammatory drugs

Nonsteroidal antiinflammatory drug overdose usually causes only minor GI upset, including mild abdominal pain, vomiting and diarrhoea. Rarely, patients have convulsions; these are usually self-limiting and seldom need treatment beyond airway protection and oxygen. Activated charcoal (within 1 hour of overdose) and symptomatic treatment are usually sufficient.

Antidepressant overdose

Tricyclic antidepressants (TCAs): cause anticholinergic, sodium channel-blocking and α-blocking effects. Severe complications include coma, hypotension and arrhythmias, such as ventricular tachycardia/fibrillation or heart block. Activated charcoal is useful within 1 hour of ingestion. ECG monitoring is needed for at least 6 hours. QRS or QT prolongation indicates risk of arrhythmia, and should be treated with IV sodium bicarbonate (8.4%).

Selective serotonin re-uptake inhibitors: cause nausea, tremor, insomnia and tachycardia, but rarely lead to serious arrhythmia, and supportive treatment is usually sufficient.

Lithium: causes nausea, diarrhoea, polyuria, weakness, ataxia, coma and convulsions. Charcoal is ineffective, and haemodialysis is used in severe cases.

Cardiovascular medications

β-Blockers: cause bradycardia and hypotension. Overdose is treated using IV fluids, with atropine or isoproterenol to counteract bradycardia.

Calcium channel blockers: cause hypotension and heart block in overdose. IV fluids and isoproterenol may be effective; insulin/dextrose infusions or pacing are also used in resistant cases.

Digoxin poisoning: is usually accidental or because of renal failure. ECG monitoring is needed, as bradycardia or ventricular arrhythmias may occur. Digoxin-specific antibody fragments should be administered if serious arrhythmias occur.

Antidiabetic agents

Sulphonylureas, meglitinides and parenteral insulins can all cause hypoglycaemia in overdose, although insulin is nontoxic if ingested.

The duration of hypoglycaemia varies, but can last for several days with the longer-acting agents such as glibenclamide, insulin zinc suspension or insulin glargine. Metformin overdose can cause lactic acidosis, which has high mortality and particularly affects elderly patients, those with renal or hepatic impairment or those who co-ingest ethanol. Hypoglycaemia should be corrected urgently using oral or IV glucose (50 mL 50% dextrose); an infusion of 10% or 20% dextrose may be required to prevent recurrence. Blood glucose and U&Es should be checked regularly.

Drugs of misuse

Benzodiazepines

Benzodiazepines (e.g. diazepam) and related substances (e.g. zopiclone) are of low toxicity when taken alone in overdose but can enhance CNS and respiratory depression when taken with other sedative agents, including alcohol. They are more hazardous in the elderly and those with chronic lung or neuromuscular disease.

The specific benzodiazepine antagonist flumazenil (0.5 mg IV, repeated if needed) increases conscious level in patients with benzodiazepine overdose, but carries a risk of seizures and is contraindicated in patients co-ingesting proconvulsants (e.g. TCAs) and those with a history of epilepsy.

Opioids

Toxicity may result from misuse of illicit drugs such as heroin or from intentional or accidental overdose of medicinal opiates such as methadone, fentanyl, pethidine and oxycodone. IV or smoked heroin gives a rapid, intensely pleasurable experience, often accompanied by heightened sexual arousal. Physical dependence occurs within a few weeks of regular high-dose use. Withdrawal can start within 12 hours, causing intense craving, rhinorrhoea, lacrimation, yawning, perspiration, shivering, piloerection, vomiting, diarrhoea and abdominal cramps. Examination reveals tachycardia, hypertension, mydriasis and facial flushing.

Opioid overdose causes respiratory depression, hypotension, slurred speech, delirium or coma, with accompanying miosis, ileus and reduced muscle tone. Needle tracks may be visible in intravenous users, and there may be drug-related paraphernalia. Methadone may also cause QT_c prolongation and torsades de pointes. Opioid poisoning can persist for up to 48 hours after long-acting agents such as methadone or oxycodone have been taken.

The specific opioid antagonist naloxone (0.4–2 mg IV in an adult, repeated if necessary) may obviate the need for intubation, although it may precipitate acute withdrawal in chronic opiate users and breakthrough pain in those receiving opioids for pain management. Repeated doses or an infusion are often required because the half-life of the antidote is short compared with that of most opiates. Patients should be monitored for at least 6 hours after the last naloxone dose.

Gamma hydroxybutyrate

Gamma hydroxybutyrate and gamma butyrolactone are sedative liquids with psychedelic and body-building effects.

Toxic features include sedation, coma, hallucinations and hypotension. Nausea, diarrhoea, vertigo, tremor, myoclonus, extrapyramidal signs, fits, metabolic acidosis, hypokalaemia and hyperglycaemia may also occur. Dependence may develop in regular users, who experience severe, prolonged withdrawal effects if use is discontinued suddenly.

Coma usually resolves spontaneously and abruptly within hours. Management is largely supportive. All patients should be monitored and supported for at least 2 hours; withdrawal symptoms are treated with benzodiazepines.

Cocaine

Cocaine is available as water-soluble hydrochloride crystals for nasal inhalation or as an insoluble free base ('crack' cocaine) that vaporises at high temperature and produces a rapid intense effect when smoked.

Effects appear rapidly after inhalation, especially after smoking, and include euphoria, agitation and aggression. Sympathomimetic effects, including tachycardia and mydriasis, are common; and serious complications, including coronary artery spasm, myocardial infarction, ventricular arrhythmias, convulsions, hypertension and stroke, may occur within 3 hours of use. All patients should be observed with ECG monitoring for at least 4 hours. ST elevation is common, and troponin T is a useful marker of myocardial damage. Benzodiazepines and IV nitrates should be used to treat chest pain or hypertension, but β-blockers should be avoided. Coronary angiography may be required, and acidosis should be corrected.

Amphetamines

These include amphetamine sulphate ('speed'), methylamphetamine ('crystal meth') and 3,4- MDMA ('ecstasy'). Tolerance is common, leading regular users to seek progressively higher doses.

Toxic features appear in minutes and last 4 to 6 hours, or longer after a large overdose. Sympathomimetic and serotonergic effects are common, and serious complications include supraventricular and ventricular arrhythmias, hyperpyrexia, rhabdomyolysis, coma, convulsions, metabolic acidosis, acute renal failure, disseminated intravascular coagulation, hepatocellular necrosis and ARDS. A small proportion of patients who have taken ecstasy develop hyponatraemia, usually through drinking excessive amounts of water in the absence of sufficient exertion to sweat it out. Management is supportive and directed at complications.

Cannabis

Cannabis (grass, pot, ganja, spliff, reefer) is commonly smoked with tobacco or eaten.

In low doses, cannabis produces euphoria, perceptual alterations and conjunctival injection, followed by relaxation and drowsiness, hypertension, tachycardia, slurred speech and ataxia. High doses can produce hallucinations and psychosis. Ingestion or smoking rarely results in serious poisoning, and supportive treatment is normally sufficient.

Synthetic cannabinoid receptor agonists

SCRAs, known colloquially as 'spice', are marketed as legal alternatives to cannabis. They are inhaled from a herbal smoking mix.

The toxic effects of SCRAs are generally more marked than those of cannabis, and include agitation, panic, delirium, hallucinations, tachycardia, ECG changes, hypertonia, dyspnoea and vomiting. Coma, respiratory acidosis, seizures, hypokalaemia and renal dysfunction also occur. Treatment is supportive.

d-Lysergic acid diethylamide (LSD)

LSD is a synthetic ergoline usually ingested as small squares of impregnated absorbent paper.

Visual perception is affected, with heightened visual awareness of colours, image distortion and hallucinations. Patients may present to hospital because of a 'bad trip', with panic, confusion, vivid visual hallucinations or self-harm caused by psychosis. Other features are delirium, agitation, aggression, dilated pupils, hypertension, pyrexia and metabolic acidosis. Patients with psychotic reactions should be observed in a quiet, dim room. Sedation with benzodiazepines may be needed.

Volatile substances

Inhalation of volatile nitrites (e.g. amyl nitrite, isobutyl nitrite, 'poppers') produces feelings of pleasure and warmth, relaxes the anal sphincter and prolongs orgasm. It also causes vasodilator effects (headache, dizziness, hypotension, tachycardia) and methaemoglobinaemia. Severe overdose is treated with methylthioninium chloride.

Volatile solvents in household products (e.g. propane, butane and trichloroethylene) have a mild euphoriant effect if inhaled. Serious toxic effects include impaired consciousness, seizures and cardiac arrhythmias.

Body packers and stuffers

Body packers smuggle large quantities of illicit cocaine, heroin or amphetamines by swallowing packages wrapped in clingfilm or condoms. Body stuffers attempt to conceal illicit drugs by swallowing them (often poorly packaged) to avoid arrest. Both risk acute severe toxicity from package rupture. Packages may be visible on x-ray, CT or ultrasound. Passage may be accelerated by whole-bowel irrigation.

Alcohol misuse and dependence

Alcohol consumption associated with social, psychological and physical problems constitutes misuse. The criteria for alcohol dependence, a more restricted term, are shown in Box 3.3. Approximately one-quarter of male patients in general hospital medical wards in the UK have a current

3.3 Criteria for alcohol dependence

- Narrowing of the drinking repertoire
- Priority of drinking over other activities (salience)
- Tolerance of effects of alcohol
- Repeated withdrawal symptoms
- Relief of withdrawal symptoms by further drinking
- Subjective compulsion to drink
- Reinstatement of drinking behaviour after abstinence

or previous alcohol problem. Availability of alcohol and social patterns of use are the most important factors. Genetic factors predispose to dependence. The majority of alcoholics do not have an associated psychiatric illness, but a few drink heavily in an attempt to relieve anxiety or depression.

Consequences of alcohol misuse

Acute and chronic effects of alcohol are summarised in Box 3.4.

Social problems: Include absenteeism, unemployment, marital tensions, child abuse, financial difficulties and legal problems such as violence and traffic offences.

Psychological problems: Alcohol has acute depressant effects, and chronic depression is common. Alcohol misuse is often implicated in suicide attempts. People who are anxious may use alcohol to relieve anxiety and then go on to develop dependence. Alcoholic hallucinosis is a rare condition in which patients experience auditory hallucinations in clear consciousness.

Alcohol withdrawal: Symptoms (see Box 3.4) usually appear 2 to 3 days after the last drink. Delirium tremens is a severe withdrawal syndrome featuring delirium, visual hallucinations and physiological hyper-arousal. It has a significant mortality and morbidity.

Effects on the brain: Acute effects include ataxia, slurred speech, aggression and amnesia after heavy drinking. Established alcoholism may cause alcoholic dementia, a global cognitive impairment that resembles Alzheimer's disease but does not progress with abstinence. Indirect effects on brain function can result from head injury, hypoglycaemia and portosystemic encephalopathy. Wernicke-Korsakoff syndrome is a rare brain disorder caused by thiamin (vitamin B_1) deficiency that results from damage to the mamillary bodies, dorsomedial nuclei of the thalamus and adjacent grey matter. The most common cause is long-standing heavy drinking with inadequate diet. Without prompt treatment, acute Wernicke's encephalopathy (nystagmus, ophthalmoplegia, ataxia and confusion) can progress to the irreversible Korsakoff's syndrome (severe short-term memory deficits and confabulation).

Diagnosis

Alcohol excess may emerge from the history, but patients commonly lie about alcohol intake. Alcohol misuse may also present through its social

3.4 Consequences of alcohol misuse

Acute intoxication

- Emotional and behavioural disturbance
- Medical problems—hypoglycaemia, aspiration of vomit, respiratory depression; accidents and injuries sustained in fights

Withdrawal effects

- Psychiatric—restlessness, anxiety, panic attacks
- Autonomic—tachycardia, sweating, pupil dilatation, nausea, vomiting
- Delirium tremens—agitation, hallucinations, illusions, delusions; seizures

Medical

- Neurological—peripheral neuropathy; cerebral haemorrhage; cerebellar degeneration; dementia
- Hepatic—fatty change, cirrhosis, hepatoma
- Gastrointestinal—oesophagitis, gastritis, pancreatitis, oesophageal cancer, Mallory-Weiss syndrome, malabsorption, oesophageal varices
- Respiratory—pulmonary tuberculosis; pneumonia, aspiration
- Skin—spider naevi; palmar erythema; Dupuytren's contractures; telangiectasis
- Cardiac—cardiomyopathy; hypertension
- Musculoskeletal—myopathy; fractures
- Endocrine/metabolic—pseudo-Cushing's syndrome; gout; hypoglycaemia
- Reproductive—hypogonadism; infertility; fetal alcohol syndrome

Psychiatric and cerebral

- Depression
- Hallucinosis
- 'Blackouts'
- Wernicke's encephalopathy
- Korsakoff's syndrome

consequences (see previously) or with withdrawal symptoms on hospital admission, when patients cannot maintain high alcohol intake.

Management

Advice about the harmful effects of alcohol and safe levels of consumption is often sufficient. Altering leisure activities or changing jobs may help, if these are contributing. Psychological treatment at specialised centres is used for patients with recurrent relapses. Support is also provided by voluntary organisations such as Alcoholics Anonymous in the UK. Withdrawal syndromes can be prevented or treated with benzodiazepines. Large doses may be required (e.g. diazepam 20 mg four times daily), tailed off over 5 to 7 days as symptoms subside. Prevention of Wernicke-Korsakoff syndrome requires immediate high doses of thiamin (IV Pabrinex). There is no treatment for established Korsakoff's syndrome. Acamprosate may help sustain abstinence by reducing craving. Disulfiram is used with psychological support to deter patients from relapsing. Antidepressants and antipsychotics may be needed to treat complications. Relapse is common after treatment.

Chemicals and pesticides

Carbon monoxide

CO is a colourless, odourless gas produced in faulty appliances burning organic fuels, house fires and vehicle exhausts. CO binds to haemoglobin and cytochrome oxidase, reducing oxygen delivery and inhibiting cellular respiration. CO poisoning is frequently fatal, often before the patient reaches hospital.

Clinical features

Early features are misleadingly nonspecific: headache, nausea, irritability, weakness and tachypnoea. Late features include lethargy, ataxia, nystagmus, drowsiness, hyperventilation and hyper-reflexia progressing to coma, convulsions, hypotension, respiratory depression and cardiovascular collapse. Myocardial infarction, arrhythmias, cerebral oedema, rhabdomyolysis and renal failure also occur.

Management

High-flow oxygen reduces the half-life of COHb from 4 to 6 hours to around 40 minutes, and should be given as soon as possible. A COHb concentration of greater than 20% confirms significant exposure but does not correlate well with the clinical severity of poisoning. Pulse oximetry is misleading, as it measures both COHb and oxyhaemoglobin. ECG should be checked in all patients, and ABGs in serious cases. Hyperbaric oxygen reduces the half-life of COHb further, but the logistical difficulties of transporting sick patients to hyperbaric chambers are considerable, and benefit has not been proven.

Organophosphorus insecticides and nerve agents

OP compounds are widely used as pesticides (e.g. malathion, fenthion), especially in developing countries, and also as chemical warfare agents (e.g. sarin). OPs inactivate acetylcholinesterase (AChE), leading to accumulation of acetylcholine at cholinergic synapses. The fatality rate following deliberate ingestion of OP pesticides in developing countries is 5% to 20%.

OP poisoning causes an acute cholinergic phase, occasionally followed by the intermediate syndrome of OP-induced delayed polyneuropathy.

Acute cholinergic syndrome: Occurs within minutes of exposure. Vomiting and profuse diarrhoea typically follow ingestion. Bronchoconstriction, bronchorrhoea and salivation cause respiratory compromise. Sweating, miosis and muscle fasciculation are typical, followed by generalised flaccid paralysis affecting respiratory and sometimes ocular muscles, causing respiratory failure. Coma, convulsions and arrhythmias can complicate severe cases.

Management: • The airways should be cleared and maintained • Decontamination: clothing should be removed, eyes irrigated, skin washed and activated charcoal given if within 1 hour of ingestion • Early use of sufficient atropine (2 mg IV, doubled every 5–10 minutes until clinical improvement occurs) is life saving • Oximes such as pralidoxime can reactivate phosphorylated AChE and prevent muscle weakness, convulsions or coma if given early • Intensive cardiorespiratory support is usually required for 48 to 72 hours. Exposure is confirmed by plasma or red blood cell cholinesterase measurements, but antidotes should not be withheld pending results.

Intermediate syndrome: Occurs in 20% of cases 1 to 4 days after poisoning. Progressive muscle weakness spreads from the ocular and facial muscles to involve the limbs, and ultimately causes respiratory failure. Onset is often rapid, but complete recovery is possible with ventilatory support.

Organophosphate-induced delayed polyneuropathy: This rare complication occurs around 2 to 3 weeks after acute exposure. Degeneration of long myelinated nerve fibres leads to a mixed sensory/motor polyneuropathy causing paraesthesia and progressive flaccid weakness, which may progress to paraplegia. Recovery is prolonged and often incomplete.

Paraquat

Paraquat is a herbicide used in many countries, although it has been banned in the European Union. It is highly toxic (commonly fatal) if ingested, causing oral burns, vomiting, diarrhoea, pneumonitis, pulmonary fibrosis and multiorgan failure.

Methanol and ethylene glycol

Ethylene glycol is used in antifreeze, and methanol is found in a number of solvents. Both cause ataxia, drowsiness, coma and fits. Methanol causes blindness. Ethanol and fomepizole are used as antidotes to block the formation of toxic metabolites. Dialysis speeds elimination in severe poisoning.

Food-related poisoning

Plant toxins: A variety of plants and fungi produce toxins capable of causing GI and neurotoxic effects, hypotension and shock.

Chemical toxins: Ciguatera toxin, originating in dinoflagellates and concentrated by shellfish or fish, can cause GI symptoms and paralysis. Scombrotoxic fish poisoning causes acute flushing, hypotension and bronchospasm and results from eating contaminated tuna, mackerel or sardines.

Drinking water contamination

In large parts of the Middle East, South-East Asia and South America, poisoning from contaminated drinking water is endemic. Arsenic causes chronic neuropathy with wasting; excessive fluoride causes tooth, bone and joint disease. Control of drinking water content is the key intervention.

Envenoming

A variety of species use venom either to acquire prey or to defend themselves. Accidental envenoming is common in the rural tropics; however, cases may occur anywhere, caused by exotic venomous pets. Snake and scorpion bites are numerically the most important, but even bee and wasp stings can cause lethal anaphylaxis. Details of individual venoms are available at www.toxinology.com.

The clinical effects of a bite or sting vary widely, and some bites contain no venom ('dry bites').

Local effects: Vary from trivial to severe pain, swelling and necrosis. Lethal systemic effects may accompany trivial local symptoms.

General systemic effects: Include headache, nausea, shock, collapse, fits, pulmonary oedema and cardiac arrest.

Specific systemic effects: Depend on the toxin present, and may be:

- Neurotoxic—flaccid paralysis or excitatory paralysis causing 'autonomic storm'.
- Cardiotoxic—usually nonspecific.
- Myotoxic—muscle pain, myoglobinuria, renal failure, raised CK.
- Renotoxic—secondary to hypotension or myoglobin, or direct. May cause hyperkalaemic cardiotoxicity.
- Coagulopathy—bruising, bleeding or thrombosis.

Management

Rapid and accurate history, examination and early initiation of treatment are all vital. Multiple bites or stings are more likely to cause major envenoming.

- In the field: effective cardiopulmonary resuscitation is crucial.
- Avoid harmful 'treatments', for example, cut and suck, tourniquets.
- Accurate identification of the organism.
- For snake bites: immobilisation of the bitten limb to limit venom spread.
- For nonnecrotic snake and spider bites: pressure bandage plus immobilisation.
- For fish/jellyfish stings: local heat (45°C water immersion).
- ECG, O_2 saturation, blood count, U&Es, CK and coagulation screen.
- In remote locations: it may be useful to check blood held in a glass container for clotting at 20 minutes.
- Cardiovascular, respiratory and renal support take precedence over antivenom administration.
- Rapid administration of the species-appropriate antivenom.
- Treatment of specific coagulopathy.

Acute medicine and critical illness

With increasing life expectancy, patients now commonly suffer multiple chronic illnesses, creating the need for experts in undifferentiated presentation. Against this background, acute illness can present in many ways, depending on the cause, the patient's underlying health, and his or her cultural and religious background. Prompt diagnosis and treatment rely on the integration of new information from multiple sources, with knowledge of prior health problems.

Patients who deteriorate in hospital are a small but important cohort. When well managed, their in-hospital mortality will be low. Key elements include: early recognition of deterioration by ward teams, appropriate end-of-life decision making, prompt resuscitation and initial management by a rapid response team.

Acute medicine

Acute medicine concerns the immediate and early management of medical patients requiring urgent care. It is closely allied to emergency medicine and intensive care medicine, but firmly rooted within general medicine. Acute physicians manage the adult medical take and lead the development of acute care pathways that aim to improve and standardise care and reduce admissions.

The decision to admit to hospital

An experienced clinician should evaluate each patient's requirement for admission based on the severity of illness, the physiological reserve, the need for urgent investigations, the nature of proposed treatments and the patient's social circumstances. In many cases, it is obvious that a patient requires admission, and a move into a medical receiving unit should be arranged immediately after the initial assessment. In hospitals without such units, patients should be moved to a downstream ward once treatment has been started and they are stable. Following initial assessment, stable patients may be discharged home with early follow-up (e.g. a rapid-access specialist clinic appointment).

Ambulatory care

It is increasingly possible to manage some problems outside hospital, avoiding admission. In acute medicine, ambulatory care offers, for a defined set of conditions (Box 4.1), prompt clinical assessment by a competent decision maker with access to appropriate investigations. The patient may return repeatedly for investigation, observation, consultation or treatment. Successful ambulatory care requires careful patient selection; although many patients are keen to return home, others may find frequent hospital visits impossible because of frailty, mobility or transport difficulties.

Presenting problems in acute medicine

Chest pain

This common presenting symptom has a wide differential diagnosis, and a detailed history and thorough clinical examination are crucial to accurate diagnosis.

Presentation

Chest 'pain' is subjective and may be described by patients in many ways. Whether the patient reports 'pain', 'discomfort' or 'pressure' in the chest, key features that must be elicited from the history include:

Site and radiation: Chest pain in myocardial ischaemia is typically central, radiating to the neck, jaw and upper or lower arms. Occasionally, it is felt only at the sites of radiation or in the back. The pain of myocarditis or pericarditis is

i	**4.1 Groups of patients who are potentially suitable for ambulatory care**	
Group	Example(s)	Quality and safety issues
Diagnostic exclusion group	Chest pain—possible myocardial infarction; breathlessness—possible pulmonary embolism	Even when a specific condition has been excluded, there is still a need to explain the patient's symptoms through the diagnostic process
Low-risk stratification group	Nonvariceal upper gastrointestinal bleed with low Blatchford score; community-acquired pneumonia with low CURB-65 score (Fig. 9.6)	Appropriate treatment plans should be in place
Specific procedure group	Replacement of PEG tube; drainage of pleural effusion/ascites	The key to implementation is how ambulatory care for this group of patients can be delivered when they present out of hours
Outpatient group with supporting infrastructure	DVT; cellulitis	These are distinct from the conditions listed above because the infrastructure required to manage them is quite different

characteristically felt retrosternally, to the left of the sternum or in either shoulder. Aortic dissection (p. 289) typically causes severe, central pain radiating to the back. Central chest pain also occurs with tumours affecting the mediastinum, or in oesophageal disease (p. 464). Pain in the left anterior chest radiating laterally is unlikely to represent cardiac ischaemia, and often indicates pleural or lung disorders, musculoskeletal problems or anxiety. Rarely, sharp, left-sided chest pain is a feature of mitral valve prolapse (p. 298).

Characteristics: Pleurisy, a sharp or 'catching' chest pain aggravated by deep breathing or coughing, indicates respiratory pathology, particularly pneumothorax, pulmonary infection or infarction. However, the pain of myocarditis or pericarditis may also be 'sharp' and may 'catch' during inspiration, coughing or lying flat. A tumour invading the chest wall or ribs can cause gnawing, continuous local pain. The pain or 'discomfort' of myocardial ischaemia is typically dull, constricting, choking or 'heavy', and is usually described as squeezing, crushing, burning or aching. Angina most commonly occurs during exertion and is promptly (<5 minutes) relieved by rest. It may also be precipitated by emotion, a large meal or a cold wind. In crescendo or unstable angina, pain occurs on minimal exertion or at rest. Increased venous return on lying down provokes pain in decubitus angina. Patients with asthma also describe chest tightness provoked by exercise, but this commonly comes on after exercise and persists during recovery, unlike myocardial ischaemia, and may be associated with wheeze, atopy and cough (p. 322). Musculoskeletal chest pain is variable in site and intensity but lacks any of the typical patterns described earlier. The pain may vary with posture or a specific movement, and local tenderness is typical. Minor soft tissue injuries are common with driving, manual work and sport.

Onset: The pain of MI typically takes several minutes to reach maximal intensity; similarly, angina increases in proportion to exertion. Pain occurring after (not during) exertion is usually musculoskeletal or psychological. The pain of aortic dissection, massive PE or pneumothorax is usually very sudden in onset. Other causes of chest pain tend to develop more gradually.

Associated features: The pain of MI, massive PE or aortic dissection is often accompanied by autonomic disturbance, including sweating, nausea and vomiting. Some patients describe a feeling of impending death, referred to as 'angor animi'. Breathlessness, attributed to left ventricular dysfunction causing pulmonary congestion, often accompanies myocardial ischemia. Breathlessness may also accompany any of the respiratory causes of chest pain, often together with cough or wheeze. Patients with myocarditis or pericarditis may describe a prodromal viral illness. Gastro-esophageal reflux or peptic ulceration may present with chest pain mimicking myocardial ischaemia, which may even be precipitated by exercise and be relieved by nitrates. However, the history often reveals that symptoms are associated with eating, drinking or oesophageal reflux. Reflux pain often radiates to the interscapular region, and dysphagia may be present. Chest pain after severe vomiting or following gastroscopy may indicate oesophageal perforation.

Anxiety-induced chest pain may be associated with breathlessness (without hypoxaemia), throat tightness, perioral tingling and other symptoms of emotional distress. However, chest pain can itself be extremely frightening, so psychological and organic features often coexist.

Clinical assessment

Cardiorespiratory examination may reveal diagnostic signs. In suspected myocardial ischaemia, a 12-lead ECG is essential. Ongoing chest pain with shock, pulmonary oedema or ventricular arrhythmia or heart block on ECG should prompt urgent cardiology review and transfer to higher level care.

Chest pain with signs of increased intracardiac pressure (especially raised JVP) increases the likelihood of myocardial ischaemia or massive PE. The legs should be examined for signs of DVT.

A large pneumothorax should be evident on clinical examination, with absent breath sounds despite resonant percussion on the affected side. Unilateral bronchial breathing or crackles usually indicate respiratory infection, and a CXR should be expedited. Pleural disease may restrict rib movement, with a pleural rub on the affected side. Local chest wall tenderness usually indicates musculoskeletal pain, but also occurs in pulmonary infarction.

Pericarditis may be accompanied by a pericardial friction rub. In aortic dissection, there may be syncope, neurological deficit, asymmetrical pulses, features of Marfan's syndrome (p. 290) or an early diastolic murmur representing aortic regurgitation.

Subdiaphragmatic inflammation (e.g. liver abscess, cholecystitis or ascending cholangitis) can mimic pneumonia by causing fever, pleuritic pain and a sympathetic right pleural effusion. Likewise, acute pancreatitis can present with thoracic symptoms, and an amylase or lipase level may be diagnostic. The abdomen must be examined in all patients with pleuritic chest pain.

Initial investigations

These are guided by the history and examination findings, but a CXR and ECG should be performed in most patients presenting to hospital with chest pain.

The CXR may reveal pneumonia, pneumothorax, rib fractures or metastatic deposits. Careful review is needed to avoid missing small abnormalities. A widened mediastinum suggests aortic dissection, but a normal CXR does not exclude this. In oesophageal rupture, more than 1 hour after symptom onset, the X-ray may show subcutaneous emphysema, pneumomediastinum or pleural effusion.

Acute chest pain with ECG changes of STEMI should trigger immediate reperfusion therapy. A history of cocaine or amphetamine use should be sought. If the history suggests MI but the ECG shows ischaemic changes not meeting STEMI criteria, regular repeat ECGs and treatment for NSTEMI/ unstable angina should begin. Serum troponin on admission is often helpful in unclear cases; however, if negative, it should be repeated 6 to 12 hours after maximal pain. Acute coronary syndrome may be diagnosed in patients with a convincing history of ischaemic pain and either ECG evidence of ischaemia or elevated serum troponin. Elevated serum troponin in a patient with an atypical history or a low risk of cardiac ischaemia may indicate myocarditis, PE, sepsis, hypotension, stroke or renal failure.

In chest pain without myocardial ischaemia, causes such as aortic dissection, massive PE and oesophageal rupture should be considered. Thoracic CT or transoesophageal echocardiography are useful in suspected dissection. In massive PE, the CXR and ECG are commonly normal; the classic $S_1Q_3T_3$ ECG pattern is rare. If massive PE is suspected and the patient is haemodynamically unstable, a transthoracic ECG may confirm right heart strain and exclude alternative diagnoses such as tamponade.

In patients at low risk of PE, a negative D-dimer effectively excludes the diagnosis. The D-dimer should be measured only if there is clinical suspicion of PE because false-positive results encourage unnecessary investigations. If the D-dimer is positive, there is high clinical suspicion or there is other convincing evidence of PE (e.g. right heart strain on ECG), prompt CT pulmonary angiography should be arranged (p. 356 and Fig. 9.13).

Acute breathlessness

In acute breathlessness, a careful history and examination will usually suggest a diagnosis that can be confirmed by CXR, ECG and ABG (Box 4.2).

Presentation

An important clue is the speed of onset. Acute severe breathlessness (onset in minutes to hours) has a different differential diagnosis to chronic exertional breathlessness (covered on p. 312). Associated cardiovascular or respiratory symptoms or a previous history of left ventricular dysfunction, asthma or COPD can narrow the differential diagnosis. In severely ill patients, history from a witness may be helpful. Remember that there is often more than one underlying diagnosis, and continued re-evaluation is needed.

Clinical assessment

Upper airway obstruction, anaphylaxis and tension pneumothorax require immediate identification and treatment, which should not await investigation; urgent anaesthetic airway support is usually required. In the absence of these life-threatening causes, document the following: level of consciousness, degree of central cyanosis, work of breathing (rate, depth, pattern, use of accessory muscles), oxygenation (SpO_2), ability to speak (single words/ sentences) and cardiovascular status (HR, BP, JVP, perfusion).

Pulmonary oedema is suggested by a raised JVP and bibasal crackles, whereas asthma or COPD are characterised by wheeze and prolonged expiration. A resonant hemithorax with absent breath sounds indicates pneumothorax, whereas severe breathlessness with normal breath sounds suggests PE. Leg swelling may suggest cardiac failure or, if asymmetrical, venous thrombosis.

Although wheeze usually accompanies bronchospasm, it can also be found in acute left heart failure because of bronchial mucosal congestion ('cardiac asthma'). In heart failure, pulmonary oedema stimulates breathing through vagal lung afferents, producing rapid, shallow breathing. An upright posture may ease the breathlessness. The patient may be unable to speak, distressed, agitated, sweaty and pale. Cough may yield frothy, blood-streaked or pink sputum. Crackles and wheezes are usually audible in the chest, and there may also be signs of right heart failure.

Any arrhythmia may cause breathlessness if the heart is structurally abnormal, for example, new atrial fibrillation in a patient with mitral stenosis. Patients sometimes describe chest tightness as 'breathlessness'.

4.2 Clinical features in acute breathlessness

Condition	History	Signs	Chest X-ray	ABG	ECG
Pulmonary oedema	Chest pain, palpitations, orthopnoea, cardiac history[a]	Central cyanosis, ↑JVP, sweating, cool extremities, basal crackles[a]	Cardiomegaly, oedema/pleural effusions[a]	↓PaO_2, ↓$PaCO_2$	Sinus tachycardia, ischaemia[a], arrhythmia
Massive pulmonary embolus	Risk factors, chest pain, pleurisy, syncope[a], dizziness[a]	Central cyanosis, ↑JVP[a], absence of signs in the lung[a], shock (tachycardia, hypotension)	Often normal. Prominent hilar vessels, oligaemic lung fields[a]	↓PaO_2, ↓$PaCO_2$	Sinus tachycardia, RBBB, $S_1Q_3T_3$ pattern ↑T(V_1–V_4)
Acute severe asthma	History of asthma, asthma medications, wheeze[a]	Tachycardia, pulsus paradoxus, cyanosis (late), →↓JVP[a], ↓peak flow, wheeze[a]	Hyperinflation only (unless complicated by pneumothorax)[a]	↓PaO_2, ↓$PaCO_2$ (↑$PaCO_2$ in extremis)	Sinus tachycardia (bradycardia in extremis)
Acute exacerbation of COPD	Previous episodes[a], smoker. If in type II respiratory failure, may be drowsy	Cyanosis, hyperinflation[a], signs of CO_2 retention (flapping tremor, bounding pulses)[a]	Hyperinflation[a], bullae, complicating pneumothorax	↓ or ↓↓PaO_2, ↑$PaCO_2$ in type II failure ± ↑H+, ↑HCO_3^- in chronic type II failure	Normal, or signs of right ventricular strain
Pneumonia	Prodromal illness[a], fever[a], rigors[a], pleurisy[a]	Fever, delirium, pleural rub[a], consolidation[a], cyanosis (if severe)	Pneumonic consolidation[a]	↓PaO_2, ↓$PaCO_2$ (↑ in extremis)	Tachycardia
Metabolic acidosis	Evidence of diabetes mellitus or renal disease, aspirin or ethylene glycol overdose	Fetor (ketones), hyperventilation without heart or lung signs[a], dehydration[a], air hunger	Normal	PaO_2 normal. ↓↓$PaCO_2$, ↑H+, ↓HCO_3^-	
Psychogenic	Previous episodes, digital or perioral dysaesthesia	No cyanosis, no heart or lung signs, carpopedal spasm	Normal	PaO_2 normal[a]. ↓↓$PaCO_2$, ↓H+[a]	

[a]Valuable discriminatory feature.

However, myocardial ischaemia may induce breathlessness by provoking transient left ventricular dysfunction. Breathlessness as the dominant feature of myocardial ischaemia is known as 'angina equivalent'.

Initial investigations

Box 4.2 outlines how clinical features, ECG, CXR and ABG are used to distinguish the common causes of acute breathlessness. Serial peak expiratory flow is used to assess the severity of asthma. In COPD, ABG is more useful than SpO_2 alone, as the $PaCO_2$, arterial H^+ and HCO_3^- indicate whether there is new or chronic type II respiratory failure (p. 320). ABG measurement is also useful in the assessment of asthma severity, metabolic acidosis and psychogenic hyperventilation.

If 'angina equivalent' is suspected, stress testing may reveal myocardial ischaemia.

Syncope/Presyncope

Syncope means sudden loss of consciousness as a result of reduced cerebral perfusion. Presyncope means lightheadedness, when the patient feels they may 'black out'.

The main causes are:
- *Cardiac syncope* — arrhythmia or mechanical cardiac dysfunction
- *Neurocardiogenic (vasovagal or reflex) syncope* — an abnormal autonomic reflex that causes bradycardia and hypotension
- *Postural hypotension* — impaired physiological peripheral vasoconstriction on standing that causes hypotension

Differentiating syncope from seizure is important. Psychogenic blackouts (nonepileptic seizures or pseudoseizures) should also be considered in the differential diagnosis.

Presentation

The terms used by patients should be clarified: for example, 'blackout' may be used for purely visual symptoms rather than loss of consciousness, and 'dizziness' may mean an abnormal perception of movement (vertigo). Fig. 4.1 shows the differential diagnoses of syncope and presyncope from symptoms.

The history from the patient and a witness is important for diagnosis. Establish whether there has been full consciousness, altered consciousness, vertigo, transient amnesia or something else. Ask about potential triggers (e.g. medication, micturition, exertion, prolonged standing), any pallor or seizure activity, the duration of the episode and the speed of recovery (Box 4.3).
- Cardiac syncope is usually sudden, but is occasionally preceded by lightheadedness, palpitation or chest discomfort. The syncope is usually brief, and recovery rapid.
- Exercise-induced syncope can be the presenting feature of aortic stenosis, obstructive cardiomyopathy or exercise-induced arrhythmia, and always requires investigation.
- Neurocardiogenic syncope is often triggered by circumstances (e.g. pain or emotion). Brief stiffening and limb-twitching may occur. Recovery is usually quick and without delirium (provided the patient is

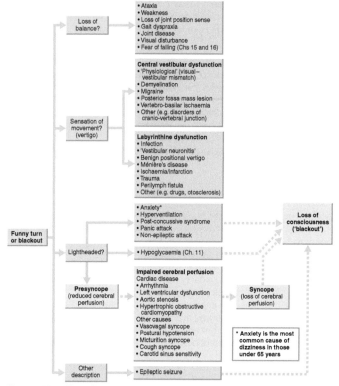

Fig. 4.1 The differential diagnosis of syncope and presyncope.

lying down), but flushing, nausea, malaise and clamminess may persist for several minutes afterwards. It rarely causes injury or amnesia on recovery.

- Seizures do not cause pallor, often cause abnormal movements, usually take more than 5 min to recover from and leave the patient confused.
- Psychogenic blackout (nonepileptic seizure, pseudoseizure) is suggested by specific emotional triggers, dramatic movements or vocalisation or very prolonged duration (hours).
- Rotational vertigo suggests a labyrinthine or vestibular disorder (p. 673).
- Postural hypotension is normally obvious from the history. Predisposing medications (diuretics, vasodilators, antidepressants) and conditions (such as diabetes mellitus and Parkinson's disease) should be sought.

		Neurocardiogenic	
	Cardiac syncope	syncope	Seizures
Premonitory symptoms	Often none Lightheadedness Palpitation Chest pain Breathlessness	Nausea Lightheadedness Sweating	Delirium Hyperexcitability Olfactory hallucinations 'Aura'
Unconscious period	Extreme 'death-like' pallor	Pallor	Prolonged (>1 min) unconsciousness Motor seizure activity[a] Tongue-biting Urinary incontinence
Recovery	Rapid (<1 min) Flushing	Slow Nausea Lightheadedness	Prolonged delirium (>5mins) Headache Focal neurological signs

4.3 Typical features of cardiac syncope, neurocardiogenic syncope and seizures

[a]Cardiac syncope can also cause convulsions by inducing cerebral anoxia.

Clinical assessment

Examination may be normal but may reveal clinical signs of an underlying cause. The systolic murmurs of aortic stenosis or obstructive cardiomyopathy are important in those with exertional syncope. Supine and standing BP measurements may confirm postural hypotension.

A hypersensitive carotid sinus baroreceptor may cause neurocardiogenic syncope. In these patients (in the absence of carotid bruit or cerebrovascular disease), carotid sinus pressure may cause a sinus pause of 3 seconds or more on ECG and/or a fall in systolic BP of more than 50 mmHg. This test will be positive in 10% of elderly individuals, of whom fewer than 25% experience spontaneous syncope. Symptoms should therefore not be attributed to carotid sinus hypersensitivity unless they are reproduced by carotid sinus pressure.

Initial investigations

An ECG is essential in all patients with syncope or presyncope. Lightheadedness may occur with many arrhythmias, but cardiac syncope (Stokes–Adams attacks, p. 270) is usually caused by profound bradycardia or malignant ventricular tachyarrhythmias. The key to diagnosis is an ECG during symptoms. Ambulatory ECG recordings are helpful only if symptoms occur several times per week. Patient-activated ECG recorders are useful for examining the rhythm in patients with recurrent dizziness, but not in sudden blackouts. When these investigations are inconclusive, an implantable ECG recorder activated automatically by extreme bradycardia or tachycardia can be used. Symptoms can be marked on the ECG using a patient-held activator. Some systems allow online home monitoring.

| **i** | **4.4 Risk factors for delirium** |

Predisposing factors

Old age	Sensory impairment
Dementia	Polypharmacy
Frailty	Renal impairment

Precipitating factors

Intercurrent illness	Dehydration
Surgery	Pain
Change of environment or ward	Constipation
Sensory deprivation (e.g. darkness) or overload (e.g. noise)	Urinary catheterisation
	Acute urinary retention
Medications (e.g. opioids, psychotropics)	Hypoxia
	Fever
	Alcohol withdrawal

A tilt-table provocation test can be used to test for vasovagal syncope. A positive test is characterised by bradycardia and/or hypotension associated with typical symptoms after tilt from supine to 60 to 70 degrees, head up.

Delirium

Delirium denotes transient, reversible cognitive dysfunction and is more common in old age. It is associated with high rates of mortality, complications, institutionalisation and longer lengths of stay. Recognised risk factors are shown in Box 4.4.

Presentation

There is a disturbance of arousal with global cognitive impairment, drowsiness, disorientation, perceptual errors and muddled thinking. Delirium may be hypoactive (with lethargy), hyperactive (with agitation) or mixed. Fluctuation is typical, and delirium is often worse at night, complicating management. Emotional disturbance (anxiety, irritability or depression) is common. The history is frequently unobtainable from the patient, and collateral history from a friend or relative is important. As delirium commonly accompanies dementia, the collateral history should establish the patient's normal functioning, as well as the onset and course of delirium.

Clinical assessment

Accurate diagnosis is the first step. Tools such as the 4AT (Box .4.5) are used to detect delirium and differentiate it from dementia. Once delirium has been diagnosed, reversible precipitating factors should be sought. Check for symptoms of infection or stroke. Review medication, in particular any drugs recently stopped or started. Consider possible alcohol withdrawal. A full physical examination of all delirious patients should then be attempted, noting: • pyrexia/signs of infection in the chest, skin, abdomen or urine

• oxygen saturation/signs of CO_2 retention • signs of alcohol withdrawal or psychoactive drug use, such as tremor or sweating • focal neurological signs.

Certain psychiatric conditions, such as depressive pseudodementia and dissociative disorder, can be mistaken for delirium. Look for and record associated mood disorder, hallucinations, delusions or behavioural abnormalities.

4

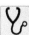

4.5 How to make a diagnosis of delirium: the 4AT score

1. Alertness
   Observe the patient. If asleep, attempt to wake with speech or gentle touch on shoulder. Ask the patient to state his or her name and address to assist rating:

• Normal (fully alert, but not agitated, throughout assessment)	0
• Mild sleepiness for <10 secs after waking, then normal	0
• Clearly abnormal	4

2. AMT4
   Age, date of birth, place (name of the hospital or building), current year:

• No mistakes	0
• 1 mistake	1
• ≥2 mistakes/untestable	2

3. Attention
   Say: 'Please tell me the months of the year in backwards order, starting at December'. To assist understanding, one prompt of 'What is the month before December?' is permitted:

• Achieves ≥7 months correctly	0
• Starts but scores <7 months/refuses to start	1
• Untestable (cannot start because unwell, drowsy, inattentive)	2

4. Acute change or fluctuating course
   Evidence of significant change or fluctuation in: alertness, cognition, other mental function (e.g. paranoia, hallucinations) arising over the last 2 weeks and still evident in last 24 hours:

• No	0
• Yes	4

Total 4AT score (maximum possible score 12)
   ≥4: possible delirium ± cognitive impairment
   1–3: possible cognitive impairment
   0: delirium or severe cognitive impairment unlikely (but delirium still possible if information in 4 incomplete)

AMT4, Abbreviated Mental Test 4.

Investigations and management

Investigate for the common causes of delirium:

1. Infection: FBC, CRP, CXR, urinalysis, blood culture.
2. Metabolic disturbance: U&E, calcium, glucose, LFTs, thyroid function, B_{12}.
3. Toxicity: Review drugs, drug levels if indicated.
4. Acute neurological conditions: CT brain if focal signs or head injury, LP if meningitis suspected.
5. Cardiorespiratory conditions: Oxygen saturation ± ABGs. If hypoxic consider PE, pneumonia, respiratory failure, pulmonary oedema; investigate as appropriate.

Nurse the patient in a well-lit and quiet environment, with hearing aids and glasses available. Prevent pressure sores and falls, and maintain hydration, nutrition and continence. Sedatives may worsen delirium and are a last resort. Resolution of delirium, particularly in the elderly, may be slow and incomplete.

Headache

Headache is common and worries patients and clinicians, but rarely represents sinister disease. The causes include:

Primary: • Migraine (± aura) • Tension-type headache • Trigeminal autonomic cephalalgia (including cluster headache) • Primary stabbing/coughing/exertional/sex-related headache • Thunderclap headache • New daily persistent headache syndrome.

Secondary (much less common): • Medication overuse headache • Intracranial haemorrhage (subdural, subarachnoid or intracerebral) • Raised ICP (brain tumour, idiopathic) • Infection (meningitis, encephalitis, brain abscess) • Inflammatory disease (temporal arteritis, vasculitis, arthritis) • Referred pain (orbit, temporomandibular joint, neck).

Presentation

In patients with headache, the history and examination aim to identify the small minority with serious underlying pathology. Red flag features include:

- Sudden onset (maximal within 5 min) — subarachnoid haemorrhage or meningitis
- Focal neurological signs (other than migrainous) — intracranial mass
- Constitutional symptoms (pyrexia, weight loss, meningism, rash) — meningitis, neoplasia
- Raised ICP (worse when supine) — intracranial mass
- Onset over 60 years of age — temporal arteritis

Establish whether the headache comes and goes (usually migraine) or is constant. Preceding visual symptoms, nausea/vomiting or photophobia/phonophobia suggest migraine. Headache resulting from cerebral venous thrombosis may be 'throbbing' or 'band-like' and associated with nausea, vomiting or hemiparesis. Raised ICP headache is usually worse supine, in the morning and when coughing, and associated with nausea and/or vomiting.

Neck stiffness together with headache and photophobia suggests meningitis. Check for other features including fever, Kernig's sign, signs of shock and rash because prompt recognition and treatment are vital in bacterial meningitis. Patient behaviour during headache is often instructive; migraine patients typically seek darkness and sleep, whereas a cluster headache often induces agitated restlessness.

Headaches lasting months or years are almost never sinister, whereas new-onset headache, especially in the elderly, is more concerning. In a patient older than 60 years of age with temporal pain, scalp tenderness or jaw claudication, consider temporal arteritis (p. 718).

Clinical assessment

Conscious level should be assessed early and monitored using the GCS (Box 4.6). Decreased conscious level suggests raised ICP requiring urgent

i 4.6 GCS	
Eye-opening (E)	
• Spontaneous	4
• To speech	3
• To pain	2
• Nil	1
Best motor response (M)	
• Obeys commands	6
• Localises to painful stimulus	5
• Flexion to painful stimulus or withdraws hand from pain	4
• Abnormal flexion (internal rotation of shoulder, flexion of wrist)	3
• Extensor response (external rotation of shoulder, extension of wrist)	2
• Nil	1
Verbal response (V)	
• Orientated	5
• Confused conversation	4
• Inappropriate words	3
• Incomprehensible sounds	2
• Nil	1
Coma score = E + M + V	
Always present GCS as breakdown, not a sum score (unless 3 or 15)	
• Minimum sum	3
• Maximum sum	15

GCS, Glasgow Coma Score.
Record the best score observed. When the patient is intubated, there can be no verbal response. The suffix 'T' should replace the verbal component of the score, and the remainder of the score is therefore a maximum of 10.

CT scanning. Neurological examination may reveal localising signs of an underlying lesion; however, false localising signs may occur with large subarachnoid haemorrhage or bacterial meningitis. Conjunctival injection is typical of cluster headache, but also occurs in acute glaucoma, accompanied by peri-/retroorbital pain, corneal clouding and decreased acuity.

Initial investigations

Urgent head CT is indicated for altered conscious level, focal neurological signs, new-onset seizures or head injury. Intracranial haemorrhage or space-occupying lesion should prompt urgent neurosurgical referral. If bacterial meningitis is suspected, LP is required; this should be preceded by CT scanning only if raised ICP is suspected. Antibiotics should not be delayed for LP. In thunderclap headache, a normal CT should be followed by an LP more than 12 hours after headache onset, looking for xanthochromia. A negative CT scan within 6 hours of headache onset is so sensitive for excluding subarachnoid haemorrhage that LP is generally considered unnecessary. In such circumstances, a CT angiogram should be considered to exclude arterial dissection. For specific causes, involve a specialist early (e.g. ophthalmologist for acute glaucoma, rheumatologist for temporal arteritis). Features of raised ICP without a mass on neuroimaging may indicate idiopathic intracranial hypertension; CSF opening pressure is likely to be informative.

Unilateral leg swelling

Most leg swelling is caused by interstitial oedema as a result of increased hydrostatic pressure, reduced intravascular oncotic pressure or lymphatic obstruction. Unilateral swelling usually indicates localised venous or lymphatic obstruction, whereas bilateral oedema, which is occasionally asymmetrical, often represents generalised fluid overload combined with the effects of gravity. Fluid overload may complicate cardiac failure, pulmonary hypertension, renal failure, hypoalbuminaemia or drug use (calcium channel blockers, glucocorticoids, mineralocorticoids, NSAIDs, and others).

Presentation

In all cases of unilateral leg swelling, underlying DVT should be considered. The pain and swelling of DVT usually develops over hours or even days. Sudden pain in the calf is more consistent with gastrocnemius muscle tear (traumatic or spontaneous) or ruptured Baker's cyst.

Clinical assessment

Lower limb DVT characteristically starts in the distal veins, causing an increase in temperature of the limb and dilatation of the superficial veins. Often, however, symptoms and signs are minimal. Consider underlying risk factors for venous thrombosis (Box 14.5, p. 560). Malignancy predisposes to thrombosis, but pelvic or abdominal masses can also produce leg swelling by venous or lymphatic obstruction. Alternative diagnoses are distinguished by the clinical features:

- Cellulitis—a well-demarcated area of erythema and skin warmth ± a visible entry site for infection (e.g. leg ulcer or insect bite). The patient may be febrile and systemically unwell.

- Superficial thrombophlebitis—localised erythema and tenderness along a firm, palpable vein.
- Compartment syndrome—swollen, extremely tender limb with altered sensation with or without loss of peripheral pulses. CK is raised, and surgical treatment is needed urgently.

Early lymphoedema is indistinguishable from other causes of oedema. Chronic lymphoedema is firm and nonpitting, with a thickened 'cobblestone' appearance of the skin.

Chronic venous insufficiency causes chronic oedema with characteristic skin changes (haemosiderin deposition, hair loss, varicose eczema, ulceration) and prominent varicosities.

Investigations and management

Clinical criteria can be used to rank patients according to their likelihood of DVT, by using scoring systems such as the Wells score (Box 4.7). Fig. 4.2 gives an algorithm for investigation of suspected DVT based

i 4.7 Predicting the pretest probability of DVT—Wells score	
Clinical characteristic	**Score**
Active cancer (patient received treatment for cancer within previous 6 months or is currently receiving palliative treatment)	1
Paralysis, paresis or recent plaster immobilisation of lower extremities	1
Recently bedridden for ≥3 days, or major surgery within previous 4 weeks	1
Localised tenderness along distribution of deep venous system	1
Entire leg swollen	1
Calf swelling ≥3 cm larger than that on asymptomatic side (measured 10 cm below tibial tuberosity)	1
Pitting oedema confined to symptomatic leg	1
Collateral superficial veins (nonvaricose)	1
Previous documented DVT	1
Alternative diagnosis at least as likely as DVT	−2
Clinical probability	**Total score**
DVT low probability	<1
DVT moderate probability	1–2
DVT high probability	>2
(From Wells PS. Evaluation of D-dimer in the diagnosis of suspected deep-vein thrombosis. N Engl J Med 2003; 349:1227; copyright © 2003 Massachusetts Medical Society.)	

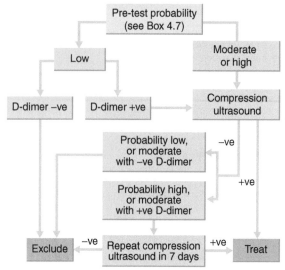

Fig. 4.2 Investigation of suspected deep vein thrombosis.

on pretest probability. In pregnancy, the D-dimer test should not be used, and there should be a low threshold for imaging, as pregnancy predisposes towards DVT.

In suspected cellulitis, serum inflammatory markers, skin swabs and blood cultures should be arranged. Ruptured Baker's cyst and calf muscle tear are diagnosed on ultrasound. If pelvic or lower abdominal malignancy is suspected, prostate-specific antigen level should be measured in males, and ultrasound or CT scans should be undertaken.

Management of DVT is by anticoagulation (p. 563).

Identification and assessment of deterioration

Early warning scores and the role of the medical emergency team

Rapid response systems aim to rapidly identify and manage physiological deterioration. One example is a medical emergency team (MET), which is called when a patient reaches a particular early warning score on monitoring (e.g. NEWS, Fig. 4.3). The MET may start treatment, advise the parent clinical team or escalate the patient to critical care.

Although the MET system makes expertise in deteriorating patients available rapidly, the team may not know the patient's background, and there is a risk that local teams become de-skilled in emergency management.

Immediate assessment of the deteriorating patient

The mnemonic 'C-A-B-C-D-E' may be useful:

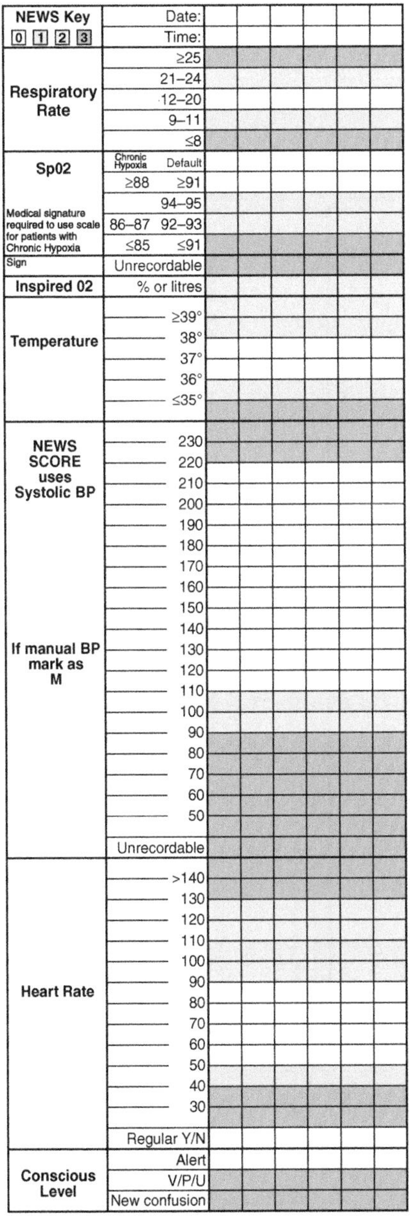

NEWS Key 0 1 2 3	Date:						
	Time:						
Respiratory Rate	≥25						
	21–24						
	12–20						
	9–11						
	≤8						
SpO2	Chronic Hypoxia / Default						
	≥88 / ≥91						
Medical signature required to use scale for patients with Chronic Hypoxia	94–95						
	86–87 / 92–93						
	≤85 / ≤91						
Sign	Unrecordable						
Inspired 02	% or litres						
Temperature	≥39°						
	38°						
	37°						
	36°						
	≤35°						
NEWS SCORE uses Systolic BP	230						
	220						
	210						
	200						
	190						
	180						
	170						
	160						
	150						
	140						
If manual BP mark as M	130						
	120						
	110						
	100						
	90						
	80						
	70						
	60						
	50						
	Unrecordable						
Heart Rate	>140						
	130						
	120						
	110						
	100						
	90						
	80						
	70						
	60						
	50						
	40						
	30						
	Regular Y/N						
Conscious Level	Alert						
	V/P/U						
	New confusion						

Fig. 4.3 Identifying and responding to physiological deterioration. A An example of an early warning score chart. *NEWS*, National Early Warning Score; *V/P/U*, Verbal/Pain/Unresponsive.

*Regardless of NEWS always escalate if concerned about a patient's condition

NEWS Score	Frequency of Observations	Clinical Response
Total 0*	Minimum 12 hourly/4 hourly in admission areas	• Continue routine NEWS monitoring with every set of observations
Total 1–4*	Minimum 4 hourly Consider Structured Response Tool Consider Fluid Balance Chart	• Inform registered nurse • Registered nurse assessment using ABCDE • Review frequency of observations • Inform Nurse in Charge • **If ongoing concern, escalate to Medical Team**
Total 5–6* Or 3 in one parameter	Increase frequency to a minimum of 1 hourly Start Structured Response Tool Start Fluid Balance Chart	• Registered nurse assessment • Inform Nurse in Charge • Escalate to Medical Team as per local escalation • Urgent medical assessment • Management plan to be discussed with Senior Trainee or above • Consider level of monitoring required in relation to clinical care
Total 7* or more	Continuous monitoring of vital signs Start Structured Response Tool Start Fluid Balance Chart	• Registered nurse to assess immediately • Inform Nurse in Charge • Request immediate assessment by Senior Trainee or above • Case to be discussed with supervising Consultant • If appropriate contact Critical Care for review

B

Fig. 4.3, cont'd **B** Responses to physiological deterioration. A and B, From Royal College of Physicians. *National Early Warning Score (NEWS); standardising the assessment of acute-illness severity in the NHS. Report of a working party.* London: RCP; 2012.

C—Control of obvious problem

For example, if the patient has ventricular tachycardia or significant bleeding, take immediate action.

A and B—airway and breathing

If the patient is talking in full sentences, the airway is clear and breathing is adequate, a rapid history should be followed by a focused respiratory examination. Oxygen saturation and ABGs should be checked.

C—circulation

A focused cardiovascular examination should include heart rate and rhythm, abnormal heart sounds, blood pressure, JVP and evidence of bleeding or shock. The carotid pulse should be palpated in the collapsed or unconscious patient; in circulatory compromise the peripheral pulses may be impalpable.

D—disability

Assess conscious level using the GCS (Box 4.6), and perform a brief neurological examination. Capillary blood glucose should be measured to exclude hypoglycaemia or severe hyperglycaemia.

E—exposure and evidence

'Exposure' indicates targeted clinical examination of the remaining body systems. 'Evidence' is gathered via collateral history from staff or family, investigations, prescriptions or charts.

Deciding where to manage the patient

Critical care benefits those patients with organ dysfunction severe enough to require organ support, those whose disease is clearly deteriorating and those in whom aggressive management may alter the outcome. The choice of an ICU/HDU will depend on local arrangements. The 'level of care' required is a useful guide to placement:

Level 3: Require intubation and ventilation or support of two or more organ systems—ICU

Level 2: Require detailed observation and monitoring beyond ward level, or support for one failing organ system—HDU

Level 1: Require intermittent observation that can be provided at ward level—General Ward

Common presentations of deterioration

Tachypnoea

Pathophysiology

Tachypnoea may be caused by cardiopulmonary causes (see previously, p. 61) or secondary to a metabolic acidosis (see also p. 198), most commonly in sepsis, haemorrhage, ketoacidosis or visceral ischaemia.

Assessment and management

Assess chest expansion, breath sounds and the presence of added sounds such as wheeze.

Arterial blood analysis is helpful in narrowing the differential diagnosis and indicating the severity of derangement. The 'base excess' provides quantification of the component of disease that is metabolic in origin. A base excess lower than -2 mEq/L (i.e. a 'base deficit' of >2 mEq/L) is likely to represent a metabolic acidosis. A lactate level of greater than 4 mmol/L or a base deficit greater than 10 mEq/L should trigger escalation to a higher level of care. In addition to examination, CXR and bedside ultrasound can help to identify consolidation, effusion and pneumothorax.

Hypoxaemia

Pathophysiology

Low PaO_2 is common in deteriorating patients. Tissue hypoxia may be caused by hypoxaemia or may be secondary to impaired cardiac output, inadequate/dysfunctional haemoglobin or impaired cellular oxygen utilisation, for example, cyanide poisoning.

The haemoglobin–oxygen dissociation curve relates the percentage saturation of haemoglobin with oxygen (SO_2) to the PO_2 in the blood. Raised capillary PCO_2 shifts the curve to the right, increasing oxygen release in the tissues (Bohr effect). In PE, tachypnoea may reduce $PaCO_2$, causing a left shift of the curve with preserved saturation despite a low PaO_2.

Relative hypoxaemia is present if the PaO_2 is lower than that expected for a given FiO_2. With the patient breathing air, a PaO_2 of 12 to 14 kPa (90–105 mmHg) would be expected; with the patient breathing 100% oxygen, a PaO_2 of more than 60 kPa (450 mmHg) would be normal.

Assessment and management

Oxygen therapy should be titrated against saturation:

- Target saturation 94% to 98% for most critically unwell patients
- 88% to 92% is the target range in patients with COPD at risk of hypercapnic respiratory failure

Too high a PaO_2 may cause free radical–induced tissue damage, inefficient haemoglobin buffering of CO_2, loss of hypoxic vasoconstriction in under-ventilated lung and decreased hypoxic drive in patients with chronic hypercapnia.

In considering the cause of hypoxaemia, the $PaCO_2$ level is helpful. Hypoxia with normal $PaCO_2$ indicates shunting of venous blood to the arterial system either in the heart or through localised regions of underventilated lung (e.g. lobar pneumonia). Hypoxia with high $PaCO_2$ represents insufficient overall alveolar ventilation and can occur with poisoning, neurological disease, myopathies, spinal deformity or severe COPD (see p. 326).

Tachycardia

Pathophysiology

A heart rate of more than 110 beats per minute in an adult should not be attributed to anxiety until other causes have been excluded. Cardiac causes of tachycardia (atrial fibrillation or flutter, SVT and ventricular dys-rhythmias) are rarer in inpatients than secondary causes.

Firstly, establish the rate and rhythm with a 12-lead ECG. A heart rate greater than 160 beats per minute should prompt escalation to higher level of care. Possible findings include:

- AF with a rapid ventricular response—usually secondary (mostly commonly to infection).
- Hypovolaemia—consider concealed bleeding (e.g. pleural, gastrointestinal or retroperitoneal). Note: in acute haemorrhage the immediate Hb can be misleadingly high.
- Sepsis—may present with tachycardia with tachypnoea, peripheral vasodilatation and raised temperature.

Other organ dysfunction should be noted from a brief history and examination.

Assessment and management

Focus on treating the cause. Treating the heart rate alone with β-blockade in a deteriorating patient should be done only under specialist guidance. Management of cardiac dysrhythmias is discussed on p. 262.

Hypotension

Pathophysiology

Mean arterial pressure (MAP; diastolic + [systolic − diastolic/3]) is a useful reference value. A MAP of greater than 65 mmHg will maintain renal perfusion in most patients, although a MAP of 80 mmHg may be required in patients with chronic hypertension.

Assessment and management

First decide if the hypotension is physiological or pathological. Even with low systolic pressures, it is rare to see a physiological MAP of less than 65 mmHg. Oliguria suggests action is needed to increase MAP (p. 88).

Shock: Shock means 'circulatory failure'. It can be defined as a level of oxygen delivery (DO_2 = oxygen content of blood × cardiac output) that fails to meet the metabolic requirements of the tissues. Hypotension and shock are not synonymous: patients can be hypotensive but not shocked, and DO_2 can be critically low despite a normal BP.

In hypotension with high cardiac output, the patient has warm hands, a high-volume pulse and low venous pressure. Causes include sepsis, allergy, drug overdose, ketoacidosis and thyrotoxicosis.

Hypotension with low cardiac output causes cold, cyanotic peripheries with raised venous pressure, and occurs with bleeding, arrhythmia, tamponade and heart failure.

Objective markers of inadequate tissue oxygen delivery (increased base deficit and lactate, oliguria) can aid identification. If shock is suspected, prompt resuscitation (p. 88) is required.

Hypotensive patients without shock are still at risk of organ dysfunction. Organ failure can occur in these patients despite having a normal or elevated DO_2, so full assessment is indicated. Any medication with antihypertensive effects or side effects should be stopped.

Hypertension

Pathophysiology

Hypertension is common and usually benign in a critical care context but can be the presenting feature of a serious disease. Furthermore, acute hypertension increases left ventricular end-systolic pressure and can cause acute pulmonary oedema.

Assessment and management

Important underlying causes to be considered include:

- *Intracranial event.* Brainstem ischaemia (commonly secondary to raised ICP) may increase BP acutely. Perform neurological examination and consider head CT.
- *Fluid overload.* This can originate from myocardial dysfunction or impaired renal clearance and may cause hypertension in younger patients without peripheral oedema.
- *Underlying medical problems.* Renal disease, spinal injury and rarer causes, for example, phaeochromocytoma, should be considered. In women, consider pregnancy-induced hypertension.
- *Primary cardiac problems.* Myocardial ischaemia, acute heart failure and aortic dissection can present with hypertension.
- *Drug-related problems.* Missed antihypertensive medication is the common cause, but drugs such as cocaine and amphetamines can raise BP.

The management of hypertension is discussed on p. 290.

Decreased conscious level

Assessment

Decreased conscious level should prompt an urgent search for the cause and an evaluation of the risk to the airway. The GCS (Box 4.6) is the most widely used tool for assessment of conscious level; however, disorders affecting language or limb function (e.g. left hemisphere stroke) may reduce its usefulness.

Serial GCS scores can track improvement or deterioration and indicate prognosis. A motor score of less than 5 suggests significant risk to the airway.

Coma is defined as a persisting state of deep unconsciousness (sustained GCS of ≤8) and has many causes (Box 4.8). The mode of onset and any precipitating event are crucial to establishing the cause and should be obtained from witnesses. A sudden onset suggests a vascular cause.

A thorough examination should include GCS and a search for needle tracks indicating drug abuse, rashes, fever and focal signs of infection, including neck stiffness or evidence of head injury. Focal neurological signs may suggest a stroke or tumour or may be falsely localising (e.g. 6th nerve palsy in raised ICP). It is vital to exclude biochemical causes of coma, as acute hyponatraemia (p. 190) and hypoglycaemia (p. 430) are easily corrected and can cause irreversible brain injury if missed.

i	4.8 Causes of coma

Metabolic disturbance

Drug overdose	Inborn errors of metabolism causing
Diabetes mellitus:	hyperammonaemia
Hypoglycaemia	Hyperammonaemia on re-feeding following
Ketoacidosis	profound anorexia
Hyperosmolar coma	Respiratory failure
Hyponatraemia	Hypothermia
Uraemia	Hypothyroidism
Hepatic failure (hyperammonaemia)	

Trauma

Cerebral contusion	Subdural haematoma
Extradural haematoma	Diffuse axonal injury

Vascular disease

Subarachnoid haemorrhage	Intracerebral haemorrhage
Brainstem infarction/haemorrhage	Cerebral venous sinus thrombosis

Infections

Meningitis	Cerebral abscess
Encephalitis	Systemic sepsis

Others

Epilepsy	Functional ('pseudo-coma')
Brain tumour	

CT imaging of the brain is often needed for accurate diagnosis. Meningitis or encephalitis may be suggested by the history, clinical signs or imaging. Broad-spectrum antibiotics and antivirals should be started immediately while awaiting definitive results in this situation.

Other drug-based, metabolic and hepatic causes of impaired consciousness are dealt with in the relevant chapters. Psychiatric conditions such as catatonic depression or neurological conditions such as the autoimmune encephalitides can impair consciousness but are diagnoses of exclusion and require specialist input.

Management
Move the unconscious patient into the recovery position to protect the airway pending escalation and definitive treatment. Intubation may be required to protect the airway from obstruction or aspiration.

Oliguria/deteriorating renal function

Assessment
A urine output of 0.5 mL/kg/hour is a commonly quoted target. Lower volumes signify the possibility of suboptimal renal perfusion.

Oliguria with hypotension or increased serum creatinine should prompt a search for the underlying cause. Prerenal causes predominate in inpatients, so optimising the MAP using intravenous fluids (± vasopressors) is the priority. If the MAP is normal, high volumes (>30 mL/kg) of intravenous fluid are not indicated. Exceptions include clinically dehydrated patients and those with high fluid losses from burns, uncontrolled diabetes (p. 427) or diabetes insipidus (p. 416).

Diagnosis and management

The management of oliguria is covered on p. 207. Two other important causes of acute renal impairment are abdominal compartment syndrome and rhabdomyolysis.

Abdominal compartment syndrome: This occurs when raised abdominal pressure reduces perfusion to the abdominal organs. It occurs in surgical patients or patients with extreme fluid retention (e.g. in cirrhosis). Urgent decompression of the stomach, bladder or peritoneum (if ascites present) is required.

Rhabdomyolysis: Rhabdomyolysis occurs following injury to a large volume of skeletal muscle, either from ischaemia of a limb or muscle compartment, from trauma, after intense physical exercise or in the context of complicating malignant hyperpyrexia.

A CK level of greater than 1000 U/L is highly suggestive. Management involves addressing the cause and providing organ support. Forced alkaline diuresis (intravenous bicarbonate and furosemide) is used to reduce tubular myoglobin precipitation.

Disorders causing critical illness

Sepsis and the systemic inflammatory response

Sepsis is a common cause of multiorgan failure. Infection and the resulting systemic inflammatory state combine to cause organ dysfunction.

The diagnosis is made when patients with suspected infection have two or more of the following:

- *Hypotension*—systolic blood pressure less than 100 mmHg
- *Altered mental status*—GCS score of 14 or lower
- *Tachypnoea*—respiratory rate 22 or more breaths per minute

Septic shock refers to patients with sepsis who also have (after fluid resuscitation) persistent hypotension requiring vasopressors to maintain a MAP greater than 65 mmHg and a serum lactate greater than 2 mmol/L (18 mg/dL).

Pathophysiology: Inflammation may be triggered by localised infection (bacterial, viral or fungal), which may progress to systemic infection if there is: • a genetic predisposition to sepsis • a large microbiological load • a virulent or resistant organism • a delay in treatment • immune compromise, malnutrition or frailty.

Noninfective processes, for example, pancreatitis, burns, trauma, surgery and drug reactions, can also initiate systemic inflammation.

Activated immune cells release cytokines that activate neutrophils, thereby causing vasodilatation, endothelial damage and passage of neutrophils, fluid and proteins into the interstitium. Damaged endothelium triggers intravascular coagulation with microvascular occlusion, which may become disseminated in severe cases (DIC, see p. 590) with multiorgan failure.

4

Lactate physiology: Tissue hypoxia, adrenergic stimulation and reduced hepatic clearance may increase lactate levels in all types of shock, not just in sepsis. Hyperlactataemia (serum lactate >2.4 mmol/L or 22 mg/dL) is an excellent marker of severity in sepsis. A lactate level of greater than 8 mmol/L (>73 mg/dL) is associated with extremely high mortality and should trigger immediate escalation. Measures to optimise oxygen delivery should be sought, and the adequacy of resuscitation measured by lactate clearance.

The antiinflammatory cascade: Alongside developing inflammation, a compensatory antiinflammatory system is activated as immune cells release antiinflammatory cytokines. This keeps the inflammatory response in check, but may cause relative immunosuppression after sepsis, predisposing to secondary infections.

Management

Always consider sepsis as a cause of a patient's deterioration, alongside alternatives including haemorrhage, PE, anaphylaxis or a low cardiac output state.

Resuscitation in sepsis: General resuscitative measures are discussed on p. 88. In sepsis, a useful guide is the 'Sepsis Six' (Box 4.9). Anaemia should be corrected by red cell transfusion to a haemoglobin level of 70 to 90 g/L (7–9 g/dL). Albumin 4% can be infused as a colloid solution, which remains in the intravascular space longer than crystalloid. Early intubation is recommended in severe cases to facilitate further management and reduce oxygen demand.

Antibiotics should be administered as early as possible, as every hour of delay carries a 5% to 10% increase in mortality. The antibiotic choice will depend on local resistance patterns, patient risk factors and the likely source of infection. Microbiological cultures of blood, urine or CSF should be taken, but should not delay antibiotic administration.

Early source control: CT scanning of the chest and abdomen has a high yield for revealing the source of sepsis. The history should be reviewed, including risk factors for HIV, contact with tuberculosis and underlying immune status. Immunocompromised patients are susceptible to a much wider range of organisms (p. 105).

Noradrenaline (norepinephrine) for refractory hypotension: Central venous access should be established early during resuscitation, and a noradrenaline infusion commenced. In severe hypotension, start noradrenaline without waiting for fluid challenge, as early vasopressor use may limit acute kidney injury.

Other therapies for refractory hypotension: Refractory hypotension is caused by either inadequate cardiac output or inadequate systemic

4.9 The 'Sepsis Six'

1. Deliver high-flow oxygen
2. Take blood cultures
3. Administer intravenous antibiotics
4. Measure serum lactate and send full blood count
5. Start intravenous fluid replacement
6. Commence accurate measurement of urine output

International recommendations for the immediate management of suspected sepsis from the Surviving Sepsis Campaign (all to be delivered within 1 hour of the initial diagnosis of sepsis).

vascular resistance (vasoplegia). Vasopressin (antidiuretic hormone) is a potent vasoconstrictor that may be added if vasoplegia is suspected. Intravenous glucocorticoids may lead to a more rapid reversal of shock; however, they do not improve overall outcome, and may slightly increase the risk of secondary infection.

Septic cardiomyopathy: This may present as acute left or right ventricular dysfunction. An echocardiogram is particularly useful for confirmation because the ECG is usually nonspecific. Dobutamine or adrenaline (epinephrine) are used to augment cardiac output, and IV calcium should be given if levels are low.

Other interventions such as IV bicarbonate in severe metabolic acidosis, high-volume haemofiltration/haemodialysis and extracorporeal support are sometimes used, but currently lack evidence.

Review of the underlying pathology: Although sepsis is the most common cause of acute systemic inflammation, up to 20% of patients will have a noninfectious cause. These include: pancreatitis, drug reactions, vasculitis, autoimmune diseases (e.g. systemic lupus), malignancy and haematological conditions (e.g. thrombotic thrombocytopenic purpura).

These 'sepsis mimics' should be considered early when the clinical picture is atypical, no source of sepsis is found or the inflammatory response is excessive for local infection.

Acute respiratory distress syndrome

Aetiology and pathogenesis

ARDS is a diffuse neutrophilic alveolitis caused by a range of conditions and characterised by:

- Onset within 1 week of a known clinical insult, or new or worsening respiratory symptoms
- Bilateral CXR opacities not explained by effusions, lobar/lung collapse or nodules
- Respiratory failure not fully explained by cardiac failure or fluid overload
- Impaired oxygenation

The pathophysiology is inflammation, as described in 'Sepsis' earlier, with similar infective and noninfective triggers. There is exudation of protein-rich fluid into alveoli with the formation of characteristic 'hyaline membranes'. Cytokines and chemokines cause progressive recruitment of inflammatory cells, with loss of surfactant, alveolar collapse, reduced lung compliance and impaired gas exchange with hypoxaemia and hypercapnia.

Diagnosis and management

4

ARDS can be difficult to distinguish from fluid overload, cardiac failure and interstitial pneumonia. Classic CXR appearances are shown in Fig. 4.4. Management is supportive, including treatment of the underlying cause, lung-protective ventilation, negative fluid balance and extracorporeal membrane oxygenation (ECMO) for severe cases.

Severity of hypoxaemia is categorised using the ratio of the arterial PaO_2 divided by the FiO_2:

- Mild: 40 to 26.6 kPa (300–200 mmHg)
- Moderate: 26.6 to 13.3 kPa (200–100 mmHg)
- Severe: 13.3 or less kPa (≤100 mmHg)

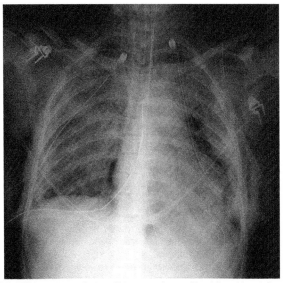

Fig. 4.4 CXR in acute respiratory distress syndrome. Note bilateral lung infiltrates, pneumomediastinum, pneumothoraces with chest drains, surgical emphysema and multiple fractures of the ribs.

Acute circulatory failure (cardiogenic shock)

Definition and aetiology

Cardiogenic shock is defined as hypoperfusion caused by inadequate cardiac output. The primary causes of cardiogenic shock are left or right ventricular infarction, PE, tamponade, endocarditis and tachyarrhythmia, but it may also complicate many other diseases (e.g. sepsis, anaphylaxis or haemorrhage).

Myocardial infarction: Cardiogenic shock following acute MI is usually caused by left ventricular dysfunction. However, it may also be attributed to right ventricular infarction, tamponade (ventricular rupture), ventricular septal defect or papillary muscle rupture causing acute mitral regurgitation.

Severe LV dysfunction reduces cardiac output, BP and coronary perfusion. Increased LV end-diastolic pressure, pulmonary congestion and oedema cause hypoxaemia that worsens myocardial ischaemia, further exacerbating cardiogenic shock. Hypotension, oliguria, delirium and cold peripheries indicate low cardiac output, whereas breathlessness, hypoxaemia, cyanosis and basal inspiratory crackles reveal pulmonary oedema. A Swan–Ganz catheter can be used to measure pulmonary artery pressure and cardiac output to quantify dysfunction and target treatment.

In cardiogenic shock complicating acute MI, immediate percutaneous coronary intervention (p. 278) should be performed to limit damage to adjacent injured myocardium.

Acute massive pulmonary embolism: Massive PE may complicate deep vein thrombosis, and usually presents with sudden collapse. Echocardiography may demonstrate a small, under-filled, vigorous left ventricle with a dilated right ventricle, or even thrombus in the RV outflow tract or pulmonary artery. CT pulmonary angiography provides a definitive diagnosis.

Acute valvular pathology, aortic dissection and cardiac tamponade: These may all cause sudden onset shock. They are discussed in Chapter 8.

Postcardiac arrest

Following successful resuscitation from cardiac arrest (p. 252), most survivors need intensive care management.

Acute management

A MAP of greater than 70 mmHg should be maintained to optimise cerebral perfusion. Shock is common following arrest, and support with inotropes, vasopressors and occasionally an intraaortic balloon pump or ECMO (p. 88) may be required. Specific cardiac interventions are described in Chapter 8. Other physiological targets include maintenance of normal temperature, blood glucose, arterial PO_2 and PCO_2.

Prognosis

Predicting recovery from brain injury after cardiac arrest is difficult. Indicators of poor outcome include: • Multiple organ failure co-morbidities • Absent pupillary and corneal reflexes • Absent motor response, persistent myoclonic jerking • A neuron-specific enolase greater than 33 µg/L • Brain CT showing loss of grey–white differentiation or other pathology • EEG signs of brain injury • Bilateral absence of somato-sensory evoked potentials.

Prognostication should ideally be delayed until after 72 hours of intensive stabilisation. This, together with the best judgement of the level of disability the individual would be prepared to accept, should inform decisions regarding treatment.

Other causes of multiorgan failure

Sepsis is the most common cause of multiorgan failure; however, single-organ cardiac, liver, renal or respiratory failure may also cause multi-organ failure, probably via the release of systemic toxins by the failing organ.

Multiorgan failure can also be caused by toxins (e.g. envenomation) and intrinsic factors such as myoglobin in rhabdomyolysis (p. 80). It can also be caused by severe physical injury from radiation, heat or blast trauma.

Critical care medicine

Decisions around intensive care admission

Being a patient in intensive care is stressful, as well as emotionally and physically invasive, even with high-quality care and analgesia. It is generally agreed that intensive treatment is only morally 'right' if there is a realistic hope that patients will regain a quality of life that justifies the pain and suffering they experience in intensive care. Few patients comprehend the implications of critical illness, so the physician must lead the process of selection for intensive care.

The decision-making process should include the likelihood of reversibility of the disease, the magnitude of the interventions required, the level of frailty and the patient's beliefs and wishes (commonly expressed through family).

Improving technology and science have prolonged survival in many conditions previously regarded as terminal. For congenital conditions, decisions on the appropriate level of intensive support should be guided by the best expert opinion and fully discussed with parents and, where possible, with the patient. Famous examples of the success of intervention or of survival, but with profound disability, shape public views and expectations, further complicating decisions in this area. Some useful decision-making techniques are listed in Box 4.10.

Stabilisation and institution of organ support

Firstly, treat the primary problem, for example, the source of sepsis or bleeding. Definitive treatment, such as laparotomy for a perforated viscus, should not be delayed after immediate resuscitation. When definitive treatment is unclear, unavailable or slow to act, organ support to stabilise the patient becomes the main goal of care.

4.10 Techniques to improve admission decision making

- Always act in the best interests of the patient
- Maximise patient capacity: if possible, consult the patient about escalation/resuscitation
- Communicate clearly and honestly with the next of kin: for example, 'If we had 100 patients with your mother's illness, only 10 would survive'
- Reach mutual agreement with the next of kin regarding the most appropriate course of action
- Seek additional opinions: involve other clinicians and err on the side of escalation where the most appropriate management is unclear. Mediation or a court ruling may rarely be needed if agreement cannot be reached.
- Plan ahead: documented advance planning in chronic, progressive disease can make decisions easier.

Respiratory support

Noninvasive respiratory support

Noninvasive respiratory support provides a bridge between simple oxygen delivery and invasive ventilation. It can be used in patients who are in respiratory distress but who lack an indication for invasive ventilation, or in those unsuitable for intubation for other reasons. Patients must be cooperative, able to protect their airway and have preserved respiratory drive and cough. Noninvasive respiratory support should not be used to prolong the dying process in end-stage disease. Likewise, a failure to respond to treatment or further deterioration should trigger a decision regarding intubation, as delayed invasive ventilation in this context is associated with a worse outcome.

High-flow nasal cannulae

These provide very high flows of fully humidified oxygen and air. They are useful in selected patients with type I respiratory failure (particularly pneumonia) who do not meet criteria for invasive ventilation. They allow patient comfort and increased expectoration and provide some PEEP and high oxygen levels, which can be titrated to SO_2.

Continuous positive airway pressure (CPAP)

CPAP involves positive pressure (5–10 cm H_2O) applied throughout the breathing cycle. Used mainly for atelectasis and pulmonary oedema, it helps to recruit collapsed alveoli and enhances clearance of alveolar fluid.

Noninvasive (bi-level) ventilation

NIV provides ventilatory support via a tight-fitting nasal or facial mask. The ventilator delivers a higher pressure (approximately 15–25 cm H_2O) during inspiration and a lower pressure (usually 4–10 cm H_2O) during expiration. Ventilation can be triggered by a patient's breaths or timed. Systems that synchronise with a patient's efforts are better tolerated and more effective in respiratory failure. Timed breaths are used for patients with central apnoea. NIV is first-line therapy in patients with type II respiratory failure secondary to acute exacerbation of COPD, because it reduces the work of breathing. It is also useful in pulmonary oedema, obesity hypoventilation syndromes and some neuromuscular disorders. It should be initiated early, especially when hypercapnic respiratory acidosis is present. Evidence for NIV in pneumonia with hypercapnia is less certain; early intubation is probably more beneficial.

Intubation and intermittent positive pressure ventilation (IPPV)

4

Intubation in a critically ill patient is risky because the patient is often exhausted or deteriorating rapidly, and cardiovascular collapse may be precipitated by the drugs used to induce anaesthesia and the apnoea invoked to facilitate intubation. Risks can be minimised by early intervention, preoxygenation, expert anaesthesia and an experienced intubator.

The main aims of IPPV are to avoid critical hypoxaemia and hypercapnia while minimising damage to the alveoli and encouraging the patient to breathe spontaneously once it is safe to do so. The physiological goal depends on the clinical context. For example, a patient with raised ICP will have a strong indication for normocapnia (because hypercapnia increases ICP). Unfortunately, achieving sufficient minute volume to maintain normocapnia can, itself, cause lung damage (see below).

Ventilator modes

Following intubation, most patients require mandatory ventilation (where the ventilator delivers a set tidal volume or inspiratory pressure) because they are paralysed as a result of the administration of muscle relaxants. The duration of mandatory ventilation depends on the severity of the lung injury, the underlying disease and the patient's condition. With pressure support, additional patient efforts between mandatory breaths can 'trigger' the ventilator to deliver a synchronised breath. Other settings that must be controlled during IPPV include the fractional inspired oxygen, respiratory rate, minute volume and the inspiratory and end-expiratory pressures.

As illness resolves, periods of spontaneous breathing with pressure support are commenced. Although spontaneous breathing is preferable to mandatory ventilation, the shearing forces of patient effort can exacerbate lung injury in severe lung damage, so weaning must be attempted cautiously.

Ventilator-induced lung injury

Positive-pressure breaths may cause alveolar damage through:

- Tidal volume distension, 'volutrauma'
- Inflation pressure, 'barotrauma'
- Alveolar collapse at end expiration, 'atelectotrauma'
- Cytokine release in response to cyclical distension, 'biotrauma'

The threshold for VILI varies between patients, and settings that would not injure healthy lungs may cause severe VILI in patients with disease. VILI may be reduced by:

- Permissive hypercapnia—limiting ventilation and tolerating moderate hypercapnia

- Preventing atelectasis using PEEP together with low tidal volumes, and occasional 'recruitment' periods of high airway pressure
- Paralysis with a muscle relaxant; poorly synchronised patient effort may worsen VILI in respiratory failure.

Extracorporeal respiratory support

Sometimes, despite optimal IPPV, it is impossible to maintain adequate oxygenation or to prevent profound respiratory acidosis. If the cause of respiratory failure is reversible extracorporeal, respiratory support may be considered. Options include:

Venous-venous ECMO

Using large-bore catheters, blood is pumped from the vena cava through a membrane oxygenator, which adds oxygen and removes carbon dioxide. Oxygenated blood is returned to the right atrium. Even if the lungs are not contributing to gas exchange, VV ECMO can keep a patient well-oxygenated and normocapnic.

Venous-arterial ECMO

VA ECMO can be life saving in profound cardiogenic shock, and may even be effective in refractory cardiac arrest; however, treatment may be futile unless a definitive solution, such as cardiac transplantation or a ventricular assist device, is available. The principles are similar to VV ECMO, except that oxygenated blood is returned to the arterial system rather than the right atrium.

Extracorporeal carbon dioxide removal

If oxygenation is good but there is refractory hypercapnia compromising care (e.g. patients with raised ICP), devices are available that can remove carbon dioxide using a much lower blood flow and smaller cannulae than VV ECMO. The technique can also be used to reduce the necessary minute ventilation to protect the lungs against VILI, or to facilitate early extubation.

Cardiovascular support

Initial resuscitation

Briefly assess whether a patient is at risk of imminent cardiac arrest. If the patient is obtunded and lacks a palpable major pulse, treatment is described on p. 252.

In anaphylactic shock or undifferentiated shock in a periarrest situation, a single dose of intramuscular adrenaline (epinephrine) 0.5 mg (0.5 mL of 1:1000) can be life saving. A small dose of intravenous adrenaline (e.g. 50 µg; 0.5 mL of 1:10000) can delay cardiac arrest long enough to identify the cause of shock and institute other support. If haemorrhage is likely, a 'major haemorrhage' alert should be issued, facilitating rapid access to large volumes of blood and blood products. A classification of shock is shown in Box 4.11.

Venous access with wide-bore cannulae for the administration of drugs and fluids is vital, but may be difficult. In extremis, the external jugular vein can be cannulated; it is often prominent in low cardiac output states and readily visible on the lateral aspect of the neck. Occluding the vein using

i	4.11 Categories of shock	
Category	**Description**	
Hypovolaemic	Either haemorrhagic or nonhaemorrhagic (e.g. hyperglycaemic hyperosmolar state (p. 430) and burns)	
Cardiogenic	See p. 84	
Obstructive	Circulatory obstruction, e.g. major pulmonary embolism, cardiac tamponade, tension pneumothorax	
Septic	See p. 80	
Anaphylactic	Inappropriate vasodilatation triggered by allergen (e.g. bee sting), often with endothelial disruption and capillary leak (p. 88)	
Neurogenic	Caused by major brain or spinal injury, which disrupts brainstem and neurogenic vasomotor control	
Others	For example, drug-related such as calcium channel blocker over-dose; Addisonian crisis	

4

finger pressure makes it easier to cannulate, but stay high in the neck to avoid accidental pneumothorax. Intra-osseous or central venous access can be established if peripheral access fails. Ultrasound may aid rapid and safe venous cannulation. Rapid infusion devices should be used to deliver warmed fluid and blood products.

Fluid and vasopressor use

Resuscitation of the shocked patient should include a 10 mL/kg fluid challenge using colloid or crystalloid; starch solutions should be avoided. The challenge can be repeated up to a maximum total of 30 mL/kg if shock persists; however, vasopressor therapy should also be considered early. Vasopressors induce venoconstriction, effectively mobilising more fluid into the circulation.

If shock persists after 30 mL/kg of fluid challenge, reconsider concealed haemorrhage or circulatory obstruction. An echocardiogram is useful to evaluate cardiac output and exclude tamponade. Noradrenaline (norepinephrine) should be commenced in most cases. However, in cardiogenic shock with low cardiac output, adrenaline (epinephrine) or dobutamine should be commenced. Both agents are equally effective, but dobutamine causes more vasodilatation, and additional noradrenaline may be required to maintain MAP. Vasopressin is added if hypotension persists despite high doses of noradrenaline and cardiac output is adequate.

In emergency situations, inotrope infusions may be given through a large-bore peripheral cannula, although central venous and arterial lines should be inserted as soon as possible.

Advanced haemodynamic monitoring

Cardiac output monitoring (using ultrasound, thoracic impedance or thermodilution) may be used where the aetiology of shock is unclear or the treatment response is poor. Portable echocardiography may reveal useful structural information, for example, aortic stenosis or regional ventricular abnormality.

In complex cases, pulmonary artery (Swan–Ganz) catheters enable measurement of pulmonary pressures, cardiac output and mixed venous oxygen saturations, indicating whether shock is caused by vasodilatation or pump failure. Complications include lung infarction, pulmonary artery rupture and catheter thrombosis.

Mechanical cardiovascular support

When shock is so severe that organ perfusion is compromised despite fluids and inotropes, it may be necessary to augment cardiac output mechanically.

Intraaortic balloon pump

A balloon-tipped tube is inserted into the femoral artery and fed into the thoracic aorta. The balloon is inflated in diastole and deflated in systole, improving diastolic pressure, abdominal and coronary perfusion. Despite these physiological benefits, it does not improve survival in cardiogenic shock. Risks include thrombosis on the balloon, mesenteric ischaemia and femoral artery pseudo-aneurysm following removal.

Renal support

RRT is covered on page 233. In an intensive care context:

- Haemodynamic instability is common. Continuous therapies tend to cause less instability than intermittent dialysis.
- Haemodialysis and haemofiltration are equally good. Although in theory haemofiltration can remove inflammatory cytokines, this does not translate into improved survival.
- Anticoagulation is usually achieved using citrate or heparin. Citrate effectively anticoagulates the extracorporeal circuit without inducing increased bleeding risk, but may accumulate in multi-organ failure and should be avoided in very unstable patients.
- Most patients who survive intensive care will regain adequate renal function to live without long-term renal support.
- A thorough investigation for reversible causes of renal dysfunction (Fig. 7.4) is essential.
- Shock appears to reverse more rapidly when renal support is instituted early.

Neurological support

Neurological conditions requiring intensive care management include coma, spinal cord injury, peripheral neuromuscular disease and prolonged seizures.

The goals of care include:

- Protecting the airway, if necessary by intubation
- Correcting hypoxaemia and hypercapnia

- Treating circulatory problems, for example, spinal shock following high spinal cord injuries
- Managing acute brain injury with control of ICP
- Controlling epileptic seizures

In acute brain injury, the goal is to optimise cerebral oxygen delivery by maintaining normal arterial oxygen content and a cerebral perfusion pressure of >60 mmHg. Secondary brain injury from hyper-/hypoglycaemia and prolonged seizures must be avoided. Raised ICP in brain injury (from haematoma, contusions, oedema or ischaemic swelling) causes direct damage to the brainstem and motor tracts owing to herniation through the tentorium and foramen magnum, and indirect damage by reducing CPP.

ICP can be measured using pressure transducers inserted directly into the brain tissue. Normal ICP is less than 15 mmHg, and an upper limit of 20 mmHg is usually adopted in intensive care. Sustained pressures of more than 30 mmHg carry a poor prognosis. ICP can be reduced by maintaining normocapnia, relieving any obstruction to cerebral venous drainage, administering intravenous mannitol or hypertonic saline, inducing hypothermia or performing decompressive craniectomy.

Complex neurological monitoring must be combined with frequent assessment of GCS, pupillary light reflexes and focal neurological signs.

Daily clinical management in intensive care

Clinical review

In intensive care, twice-daily ward rounds are usual, with detailed clinical examination and results review. The mnemonic 'FAST HUG' lists interventions that reduce intensive care complications: feeding, analgesia, sedation, thromboprophylaxis, head of bed elevation (to minimise aspiration), ulcer prophylaxis and glucose control.

Clinical review aims to identify and address any issues impeding recovery, to define specific goals for each relevant organ system and to titrate therapy accordingly. An example daily goal might be: 'Titrate the noradrenaline (norepinephrine) to achieve a MAP of 65 mmHg, aim for a negative fluid balance, titrate FiO_2 to achieve oxygen saturations of 92% to 95%'.

Sedation and analgesia

Most patients require sedation and analgesia to ensure comfort, relieve anxiety and tolerate mechanical ventilation. Deep sedation is required for critically high ICP or critical hypoxaemia, to reduce tissue oxygen requirements and to protect the brain from the peaks in ICP associated with coughing or gagging. In most cases, however, optimal sedation is an awake and lucid patient who is comfortable and able to tolerate an endotracheal tube.

Over-sedation is associated with delirium, prolonged ventilation and ICU stays and an increased incidence of ICU-acquired infection. The patient should primarily receive analgesia, rather than anaesthesia, using a balance of analgesic and sedative drugs. Beware of drugs that accumulate in patients with hepatic and renal dysfunction.

Monitoring sedation with clinical sedation scales (e.g. the Richmond Agitation–Sedation Scale) is associated with shorter ICU stay. Many ICUs use a daily 'sedation break', commonly combined with a trial of spontaneous breathing aiming to shorten the duration of mechanical ventilation.

Delirium in intensive care

Delirium is discussed on p. 66. It is common in critically ill patients, and often appears as sedation is reduced. Hypoactive delirium is more common than hyperactive delirium but is easily missed. Bedside assessment is important: the patient is asked to squeeze the examiner's hand in response to instruction and questions, aiming to detect disordered thought or sensory inattention.

Delirium is associated with poorer outcome. Management is focused on nonpharmacological interventions such as early mobilisation, reinstatement of day–night routine, noise reduction, cessation of drugs causing delirium and treatment of underlying causes (e.g. thiamin replacement in alcohol dependency). Patients with agitated delirium refractory to verbal de-escalation should initially receive small doses of intramuscular antipsychotics, changed to oral medication once control is established. Antipsychotics such as olanzapine and quetiapine are superior to haloperidol. These drugs are not useful as prophylaxis or in hypoactive delirium.

Weaning from respiratory support

Spontaneous breathing trials

This involves the removal of respiratory support followed by observation of how long the patient can breathe unassisted. Ideally, sedation is reduced, and PEEP and pressure support are either reduced to low levels or patients are disconnected from the ventilator and breathe oxygen or humidified air through the endotracheal tube. Signs of failure include rapid shallow breathing, hypoxaemia, rising $PaCO_2$, sweating and agitation. Patients who do well are next assessed for possible extubation.

Progressive reduction in pressure support ventilation

PSV is progressively reduced over a period of hours or days, according to patient response. A useful guide to weaning is the rapid shallow breathing index (= respiratory rate/tidal volume), a numerical indication of respiratory difficulty. An index of >100 suggests that spontaneous breathing would be unsustainable for long periods.

Extubation

A patient's readiness to be extubated cannot be predicted accurately; clinical judgement is needed. At the least, patients must have stable ABGs with resolution of hypoxaemia and hypercapnia despite minimal ventilator pressure support and a low FiO_2. Conscious level must be adequate to protect the airway, comply with physiotherapy and cough. The patient must also be able to sustain the required minute volume without ventilator support. This depends on the condition of the lungs, muscle strength, temperature

4.12 Advantages and disadvantages of tracheostomy

Advantages

Patient comfort
Improved oral hygiene
Access for tracheal toilet
Ability to speak with cuff deflated and a
speaking valve attached

Reduced equipment 'dead space' (the
volume of tubing)
Earlier weaning and intensive care unit
discharge
Reduced sedation requirement
Reduced vocal cord damage

Disadvantages

Immediate complications: hypoxaemia,
haemorrhage
Tracheostomy site infection

Tracheal damage; late stenosis

and metabolic rate. Re-intubation following extubation is associated with poorer outcome, but patients who are not given the opportunity to wean are at increased risk of complications such as pneumonia and myopathy.

Tracheostomy

A tracheostomy is a tube passed percutaneously into the upper trachea to facilitate longer-term ventilation. The advantages and disadvantages of tracheostomy are listed in Box 4.12. When weaning has been unsuccessful, tracheostomy facilitates further trials of ventilator withdrawal, as support is easily reinstated. In patients who have undergone laryngectomy, the tracheal stoma is the only access to the airway, and blockage is life threatening.

Nutrition

Critically ill patients must receive adequate calories, protein and essential vitamins and minerals. Requirements should be assessed by a dietitian. Under-feeding leads to muscle wasting and delayed recovery, whereas over-feeding can lead to biliary stasis, jaundice and steatosis. Enteral feeding is preferred where possible, because it avoids the infective complications of TPN and helps to maintain gut integrity. TPN is reserved for patients who suffer a sustained period without effective enteral feeding.

Other essential components of intensive care

The prevention of medical complications during recovery from the primary insult is a key factor determining survival.

Thromboprophylaxis

DVT, venous catheter-related thrombosis and PE are common in critically ill patients. Low-molecular-weight heparin should always be given, unless there is a contraindication, in which case risk/benefit evaluation is needed. Intermittent calf compression devices are useful adjuvants in high-risk patients.

Glucose control

Hyperglycaemia may occur in people with pre-existing or undiagnosed diabetes, following administration of glucocorticoids or as a consequence of stress. It is commonly managed using an insulin infusion titrated using a 'sliding scale' to achieve a blood glucose of 6 to 10 mmol/L (108–180 mg/dL).

Blood transfusion

Many critically ill patients become anaemic because of reduced red cell production and red cell loss through bleeding and blood sampling. However, transfusion carries risks including immunosuppression, fluid overload, microemboli and transfusion reactions. In stable patients, 70 g/L (7 g/dL) is a safe compromise haemoglobin level, although a higher threshold may be appropriate with myocardial ischaemia.

Peptic ulcer prophylaxis

Proton pump inhibitors or histamine-2 receptor antagonists are effective at preventing stress ulceration during critical illness. However, these agents, particularly when given with antibiotics, may increase the incidence of nosocomial infection, especially infection with *Clostridium difficile*, so ulcer prophylaxis is usually stopped once enteral feeding is re-established.

Complications and outcomes of critical illness

The majority of patients survive their episode of critical illness. Although some return to full, active lives, many have ongoing physical, emotional and psychological problems.

Adverse neurological outcomes

Brain injury

Head injury, hypoxic–ischaemic injury, infection and inflammatory and vascular pathologies can all irreversibly injure the brain. If treatment is unsuccessful, patients may die or suffer residual disability, and the decision to continue organ support will depend on the severity of the injury, the prognosis and the wishes of the patient (usually via relatives). Brain death is a state in which cortical and brainstem function is irreversibly lost. Diagnosing brain death may allow physicians to withdraw active treatment and discuss the potential for organ donation. Confirming brain death is complex and should be done only by experienced physicians. It is vital first to exclude reversible causes of coma such as drugs, hypothermia, hypoglycaemia or other biochemical disorder. Other types of reduced consciousness such as vegetative state, minimally conscious state and locked-in syndrome must be excluded. A range of specific neurological tests is performed by two physicians and repeated after an interval before the diagnosis of brain death is made.

ICU-acquired weakness

Weakness is common among survivors of critical illness. It is usually symmetrical, proximal and worst in the legs. Critical illness polyneuropathy and myopathy may coexist and can be hard distinguish. Risk factors for both include the severity of multiorgan failure, poor glycaemic control and the use of muscle relaxants and glucocorticoids.

Critical illness polyneuropathy: This presents as proximal muscle weakness with preserved sensation, or as failure to wean from a ventilator because of respiratory muscle weakness. Electrophysiological studies help to rule out other causes such as Guillain–Barré syndrome. Weakness may persist long into convalescence, and there are no specific treatments aside from those of the underlying cause and rehabilitation.

Critical illness myopathy: Immobility and the catabolic state are among the many causes of critical illness myopathy. Typically, CK is normal or only mildly elevated. Myopathy is usually a clinical diagnosis, but nerve conduction studies and electromyography may help to rule out other pathology. Muscle biopsy shows selective loss of thick myofibrils and muscle necrosis. Management is conservative, and the prognosis is good.

Other long-term problems

The experience of critical illness and invasive management can have psychological sequelae akin to post–traumatic stress syndrome. Sometimes recovering patients benefit from returning to the ICU to understand better the experiences that haunt them.

Physical sequelae are also common. Organ damage often persists, and diseases may recur; for example, patients with sepsis are far more likely than others to suffer from it again. Iatrogenic complications, for example, tracheal stenosis caused by the endotracheal tube, are common. Intensive care follow-up clinics are useful for addressing such issues.

The older patient

The ability to make a full recovery depends on frailty rather than age, so it can be helpful to use a validated frailty scoring system to inform decision making. Rehabilitation has much to offer survivors of critical illness, and an early referral is beneficial when it is clear that a patient is likely to survive with significant morbidity.

Withdrawal of active treatment and death in intensive care

Futility

Hippocrates stated that physicians should 'refuse to treat those who are overmastered by their disease, realising that in such cases medicine is powerless'. In intensive care, where futility is often used as a criterion to limit or withdraw treatment, a helpful working definition on which families and physicians can agree is 'the point at which recovery to a quality of life that the patient would find acceptable has passed'.

Death

Although most patients prefer to die at home, many die in hospital. Moving to a palliative care strategy should not change care intensity, only the over-arching objective. Only interventions that improve the quality of a patient's remaining life should be offered. In the ICU, this may include infusions of sedatives and analgesics, as stopping them may cause unnecessary pain and agitation. Measures to prolong life should be withdrawn (e.g. inotropes and extubation) to allow patients to die peacefully with their family and friends present.

Organ donation

Donation after brain death

Once brain death has been confirmed (p. 94), organ donation should be considered, termed 'donation after brain death'. Time of death is recorded as the time when the first series of brain death tests are undertaken, although the deceased patient continues to be ventilated.

Organ donation specialists can facilitate communication with relatives and coordination of any donation. Many patients will have expressed their wishes through an organ donor register, but agreement of family and next of kin is a moral (and sometimes legal) prerequisite before proceeding.

Donation after cardiac death

If a patient does not meet brain death criteria but withdrawal of treatment has been agreed, donation of organs with residual function may still be possible. This is termed 'donation after cardiac death'. If the patient dies with a short 'warm ischaemic time' (the period of physiological derangement between the withdrawal of active treatment and asystole), then donation after cardiac death can proceed, with the appropriate permissions as outlined above.

Postmortem examination

There are several indications for a postmortem examination. A coroner (or legal equivalent) may require one if death is unexpected, violent or has occurred in suspicious circumstances. The physician may request one if the cause of death is unclear, or if it may yield information valuable to the family or clinical team.

Discharge from intensive care

When the original indication for admission has resolved and the patient has sufficient reserve to recover outside intensive care, 'step-down' to the HDU is usual. ICU discharge is stressful for patients and families, and clear communication with the receiving clinical team is vital. Nursing ratios change from 1:1 (one nurse per patient) or 1:2 to much lower staffing levels. Discharge from the ICU or HDU to standard wards should take place within normal working hours to ensure adequate medical and nursing handover. The receiving team should be provided with a comprehensive written summary, including the escalation plan in the event of deterioration.

Critical care scoring systems

Clinical scores are used to define the severity of illness to assess the effects of care on the outcomes achieved. Two widely used systems are

> ### 4.13 Intensive care scoring systems: APACHE II and SOFA
>
> #### APACHE II score
>
> - An assessment of admission characteristics (e.g. age and preexisting organ dysfunction) and the maximum/minimum values of 12 routine physiological measurements taken during the first 24 hours of admission (e.g. temperature, blood pressure, GCS) that reflect the physiological impact of the illness
> - Composite score out of 71
> - Higher scores are given to patients with more serious underlying diagnoses, medical history or physiological instability; higher mortality correlates with higher scores
>
> #### SOFA score
>
> - A score of 1–4 is allocated to six organ systems (respiratory, cardiovascular, liver, renal, coagulation and neurological) to represent the degree of organ dysfunction, e.g. platelet count >150 × 10^9/L scores 1 point, <25 × 10^9/L scores 4 points
> - Composite score out of 24
> - Higher scores are associated with increased mortality

APACHE II: Acute Physiology Assessment and Chronic Health Evaluation and *SOFA score*: Sequential Organ Failure Assessment tool (Box 4.13).

When combined with the admission diagnosis, scores have been shown to correlate well with in-hospital mortality. Such outcome predictions are useful at a population level but lack the specificity to be of use in individual patients. This is in contrast to well-validated, disease-specific tools, such as the CURB-65 tool for pneumonia, which can be helpful in guiding individual management (see Fig. 9.6).

SMRs for common diagnoses have been calculated from large databases involving many ICUs. These allow a particular unit to evaluate its performance compared with other ICUs. If a unit has a high SMR in a certain diagnostic category, it should prompt an audit of the management of patients with that diagnosis.

Infectious disease

'Infection' occurs when infectious agents become established in the host's tissues, replicate, cause harm and induce a host response. If a microorganism survives and replicates on a mucosal surface without causing illness, the host is said to be 'colonised'. If a microorganism lies dormant after invading host tissues, the infection is said to be 'latent'. When the infectious agent, or the host response to it, is sufficient to cause illness, then the process is termed an 'infectious disease'. Not all infections are 'infectious', that is, transmissible from person to person. Infectious diseases transmitted between hosts are called communicable diseases, whereas those caused by organisms that are already colonising the host are described as endogenous.

Principles of infectious disease

Infectious agents are divided into the following categories:

- Viruses—RNA- or DNA-containing pathogens that rely on host cells for replication.
- Prokaryotes: bacteria—capable of independent replication but lacking a nucleus.
- Eukaryotes—fungi, protozoa and helminths.
- Prions—not microorganisms but misfolded proteins without nucleic acids; cause transmissible encephalopathies (see p. 694).

The human body is colonised by large numbers of bacteria (termed the human microbiota or normal flora), which have a profound influence on human health. Some benefit the host (e.g. gut flora producing vitamins K and B_{12}). In contrast, disease results when pathogenic organisms produce virulence factors that damage host cells. Primary pathogens cause disease in healthy hosts, whereas opportunistic pathogens cause disease only in the immune-compromised host.

Clinical examination of patients with infectious disease

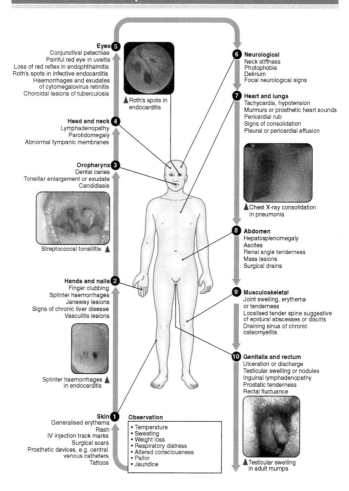

Eyes ⑤
Conjunctival petechiae
Painful red eye in uveitis
Loss of red reflex in endophthalmitis
Roth's spots in infective endocarditis
Haemorrhages and exudates
of cytomegalovirus retinitis
Choroidal lesions of tuberculosis

▲ Roth's spots in endocarditis

Head and neck ④
Lymphadenopathy
Parotidomegaly
Abnormal tympanic membranes

Oropharynx ③
Dental caries
Tonsillar enlargement or exudate
Candidiasis

Streptococcal tonsillitis ▲

Hands and nails ②
Finger clubbing
Splinter haemorrhages
Janeway lesions
Signs of chronic liver disease
Vasculitis lesions

Splinter haemorrhages ▲
in endocarditis

Skin ①
Generalised erythema
Rash
IV injection track marks
Surgical scars
Prosthetic devices, e.g. central
venous catheters
Tattoos

Observation
• Temperature
• Sweating
• Weight loss
• Respiratory distress
• Altered consciousness
• Pallor
• Jaundice

⑥ **Neurological**
Neck stiffness
Photophobia
Delirium
Focal neurological signs

⑦ **Heart and lungs**
Tachycardia, hypotension
Murmurs or prosthetic heart sounds
Pericardial rub
Signs of consolidation
Pleural or pericardial effusion

▲ Chest X-ray consolidation
in pneumonia

⑧ **Abdomen**
Hepatosplenomegaly
Ascites
Renal angle tenderness
Mass lesions
Surgical drains

⑨ **Musculoskeletal**
Joint swelling, erythema
or tenderness
Localised tender spine suggestive
of epidural abscesses or discitis
Draining sinus of chronic
osteomyelitis

⑩ **Genitalia and rectum**
Ulceration or discharge
Testicular swelling or nodules
Inguinal lymphadenopathy
Prostatic tenderness
Rectal fluctuance

▲ Testicular swelling
in adult mumps

Detection of infection

A variety of methods are used:

Direct detection of organisms: Microscopy (e.g. for mycobacteria) can be used to directly identify organisms that are slow or impossible to grow in culture.

Nucleic acid amplification tests (NAAT): Can not only identify viruses and bacteria, but also detect strain types and toxin or resistance genes.

Culture: Largely supplanted by NAAT for viruses. Bacterial culture is still widely used for identification and antibiotic sensitivity testing, but can be slow, and not all organisms grow in culture. Specialised mass spectrometers can be used for rapid identification of organisms in blood cultures.

Immunological tests: Host antibodies can be detected using *in vitro* immunological assays. A rise in titre between acute and convalescent serum indicates recent infection, but tests may be negative in the immunocompromised. Interferon-gamma release assays detect infection through the release of interferon from sensitised host T cells exposed to bacterial peptides.

Reservoirs of infection

Human reservoirs: Colonised or infected individuals may act as reservoirs, carrying organisms on the skin or in the throat (e.g. meningococci), nose, bowel (e.g. *Salmonella*) or blood (e.g. HBV).

Animal reservoirs: Animals are a source of human infections (zoonoses), for example, *Salmonella* from poultry, TB from milk. Spread may continue from human cases to other humans (e.g. Q fever).

Environmental reservoirs: Many infective pathogens are acquired from an environmental source. However, some of these are maintained in human or animal reservoirs, with the environment acting only as a conduit for infection.

Transmission of infection

Communicable diseases spread by several routes:

- Respiratory—inhalation.
- Faecal–oral—ingestion.
- Sexually transmitted—mucous membrane contact.
- Blood-borne—inoculation.
- Via vector or fomite—an animal or object bridges the gap between host and reservoir.

Healthcare associated infections

HAIs affect around 10% of all hospital admissions, causing significant clinical and economic burden. The close proximity of hospital inpatients, the widespread use of antibiotics and the ease of transmission by health-care workers have led to the selection of multidrug-resistant organisms such as MRSA and glycopeptide-resistant enterococci (GRE). Spread of these organisms, plus infection with organisms such as *Clostridium difficile* and norovirus, leads to outbreaks that necessitate ward or hospital closure

Prevention of infection

HAIs are managed by comprehensive antibiotic policies and strict adherence to infection prevention and control protocols. Although clean clothing and environment are important, recent evidence has confirmed the absolute importance of hand hygiene in the control of HAIs. The use of alcohol hand lotion by all health-care workers between every patient contact is an effective alternative to soap and water in the prevention of most HAIs, but not of *Clostridium difficile*.

Outbreak control

An outbreak of infection is defined as the occurrence of any disease clearly in excess of normal expectancy. Confirmation requires evidence of identical phenotypic and/or genotype in the causal organisms. Cases are sought by testing, then plotted on an outbreak curve. Case-control studies may be used to establish the source. Good communication of data to health-care workers is needed to achieve control. Many countries have systems for compulsory notification of contagious conditions to public health authorities to assist outbreak control.

Immunisation

Passive immunisation means administering antibodies targeting a specific pathogen. This gives temporary protection after exposure but, as antibodies are obtained from blood, there is a risk of blood-borne infection.

Active immunisation is achieved by vaccination with whole organisms or organism components. Vaccination may be applied to entire populations or to subpopulations at specific risk through travel or occupation. Usually the goal is to prevent infection, but vaccination against HPV was introduced to prevent cervical cancer. Vaccination is successful when the number of susceptible hosts in a population becomes too low to sustain transmission (herd immunity). Naturally acquired smallpox was eradicated by vaccination in 1980. A similar programme aims to eradicate poliomyelitis.

Presenting problems in infectious diseases

Fever

Fever implies an elevated core temperature of greater than 38°C. Clinical features are used to guide appropriate investigations, which include:
• FBC and differential • U&Es, liver function, glucose and muscle enzymes • ESR and CRP • HIV antibodies • Autoantibodies • CXR and ECG • Urinalysis and culture • Blood culture • Throat swab

Additional tests are indicated by local symptoms and if the patient is immunocompromised.

Pyrexia of unknown origin

PUO is a common presenting problem and is defined as a temperature of greater than 38°C on multiple occasions persisting for more than 3 weeks with no diagnosis after initial investigation. Many causes of PUO are listed in Box 5.1. Two or more causes may coexist. Fever in old age merits special attention (Box 5.2).

Detailed history should include:

Recent travel: Malaria, respiratory infections, viral hepatitis, typhoid and dengue are the most common causes of imported fever in the UK.

Personal and social history: Exposure to STI, illicit drug use.

Occupational or recreational history: Animal exposure, unpasteurised milk consumption, watersports (leptospirosis).

5.1 Aetiology of pyrexia of unknown origin

Infections (~30%)

- Specific locations: abscess at any site, cholecystitis/cholangitis, UTI, prostatitis, dental, sinus, bone and joint infections, endocarditis
- Specific organisms: TB (esp. extrapulmonary), brucellosis, *Tropheryma whipplei*, viruses (CMV, EBV, HIV-1), fungi (*Aspergillus, Candida*)
- Specific patient groups: imported infections, for example, malaria, dengue, leishmaniasis, enteric fevers, *Burkholderia pseudomallei*, nosocomial infections, HIV-related infections, for example, *Pneumocystis jirovecii*, disseminated *Mycobacterium avium*, CMV

Malignancy (~20%)

- Lymphoma, myeloma and leukaemia
- Solid tumours (renal, liver, colon, stomach, pancreas)

Connective tissue disorders (~15%)

- Older patients: temporal arteritis/polymyalgia rheumatica
- Younger patients: SLE, Still's disease, polymyositis, vasculitis, Behçet's disease
- Rheumatic fever

Miscellaneous (~20%)

- Inflammatory bowel disease, alcoholic liver disease, granulomatous hepatitis, pancreatitis
- Myeloproliferative disease, haemolytic anaemia
- Sarcoidosis, atrial myxoma, thyrotoxicosis, hypothalamic lesions
- Familial Mediterranean fever, drug reactions, factitious fever

No diagnosis or resolves spontaneously (15%)

 5.2 Fever in old age

- **Temperature measurement**: fever may be missed because oral temperatures are unreliable. Rectal measurement may be needed, but core temperature is increasingly measured using eardrum reflectance.
- **Delirium**: common with fever, especially in those with underlying cerebrovascular disease or dementia.
- **Prominent causes of PUO**: TB, intraabdominal sepsis, UTI and endocarditis. Noninfective causes include polymyalgia rheumatica, temporal arteritis and tumours.
- **Common infective causes in the very frail** (e.g. nursing home residents): pneumonia, urinary infection, soft tissue infection and gastroenteritis.

Investigations and management

Regularly review and expand history taking; this helps to select appropriate tests. Repeat physical examination regularly for emerging signs (e.g. murmurs, lymphadenopathy, rashes). Initial investigations are listed above. If these are inconclusive, those in Box 5.3 should be considered.

Lesions on imaging should normally be biopsied to detect pathogens by culture or nucleic acid detection.

5.3 Additional investigations in PUO

- Serological tests: autoantibodies, complement, immunoglobulins, cryoglobulins
- Echocardiography
- USS of abdomen
- CT/MRI of thorax, abdomen and/or brain
- Skeletal imaging: X-rays, CT/MRI spine, isotope bone scan
- Labelled white-cell scan
- PET scan
- Biopsy: bronchoscopic, lymph node, liver, bone marrow, temporal artery, laparoscopic

Liver biopsy: May reveal TB, lymphoma or granulomatous disease, including sarcoidosis. It is unlikely to help unless the liver is biochemically or radiologically abnormal.

Bone marrow biopsy: Has a diagnostic yield in PUO of around 15%, the most common abnormalities being myelodysplasia, other haematological malignancies and TB. More rarely, brucellosis, typhoid fever or visceral leishmaniasis may be detected, emphasising the importance of culture as well as microscopy of samples.

Temporal artery biopsy: Should be considered in patients over 50 years of age, even if the ESR is not significantly elevated. Because arteritis is patchy, diagnostic yield is increased if a 1.5-cm section of artery is biopsied.

Prognosis

No cause is found in approximately 10% of PUO cases, but as long as there is no significant weight loss or signs of another disease, the long-term mortality is low.

Fever in the injection drug user

Infection is introduced by nonsterile (often shared) equipment. Risks increase with prolonged drug use and central injection in large veins, necessitated by thrombosis of peripheral veins. Fever is usually caused by soft tissue or respiratory infections.

Clinical assessment

Site: Femoral vein injections may cause DVT, of which 50% are septic. Arterial injection may cause false aneurysm formation and compartment syndrome. Psoas abscess and septic arthritis also occur. *Clostridium* infection has been recorded with SC or IM injection of heroin.

Technical details: Sharing of needles and spoons, and use of contaminated drugs or solvents increase the risk of infection (e.g. HIV, HBV or HCV). Establish what has been injected, including what solvents were used.

Blood-borne viral test status: Check recent results and vaccinations. Surreptitious self-treatment with antibiotics: May mask culture results.

Other symptoms: Breathlessness, myalgia, confusion and tachycardia may be caused by infection or to drug withdrawal.

Signs: These include:

- Rashes.
- Injection site abscess.

- Joint pain or swelling from injection.
- DVT or compartment syndrome in the legs.
- Local tenderness or referred pain from an abscess site, for example, flexion at the hip eliciting back pain suggests ilio-psoas abscess.
- New murmurs or evidence of cardiac decompensation: may suggest either right- or left-sided endocarditis (check nails for splinter haemorrhages) or the cardiomyopathy of generalised sepsis. The jugular venous pressure may show V waves in tricuspid endocarditis.
- Pleural rub or effusion is seen in DVT with pulmonary embolism, or septic emboli from endocarditis or infected DVT.
- Stupor: occurs in drug overdose or hepatic encephalopathy; agitation with drug withdrawal; headache and drowsiness in meningitis or encephalitis; local paralysis or spasms with tetanus or botulism.

Management

Management is that of the underlying condition. Flucloxacillin is useful against *Staphylococcus aureus*, although vancomycin may be needed if MRSA is present. Nonadherence to prescribed antimicrobial regimens leads to a high rate of complications.

Fever in the immunocompromised host

Immunosuppression may be congenital; acquired through infection or haematological disease; or iatrogenic, induced by chemotherapy or immunosuppression for autoimmune diseases or transplantation. These may be distinguished by history, and careful examination may reveal where infection has breached the skin or mucosal barriers.

Initial tests are as described earlier (p. 102). Immunocompromised patients often have attenuated physical signs, such as neck stiffness with meningitis. Chest and/or abdominal CT should be considered in addition to CXR according to symptoms. Cultures of blood, urine and stool are often helpful. Nasopharyngeal aspirates are sometimes diagnostic, as immunocompromised hosts may shed respiratory viruses for prolonged periods. Skin nodules should be biopsied and stained for fungi. PCR should be performed for CMV and *Aspergillus* DNA, and antigen assays should be performed for *Cryptococcus* or *Aspergillus* in blood, and for *Aspergillus* and other invasive fungi or *Legionella* in urine. Antibody detection is unhelpful in immunocompromised patients. Patients with respiratory symptoms should be considered for bronchoalveolar lavage to detect *Pneumocystis jirovecii*, other fungi, bacteria and viruses.

Neutropenic fever is defined as a neutrophil count of less than 0.5×10^9/L, with fever greater than 38.5°C, and is covered on p. 797. Sepsis is discussed on p. 80.

Severe skin and soft tissue infections

Necrotising fasciitis

There are two common types of necrotising fasciitis:

Type 1: Mixed infection with Gram-negative bacteria and anaerobes, often seen following surgery or in diabetic or immunocompromised patients.

Type 2: Caused by group A or other streptococci. About 60% of cases are associated with streptococcal toxic shock syndrome (p. 129).

Rarer types caused by *Aeromonas hydrophila*, *Vibrio vulnificus* or mucoraceous moulds are seen in tropical and subtropical regions.

In necrotising fasciitis, cutaneous erythema and oedema progress to bullae or areas of necrosis. Unlike in cellulitis, pain is disproportionately intense relative to the visible cutaneous features, or may spread beyond the zone of erythema. Infection spreads quickly along the fascial plane. Treatment is with emergency surgical debridement and broad-spectrum antibiotics, for example, piperacillin/tazobactam or meropenem together with clindamycin, plus antifungals if fungal necrotising fasciitis is suspected.

Gas gangrene

Although *Clostridia* may colonise or contaminate wounds, no action is required unless spreading infection occurs. In anaerobic cellulitis, usually caused by *C. perfringens*, gas forms locally and extends along tissue planes, but bacteraemia does not occur. Prompt surgical debridement, along with penicillin or clindamycin therapy, is usually effective.

Gas gangrene is defined as acute invasion of healthy living muscle undamaged by previous trauma by *C. perfringens*. It develops following deep penetrating injury sufficient to create an anaerobic environment and allow clostridial introduction and proliferation.

Severe pain at the site of injury progresses rapidly over 18 to 24 hours. Bronze/purple discoloration develops in tense and exquisitely tender skin. Gas in tissues may cause crepitus on examination or be visible on X-ray, CT or USS. Systemic toxicity develops rapidly with high leucocytosis, multi-organ dysfunction, raised creatine kinase and disseminated intravascular haemolysis. High-dose IV penicillin, clindamycin, cephalosporins and metronidazole therapy is very effective, coupled with aggressive surgical debridement of affected tissues. Use of hyperbaric oxygen is controversial.

Acute diarrhoea and vomiting

Acute diarrhoea, sometimes with vomiting, is a common presenting problem, and may result from both infectious and noninfectious causes (Box 5.4). Infectious diarrhoea is caused by transmission of viruses, bacteria or protozoa, either by the faecal–oral route or via infected fomites, food or water. Antimicrobial-associated diarrhoea is common in the elderly. Some 20% to 25% of cases are caused by *C. difficile* (p. 139), *C. perfringens* and *Klebsiella oxytoca* are rarer causes. Psychological or physical stress may also precipitate diarrhoea. Occasionally, diarrhoea may be the presenting feature of another systemic illness, such as pneumonia.

Some organisms, for example, *Bacillus cereus*, *Staphylococcus aureus* and *Vibrio cholerae*, produce exotoxins causing vomiting and/or 'secretory' watery diarrhoea. Organisms that invade the mucosa, such as *Shigella*, *Campylobacter* and enterohaemorrhagic *E. Coli* (EHEC), have longer incubation periods and may also cause systemic upset and prolonged bloody

5.4 Causes of acute diarrhoea

Infectious

- **Toxin-mediated**: *Bacillus cereus*, *Clostridium* spp. enterotoxin, *Staphylococcu aureus*
- **Bacterial**: *Shigella*, *Campylobacter*, *Clostridium difficile*, *Salmonella*, enterotoxigenic *Escherichia coli*, enteroinvasive *E. coli*, *Vibrio cholerae*
- **Viral**: rotavirus, norovirus
- **Protozoal**: *Giardia*, *Cryptosporidium*, microsporidiosis, amoebic dysentery, isosporiasis
- **Systemic**: Acute diverticulitis, sepsis, pelvic inflammatory disease, meningococcaemia, atypical pneumonia, malaria

Noninfectious

- **GI**: inflammatory bowel disease, bowel malignancy, overflow from constipation, enteral tube feeding
- **Metabolic**: diabetic ketoacidosis, thyrotoxicosis, uraemia, neuroendocrine tumours releasing 5-HT or vasoactive intestinal peptide
- **Drugs and toxins**: NSAIDs, cytotoxic agents, PPIs, antibiotics, dinoflagellates, plant toxins, heavy metals, ciguatera or scombrotoxic fish poisoning

5.5 Foods associated with infection, including gastroenteritis

- **Raw seafood**: norovirus, *Vibrio*, hepatitis A
- **Raw eggs**: *Salmonella*
- **Undercooked meat/poultry**: *Salmonella*, *Campylobacter*, EHEC, *Clostridium perfringens*
- **Unpasteurised milk or juice**: *Salmonella*, *Campylobacter*, EHEC, *Yersinia enterocolitica*
- **Unpasteurised soft cheeses**: *Salmonella*, *Campylobacter*, enterotoxigenic *E. coli*, *Y. enterocolitica*, *Listeria*
- **Home-made canned foods**: *Clostridium botulinum*
- **Raw hot dogs, pâté**: *Listeria*

diarrhoea. *Salmonella typhi* and *Salmonella paratyphi* can cause both secretory and invasive features.

Clinical assessment

The history should address foods ingested (Box 5.5), duration and frequency of diarrhoea, presence of blood or steatorrhoea, abdominal pain and tenesmus, and whether other people have been affected.

Fever and bloody diarrhoea suggest an invasive, colitic, dysenteric process. An incubation period of less than 18 hours suggests a toxin-mediated food poisoning; more than 5 days suggests protozoal or helminthic infection.

On examination, look for dehydration (reduced skin turgor, dry mouth, sunken eyes) and chart serial blood pressure (BP), pulse rate, urine output and stool frequency and appearance. Examine the abdomen regularly.

Investigations
• Stool microscopy (for cysts, ova and parasites), culture and *C. difficile* toxin assay. • FBC, U&Es. • Blood film for malaria if patient has been in an affected area. • Blood/urine culture and CXR: may reveal an underlying diagnosis.

Management of acute diarrhoea
Isolation: All patients with acute, potentially infective diarrhoea should be isolated to minimise spread of infection.

Fluid replacement: Replace established and ongoing losses, as well as normal daily requirements. This may be done with IV fluid or oral rehydration solution (ORS). Initial replacement of 2 to 4 L is usual. Thereafter, one sachet of commercial ORS made up to 200 mL is given for each diarrhoea stool, plus the normal daily requirement of 1 to 1.5 L.

Antimicrobial therapy: Not generally beneficial, except in severe cases (e.g. immunocompromise, comorbidity or systemic involvement, as in *Shigella* and *Salmonella*). Antibiotics may limit infective spread in cholera, but are contraindicated in EHEC infection, as they may precipitate haemolytic uraemic syndrome.

Antidiarrhoeal therapy: Antimotility drugs are not generally recommended, and are potentially dangerous in childhood dysentery, causing intussusception.

Infections acquired in the tropics

Most travel-associated infections can be prevented by:
• Avoidance of insect bites • Sun protection • Food and water hygiene ('Boil it, cook it, peel it or forget it!') • Seeking medical advice if diarrhoea is bloody or lasts for more than 48 hours • Condom use

Fever acquired in the tropics

Fever is common in travellers to the tropics or local inhabitants who lack or lose immunity to tropical pathogens. Frequent final diagnoses are:
• Malaria • Typhoid fever • Viral hepatitis • Dengue fever • Travellers to affected areas may have viral haemorrhagic fever (VHF, e.g. Ebola or Lassa), avian influenza (H5N1) or Middle Eastern respiratory syndrome (MERS); all these require special isolation.

Clinical assessment
History should cover:
• Countries and environments visited. • Travel dates. • Exposures: ill people, animals, insect bites, freshwater swimming. • Dietary history. • Sexual history. • Malaria prophylaxis—what was taken and local

i	5.6 Differential WCC in tropically-acquired acute fever without localising signs		

WCC differential	Potential diagnoses	Further investigations
Neutrophil leucocytosis	Bacterial sepsis	Blood culture
	Leptospirosis	Culture of blood and urine, serology
	Borreliosis: tick or louse-borne relapsing fever	Blood film
	Amoebic liver abscess	USS
Normal WCC and differential	Malaria (may be anaemic)	Blood film, antigen test
	Typhoid fever	Blood and stool culture
	Typhus	Serology
Lymphocytosis or atypical lymphocytes	Viral fevers including VHF	Serology, PCR
	Infectious mononucleosis	Monospot, serology
	Rickettsial fevers	Serology
	Hepatitis viruses	Serology, antigen, PCR
	Malaria, trypanosomiasis	Blood film, antigen, PCR
	HIV (acute retroviral syndrome)	Serology, antigen

resistance. • Any local medicines/remedies taken. • Vaccination history—if the patient was vaccinated against yellow fever and hepatitis A and B, this virtually rules out these infections. Oral and injectable typhoid vaccinations are 70% to 90% effective.

The incubation period can aid diagnosis: *Falciparum* malaria presents 7 to 28 days after exposure, whereas VHF, dengue and rickettsial infections can be excluded if starting more than 21 days after exposure.

Examination: This is summarised on p. 100. Particular attention should be paid to the skin, throat, eyes, nail beds, lymph nodes, abdomen and heart. Patients may be unaware of tick bites or eschars. Temperature should be measured at least twice daily.

Investigations

Initial investigations should start with blood films for malaria parasites, FBC, urinalysis and CXR if indicated. Box 5.6 lists the main diagnoses to be considered in tropically acquired acute fever with no localising signs, grouped by differential WCC.

Management and appropriate isolation precautions depend on the identified cause.

i 5.7 Parasitic causes of eosinophilia		
Infestation	**Pathogen**	**Clinical syndrome**
Strongyloidiasis	*Strongyloides stercoralis*	Larva currens
Helminth infections	Hookworm, *Ascaris*, *Toxocara*	Anaemia Visceral larva migrans
Schistosomiasis	*Schistosomiasis haematobium* *S. mansoni, S. japonicum*	Katayama fever Chronic infection
Filariases	*Loa* *Wuchereria bancrofti* *Onchocerca volvulus*	Skin nodules Elephantiasis Visual disturbance
Other nematode infections	*Trichinella*	Myositis
Cestode infections	*Taenia saginatum, T. solium,* *Echinococcus granulosus*	Asymptomatic, lesions in liver
Liver fluke infections	*Fasciola hepatica*	Hepatic symptoms
Lung fluke infections	*Paragonimus westermani*	Lung lesions

Diarrhoea acquired in the tropics

Common causes include *Salmonella*, *Campylobacter* and *Cryptosporidia* infections. *Shigella* spp. and *Entamoeba histolytica* (amoebiasis) usually occur in visitors to or residents of the Indian subcontinent and sub-Saharan Africa. Other causes to be considered are tropical sprue (p. 481), giardiasis and HIV enteropathy.

Eosinophilia acquired in the tropics

Nonparasitic causes of eosinophilia include haematological conditions (p. 573), allergic reactions and HIV-1 or human T-cell lymphotropic virus-1 infection. However, eosinophils are also raised in parasitic infections, particularly those with a tissue migration phase. In travellers to or residents of the tropics, an eosinophil count of greater than 0.4×10^9/L should be investigated for both parasitic (Box 5.7) and nonparasitic causes. Long-infected residents may no longer have eosinophilia.

Clinical assessment

Take a travel history as for fever (above), noting which infections are endemic in the visited areas. Specific clinical features are listed in Box 5.8.

Investigations

Direct visualisation of adult worms, larvae or ova provides the best evidence. Box 5.9 lists the initial investigations for eosinophilia.

i 5.8 Clinical features of parasitic infections

System affected	Symptom or sign	Parasitic disease
Skin	Rashes	Schistosomiasis, strongyloidiasis
	Migratory swellings	Loiasis
	Pruritis	Onchocerciasis
Respiratory	Haemoptysis	Paragonimiasis
	Cough, wheeze, infiltrates	Nematodes, filariae
	Pulmonary hypertension	Chronic schistosomiasis
Abdominal	Hepatosplenomegaly	Schistosomiasis, fasciolasis, toxocariasis
	Intestinal obstruction or diarrhoea	Ascaris, strongyloidiasis
Neuromuscular	Eosinophilic meningitis	Angiostrongyliasis, gnathostomiasis
	Myosistis	Trichinosis, cysticercosis
Urogenital	Haematuria, haemato-spermia	Schistosomiasis
Ocular	Visual field defects	Toxocariasis

i 5.9 Initial investigation of eosinophilia

Investigation	Pathogens sought
Stool microscopy	Ova, cysts and parasites
Terminal urine	Ova of *Schistosoma haematobium*
Duodenal aspirate	Filariform larvae of *Strongyloides*, liver fluke ova
Day bloods	Microfilariae of *Brugia malayi, Loa*
Night bloods	Microfilariae of *Wuchereria bancrofti*
Skin snips	*Onchocerca volvulus*
Serology	*Schistosoma, Filaria, Strongyloides*, hydatid, trichinosis, etc.

Skin conditions acquired in the tropics

The most common skin problems in the tropics are bacterial and fungal skin infections, scabies and eczema. These are described in Chapter 17. In travellers, infected insect bites and cutaneous larva migrans are common. Box 5.10 summarises the types of rash commonly seen in tropical travellers/residents. Skin biopsy and culture may be required to achieve a firm diagnosis.

 5.10 Rash in tropical travellers/residents

Maculopapular

- Dengue, HIV-1, typhoid, *Spirillum minus*, rickettsial infections, measles

Petechial or purpuric

- Viral haemorrhagic fevers, yellow fever, meningococcal sepsis, leptospirosis, rickettsial spotted fevers, malaria

Urticarial

- Schistosomiasis, toxocariasis, strongyloidiasis, fascioliasis

Vesicular

- Monkeypox, insect bites, rickettsial pox

Ulcers

- Leishmaniasis, *Mycobacterium ulcerans* (Buruli ulcer), dracunculosis, anthrax, rickettsial eschar, tropical ulcer, ecthyma

Papules

- Scabies, insect bites, prickly heat, ringworm, onchocerciasis

Nodules or plaques

- Leprosy, chromoblastomycosis, dimorphic fungi, trypanosomiasis, onchocerciasis, myiasis, tungiasis

Migratory linear rash

- Cutaneous larva migrans, *Strongyloides stercoralis*

Migratory papules/nodules

- *Loa*, gnathosomiasis, schistosomiasis

Thickened skin

- Mycetoma, elephantiasis

Infection issues in adolescence

These are summarised in Box 5.11.

5.11 Infection issues in adolescence	
Common infectious syndromes	Infectious mononucleosis, bacterial pharyngitis, whooping cough, staphylococcal skin/soft tissue infection, UTI, gastroenteritis
Life-threatening infections	Meningococcal meningitis, bacterial sepsis
STIs	HIV-1, hepatitis B, chlamydia
Travel-related infections	Diarrhoea, malaria
Infections in susceptible groups	For example, those with cystic fibrosis, congenital immunodeficiency, acute leukaemia
Adherence to prolonged treatment	For example, TB, antiretroviral therapy, osteomyelitis–adherence often hard to achieve in adolescence
Vaccination	HPV
Risk reduction	Education on sexual health, alcohol and recreational drug use important

Infection issues in pregnancy

These are summarised in Box 5.12.

5.12 Infection issues in pregnancy		
Infection	**Consequence**	**Prevention/management**
Rubella	Congenital malformation	Vaccination of nonimmune mothers
CMV	Congenital malformation	Limited prevention strategies
Varicella zoster	Congenital malformation, neonatal infection	VZ immune globulin or aciclovir if exposure > 4 days previously
Herpes simplex	Congenital or neonatal infection	Aciclovir and consider caesarean delivery if genital HSV. Aciclovir for infant
Hepatitis B	Chronic infection of neonate	Hep B immune globulin/vaccinate newborn
HIV-1	Chronic infection of neonate	Antiretrovirals for mother and child. Consider caesarean delivery if viral load detectable. Avoid breastfeeding

5.12 Infection issues in pregnancy—cont'd

Infection	Consequence	Prevention/management
Parvovirus B19	Hydrops fetalis	Avoid infected persons during pregnancy
Measles	Infection of mother/neonate	Immunisation of mother
Dengue	Neonatal dengue	Vector (mosquito) control
Syphilis	Congenital malformation	Serology and treatment of mothers
Gonorrhoea and chlamydia	Neonatal conjunctivitis	Treatment of mother and neonate
Listeriosis	Neonatal meningitis/sepsis, maternal sepsis	Avoid unpasteurised cheeses/other dietary sources
Brucellosis	Possibly increased fetal loss	Avoid unpasteurised dairy products
Group B streptococcus	Neonatal meningitis/sepsis, maternal postpartum sepsis	Risk-based antibiotic prophylaxis
Toxoplasmosis	Congenital malformation	Avoid undercooked meat
Malaria	Fetal loss, growth retardation, maternal malaria	Avoid insect bites. Intermittent preventative treatment in high-risk areas

Viral infections

Systemic viral infections with exanthem

Childhood exanthems are characterised by fever and widespread rash. Maternal antibodies protect for the first 6 to 12 months. Although the incidence of exanthems has diminished as a result of vaccination, incomplete uptake results in infections in later life.

Measles

The WHO has set the objective of eradicating measles, but vaccination of 95% of a population is required to prevent outbreaks. Natural illness produces lifelong immunity.

Clinical features

Infection is by respiratory droplets with an incubation period of 6–19 days to onset of rash. A prodromal illness occurs 1 to 3 days before the rash, with upper respiratory symptoms, conjunctivitis and the presence of 'Koplik's spots' (small white spots surrounded by erythema) on the internal buccal mucosa (Fig. 5.1). As natural antibodies develop, the maculopapular rash appears (Fig. 5.2), spreading from face to extremities. Lymphadenopathy and diarrhoea are common.

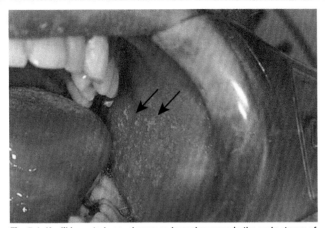

Fig. 5.1 Koplik's spots (arrows) seen on buccal mucosa in the early stages of clinical measles.

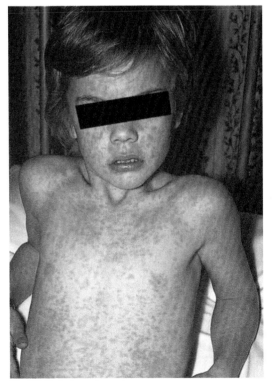

Fig. 5.2 Typical measles rash.

Complications include:
• Otitis media. • Bacterial pneumonia. • Encephalitis/convulsions. • Subacute sclerosing panencephalitis (rare, late and serious).

Management

In the immunocompetent, measles is self-limiting; however, severity and complications are increased in the malnourished and immuno-suppressed. Disease is attenuated in the immunocompromised and in nonimmune pregnant women by immunoglobulin treatment. All children aged 12 to 15 months should receive measles vaccination as a combined vaccine with mumps and rubella, with a further dose at age 4 years.

Rubella (German measles)

Rubella is transmitted by respiratory droplets, with infectivity from up to 10 days before to 2 weeks after the onset of the rash. The incubation period is 15 to 20 days. Most childhood cases are subclinical, although disease can present with fever, lymphadenopathy and a maculopapular rash that spreads from the face to the trunk. Complications include arthralgia, thrombocytopenia, hepatitis and rarely encephalitis.

If transplacental infection takes place in the first trimester or later, viral persistence is likely, and severe congenital disease may result. Following exposure during pregnancy, confirmation of infection is provided either by rubella IgM antibodies in serum or by IgG seroconversion. In an exposed pregnant woman, absence of rubella IgG confirms the potential for congenital infection. All children should be immunised with MMR to prevent rubella. Prepregnancy MMR is now considered the best way of protecting pregnant women.

Parvovirus B19

This air-borne virus causes mild or subclinical infection in normal hosts. Around 50% of children and 60% to 90% of adults are seropositive. In addition to the clinical manifestations summarised in Box 5.13, there may be a transient block in erythropoiesis, which is insignificant unless haemoglobinopathy or haemolysis is also present. Parvovirus B19 DNA may be detected in the serum by PCR; however, as illness is usually mild or subclinical and self-limiting, confirmatory blood tests are not always required. If infection occurs during pregnancy, the fetus should be monitored closely for signs of hydrops.

Human herpesvirus 6 and 7

These viruses are associated with a benign febrile illness of children with a maculopapular erythematous rash: 'exanthem subitum'. In the immunocompromised, they cause an infectious mononucleosis-like syndrome. Around 95% of children are infected by age 2 years.

Chickenpox

Varicella zoster virus (VZV) is a dermotropic and neurotropic virus causing primary infection, usually in childhood, which may reactivate in later life. It

5.13 Clinical features of parvovirus B19 infection	
Syndrome/affected age group	**Clinical manifestations**
Fifth disease (erythema infectiosum) Small children	Three clinical stages: a 'slapped cheek' appearance (Fig. 5.3), reticulate eruption on the body and limbs then resolution. Often the child is quite well throughout
Gloves and socks syndrome Young adults	Fever and an acral purpuric eruption with a clear margin at the wrists and ankles. Mucosal involvement also occurs
Arthropathies Adults, occasionally children	Polyarthropathy of small joints. In children it tends to involve the larger joints in an asymmetrical distribution
Impaired erythropoiesis Adults, those with haematological disease, the immunosuppressed	Can cause a mild anaemia, but in an individual with underlying haematological abnormality can precipitate an aplastic crisis
Hydrops fetalis Transplacental fetal infection	Asymptomatic or symptomatic maternal infection can cause fetal anaemia with aplastic crisis leading to nonimmune hydrops fetalis and spontaneous abortion

is spread by aerosol and direct contact and is highly infectious. Disease in children is usually better tolerated than in adults, pregnant women and the immunocompromised.

The incubation period is 11 to 20 days, after which a vesicular eruption begins (Fig. 5.4), often on mucosal surfaces first, followed by rapid dissemination in a centripetal fashion. New lesions occur in crops every 2 to 4 days, accompanied by fever. The rash progresses within 24 hours from small pink macules to vesicles and pustules, which then crust. Infectivity lasts from 2 to 4 days before the rash appears until the last crusts separate. Diagnosis is clinical but may be confirmed by PCR of vesicular fluid.

Complications include:
• Secondary bacterial infection of rash (caused by scratching). • Self-limiting cerebellar ataxia. • Congenital abnormalities if maternal disease is contracted in the first trimester. • Pneumonitis, which may be fatal.

Antiviral agents such as aciclovir and famciclovir are not required for uncomplicated childhood chickenpox. They are used in adults when patients present within 24 to 48 hours of vesicle onset, and in all patients with complications, pregnant women and the immunosuppressed. More severe cases require prolonged treatment, initially parenteral. Human VZV immunoglobulin may attenuate infection in highly susceptible contacts of chickenpox sufferers such as the immunosuppressed and pregnant women. VZV vaccine, now in use in the United States, offers effective protection.

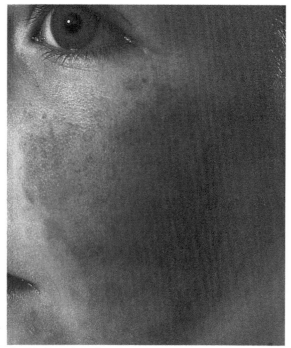

Fig. 5.3 Slapped cheek syndrome. The typical facial rash of human parvovirus B19 infection.

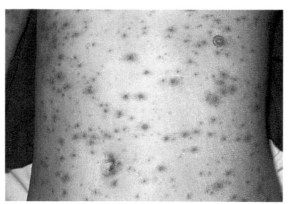

Fig. 5.4 Chickenpox.

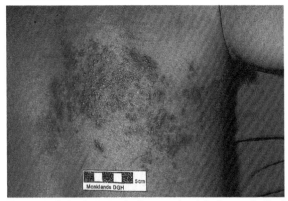

Fig. 5.5 Typical 'shingles' varicella zoster virus infection reactivating in a thoracic dermatome: 'a band of roses from Hell'.

Shingles (herpes zoster)

This is produced by reactivation of latent VZV from the dorsal root ganglion of sensory nerves, and most commonly involves the thoracic dermatomes (Fig. 5.5) and the ophthalmic division of the trigeminal nerve.

Burning discomfort develops in the affected dermatome, followed 3 to 4 days later by a vesicular rash. There may be viraemia and distant 'satellite' lesions. Severe, extensive or prolonged disease suggests underlying immunosuppression, for example, HIV. Chickenpox may be caught from shingles, but not vice versa.

Complications

• Ophthalmic trigeminal involvement: may lead to corneal ulceration, and requires ophthalmology review. • Ramsay Hunt syndrome: facial palsy, ipsilateral loss of taste and buccal ulceration and a rash in the external auditory canal. • Postherpetic neuralgia: can be difficult to treat, but may respond to amitriptyline or gabapentin. • Myelitis/encephalitis: rare.

Early therapy with aciclovir helps to limit early- and late-onset pain and to prevent the development of postherpetic neuralgia. VZV vaccination is now offered to patients aged 70 and 78 years in the UK to prevent shingles.

Systemic viral infections without exanthem

Mumps

Mumps is a systemic viral infection causing swelling of the parotid glands. It is endemic worldwide and peaks at 5 to 9 years of age. Vaccination has reduced childhood incidence but, if incomplete, leads to outbreaks in young adults. Infection is by respiratory droplets. Incubation lasts 15 to 24 days, and tender parotid swelling (bilateral in 75%) develops after a prodrome of pyrexia and headache. Diagnosis is clinical.

Complications

• Epididymo-orchitis: occurs in 25% of postpubertal males, with testicular atrophy, although sterility is unlikely. Oophoritis is less common. • Mumps meningitis: complicates 10% of cases, with lymphocytes in the CSF. • Encephalitis. • Transient hearing loss and labyrinthitis: uncommon. • Spontaneous abortion.

Management and prevention

Analgesia for symptoms is sufficient. There is no evidence that glucocorticoids are of value in orchitis. Mumps vaccine is one of the components of the combined MMR vaccine.

Influenza

This is an acute systemic viral illness predominantly affecting the respiratory system, caused by influenza A or B viruses. Seasonal changes in haemagglutinin (H) and neuraminidase (N) glycoproteins allow the organism to evade natural immunity and cause outbreaks or epidemics of varying severity.

Clinical features

Influenza is highly infectious by respiratory droplet spray from the earliest stages of infection. Incubation is 1 to 3 days, and onset is with fever, malaise, myalgia and cough. Viral or superadded bacterial pneumonia is an important complication. Myositis, myocarditis, pericarditis and encephalitis are rare complications.

Acute infection is diagnosed by viral antigen or RNA detection in a nasopharyngeal sample.

Management involves early diagnosis, scrupulous hand hygiene and infection control to limit spread by coughing and sneezing. Neuraminidase inhibitors such as oseltamivir (75 mg twice daily for 5 days) can reduce the severity of symptoms if started within 48 hours of symptom onset.

Prevention involves seasonal vaccination of vulnerable groups, for example, people over 65 years, children aged 2 to 7 years, the immunosuppressed and those with chronic illnesses.

Avian influenza is the transmission of avian influenza A from sick poultry to humans, causing severe disease. Human–human spread is rare. Swine influenza, caused by a H1N1 strain infecting humans, spread around the world from Mexico in 2009.

Infectious mononucleosis and Epstein-Barr virus

Infectious mononucleosis is a syndrome of pharyngitis, cervical lymphadenopathy, fever and lymphocytosis (also known as glandular fever), most often caused by EBV, a gamma herpesvirus. In developing countries, subclinical infection in childhood is virtually universal. In developed countries, primary infection may be delayed until adolescence or later. Saliva from asymptomatic excreters is the main means of spread, either by droplet infection or environmental contamination in childhood, or by kissing among adolescents and young adults. Infectious mononucleosis is not highly contagious, so case isolation is unnecessary.

In addition to EBV, an infectious mononucleosis syndrome may result from infection with CMV, herpesvirus 6 or 7, HIV-1 or toxoplasmosis.

Clinical features

• Prolonged prodrome of fever, malaise and headache. • Lymphade-nopathy, especially posterior cervical. • Pharyngeal inflammation or exudates. • Persisting fever and fatigue. • Splenomegaly. • Palatal petechiae. • Periorbital oedema. • Clinical or biochemical hepatitis. • A nonspecific rash.

Complications

Common: Include an antibiotic-induced rash (classically amoxicillin), severe laryngeal oedema and postviral fatigue.

Less common: Cranial nerve palsies, meningoencephalitis, haemolytic anaemia, splenic rupture, glomerulonephritis, pericarditis, pneumonitis and thrombocytopenia.

Long-term: Some forms of Hodgkin's lymphoma, Burkitt's lymphoma, lymphoproliferative disease in the immunosuppressed and nasopharyngeal carcinoma (in China and Alaska).

Investigations

• Atypical lymphocytes on blood film. • Monospot test (heterophile anti-body absorption test): may initially be negative, so should be repeated if clinical suspicion is high. • EBV IgM antibodies.

Management

Treatment is symptomatic, for example, aspirin gargles to relieve a sore throat. Oral glucocorticoids may be required to relieve laryngeal oedema. Chronic fatigue may respond to graded exercise programmes. Contact sports should be avoided until splenomegaly has resolved, to avoid splenic rupture.

Cytomegalovirus

CMV circulates readily among children. There is a second period of virus acquisition in teenagers and adults up to 35 years of age, with significant sexual and oral spread. The infection is transferred by contact with an excreter, who sheds virus in saliva, urine and genital secretions.

Most postchildhood CMV infections are asymptomatic, but some adults develop an illness resembling infectious mononucleosis. Lymphadenopa-thy, pharyngitis and tonsillitis are found less often than in infectious mono-nucleosis, whereas hepatomegaly is more common. Complications include meningo-encephalitis, Guillain–Barré syndrome, autoimmune haemolytic anaemia, myocarditis and rashes. Immunocompromised patients can develop hepatitis, oesophagitis, colitis, pneumonitis, retinitis, encephalitis and polyradiculitis. CMV infection during pregnancy carries a 40% risk of fetal infection, causing rashes, hepatosplenomegaly and a 10% risk of neu-rological damage to the fetus.

Atypical lymphocytes are seen less commonly than in infectious mono-nucleosis, and the monospot test is negative. Detection of CMV-specific IgM antibodies confirms the diagnosis, and treatment is symptomatic in the immunocompetent. In immunosuppressed patients, diagnosis is by PCR virus detection and treatment is with IV ganciclovir or oral valganciclovir.

Dengue

The dengue flavivirus is spread by the vector mosquito *Aedes aegypti* and is endemic in South-East Asia, the Pacific, Africa and the Americas.

The incubation period following a mosquito bite is 2 to 7 days, with a prodrome of malaise and headache, followed by a morbilliform rash, arthralgia, pain on eye movement, headache, nausea, vomiting, lymphadenopathy and fever. The rash spreads centrifugally, spares the palms and the soles, and may desquamate on resolution. The disease is self-limiting, but convalescence is slow.

Dengue haemorrhagic fever and dengue shock syndrome: These more severe manifestations occasionally complicate infection: circulatory failure, features of a capillary leak syndrome and DIC with haemorrhagic complications such as petechiae, ecchymoses, epistaxis, GI bleeding and multiorgan failure. Other complications include encephalitis, hepatitis and myocarditis. Case fatality with this aggressive disease may approach 10%.

Investigations

• Detection of a fourfold rise in antidengue IgG antibody titres. • Amplification of dengue RNA by PCR.

Management and prevention

Management is supportive, including fluid replacement and management of shock and organ dysfunction. Insecticides that control mosquito levels help to limit transmission. Aspirin should be avoided, and steroids are ineffective. A recently licensed vaccine is available.

Yellow fever

Yellow fever is a flavivirus infection that is a zoonosis of monkeys in the tropical rainforests of West and Central Africa and South and Central America. It is transferred to humans by infected *Aedes* or *Haemagogus* mosquitoes, and is a major public health problem, causing 200 000 infections per year, mainly in sub-Saharan Africa, with a mortality of around 15%.

The incubation period is 3 to 6 days, and the acute phase is usually characterised by a mild febrile illness lasting less than a week. Fever remits, then recurs in some cases after a few hours to days. In severe cases, the disease returns with rigors and high fever, severe backache, abdominal pain, nausea, vomiting, bradycardia and jaundice. This may progress to shock, DIC, hepatic and renal failure with jaundice, petechiae, mucosal haemorrhages, GI bleeding, seizures and coma.

Diagnosis in blood is by detecting virus (RT-PCR) or IgM or rising IgG antibodies.

Management

Treatment is supportive, with careful fluid and electrolyte balance, urine output and BP measurement. Blood transfusions, plasma expanders and peritoneal dialysis may be necessary. Isolation is needed to prevent cross-infection. Vaccination prevents disease for at least 10 years.

Viral haemorrhagic fevers

The viral haemorrhagic fevers are zoonoses caused by several different viruses, and occur in rural and health-care settings in defined regions, as summarised in Box 5.14. Management is supportive; ribavirin is effective in

i 5.14 Common viral haemorrhagic fevers			
Disease (geography)	**Reservoir**	**Transmission**	**Clinical features if severe (% mortality)**
Lassa fever (West Africa)	Multimammate rats	Rat urine Body fluids	Haemorrhage, encephalopathy, ARDS (responds to ribavirin) (15%)
Ebola fever (West and Central Africa)	Fruit bats and bush meat	Body fluids Handling primates	Haemorrhage, diarrhoea hepatic failure and AKI (25%–90%)
Marburg fever (Central Africa)	Undefined	Body fluids Handling primates	Haemorrhage, diarrhoea, encephalopathy, orchitis (25%–90%)
Yellow fever (Central Africa, South and Central America)	Monkeys	Mosquitoes	Hepatic failure, AKI, haemorrhage (~15%)
Dengue (Africa, India, South Asia, South and Central America)	Humans	*Aedes aegypti*	Haemorrhage, shock (<10%)
Crimean-Congo (Africa, Asia, E Europe)	Small vertebrates	*Ixodes* tick Body fluids	Encephalopathy, haemorrhage, hepatic failure, AKI, ARDS (30%)
Bolivian and Argentinean (South America)	Rodents (*Calomys* spp.)	Urine	Haemorrhage, shock, cerebellar signs (15%–30%)
Haemorrhagic fever with renal syndrome (Hantaan fever) (North Asia, North Europe, Balkans)	Rodents	Aerosols from faeces	Acute kidney injury, stroke, pulmonary oedema, shock (5%)

some viral haemorrhagic fevers. Transmission by infected secretions can cause major outbreaks, for example, Ebola in West Africa in 2014. Case isolation and scrupulous infection control are essential.

Zika virus

Zika is a flavivirus spread from primates by *Aedes* mosquitoes, which is epidemic in the Caribbean and Central and South America. Infection is asymptomatic or mild, with fever, arthralgia, conjunctivitis and rash, but is associated with a marked increase in microcephaly in babies of infected pregnant women. Prevention involves avoiding mosquito bites and practicing safe sex, as the virus is found in semen.

Viral infections of the skin

Herpes Simplex Virus 1 and 2

Type 1 HSV typically produces mucocutaneous lesions of the head and neck, whereas type 2 predominantly affects the genital tract. Seroprevalence is 30% to 100% for HSV-1 and 20% to 60% for HSV-2.

Virus shed by an infected individual infects via a mucosal surface of a susceptible person. HSV infects sensory and autonomic nerve ganglia, and episodes of reactivation occur throughout life, precipitated by stress, trauma, illness or immunosuppression. Primary infection normally occurs as a vesiculating gingivostomatitis. It may also present as a keratitis (dendritic ulcer), viral paronychia, genital ulceration or, rarely, as encephalitis. HSV reactivation in the oral mucosa produces the classical 'cold sore' (herpes labialis). Diagnosis is by PCR, electron microscopy or culture of vesicular fluid.

Complications

• Corneal dendritic ulcers: may produce scarring. • Encephalitis: preferentially affects the temporal lobe. • HSV infection in patients with eczema: can result in disseminated skin lesions (eczema herpeticum; Fig. 5.6). • Neonatal HSV infection: may be disseminated and potentially fatal.

Management

Treatment is with antiviral agents such as acyclovir, started within 48 hours of onset.

Human herpesvirus 8

This virus, which spreads via saliva, causes Kaposi's sarcoma in both AIDS-related and endemic, non-AIDS-related forms.

Enterovirus infections

Hand, foot and mouth disease: A mild febrile illness affecting children, mainly in the summer months, and caused by coxsackieviruses or echoviruses. There is fever, lymphadenopathy, mouth ulceration and a vesicular eruption on the hands and feet.

Herpangina: Causes discrete vesicles on the palate associated with high fever, sore throat and headache.

Both of these conditions are self-limiting without treatment.

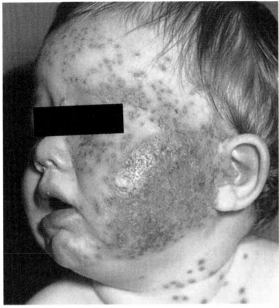

Fig. 5.6 Eczema herpeticum. Herpes simplex virus-1 infection spreads rapidly in eczematous skin.

Poxvirus infections

These DNA viruses are rare but potentially important pathogens.

Smallpox (variola): This severe disease, with high mortality, was eradicated worldwide by vaccination. The classical form comprised a centrifugal vesicular/pustular rash, worst on the face and extremities, without cropping (unlike chickenpox), and accompanied by fever, myalgia and odynophagia.

Monkeypox and cowpox: Cause vesicular rashes and are spread by contact with infected animals.

Molluscum contagiosum: Covered on p. 751.

Gastrointestinal viral infections

Norovirus (Norwalk agent)

Norovirus is the most common cause of infectious gastroenteritis in the UK, causing outbreaks in hospital wards, on cruise ships and in military camps. Food handlers also transmit norovirus. It is highly infectious by the faecal–oral route and causes prominent vomiting with diarrhoea after an incubation period of 24 to 48 hours. Diagnosis is by electron microscopy or PCR of stool samples. Case isolation and scrupulous cleaning are required to control outbreaks.

Rotavirus

Rotaviruses infect enterocytes and are a major cause of diarrhoeal illness in young children worldwide. There are winter epidemics in developed countries, particularly in nurseries. Adults in close contact with cases may develop disease. The incubation period is 48 hours, and patients present with watery diarrhoea, vomiting, fever and abdominal pain. Diagnosis is aided by commercially available enzyme immunoassay kits, which simply require fresh or refrigerated stool for effective demonstration of the pathogens. The disease is self-limiting, but dehydration needs appropriate management. Effective vaccines have been developed.

Other viruses

Adenoviruses are frequently identified from stool culture and implicated as a cause of diarrhoea.

MERS-CoV

In 2012, this novel coronavirus, related to the severe acute respiratory syndrome (SARS) coronavirus, caused several deaths with pneumonia in patients from the Middle East.

Covid-19

In late 2019, a novel strain of coronavirus emerged in Wuhan, China leading to a global pandemic with numerous fatalities from pneumonia.

Prion diseases

These primarily affect the nervous system, and are covered on p. 694.

Bacterial infections

Bacterial infections of the skin, soft tissues and bones

Staphylococcal infections

Staphylococci are normal commensals of human skin and anterior nares, but they can disseminate widely if they gain access to the blood through a cannula, a surgical incision or a primary skin condition such as eczema. Ecthyma, folliculitis, furuncles and carbuncles represent superficial skin infections with this ubiquitous organism (p. 749).

Wound- and cannula-related infections caused by *S. aureus* are important causes of inpatient morbidity. Their incidence may be lessened by good infection control techniques. If there is evidence of spreading infection such as a surrounding cellulitis, antistaphylococcal antimicrobial therapy, for example, flucloxacillin, should be instituted. IV drug users who are susceptible to skin and subcutaneous tissue infections may also develop thrombosis in the affected limb. If staphylococcal infection reaches the blood stream (staphylococcal bacteraemia), this may cause severe sepsis and complications (e.g. endocarditis or cavernous sinus thrombosis), and must be treated aggressively. Growth of *S. aureus* in blood cultures should never be dismissed as a 'contaminant' unless all possible underlying causes have been excluded and repeat cultures are negative.

S. aureus can also cause severe systemic disease by production of toxins at superficial sites, in the absence of tissue invasion by bacteria.

MRSA

Resistance to meticillin is attributed to a penicillin-binding protein mutation in *S. aureus*. Resistance to vancomycin/teicoplanin (glycopeptides) in either glycopeptide-intermediate *S. aureus* or, rarely, vancomycin-resistant strains threatens the ability to manage serious infections with such organisms. MRSA now accounts for up to 40% of staphylococcal bacteraemias in developed countries, requiring care in both control and specific therapy of these infections. Clinicians must prescribe according to sensitivity testing and take whatever infection control measures are advised locally.

Staphylococcal TSS

This serious and life-threatening disease is associated with infection by *S. aureus* that produces toxic shock syndrome toxin 1. Staphylococcal TSS is seen in women using tampons, but can also complicate any staphylococcal infection with a relevant toxin-producing strain. The toxin acts as a 'super-antigen', triggering significant T cell activation and massive cytokine release.

TSS has an abrupt onset with high fever, generalised systemic upset (myalgia, headache, sore throat and vomiting), a widespread erythematous blanching rash resembling scarlet fever and hypotension. It rapidly progresses over a few hours to multiorgan failure, leading to death in 10% to 20% of patients. The diagnosis is clinical, supported by Gram stain of menstrual fluid demonstrating typical staphylococci. Treatment is with IV fluid resuscitation and antistaphylococcal antibiotics such as flucloxacillin or vancomycin. Recovery is accompanied at 7 to 10 days by desquamation (Fig. 5.7).

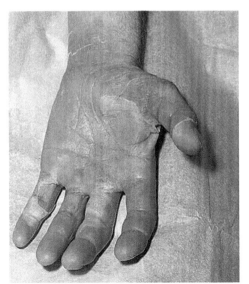

Fig. 5.7 Full-thickness desquamation after toxic shock syndrome.

Streptococcal infections

Streptococci are Gram-positive oropharyngeal and gut commensals that cause a range of human infections (Box 5.15).

Streptococcal scarlet fever

Group A (or occasionally group C and G) streptococci causing pharyngitis or tonsillitis may lead to scarlet fever if the organism produces pyogenic

---

 5.15 Streptococcal and related infections

Group A (Streptococcus pyogenes)

- Skin/tissue infection (erysipelas, impetigo, necrotising fasciitis)
- Puerperal sepsis
- Glomerulonephritis
- Bone and joint infection
- Streptococcal toxic shock syndrome
- Scarlet fever
- Rheumatic fever
- Tonsillitis

Group B streptococci (S. agalactiae)

- Neonatal infections, including meningitis
- Septicaemia
- Female pelvic infections
- Cellulitis

Group D enterococci (Enterococcus faecalis)

- Endocarditis
- Urinary tract infection

α-Haemolytic viridans streptococci (S. mitis, sanguinis, mutans, salivarius)

- Endocarditis
- Septicaemia in immunosuppressed

α-Haemolytic optochin-sensitive (S. pneumoniae)

- Pneumonia
- Meningitis
- Endocarditis
- Septicaemia
- Bacterial peritonitis
- Otitis media

Anaerobic streptococci (Peptostreptococcus spp.)

- Peritonitis
- Liver abscess
- Dental infections
- Pelvic inflammatory disease

Note: All streptococci can cause septicaemia.

exotoxin. Common in school-age children, scarlet fever can occur in young adults in contact with young children.

A diffuse erythematous rash occurs, which blanches on pressure (Fig. 5.8), classically with circumoral pallor. The tongue, initially coated, becomes red and swollen ('strawberry tongue'). The disease lasts around 7 days; the rash disappears in 7 to 10 days, followed by a fine desquamation. Residual petechial lesions in the antecubital fossa may be seen. Treatment involves IV benzylpenicillin or oral penicillin, plus symptomatic measures.

Streptococcal TSS

Group A (or occasionally C or G) streptococci can produce toxins such as pyogenic exotoxin A. Initially, an influenza-like illness occurs with signs of localised skin or soft tissue infection in 50% of cases. A faint erythematous rash, mainly on the chest, progresses rapidly to circulatory shock, then multi-organ failure.

Fluid resuscitation is essential, along with parenteral antistreptococcal antibiotics, usually benzylpenicillin with clindamycin. If necrotising fasciitis is present (p. 105), urgent debridement is required.

Cellulitis, erysipelas and impetigo

See p. 749 and 747.

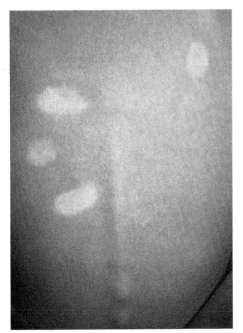

Fig. 5.8 Scarlet fever. Note blanching on pressure.

Treponematoses

Syphilis

This disease is described on p. 173.

Endemic treponematoses

Yaws: This granulomatous disease is caused by *Treponema pertenue*, which is morphologically and serologically indistinguishable from the causative organisms of syphilis and pinta. Organisms are transmitted through minor skin abrasions by bodily contact with a patient with infectious yaws. After 3 to 4 weeks, a granulomatous primary lesion develops at the site of infection. This is followed by secondary eruptions and hypertrophic periosteal bone lesions and, in late yaws, osteitis and gummas resembling tertiary syphilis.

Pinta and bejel: These two treponemal infections occur in poor rural populations with low standards of domestic hygiene but are found in separate parts of the world (pinta: South and Central America; bejel: Middle East, Central Asia). Pinta is a skin disease transmitted by contact, and bejel is a nonvenereal form of syphilis transmitted by contact and through common eating and drinking utensils.

For yaws, pinta and bejel, diagnosis is by microscopic detection of spirochaetes and serology; treatment involves a single IM dose of long-acting (e.g. benzathine) benzylpenicillin. Improvements in domestic hygiene greatly reduce these diseases.

Systemic bacterial infections

Brucellosis

Brucellosis is caused by a Gram-negative intracellular bacillus endemic in animals. The four species causing human disease are:
- *B. melitensis* (goats, sheep and camels). • *B. abortus* (cattle). • *B. suis* (pigs). • *B. canis* (dogs). *B. melitensis* causes the most severe disease.

Infected animals may excrete brucellae in their milk for long periods, and human infection is acquired by ingesting contaminated dairy products and uncooked meat or offal, or via the respiratory tract or abraded skin through splashes of infected animal secretions or excreta.

Clinical features

Acute illness is characterised by a high swinging temperature, rigors, sweating, lethargy, headache and joint and muscle pains. Occasionally, there is delirium, abdominal pain and constipation. Physical signs are nonspecific, for example, enlarged lymph nodes. Splenomegaly may cause thrombocytopenia.

Investigations

- Blood cultures are positive in up to 80% of cases; *B. melitensis* is the most readily cultured species. • CSF culture in neurobrucellosis: positive in around 30% of cases. • Serology: a single titre of more than 1/320 or a four-fold rise in antibody supports the diagnosis, but can take several weeks.

Management

Aminoglycosides show synergistic activity with tetracyclines when used against brucellae. Standard therapy therefore consists of 6 weeks of doxycycline with IV gentamicin for the first 7 days. Rifampicin is added if there is bone involvement, and ceftriaxone if there is neurobrucellosis.

Borrelia infections

Lyme disease

Lyme disease (named after the town of Old Lyme in Connecticut, USA) is caused by *Borrelia burgdorferi,* which occurs in the United States, Europe, Russia, China, Japan and Australia. In Europe, *B. afzelii* and *B. garinii* are also found. The reservoir of infection is ixodid (hard) ticks that feed on a variety of large mammals, particularly deer. The organism is transmitted to humans via infected tick bites.

Clinical features

There are three stages. Progression may be arrested at any stage.

Early localised disease: The characteristic feature is a skin reaction around the site of the tick bite, known as erythema migrans. Initially, a red 'bull's eye' macule or papule appears 2 to 30 days after the bite. It then enlarges peripherally with central clearing, and may persist for months. The rash may be accompanied by fever, headache and regional lymphadenopathy.

Early disseminated disease: Dissemination occurs via the blood stream and lymphatics. There may be a systemic reaction with malaise, arthralgia and occasionally metastatic areas of erythema migrans. Neurological involvement may follow weeks or months after infection, with lymphocytic meningitis, cranial nerve palsies (especially unilateral or bilateral facial palsy) and peripheral neuropathy. Radiculopathy, often painful, may present a year or more after initial infection. Carditis, sometimes accompanied by atrioventricular conduction defects, occurs in the United States, but is rare in Europe.

Late disease: Late manifestations include arthritis, polyneuritis and encephalopathy. Prolonged arthritis, particularly affecting large joints, and cerebral involvement may occur, but are rare in the UK. Acrodermatitis chronica atrophicans is an uncommon late complication seen more frequently in Europe than in North America. Doughy, patchy discoloration occurs on the peripheries, eventually leading to shiny, atrophic skin. The lesions are easily mistaken for those of peripheral vascular disease.

Investigations

The diagnosis of Lyme borreliosis is often clinical. Anti-*Borrelia* antibody detection is frequently negative in the early stages, but 90–100% sensitive in late disease. Culture from biopsies is slow and not generally available; it has a low yield. PCR has been used to detect DNA in blood, urine and CSF.

Management

Asymptomatic patients with positive antibody tests should not be treated. Standard therapy for erythema migrans consists of 14 days of doxycycline or amoxicillin; disseminated disease requires at least 28 days of treatment. Some 15% of patients with early disease will develop a mild Jarisch–Herxheimer reaction during the first 24 hours of therapy. Neuroborreliosis is treated with parenteral β-lactams or 3rd generation cephalosporins for

3 to 4 weeks. Protective clothing and insect repellents should be used for prevention in tick-infested areas.

Louse-borne relapsing fever

The human body louse, *Pediculus humanus*, causes itching. Borreliae (*B. recurrentis*) are liberated from the infected lice when they are crushed during scratching, which also inoculates the borreliae into the skin.

The borreliae invade most tissues of the body, including liver, spleen and meninges, causing hepatosplenomegaly, jaundice and meningism, accompanied by high fever, tachycardia and headache. Thrombocytopenia results in petechial rash, serosal haemorrhage and epistaxis. The acute illness lasts between 4 and 10 days. A proportion of patients may relapse.

Examination of thick and thin blood films or dark-ground microscopy demonstrate the organism. Treatment is with procaine penicillin followed by tetracycline. A severe Jarisch–Herxheimer reaction is seen with successful chemotherapy.

Tick-borne relapsing fever

Soft ticks (*Ornithodoros* spp.) transmit *B. duttonii* (and other *Borrelia* species) through saliva while feeding on their host. Rodents are the reservoir in all parts of the world, except in East Africa where humans are the reservoir.

Clinical manifestations are similar to the louse-borne disease, but microorganisms are detected in fewer patients on dark-field microscopy. A 7-day course of treatment with either tetracycline or erythromycin is needed.

Leptospirosis

Leptospires are tightly coiled, thread-like organisms, around 5 to 7 μm in length, which are actively motile by rotating and bending. In reservoir species they persist in the convoluted tubules of the kidney in asymptomatic animals and are shed in the urine in massive numbers. Particular leptospiral serogroups are associated with characteristic animal hosts; for example, *Leptospira icterohaemorrhagica* is a parasite of rats, and *L. canicola* of dogs.

Leptospires can enter their human hosts through intact or injured skin or mucous membranes, for example, following immersion in contaminated water.

Clinical features

The incubation period averages 1 to 2 weeks. Four main clinical syndromes can be discerned:

Bacteraemic leptospirosis: A nonspecific illness with high fever, weakness, muscle pain and tenderness (especially of the calf and back), intense headache and photophobia and sometimes diarrhoea and vomiting. Conjunctival congestion is the only notable physical sign. The illness comes to an end after around 1 week, or else merges into one of the other forms of infection.

Aseptic meningitis: Classically associated with *L. canicola*, this is very difficult to distinguish from viral meningitis. The conjunctivae may be congested, but there are no other differentiating signs.

Icteric leptospirosis (Weil's disease): A dramatic, life-threatening event, accounting for less than 10% of symptomatic infections. It is characterised by fever, haemorrhages, jaundice and acute kidney injury.

Conjunctival hyperaemia is a frequent feature. The patient may have a transient macular erythematous rash, but the characteristic skin changes are purpura and large areas of bruising. In severe cases there may be epistaxis, haematemesis and melaena, or bleeding into the pleural, pericardial or subarachnoid spaces. Thrombocytopenia is present in 50% of cases. Jaundice is deep, and the liver is enlarged, but there is usually little evidence of hepatic failure or encephalopathy. Acute kidney injury, primarily caused by impaired renal perfusion and acute tubular necrosis, results in oliguria or anuria, with albumin, blood and casts in the urine. Myocarditis, encephalitis and aseptic meningitis are other associated features. Uveitis and iritis may appear months after apparent clinical recovery.

Pulmonary syndrome: This is particularly recognised in the Far East. It is characterised by haemoptysis, patchy lung infiltrates on CXR and respiratory failure. Total bilateral lung consolidation and ARDS develop in severe cases.

Investigations

Laboratory tests show polymorphonuclear leucocytosis, thrombocytopenia and elevated creatine phosphokinase. In jaundiced patients, LFTs are mildly hepatitic in pattern, with moderately raised transaminases; the prothrombin time may be prolonged. A lumbar puncture may show a moderately elevated protein level and a normal glucose content in the CSF. Definitive diagnosis requires detection of the organism, its DNA or a rising antibody titre:
• Blood culture: most likely to be positive if taken before the 10th day of illness. • Urine culture: leptospires appear in the urine during the second week of illness. • Microscopic agglutination test: seroconversion or a fourfold rise in titre between acute and convalescent sera is confirmatory. • PCR: can detect leptospiral DNA in blood in early symptomatic disease, and is positive in urine from the 8th day and for many months afterwards.

Management and prevention

Supportive management, including the transfusion of blood and platelets, along with dialysis, is critical. Oral doxycycline or IV penicillin is effective, but may not prevent acute kidney injury. IV ceftriaxone is an effective alternative. A Jarisch–Herxheimer reaction may occur during treatment, but is usually mild. Prophylactic doxycycline 200 mg weekly can prevent infection.

Plague

Plague is caused by *Yersinia pestis*, a small Gram-negative bacillus that is spread between rodents by their fleas, which may also bite humans. In the late stages of human plague, *Y. pestis* may be expectorated and spread between humans by droplets. Epidemics of plague, such as the 'Black Death', have afflicted humans since ancient times, with a high fatality rate. Because of the possibility of person-to-person spread and the high fatality rate, it is also a potential bioweapon.

The incubation period is 3 to 6 days following access via the skin but is shorter after inhalation.

Three distinct forms are recognised.

Bubonic plague: In this, the most common form of the disease, the onset is usually sudden with a rigor, high fever, dry skin and severe headache. Soon, aching and swelling at the site of the affected lymph nodes begin. The groin is the most common site of the 'bubo' (the swollen lymph node and surrounding tissue). A rapid pulse, hypotension, and delirium develop rapidly. The spleen is usually palpable.

Septicaemic plague: In this form, common in the elderly, the patient is toxic and may have GI symptoms such as nausea, vomiting, abdominal pain and diarrhoea. DIC may occur, manifested by bleeding from various orifices or puncture sites, along with ecchymoses. Hypotension, shock, acute kidney injury and ARDS may lead to further deterioration. Meningitis, pneumonia and expectoration of blood-stained sputum may complicate the picture. There is a high mortality.

Pneumonic plague: The onset is very sudden, with cough and dyspnoea. The patient soon expectorates copious blood-stained, frothy, highly infective sputum, becomes cyanosed and dies. X-rays of the lung show bilateral nodular infiltrates progressing to ARDS.

Investigations

The organism may be cultured from blood, sputum or bubo aspirates. Characteristic bipolar coccobacilli are seen in smears of these fluids after staining with Wayson's stain or by immunofluorescence. Seroconversion or a single anti-F1 antibody titre greater than 128 confirms the diagnosis. DNA diagnosis through PCR is under evaluation. Plague is a notifiable disease.

Management

Immediate treatment is vital. Streptomycin (1 g twice daily) or gentamicin (1 mg/kg three times daily) are the drugs of choice. Tetracycline and chloramphenicol are alternatives. Treatment may also be needed for acute circulatory failure, DIC and hypoxia. The patient should be isolated for 48 hours, carers should wear protective clothing, and inadvertent exposure should prompt prophylactic treatment with doxycycline.

Listeriosis

Listeria monocytogenes is an environmental Gram-positive bacterium that can contaminate food, including cheese and undercooked meats. It outgrows other pathogens during refrigeration. It causes gastroenteritis in immunocompetent patients, but more serious invasive illness in pregnant women, adults over 55 years of age and the immunocompromised. In pregnancy, in addition to systemic symptoms like fever and myalgia, listeriosis causes chorioamnionitis, fetal deaths, abortions and neonatal infection. Meningitis is another common manifestation. Diagnosis is made by blood and CSF culture. The most effective treatment is a combination of IV ampicillin with an aminoglycoside. A sulfamethoxazole/trimethoprim combination can be used in those with penicillin sensitivity. Good food hygiene helps to prevent infection. Pregnant women should avoid high-risk foods (see Box 5.5).

Typhoid and paratyphoid (enteric) fevers

These diseases, which are transmitted by the faecal–oral route, are important causes of fever in the Indian sub-continent, sub-Saharan Africa and Latin America. Elsewhere they are relatively rare. The causative organisms are *S. typhi* and *S. paratyphi* A and B.

Clinical features

Typhoid fever: The incubation period of typhoid fever is around 10 to 14 days, and the onset may be insidious. The temperature rises in a stepladder fashion for 4 or 5 days with malaise, increasing headache, drowsiness and aching in the limbs. Constipation may be present, although in children diarrhoea and vomiting may be prominent early in the illness. There is a relative bradycardia. At the end of the first week, a rash may appear on the upper abdomen and on the back as sparse, slightly raised, rose-red spots, which fade on pressure. Cough and epistaxis occur. Around the seventh to tenth day, the spleen becomes palpable. Constipation is followed by diarrhoea and abdominal distension with tenderness. Bronchitis and delirium may develop. If untreated, by the end of the second week the patient may be profoundly ill. Following recovery, up to 5% of patients become chronic carriers of *S. typhi*.

Paratyphoid fever: The course tends to be shorter and milder than that of typhoid fever, and the onset is often more abrupt, with acute enteritis. The rash may be more abundant and the intestinal complications less frequent.

Complications

Haemorrhage from, or a perforation of, the ulcerated Peyer's patches (follicles in the small intestine where bacilli localise) may occur at 2 to 3 weeks into the illness. Additional complications include cholecystitis, myocarditis, nephritis, arthritis and meningitis. Bone and joint infection are common in children with sickle-cell disease.

Investigations

Multiple blood cultures are the most important investigations in a suspected case. Blood count typically shows leucopenia. Stool cultures are often positive during the second and third weeks.

Management

Ciprofloxacin (500 mg twice daily) is the drug of choice, although resistance is rising in the Indian subcontinent and the UK. Ceftriaxone or azithromycin are alternatives. Treatment should be continued for 14 days. Pyrexia may persist for up to 5 days into treatment. Improved sanitation and living conditions, as well as vaccination of travellers, reduce the incidence of typhoid.

Tularaemia

Tularaemia is a zoonotic disease of the northern hemisphere caused by a highly infectious Gram-negative bacillus, *Francisella tularensis*. Wild rabbits and domestic dogs or cats are the reservoirs; ticks and mosquitoes are the vectors.

Infection is introduced through insect bites or by contact with infected animals. The most common 'ulceroglandular' variety of the disease (70%–80%) is characterised by skin ulceration with regional lymphadenopathy. Inhalation of the infected aerosols may result in pulmonary tularaemia, presenting as pneumonia. Rarely, the portal of entry of infection may be the conjunctiva, leading to a nodular, ulcerated conjunctivitis with regional lymphadenopathy (an 'oculoglandular' form). Demonstration of a single high titre (≥1:160) or a fourfold rise in 2 to 3 weeks in the tularaemia tube agglutination test confirms the diagnosis. DNA detection methods to enable rapid diagnosis are in development. Treatment consists of 10 to 21 days of parenteral streptomycin or gentamicin, or oral doxycycline or ciprofloxacin.

Melioidosis

Melioidosis is caused by *Burkholderia pseudomallei,* and is common in South-East Asia and Australia. Inhalation or inoculation leads to bacteraemia with pneumonia and abscesses in the lungs, liver, spleen and subcutaneous tissues. The CXR may resemble cavitary TB. Culture of blood, sputum or pus may yield *B. psuedomallei.* Treatment is with IV ceftazidime or meropenem, followed by oral co-trimoxazole or doxycycline for 3 to 6 months. Abscesses should be drained.

Actinomycete infections

Nocardiosis

This uncommon infection is caused by aerobic actinomycetes (genus *Nocardia*), found in soil. Traumatic inoculation, inhalation or ingestion causes cutaneous ulcers or nodules, usually on the legs. In tropical countries, chronic infection can develop into actinomycetoma, involving soft tissues and occasionally bone (p. 171). In immunocompromised individuals, systemic *Nocardia* causes suppurative disease with lung and brain abscesses. Treatment of systemic infection requires imipenem with ceftriaxone, amikacin or co-trimoxazole, for 6 to 12 months or longer.

Actinomyces spp.

Actinomyces are anaerobic actinomycetes, oral commensals which can cause deep, suppurating infection in the head and neck, the lungs and the pelvis (associated with IUCDs). The most common species is *Actinomyces israelii*. Treatment requires prolonged penicillin or doxycycline.

Gastrointestinal bacterial infections

Food Poisoning

Infectious causes of acute gastroenteritis are listed in Box 5.4.

Staphylococcal food poisoning

S. aureus transmission occurs from the hands of food handlers to foodstuffs such as dairy products, including cheese, and cooked meats. Inappropriate storage permits growth and production of heat-stable enterotoxins.

Nausea and vomiting develop within 1 to 6 hours. Diarrhoea may not be marked. Most cases settle rapidly, but severe dehydration can occasionally be life-threatening. Antiemetics and fluid replacement are the mainstays of treatment. Public health authorities should be notified if food vending is involved.

Bacillus cereus

Ingestion of the preformed enterotoxins of *B. cereus* leads to rapid onset of vomiting and some diarrhoea within hours of food consumption, resolving within 24 hours. Fried rice and sauces are frequent sources; enterotoxin is formed during storage.

If viable organisms are ingested, the toxin is produced within the gut, leading to a longer incubation period of 12 to 24 hours and watery diarrhoea with abdominal cramps. The disease is self-limiting. Management consists of fluid replacement and public health notification.

Clostridium perfringens

Spores of *C. perfringens* are widespread in the guts of large animals and in soil. If contaminated meat products are incompletely cooked and stored in anaerobic conditions, *C. perfringens* spores germinate, and viable organisms multiply. Subsequent reheating of the food causes release of enterotoxin. Symptoms (diarrhoea and cramps) occur 6 to 12 hours following ingestion. The illness is usually self-limiting.

Clostridial enterotoxins are potent, and most people who ingest them will be symptomatic. 'Point source' outbreaks, in which a number of cases all become symptomatic following ingestion, classically occur after school or canteen lunches where meat stews are served.

Campylobacter jejuni

This infection is a zoonosis, although the organism can also survive in fresh water. It is the most common cause of bacterial gastroenteritis in the UK. The usual sources are chicken, beef or contaminated milk products, but contact with pet puppies has also caused cases.

The incubation period is 2 to 5 days. Colicky abdominal pain develops along with nausea, vomiting and significant diarrhoea, frequently containing blood. Most *Campylobacter* infections affect fit young adults and are self-limiting after 5 to 7 days. Some 10% to 20% have prolonged symptoms and merit treatment with a macrolide, usually azithromycin, as ciprofloxacin resistance is common. About 1% of cases will develop bacteraemia and possible distant foci of infection. *Campylobacter* spp. have been linked to Guillain-Barré syndrome and postinfectious reactive arthritis.

Salmonella spp.

Salmonella enterica serovars other than *Salmonella* Typhi and Paratyphi (p. 135) are widely distributed in animals and can cause gastroenteritis. Worldwide, the most important are *Salmonella* Enteritidis phage type 4 and *Salmonella* Typhimurium DT104. The latter may be resistant to ciprofloxacin. Transmission is by contaminated water or food, particularly poultry, egg products and minced meat; person-to-person spread; or from exotic pets, for example, salamanders, lizards or turtles.

The incubation period of *Salmonella* gastroenteritis is 12 to 72 hours, and the predominant feature is diarrhoea, sometimes containing blood. Vomiting may be present at the outset. About 5% of cases will be bacteraemic.

5.16 Most common causes of travellers' diarrhoea

- ETEC
- *Shigella* spp.
- *Campylobacter jejuni*
- *Salmonella* spp.
- *Plesiomonas shigelloides*
- Noncholera *Vibrio* spp.
- *Aeromonas* spp.

Reactive (postinfective) arthritis occurs in about 2% of cases. Antibiotics are not indicated unless there is bacteraemia, which is a clear indication for antibiotic therapy, as salmonellae are notorious for persistent infection and often colonise endothelial surfaces such as an atherosclerotic aorta or a major blood vessel.

Escherichia coli

Many serotypes of *E. coli* exist in the human gut microbiome. Clinical disease requires either colonisation with a new strain or acquisition by a colonising strain of a new pathogenicity factor (e.g. toxin production). There are five different clinico-pathological patterns of disease, all associated with diarrhoea.

Enterotoxigenic E. coli (ETEC): This is the most common among the many causes of travellers' diarrhoea in developing countries (Box 5.16). The organisms produce either a heat-labile or a heat-stable enterotoxin, causing marked secretory diarrhoea and vomiting after 1 to 2 days' incubation. The illness is usually mild and self-limiting after 3 to 4 days. Antibiotics are of questionable value.

Enteroinvasive E. coli (EIEC): This illness is very similar to *Shigella* dysentery and is caused by invasion and destruction of colonic mucosal cells. No enterotoxin is produced. Acute watery diarrhoea, abdominal cramps and some scanty blood-staining of the stool are common. The symptoms are rarely severe and are usually self-limiting.

Enteropathogenic E. coli (EPEC): These are very important in infant diarrhoea. Ability to attach to the gut mucosa is the basis of their pathogenicity. This causes destruction of microvilli and disruption of normal absorptive capacity. The symptoms vary from mild, nonbloody diarrhoea to quite severe illness.

Enteroaggregative E. coli (EAEC): These strains adhere to the mucosa and produce a locally active enterotoxin. A 'stacked brick' aggregation is seen in the small bowel. They have been associated with prolonged diarrhoea in children in South America, South-East Asia and India.

Enterohaemorrhagic E. coli (EHEC): A number of distinct 'O' serotypes of *E. coli* produce two distinct enterotoxins (verocytotoxin), which are identical to toxins produced by *Shigella* (shigatoxins 1 and 2). *E. coli* O157:H7 is perhaps the best known of these verocytotoxigenic *E. coli*, but others, including types O126 and O11, are also implicated. The organism has an extremely low infecting dose (10–100 organisms). The reservoir is in the gut of herbivores.

Contaminated vegetables, milk and meat products (especially under-cooked hamburgers) are all recognised sources. The incubation period is between 1 and 7 days. Initial watery diarrhoea becomes uniformly blood-stained in 70% of cases and is associated with severe abdominal pain. There is little systemic upset, vomiting or fever. Enterotoxins have both a local effect on the bowel and distant effects on the glomerular apparatus, heart and brain. The potentially life-threatening HUS occurs in 10% to 15% of cases, arising 5 to 7 days after the onset of symptoms. It is most likely at the extremes of age, is heralded by a high peripheral leucocyte count and may be induced, particularly in children, by antibiotics. HUS is treated by dialysis if necessary, and may be averted by plasma exchange.

Clostridium difficile infection

C. difficile is occasionally present in the gut microbiome and is the most commonly diagnosed cause of antibiotic-associated diarrhoea. Clinical infection usually follows up to 6 weeks after antibiotic therapy, which alters gut flora. Transmission is by spores, which are resistant to alcohol hand gels, and disease results from the production of two toxins. A number of different ribotypes of the organism exist, with the 027 ribotype producing particularly severe disease and significant mortality.

Infection causes diarrhoea, which may be bloody and may be complicated by pseudomembranous colitis. Around 80% of patients over 65 years of age, and many have multiple comorbidities.

C. difficile is found in the stool in 30% of cases of antibiotic-associated diarrhoea and 90% of those with pseudomembranous colitis, but also in 20% of healthy elderly patients in care. Diagnosis therefore depends on finding *C. difficile* toxin in the stool.

Precipitating antibiotics should be stopped. Treatment is with IV rehydration and oral metronidazole for 10 days or, in severe cases, oral vancomycin. Faecal transplantation is used increasingly as a treatment for relapses.

Yersinia enterocolitica

This organism, commonly found in pork, causes mild to moderate gastroenteritis and can produce significant mesenteric adenitis after an incubation period of 3 to 7 days. It predominantly causes disease in children, but adults may also be affected. The illness resolves slowly. Complications include reactive arthritis (10%–13% of cases) and anterior uveitis.

Cholera

Cholera, caused by *Vibrio cholerae* serotype O1, is the archetypal toxin-mediated bacterial cause of acute watery diarrhoea, and has caused numerous pandemics worldwide. Infection spreads via the stools or vomit of symptomatic patients or of the much larger number of subclinical cases. The microorganism survives for up to 2 weeks in fresh water and 8 weeks in salt water. Transmission is normally through infected drinking water, shellfish and food contaminated by flies, or on the hands of carriers.

Clinical features

Severe diarrhoea without pain or colic begins suddenly, followed by vomiting. Following the evacuation of normal gut faecal contents, typical 'rice-water' material is passed, consisting of clear fluid with flecks of mucus, resulting in enormous loss of fluid and electrolytes. Shock and oliguria ensue, necessitating fluid and electrolyte replacement.

Investigations and management

The diagnosis should be confirmed by visualisation of the organism on stool dark-field microscopy, which shows the 'shooting star' motility of *V. cholerae*. Rectal swab or stool cultures allow identification. Cholera is notifiable under international health regulations. Replacement of fluid and electrolyte losses is paramount. IV Ringer's lactate solution is used until vomiting stops; thereafter, oral rehydration solution is used. Up to 50 L may be needed in 2 to 5 days. Treatment with tetracycline, doxycycline or ciprofloxacin reduces the duration of excretion of *Vibrio*. Strict personal hygiene, a clean piped water supply and good food hygiene practices prevent the spread of disease.

Vibrio parahaemolyticus

This marine organism produces a disease similar to ETEC. It is very common where ingestion of raw seafood is widespread (e.g. Japan). After an incubation period of around 20 hours, explosive diarrhoea, abdominal cramps and vomiting occur. Systemic symptoms of headache and fever are frequent, but the illness is self-limiting, taking 4 to 7 days to resolve.

Bacillary dysentery (shigellosis)

Shigellae are Gram-negative rods, closely related to *E. coli*, that invade the colonic mucosa. They are often multi-resistant to antibiotics. The organism only infects humans, and its spread is facilitated by its low infecting dose of around 10 organisms. Transmission is most commonly by unwashed hands after defecation. Outbreaks occur in psychiatric hospitals, residential schools and other closed institutions. It is a common accompaniment of war and natural catastrophe.

Disease severity varies with serotype; cases caused by *Shigella sonnei* are mild, whereas those attributed to *S. dysenteriae* may be fulminating and cause death within 48 hours. Symptoms include diarrhoea, which may be bloody, colicky abdominal pain and tenesmus. Reactive arthritis or iritis may occasionally complicate bacillary dysentery (p. 620).

Oral rehydration therapy is necessary to replace water and electrolytes. Antibiotic therapy with ciprofloxacin (500 mg twice daily for 3 days) is effective; azithromycin and ceftriaxone are alternatives. Resistance to all three occurs. Hand-washing is very important.

Respiratory bacterial infections

Most of these are described in Chapter 9.

Diphtheria

Corynebacterium diphtheriae, the causative organism, is highly contagious, and spreads by droplet infection. The average incubation period is 2 to 4 days. Diphtheria was eradicated from much of the developed world by mass vaccination in the mid-20th century but remains an important cause of illness in Russia and South-East Asia. The WHO have issued international guidelines for the management of infection.

Clinical features

Acutely, the disease presents with a sore throat, modest fever and marked tachycardia. The diagnostic feature is the 'wash-leather' elevated greyish-green membrane on the tonsils. There may be swelling of the neck ('bull-neck'), tender enlargement of the lymph nodes, blood-stained nasal discharge and a high-pitched cough. Complications occur as a result of exotoxins acting on the heart or nervous system and include myocarditis and peripheral neuropathy. Laryngeal obstruction or paralysis may occur and is life-threatening.

Management

The patient should be sent to a specialist infectious diseases unit. Empirical treatment should begin after collection of appropriate swabs. The three main areas of management are:

- Diphtheria antitoxin produced from hyperimmune horse serum: neutralises any toxin not fixed to tissue but can cause anaphylaxis.
- Administration of antibiotic: penicillin or amoxicillin.
- Strict isolation procedures: cases must be isolated until cultures from three swabs 24 hours apart are negative.

Prevention

Active immunisation should be given to all children. If diphtheria occurs in a closed community, contacts should be given erythromycin, which is more effective than penicillin in eradicating the organism in carriers. All contacts should also be immunised or given a booster dose of toxoid. Booster doses are required every 10 years to maintain immunity.

Pneumococcal infection

Streptococcus pneumoniae is the leading cause of pneumonia (p. 333), but also causes otitis media, meningitis and sinusitis. Asplenic individuals are at particular risk of fulminant pneumococcal sepsis. Resistance to penicillins, macrolides, cephalosporins and quinolones is increasing, but is still uncommon in the UK. Pneumococcal vaccine is helpful in those predisposed to infection, especially the elderly and those without a functioning spleen.

Anthrax

The Gram-positive *Bacillus anthracis* usually causes infection through contact with herbivores, although its spores can survive for years in soil. There are three recognised forms of infection:

Cutaneous anthrax: When processing hides and bones, spores are inoculated into exposed skin, producing an irritated papule on an oedematous haemorrhagic base. This develops into a black eschar.

GI anthrax: This is caused by ingestion of contaminated meat. The caecum is the seat of infection, producing nausea, vomiting, anorexia and fever, followed 2 to 3 days later by abdominal pain and bloody diarrhoea.

Inhalational anthrax: Disease caused by inhalation of spores is very rare but is a potential form of bioterrorism. Fever, dyspnoea, cough, headache, pleural effusions and sepsis develop 3 to 14 days after exposure, and mortality is 50% to 90%.

Management

B. anthracis can be cultured from swabs of skin lesions. Skin lesions are readily curable with early antibiotic therapy. Treatment is with ciprofloxacin until penicillin susceptibility is confirmed; the regimen can then be changed to benzylpenicillin IM. The addition of an aminoglycoside may improve the outlook. Two months of ciprofloxacin or doxycycline is then given to eradicate spores. Prophylaxis with ciprofloxacin is recommended for anyone at high risk of exposure to biological warfare.

Bacterial infections with neurological involvement

Bacterial meningitis, botulism and tetanus are dealt with in Chapter 16.

Mycobacterial infections

Tuberculosis

This is described in Chapter 9.

Leprosy

Leprosy (Hansen's disease) is a chronic granulomatous disease affecting skin and nerve and is caused by *Mycobacterium leprae*. The clinical form of the disease is determined by the degree of cell-mediated immunity (CMI) expressed by that individual towards *M. leprae*. High levels of CMI with elimination of leprosy bacilli produce tuberculoid leprosy, whereas absent CMI results in lepromatous leprosy. Complications arise as a result of nerve damage, immunological reactions and bacillary infiltration. It affects 4 million people worldwide, 70% of whom live in India; it is also endemic in Brazil, Indonesia, Mozambique, Madagascar, Tanzania and Nepal.

Untreated lepromatous patients discharge bacilli from the nose. Infection occurs through the nose, followed by haematogenous spread to skin and nerve. The incubation period is 2 to 5 years for tuberculoid cases and 8 to 12 years for lepromatous cases.

Clinical features

The cardinal features are skin lesions with anaesthesia, thickened peripheral nerves and acid-fast bacilli on skin smear or biopsy. The features of the two principal types of leprosy are compared in Box 5.17.

Skin: The most common skin lesions are macules or plaques. Tuberculoid patients have a few hypopigmented lesions. In lepromatous leprosy, papules, nodules or diffuse infiltration of the skin occur. Confluent lesions on the face can lead to a 'leonine facies' (Fig. 5.9).

Anaesthesia: In skin lesions, the small dermal sensory and autonomic nerve fibres are damaged, causing localised sensory loss and loss of sweating. Anaesthesia can occur in the distribution of a large peripheral nerve, or in a 'glove and stocking' distribution.

Nerve damage: Peripheral nerve trunks are affected at 'sites of predilection', including the ulnar (elbow), median (wrist), radial (humerus, causing wrist drop), radial cutaneous (wrist), common peroneal (knee), posterior tibial nerves and the sural nerves at the ankle; the facial nerve as it crosses the zygomatic arch; and the great auricular nerve in the posterior triangle

	5.17 Clinical characteristics of the polar forms of leprosy	
Clinical and tissue-specific features	**Lepromatous**	**Tuberculoid**
Skin and nerves		
Number and distribution	Wide dissemination	Few sites, asymmetrical
Skin lesions		
Margin–definition	Poor	Good
–elevation	Never	Common
Colour–dark skin	Slight hypopigmentation	Marked hypopigmentation
–light skin	Slight erythema	Coppery or red
Surface	Smooth, shiny	Dry, scaly
Central healing	None	Common
Sweat, hair	Impaired late	Impaired early
Loss of sensation	Late	Early, marked
Nerve enlargement/damage	Late	Early, marked
Bacilli	Many	Absent
Natural history	Progressive	Self-healing
Other tissues	Upper respiratory mucosa, eye, testes, bone, muscle	None
Reactions	Immune complexes (type 2)	Cell-mediated (type 1)

5

of the neck. All these nerves should be examined for enlargement and tenderness, and tested for motor and sensory function. The CNS is not affected.

Eye involvement: Blindness is a devastating complication for a patient with anaesthetic hands and feet. Eyelid closure is impaired when the facial (7th) nerve is affected. Damage to the trigeminal nerve causes anaesthesia of the cornea and conjunctiva. The cornea is then susceptible to trauma and ulceration.

Other features: These include nasal collapse caused by destruction of bone and cartilage, and hypogonadism from testicular atrophy.

Borderline cases

Borderline tuberculoid (BT): The skin lesions are more numerous than in tuberculoid leprosy, and there is more severe nerve damage. These patients are prone to type 1 reactions (see later) with consequent nerve damage.

Borderline leprosy (BB): Patients have numerous skin lesions varying in size, shape and distribution. Annular lesions are characteristic, and nerve damage is variable.

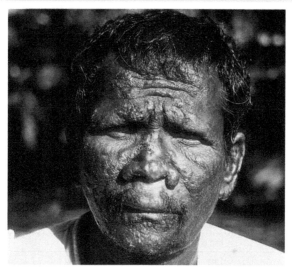

Fig. 5.9 Lepromatous leprosy. Widespread nodules and infiltration with loss of the eyebrows. This man also has early collapse of the nose.

Borderline lepromatous leprosy (BL): There are widespread small macules and nerve involvement. Patients may experience both type 1 and type 2 reactions.

Pure neural leprosy: This type occurs principally in India, and accounts for 10% of cases. Asymmetrical peripheral nerve involvement occurs without skin lesions.

Leprosy reactions

These are events superimposed on the cardinal features described above.

Type 1 (reversal) reactions: These occur in 30% of borderline patients (BT, BB, BL), and are delayed hypersensitivity reactions. Skin lesions become erythematous; peripheral nerves become tender and painful with sudden loss of nerve function. Reversal reactions may occur spontaneously, after starting treatment or after completion of multidrug therapy.

Type 2 (erythema nodosum leprosum (ENL)) reactions: Partly caused by immune complex deposition, these occur in BL and lepromatous patients who produce antibodies and have a high antigen load. Patients develop malaise, fever and crops of small pink nodules on the face and limbs. Iritis and episcleritis are common. Other signs are acute neuritis, lymphadenitis, orchitis, bone pain, dactylitis, arthritis and proteinuria. ENL may continue intermittently for several years.

Investigations

• Slit skin smears: dermal material is scraped on to a glass slide and stained, then acid-fast bacilli are counted by microscopy. • Skin biopsy: histological examination may aid diagnosis. • Neither serology nor PCR testing is sensitive or specific enough for diagnosis.

<table>
<tr><td colspan="5">i 5.18 Modified WHO-recommended multidrug therapy regimens in leprosy</td></tr>
</table>

Type of leprosy[a]	Monthly supervised treatment	Daily self-administered treatment	Duration of treatment[b]
Paucibacillary	Rifampicin 600 mg	Dapsone 100 mg	6 months
Multibacillary	Rifampicin 600 mg Clofazimine 300 mg	Clofazimine 50 mg Dapsone 100 mg	12 months
Paucibacillary single lesion	Ofloxacin 400 mg Rifampicin 600 mg Minocycline 100 mg		Single dose

[a] WHO classification for field use when slit-skin smears are not available:
- paucibacillary single lesion (1 lesion)
- paucibacillary (2–5 skin lesions)
- multibacillary (>5 skin lesions).

[b] Multibacillary patients with a high bacillary index need at least 24 moths treatment

Management

Multidrug treatment (MDT) is required for all leprosy patients (Box 5.18). Rifampicin is a potent bactericidal for *M. leprae,* but should always be given with other drugs, as a single mutation can confer resistance. Dapsone is bacteriostatic. It commonly causes mild haemolysis and, rarely, anaemia. Clofazimine is a red, fat-soluble crystalline dye that is weakly bactericidal for *M. leprae*. Skin discoloration (red to purple-black) and ichthyosis are troublesome side effects, particularly on pale skins. Newer drugs such as perfloxacin, ofloxacin, clarithromycin and minocycline are now established second-line options.

Treatment of reactions: Most reactions respond to high-dose oral prednisolone. Thalidomide may also be used, but teratogenicity limits its use in women who may become pregnant. Hydrocortisone eye drops are used for ocular symptoms.

Patient education and rehabilitation: Patients should be reassured that after 3 days of chemotherapy they are not infectious and can lead a normal social life. Additional measures include:
• Patients with anaesthetic hands or feet need to avoid and treat burns or other minor injuries. • Good footwear is important. • Ulceration: the cause of the injury should be identified, and the patient advised not to weight-bear until the ulcer has healed. • Physiotherapy: can help prevent contractures and muscle atrophy.

Prognosis

Tuberculous leprosy may self-heal, but lepromatous leprosy has high morbidity if untreated.

Most patients, especially those without nerve damage at the time of diagnosis, do well on MDT, with resolution of skin lesions. Borderline patients are at risk of developing type 1 reactions, which may result in devastating nerve damage.

Prevention and control

Programmes aimed at case detection and provision of MDT are now in place in many of the countries affected by leprosy. BCG vaccination has been shown to give good but variable protection against leprosy; adding killed *M. leprae* to BCG does not give enhanced protection.

Rickettsial and related intracellular bacterial infections

These are caused by Gram-negative organisms that occur in the intestines and saliva of ticks, mites, lice and fleas. Following an inoculating bite, the organisms multiply in capillary endothelial cells and cause fever, rash and organ damage. There are two main groups of rickettsial fevers: the spotted fever group and the typhus group.

Spotted fever group

Rocky Mountain spotted fever: Rickettsia rickettsii is transmitted by tick bites, largely in western and south-eastern states of the United States and also in Central and South America. The incubation period is around 7 days. The rash appears on about the third or fourth day, looking at first like measles, but in a few hours the typical maculopapular eruption develops. Within 24 to 48 hours the rash spreads in a centripetal fashion from wrists, forearms and ankles to the back, limbs and chest, and then to the abdomen, where it is least pronounced. Larger cutaneous and subcutaneous haemorrhages may appear in severe cases. The liver and spleen become palpable. At the extremes of life the mortality is 2% to 12%.

Other spotted fevers: R. conorii and R. africae cause Mediterranean and African tick typhus. An eschar (black, necrotic sore) is associated with a maculopapular rash on the trunk, limbs, palms and soles. Complications include delirium and meningism.

Typhus group

Scrub typhus fever: Caused by *Orientia tsutsugamushi*, transmitted by mites. It occurs in the Far East, Myanmar, Pakistan, Bangladesh, India, Indonesia, the South Pacific and Queensland. Initially the patient develops one or more eschars, surrounded by cellulitis with regional lymphadenopathy. The incubation period is around 9 days. Mild or subclinical cases are common. The onset of symptoms is usually sudden with headache (often retro-orbital), fever, malaise, weakness and cough. An erythematous maculopapular rash appears on about the fifth to seventh day and spreads to the trunk, face and limbs, including the palms and soles, with generalised painless lymphadenopathy. The rash fades by the fourteenth day. The patient develops a remittent fever that falls by the twelfth to eighteenth day. In severe infection the patient is prostrate with cough, pneumonia, delirium and deafness. Cardiac failure, renal failure and haemorrhage may develop. Convalescence is often slow, and tachycardia may persist for some weeks.

Epidemic (louse-borne) typhus: Caused by R. prowazekii and prevalent in parts of Africa, especially Ethiopia and Rwanda, and in the South American Andes and Afghanistan. Overcrowding facilitates spread, which is through scratching skin contaminated with louse faeces. The incubation period is usually 12 to 14 days. The onset is usually sudden, with rigors, fever, frontal headaches, pains in the back and limbs, constipation and bronchitis. The face is flushed and cyanotic, the eyes are congested, and the patient becomes confused. A petechial, mottled rash appears on the fourth to sixth day, first on the anterior folds of the axillae, sides of the abdomen or backs of hands, then on the trunk and forearms, sparing the neck and face. During the second week, symptoms increase, with sores on the lips and a dry, brown, shrunken and tremulous tongue. The spleen is palpable, the pulse feeble and the patient stuporous and delirious. The temperature falls rapidly at the end of the second week, and the patient recovers gradually. Fatal cases usually die in the second week from toxaemia, cardiac or renal failure or pneumonia.

Endemic (flea-borne) typhus: Flea-borne or 'endemic' typhus, caused by *R. typhi*, is endemic worldwide. Humans are infected when the faeces or contents of a crushed flea that has fed on an infected rat are introduced into the skin. The incubation period is 8–14 days. The symptoms resemble those of a mild louse-borne typhus. The rash may be scanty and transient.

Investigation of rickettsial infection

The diagnosis of rickettsial infection is essentially clinical, and may be confirmed by antibody detection or PCR in specialised laboratories. Differential diagnoses include malaria, typhoid, meningococcal septicaemia and leptospirosis.

Management of the rickettsial diseases

The different rickettsial fevers vary in severity, but all respond to tetracycline, doxycycline or chloramphenicol. Sedation may be required for delirium, and transfusion for haemorrhage. Reservoirs of the disease, such as fleas, ticks and mites, should be controlled with insecticides.

Q Fever

Q fever occurs worldwide and is caused by the rickettsia-like organism *Coxiella burnetii*, an obligate intracellular organism that survives in the extracellular environment. Cattle, sheep and goats are important reservoirs, and the organism is transmitted by inhalation of aerosolised particles, usually during meat processing. In culture, the organism undergoes antigenic shift from the infectious phase I to the noninfectious phase II form.

Clinical features

The incubation period is 3 to 4 weeks. The initial symptoms are nonspecific, with fever, headache and chills. In 20% of cases a maculopapular rash occurs. Other presentations include pneumonia and hepatitis. Chronic Q fever may present with osteomyelitis, encephalitis and endocarditis.

Investigations

Diagnosis is usually serological, and the stage of the infection can be distinguished by isotype tests and phase-specific antigens. Acute phase II IgM titres peak at 4 to 6 weeks. In chronic infections, IgG titres to phase I and II antigens may be raised.

Management

Doxycycline is the treatment of choice. Rifampicin is added in cases of Q fever endocarditis, which requires prolonged treatment with doxycycline and rifampicin and often valve surgery.

Bartonellosis

This group of diseases is caused by intracellular Gram-negative rods closely related to the rickettsiae that are found in many domestic pets. The principal human pathogens are *Bartonella quintana* and *B. henselae*. *Bartonella* is associated with the following:

Trench fever: This is a relapsing fever with severe leg pain, which is debilitating but not fatal.

Bacteraemia and endocarditis in the homeless: The endocarditis is associated with severe damage to the heart valves.

Cat-scratch disease: *B. henselae* causes this common benign lymphadenopathy in children and young adults. A vesicle or papule develops on the head, neck or arms after a cat scratch. The lesion resolves spontaneously, but lymphadenopathy may persist for up to 4 months.

Bacillary angiomatosis: This is an HIV-associated disease.

Investigations

• PCR is often used for diagnosis. • Blood cultures: specialised laboratories only. • Serological testing: possible, but cross-reactions occur with *Chlamydia* and *Coxiella*.

Management

Bartonella spp. are usually treated with macrolides or tetracyclines. Antibiotic use is guided by clinical need. Cat-scratch disease usually resolves spontaneously, but *Bartonella* endocarditis requires valve replacement and a combination of doxycycline and gentamicin.

Chlamydial infections

Three organisms cause most human chlamydial infections:
• *Chlamydia trachomatis* causes trachoma (see below), lymphogranuloma venereum and sexually transmitted genital infections (p. 175). • *C. psittaci* causes psittacosis. • *C. pneumoniae* is a cause of pneumonia (p. 333).

Trachoma

Trachoma is a chronic keratoconjunctivitis caused by *C. trachomatis* and is the most common cause of avoidable blindness. Transmission occurs in dry and dirty environments through flies, on fingers and within families. In endemic areas, the disease is most common in children.

Clinical features

The onset is usually insidious and may be asymptomatic. Early symptoms include conjunctivitis and blepharospasm, which may be difficult to distinguish from other types of conjunctivitis, but hyperaemia with pale follicles on the conjunctivae are characteristic of trachoma. Lid inversion and corneal vascularisation with opacity are important complications. Infection may not be detected until vision begins to fail.

Investigations and management

Intracellular inclusions may be demonstrated in conjunctival scrapings by staining with iodine or immunofluorescence. A single dose of azithromycin

(20 mg/kg) is first-choice treatment and is superior to tetracycline eye oint-ment. Deformity and scarring of the lids, and corneal opacities, ulceration and scarring require surgical treatment after control of local infection.

The WHO is promoting the SAFE strategy for trachoma control (**s**urgery, **a**ntibiotics, **f**acial cleanliness and **e**nvironmental improvement). Proper eye care of newborn and young children is essential.

Protozoal infections

Systemic protozoal infections

5

Malaria

Malaria is caused by *Plasmodium falciparum*, *P. vivax*, *P. ovale* and *P. malar-iae*, as well as the predominantly simian parasite *P. knowlesi*. It is transmit-ted by the bite of female anopheline mosquitoes, and occurs throughout the tropics and subtropics at altitudes below 1500 m. The WHO estimates that 214 million cases occurred in 2015, 88% of these in Africa. *P. fal-ciparum* is now resistant to chloroquine and sulfadoxine-pyrimethamine in South-East Asia and throughout Africa. Reversal of the resurgence in malaria by improved vector and disease control is a major goal of the WHO.

Travellers are susceptible to malaria. Most cases are caused by *P. fal-ciparum*, usually from Africa, and of these 1% die because of late diagno-sis. Migrants from endemic countries resident in nonendemic countries are particularly at risk if they visit relatives in their country of origin. They have lost their partial immunity and frequently do not take malaria prophylaxis. People living near airports in Europe occasionally acquire malaria from acci-dentally imported mosquitoes.

Life cycle

The female anopheline mosquito becomes infected by feeding on human blood containing malarial parasite gametocytes. Human infection starts when an infected mosquito inoculates saliva containing sporozoites into the skin during feeding; these disappear from human blood within half an hour and enter the liver. After some days merozoites leave the liver and invade red blood cells, where further multiplication takes place, producing schizonts (Fig. 5.10). Rupture of the schizont releases more merozoites into the blood and causes fever, the periodicity of which depends on the spe-cies of parasite (see below).

P. vivax and *P. ovale* may persist in liver cells as dormant forms, hypno-zoites, capable of developing into merozoites months or years later. Thus, the first attack of clinical malaria may occur long after the patient has left the endemic area, and the disease may relapse after treatment with drugs that only kill the erythrocytic stage of the parasite. *P. falciparum*, *P. knowlesi* and *P. malariae* have no persistent exo-erythrocytic phase, but recrudescence of fever may result from multiplication of parasites in red cells that have not been eliminated by treatment and immune processes.

Clinical features

The pathology in malaria is caused by haemolysis of infected red cells and adherence of infected red blood cells to capillaries.

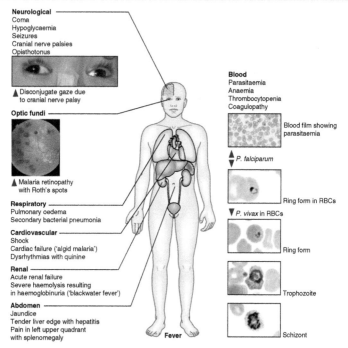

Neurological
Coma
Hypoglycaemia
Seizures
Cranial nerve palsies
Opisthotonus

▲ Disconjugate gaze due
to cranial nerve palsy

Optic fundi

▲ Malaria retinopathy
with Roth's spots

Respiratory
Pulmonary oedema
Secondary bacterial pneumonia

Cardiovascular
Shock
Cardiac failure ('algid malaria')
Dysrhythmias with quinine

Renal
Acute renal failure
Severe haemolysis resulting
in haemoglobinuria ('blackwater fever')

Abdomen
Jaundice
Tender liver edge with hepatitis
Pain in left upper quadrant
with splenomegaly

Blood
Parasitaemia
Anaemia
Thrombocytopenia
Coagulopathy

Blood film showing
parasitaemia

P. falciparum

Ring form in RBCs

▼ *P. vivax* in RBCs

Ring form

Trophozoite

Schizont

Fever

Fig. 5.10 Features of *Plasmodium falciparum* infection.

P. falciparum infection: (Fig. 5.10) This is the most dangerous of the malarias. The onset is often insidious, with malaise, headache and vomiting. Cough and mild diarrhoea are also common. The fever has no particular pattern. Jaundice is common as a result of haemolysis and hepatic dysfunction. The liver and spleen enlarge and become tender, and anaemia and thrombocytopenia develop rapidly. Complications of falciparum malaria are summarised in Box 5.19. Previous splenectomy increases the risk of severe malaria.

P. vivax and P. ovale infection: In many cases the illness starts with several days of continued fever before the development of classical bouts of fever on alternate days. Fever starts with a rigor. The patient feels cold, and the temperature rises to around 40°C. After half an hour to an hour, the hot or flush phase begins. It lasts several hours and gives way to profuse perspiration and a gradual fall in temperature. The cycle is repeated 48 hours later. Gradually the spleen and liver enlarge and may become tender. Anaemia develops slowly. Relapses are frequent in the first 2 years after leaving the malarious area.

P. malariae and P. knowlesi infection: This is usually associated with mild symptoms and bouts of fever every third day. Parasitaemia may persist for many years with the occasional recrudescence of fever, or without producing any symptoms. *P. malariae* causes glomerulonephritis and the nephrotic syndrome in children. *P knowlesi* is usually mild but can deteriorate rapidly.

✚ 5.19 Severe manifestations of *P. falciparum* malaria and their management

Cerebral malaria	
Coma	Maintain airway, exclude other causes, ventilate if necessary
Convulsions	Diazepam or paraldehyde
Hyperpyrexia	Tepid sponging, fan, paracetamol
Hypoglycaemia	Monitor blood glucose, IV dextrose infusion
Severe anaemia (PCV <15%)	Transfusion
Acute pulmonary oedema	Nurse at 45°, venesect, limit IV fluids, diuretics, CPAP, haemofilter
Acute renal failure	Exclude other causes, dialysis (peritoneal or haemodialysis)
Bleeding/coagulopathy	Transfuse screened fresh blood, or FFP, cryoprecipitate
Metabolic acidosis	Fluids, oxygen, treat sepsis and hypo-glycaemia
Shock ('algid malaria')	Suspect Gram-negative septicaemia, IV antimicrobials, fluid resuscitation
Aspiration pneumonia	IV antimicrobials, oxygen, physiotherapy
Hyperparasitaemia	Partial or full exchange transfusion, haemapheresis

(From WHO. Severe falciparum malaria. In: Severe and complicated malaria. 3rd ed. Trans R Soc Trop Med Hyg 2000; 94 (suppl. 1): S1–41.)

Investigations

Giemsa-stained thick and thin blood films should be examined. In the thick film erythrocytes are lysed, releasing all blood stages of the parasite. This facilitates the diagnosis of low-level parasitaemias. A thin film is essential to confirm the diagnosis, species and, in *P. falciparum* infections, to quantify the parasite load (by counting the percentage of infected erythrocytes).

Immunochromatographic 'dipstick' tests for *P. falciparum* antigens are now marketed and provide a useful nonmicroscopic means of diagnosing this infection. They should be used alongside blood film examination, and are especially useful when the microscopist is less experienced. PCR remains largely a research tool.

Management

Mild *P. falciparum* malaria: *P. falciparum* is now resistant to chloroquine and sulfadoxine-pyrimethamine almost worldwide, so an artemisinin-based treatment is recommended. Co-artemether (artemether and lumefantrine) is given at a dose of four tablets at 0, 8, 24, 36, 48 and 60 hours. Alternatives are quinine (600 mg quinine salt three times daily for 5–7 days), followed by doxycycline or clindamycin. Doxycycline should be avoided in pregnancy, and artemether in early pregnancy. The WHO recommends artemisinin-based combination therapy, but artemisinin resistance is appearing in South-East Asia.

Complicated P. falciparum malaria: Severe malaria (parasite count >2% in any nonimmune patient) is a medical emergency. Immediate management should include IV artesunate (2.4 mg/kg IV at 0, 12 and 24 hours, then daily for 7 days). When the patient has recovered sufficiently, oral artesunate 2 mg/kg once daily is given instead of infusions to a total cumulative dose of 17 to 18 mg/kg. IV quinine salt is an alternative, with ECG monitoring. Management of the complications of severe *P. falciparum* infection is summarised in Box 5.19.

Non-falciparum malaria: *P. vivax, P. ovale, P. knowlesi* and *P. malariae* infections should be treated with oral chloroquine (600 mg chloroquine base, followed at 6 hours by 300 mg, then 150 mg twice daily for two more days). Relapses can be prevented by taking one of the antimalarial drugs in suppressive doses. Radical cure is achieved in *P. vivax* and *P. ovale* using primaquine, which destroys the hypnozoite phase in the liver, after checking glucose-6-phosphate dehydrogenase (G6PD) status. Haemolysis may develop in those who are G6PD-deficient. Cyanosis as a result of the formation of methaemoglobin in the red cells is more common, but not dangerous.

Prevention

Clinical attacks of malaria may be preventable with chemoprophylaxis using chloroquine, atovaquone plus proguanil (Malarone), doxycycline or mefloquine. The risk of malaria in the area to be visited and the degree of chloroquine resistance guide the recommendations for prophylaxis. Updated recommendations are summarised at www.fitfortravel.nhs.uk. Many agents must be taken in advance of travel and continued after return. Mefloquine is useful in areas of multiple drug resistance, but contraindications exist. Use of insecticide-treated bed nets, insect repellents and protective clothing are also important means of reducing infection. Research to produce a fully-protective malaria vaccine is ongoing.

Babesiosis

This is caused by a tickborne intra-erythrocytic protozoon parasite. Patients present with fever 1 to 4 weeks after a tick bite. Severe illness is seen in splenectomised patients. The diagnosis is made by blood film examination. Treatment is with quinine and clindamycin.

African trypanosomiasis (sleeping sickness)

African sleeping sickness is caused by trypanosomes conveyed to humans by the bites of infected tsetse flies and is unique to sub-Saharan Africa. The disease has declined by 60% since 1990 because of improved control. *Trypanosoma brucei gambiense* has a wide distribution in West and Central Africa and accounts for 90% of cases. *T. brucei rhodesiense* is found in parts of East and Central Africa and, unlike *gambiense*, has a large reservoir in wild animals. Transmission is common at riversides and in wooded grasslands.

Clinical features

A tsetse fly bite is painful and commonly becomes inflamed; if trypanosomes are introduced, the site may again become painful and swollen around 10 days later ('trypanosomal chancre'), associated with regional lymphadenopathy. Within 2 to 3 weeks of infection the trypanosomes invade the blood stream. The early haematolymphatic stage gives way to a late encephalitic stage.

Rhodesiense infections: Acute and severe. Within days or a few weeks the patient is usually severely ill and may have developed pleural effusions and signs of myocarditis or hepatitis. There may be a petechial rash. The patient may die before there are signs of involvement of the CNS. If the illness is less acute, drowsiness, tremors and coma develop.

Gambiense infection: Slow course, with irregular bouts of fever and firm, discrete, rubbery and painless lymphadenopathy, particularly in the posterior triangle of the neck. The spleen and liver may become palpable. After some months without treatment, the CNS is invaded. Patients develop headache, altered behaviour, cognitive impairment, insomnia by night and sleepiness by day, delirium and eventually tremors, pareses, wasting, coma and death.

Investigations

• Thick and thin malaria blood films will reveal trypanosomes. • Lymph node aspirate may be more sensitive in *gambiense* infection. • The card agglutination trypanosomiasis test allows simple serological screening for *gambiense*. • Lumbar puncture: with CNS involvement, CSF will reveal raised protein, WCC and IgM, and diminished glucose.

Management

Therapeutic options for African trypanosomiasis are limited, as most antitrypanosomal drugs are toxic and expensive. The prognosis is good if treatment is begun before CNS involvement. For early *gambiense*, pentamidine 4 mg/kg IM or IV is given for 7 days. Early *rhodesiense* is treated with intravenous suramin five injections of 20 mg/kg given weekly. For those with CNS disease, eflornithine and nifurtimox are used for *gambiense,* and melarsoprol for *rhodesiense*.

American trypanosomiasis (Chagas' disease)

Chagas' disease occurs widely in South and Central America. The cause is *Trypanosoma cruzi*, transmitted to humans from the faeces of a reduviid (triatomine) bug, in which the trypanosomes develop before infecting humans. Infected faeces are rubbed in through the conjunctiva, mucosa of the mouth or nose or abrasions of the skin. Blood transfusions are responsible for up to 5% of infections, and congenital transmission may also occur.

Clinical features

Acute phase: The acute phase is seen in only 1% to 2% of infected individuals infected before the age of 15 years. Young children (1–5 years of age) are most commonly affected. The entrance of *T. cruzi* through an abrasion produces a dusky-red firm swelling and regional lymphadenopathy.

A conjunctival lesion, although less common, is more characteristic; the unilateral firm reddish swelling of the lids may close the eye, and this constitutes 'Romaña's sign'. In a few patients, an acute generalised infection soon appears, with a transient morbilliform or urticarial rash, fever, lymphadenopathy and enlargement of the spleen and liver. In a small minority of patients, acute myocarditis and heart failure or neurological features, including personality changes and signs of meningoencephalitis, may be seen. The acute infection may be fatal to infants.

Chronic phase: About 50% to 70% of infected patients become seropositive and develop an indeterminate form when no parasitaemia is detectable. They have a normal lifespan with no symptoms, but are a natural reservoir for the disease and maintain the life cycle of parasites. After a latent period of several years, 10% to 30% of chronic cases develop low-grade myocarditis and damage to conducting fibres causing a cardiomyopathy. In nearly 10% of patients, damage to Auerbach's plexus results in dilatation of various parts of the alimentary canal, especially the colon and oesophagus, so-called 'mega' disease. Dilatation of the bile ducts and bronchi are also a recognised sequelae. Reactivation of Chagas' disease can occur in patients with HIV if the CD4 count falls to less than 200 cells/mm^3 (p. 178).

Investigations

• Blood film: *T. cruzi* is easily detectable in the acute illness. • Chronic disease: xenodiagnosis- infection-free, laboratory-bred reduviid bugs feed on the patient, and the bugs' faeces are subsequently examined for parasites. • PCR: parasite DNA detection by PCR is highly sensitive in blood or in bug faeces in xenodiagnosis. • Antibody detection is also highly sensitive.

Management

Nifurtimox (10 mg/kg daily for 90 days) and benznidazole (5 mg/kg daily for 60 days), both given as divided daily doses, are parasiticidal drugs. Either can be used in the acute and early chronic phase. Adverse reactions are frequent (30%–55%), but cure rates of up to 80% result. Surgery may be required for 'mega' disease. Prevention involves destruction of the bugs with insecticides and screening of blood donors.

Toxoplasmosis

Toxoplasma gondii is an intracellular parasite. The sexual phase of its life cycle occurs in the small intestinal epithelium of the cat. Oöcysts shed in cat faeces survive in moist conditions for weeks or months and spread to intermediate hosts (pigs, sheep and also humans) through contaminated soil. Once ingested, the parasite transforms into rapidly dividing tachyzoites. Microscopic tissue cysts develop containing bradyzoites, which persist for the lifetime of the host. Cats become infected or reinfected by ingesting tissue cysts in prey.

Human infection occurs via oöcyst-contaminated soil, salads and vegetables, or by eating under-cooked meat containing tissue cysts. Sheep, pigs and rabbits are the most common meat sources. Outbreaks have occurred after consumption of unfiltered water. In developed countries, toxoplasmosis is the most common protozoal infection; around 22% of adults in the UK are seropositive.

Clinical features

In most immunocompetent individuals, including children and pregnant women, the infection goes unnoticed. In around 10% of patients it causes a self-limiting illness, most common in adults aged 25 to 35 years. The presenting feature is usually painless lymphadenopathy. Systemic symptoms, which are 'flu-like', are infrequent. Complete resolution usually occurs within a few months, although symptoms and lymphadenopathy tend to fluctuate unpredictably, and some patients do not recover completely for a year or more. Encephalitis, myocarditis, polymyositis, pneumonitis or hepatitis occasionally occur in immunocompetent patients, but are more common in the immunocompromised. Toxoplasmosis acquired in utero by vertical spread can also cause retinochoroiditis, hydrocephalus and microcephaly.

Investigations

The Sabin–Feldman indirect fluorescent antibody test is used in immunocompetent patients. A fourfold rise in IgG or the presence of IgM indicates acute infection. The presence of high-avidity IgG excludes infection in the past 3 to 4 months, which is important in pregnancy. In immunocompromised patients, *Toxoplasma* organisms can be detected histochemically in a lymph node biopsy or other tissue with *T. gondii* antiserum, or by using PCR to detect *Toxoplasma*-specific DNA.

Management

Because the disease is usually self-limiting, treatment is reserved for rare cases of severe or progressive disease, and for infection in immunocompromised patients. *T. gondii* infection responds poorly to antimicrobial therapy, but pyrimethamine, sulfadiazine and folinic acid may be used.

Leishmaniasis

Leishmaniasis is caused by unicellular flagellate intracellular protozoa belonging to the genus *Leishmania*. It comprises three broad groups of disorder:
• Visceral leishmaniasis (VL, kala-azar). • Cutaneous leishmaniasis (CL).
• Mucosal leishmaniasis (ML).

Although most clinical syndromes are caused by zoonotic transmission of parasites from animals (chiefly canine and rodent reservoirs) to humans through phlebotomine sandfly vectors, humans are the only known reservoir (anthroponotic person-to-person transmission) in major VL foci in the Indian subcontinent and injection drug users. Leishmaniasis occurs in around 100 countries, with an estimated annual incidence of 0.9 to 1.3 million new cases (25% VL).

Life cycle

Flagellar promastigotes (10–20 μm) are introduced by the feeding female sandfly (*Phlebotomus* in the eastern hemisphere, *Lutzomyia* and *Psychodopygus* in the western hemisphere). The promastigotes are taken up by neutrophils, which undergo apoptosis and are engulfed by macrophages in which the parasites transform into amastigotes (2–4 μm, Leishman-Donovan bodies). These multiply, causing macrophage lysis and infection of other cells. Sandflies pick up amastigotes when feeding on infected patients or animal reservoirs. In the sandfly, the parasite transforms into a flagellar promastigote, which multiplies in the gut of the vector and migrates to the proboscis to infect a new host.

Visceral leishmaniasis (Kala-Azar)

VL is caused by the protozoon *Leishmania donovani* complex (comprising *L. donovani*, *L. infantum* and *L. chagasi*). Rarely, a dermatotropic species (e.g. *L. tropica*) may cause visceral disease. India, Sudan, Bangladesh and Brazil account for 90% of cases of VL. Other affected regions include the Mediterranean, East Africa, China, Arabia, Israel and other South American countries. VL can present unexpectedly, for example, after blood transfusion, in immunosuppressed patients after transplantation and in HIV infection.

Clinical features

The majority of people infected remain asymptomatic. In the Indian subcontinent, adults and children are equally affected; elsewhere it is predominantly a childhood disease, except in adults with HIV.

Symptomatic cases feature:

• Fever: accompanied initially by rigor and chills, and decreasing over time with occasional relapses. • Splenomegaly: develops quickly in the first few weeks and may become massive. • Hepatomegaly. • Lymphadenopathy: common except in the Indian subcontinent. • Skin: a blackish discoloration of the skin ('kala-azar' is Hindi for 'black fever') is a feature of advanced disease, and is now rarely seen. • Pancytopenia is common. Severe anaemia can cause cardiac failure. • Thrombocytopenia may cause retinal, GI or nasal bleeding. • Oedema and ascites: secondary to low albumin. • Secondary infection: profound immunosuppression may result in TB, dysentery, gastroenteritis and chickenpox. Cellulitis, shingles and scabies are common.

Investigations

There is pancytopenia with granulocytopenia and monocytosis. There is polyclonal hypergammaglobulinaemia (IgG first, then IgM) and hypoalbuminaemia. Splenic smears demonstrate amastigotes (Leishman-Donovan bodies) with 98% sensitivity, but risk haemorrhage. PCR is performed on peripheral blood; it is sensitive especially in the immunosuppressed, but only performed in specialised laboratories. Serodiagnosis by immunofluorescence is also used in developed countries. In endemic regions, a highly sensitive and specific direct agglutination test of stained promastigotes and an equally efficient rapid immunochromatographic K39 strip test have been developed.

Differential diagnosis

This includes malaria, typhoid, TB, schistosomiasis and many other infectious and neoplastic conditions, some of which may coexist with VL. Fever, splenomegaly, pancytopenia and nonresponse to antimalarial therapy may provide clues before specific laboratory diagnosis is made.

Management

Antimony (Sb) compounds: These compounds, such as sodium stibogluconate and meglumine antimoniate, are the mainstay of treatment in most parts of the world; in the Indian subcontinent, however, almost two-thirds of cases are refractory to Sb. A daily dose of 20 mg/kg is given, IV or IM, for 28 to 30 days. Side effects are common and include arthralgia, myalgia, raised hepatic transaminases and pancreatitis, especially in patients co-infected with HIV. Severe cardiotoxicity, manifested by concave ST segment elevation, prolongation of QT_c greater than 0.5 msec, ventricular ectopics, ventricular dysrhythmias and sudden death, is not uncommon. The incidence of cardiotoxicity and death is particularly high with improperly manufactured Sb.

Amphotericin B deoxycholate: 0.75 to 1 mg/kg daily for 15 to 20 doses, is an alternative in areas where there is Sb unresponsiveness. It has a cure rate of nearly 100%. Infusion-related side effects, for example, high fever with rigor thrombophlebitis, diarrhoea and vomiting, are extremely common. Serious side effects, including renal or hepatic toxicity, hypokalaemia, thrombocytopenia and myocarditis, are not uncommon. Lipid formulations of amphotericin B are less toxic. AmBisome is first-line therapy in Europe for VL. High daily doses of the lipid formulations are well tolerated, thus reducing hospital stay and cost. AmBisome has been made available at preferential cost in developing countries.

Other drugs: Miltefosine, paromomycin and pentamidine have also been used to treat VL. Multidrug therapy is likely to increase to prevent the emergence of resistance.

Response to treatment

A good response results in abatement of fever, improved well-being, reduction in splenomegaly, weight gain and recovery of blood counts. Patients should be followed regularly for 6 to 12 months because some may relapse.

HIV–visceral leishmaniasis co-infection

This is declining in Europe because of ART, but is increasing in Africa, South America and the Indian subcontinent.

The clinical triad of fever, splenomegaly and hepatomegaly is found in most co-infected cases, but those with a low CD4 count may have atypical clinical presentations. VL may present with GI involvement (stomach, duodenum or colon), ascites, pleural or pericardial effusion or involvement of lungs, tonsil, oral mucosa or skin. Diagnostic principles remain the same as for non-HIV patients, based on the detection of amastigotes in body fluids or PCR of the blood.

Treatment of VL in a setting of HIV co-infection is essentially the same as in immunocompetent patients, using amphotericin B or Sb, but there are some differences in outcome. There is a tendency to relapse within a year, and monthly maintenance liposomal amphotericin B is useful.

Post-kala-azar dermal leishmaniasis

After treatment and recovery from VL in India and Sudan, some patients develop dermatological manifestations. In India, dermatological changes occur in a small minority of patients aged 6 months to 3 years or older after the initial infection. Diagnosis is clinical, based on the characteristic appearance of macules, papules, nodules (most frequently) and plaques on the face, especially around the chin. The face often appears erythematous. Hypopigmented macules can occur, and are highly variable in extent and location. There are no systemic symptoms, and little spontaneous healing occurs.

In Sudan, 50% of patients with VL (usually children) develop PKDL rapidly (within 6 months), and three–quarters undergo spontaneous healing. Treatment of Indian PKDL is difficult—Sb for 120 days, several courses of amphotericin B infusions or miltefosine for 12 weeks is required. In Sudan, Sb for 2 months is considered adequate.

Prevention and control

Insecticides, as well as physical barriers such as mosquito nets and protective clothing, help prevent disease transmission to humans. In endemic areas, infected or stray dogs should be destroyed. Early detection and adequate treatment of cases reduce the human reservoir of the disease.

Cutaneous and mucosal leishmaniasis

Cutaneous leishmaniasis

CL (oriental sore) occurs in both the Old World and the New World, causing two distinct types of leishmaniasis:

Old World CL: A mild disease found around the Mediterranean basin; throughout the Middle East and Central Asia as far as Pakistan; and in sub-Saharan West Africa and Sudan. It is caused by *Leishmania major*, *L. tropica* and *L. aethiopica*.

New World CL: A disfiguring disease, largely found in Central and South America. It is caused by the *Leishmania mexicana* complex (*L. mexicana*, *L. amazonensis* and *L. venezuelensis*) and by the *Viannia* subgenus *L. (V.) brasiliensis* complex (*L. (V.) guyanensis*, *L. (V.) panamensis*, *L. (V.) brasiliensis* and *L. (V.) peruviana*).

The incubation period is 2 to 3 months (range: 2 weeks to 5 years). In all types of CL, a small, red papule develops at the site of the vector bite. The papules may be single or multiple, and increase gradually in size, reaching 2 to 10 cm in diameter. A crust forms, overlying an ulcer with raised borders (Fig. 5.11). There can be satellite lesions, especially in *L. major* and occasionally in *L. tropica* infections. Regional lymphadenopathy, pain, pruritus and secondary bacterial infections may occur. *L. mexicana* is responsible for chiclero ulcers, self-healing sores seen in Mexico. If immunity is good, there is usually spontaneous healing in *L. tropica*, *L. major* and *L. mexicana* lesions. In some patients with anergy to *Leishmania*, the skin lesions of *L. aethiopica*, *L. mexicana* and *L. amazonensis* infections progress to the development of diffuse CL; this is characterised by spread of the infection from the initial ulcer, usually on the face, to involve the whole body with nonulcerative nodules. Occasionally, in *L. tropica* infections, sores that have apparently healed relapse persistently (recidivans or lupoid leishmaniasis).

Mucosal leishmaniasis

The *Viannia* subgenus (New World CL) extends from the Amazon basin to Paraguay and Costa Rica, and is responsible for deep sores and ML. Young men with chronic lesions are particularly at risk, and 2% to 40% of infected persons develop 'espundia', metastatic lesions in the mucosa of the nose or mouth. This is characterised by thickening, erythema and later ulceration of the nasal mucosa, typically starting at the junction of the nose

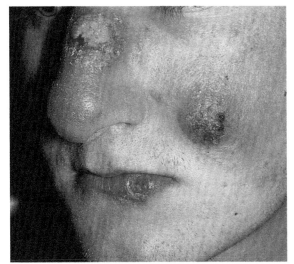

Fig. 5.11 Cutaneous leishmaniasis.

and upper lip. The lips, soft palate, fauces and larynx may also be invaded and destroyed. There is no spontaneous healing, and death may result from severe respiratory tract infections as a result of massive destruction of the pharynx.

Investigations in CL and ML

• Parasitological confirmation of the clinical diagnosis is important. • Slit skin smear: amastigotes identified using Giemsa stain. • Culture: material obtained from sores or fine needle aspiration. • PCR: increasingly used for diagnosis and speciation, especially in ML.

Management of CL and ML

Treatment of CL should be individualised on the basis of the causative organism, severity of the lesions, availability of drugs, tolerance of the patient for toxicity and local resistance patterns.

Topical application of paromomycin 15% plus methylbenzethonium chloride 12% is beneficial in CL. Intralesional antimony is also rapidly effective and generally well tolerated in CL. For CL with multiple lesions and for ML, parenteral Sb (20 mg/kg/day) should be used. CL requires 20 days of systemic Sb; ML is treated for 28 days. Refractory CL or ML should be treated with amphotericin B. Other effective drugs include pentamidine, fluconazole, ketoconazole and itraconazole.

Prevention of CL and ML

Personal protection against sandfly bites is important. No effective vaccine is yet available.

Gastrointestinal protozoal infections

▌Amoebiasis

Amoebiasis is caused by *Entamoeba histolytica*; it is common throughout the tropics and is occasionally acquired in nontropical countries. Infection can give rise to amoebic dysentery or extra-intestinal amoebiasis, for example, amoebic liver abscess.

Clinical Features

Intestinal amoebiasis or amoebic dysentery: Cysts of *E. histolytica* are ingested in water or uncooked food contaminated by human faeces. The parasite invades the mucous membrane of the colon, producing ulceration. The incubation period of amoebiasis ranges from 2 weeks to many years, followed by a chronic course with grumbling abdominal pains (often in the right lower quadrant, mimicking appendicitis) and two or more unformed stools a day. Diarrhoea alternating with constipation is common, as is mucus, sometimes with streaks of blood. There is a dysenteric presentation, with passage of blood and mucus simulating bacillary dysentery or ulcerative colitis, especially in the elderly and those with superadded pyogenic infection.

Amoebic liver abscess: This occurs when trophozoites enter the liver via the portal vein. In the liver, usually the right lobe, they multiply rapidly and destroy the parenchyma, forming an amoebic abscess. Local symptoms of an enlarged, tender liver, cough and pain in the right shoulder are characteristic, but symptoms may remain vague and signs minimal. A high swinging fever without much systemic upset is sometimes seen. A large abscess may rupture through the diaphragm into the lung, and its contents may be coughed up. Rupture into the pleural cavity, the peritoneal cavity or pericardial sac is less common but more serious.

Investigations

• Fresh stool sample: may reveal motile trophozoites on microscopy. • Sigmoidoscopy: typical flask-shaped ulcers may be seen, and should be scraped for microscopy. • Antibodies: detectable by immunofluorescence in 95% of patients with hepatic amoebiasis and intestinal amoeboma, but in only around 60% of cases of dysenteric amoebiasis. • PCR: also sensitive, but not widely available.

In suspected amoebic liver abscess, there may be a neutrophil leucocytosis and a raised right hemidiaphragm on CXR. Confirmation is by liver USS.

Management

Intestinal and early hepatic amoebiasis respond quickly to oral metronidazole (800 mg three times daily for 5–10 days). Diloxanide furoate should be given orally for 10 days after treatment to eliminate luminal cysts. Drainage/aspiration may be required to prevent abscess rupture; this yields characteristic chocolate-brown liquid that rarely contains free amoebae. Surgical drainage is needed if rupture occurs.

▌Giardiasis

Infection with *Giardia lamblia* is found worldwide and is common in the tropics. It particularly affects children, tourists and immunosuppressed individuals, and is the parasite most commonly imported into the UK. The cysts remain viable in water for up to 3 months, and infection occurs by ingesting contaminated water. The parasites attach to the duodenal and jejunal mucosa, causing inflammation.

After an incubation period of 1 to 3 weeks, there is diarrhoea, abdominal pain, weakness, anorexia, nausea and vomiting. Malabsorption with steatorrhoea may develop. Examination may reveal abdominal distension and tenderness. Microscopy of stool or duodenal aspirate reveals cysts. Treatment is with a single dose of tinidazole 2 g, or metronidazole 400 mg three times daily for 10 days.

Cryptosporidiosis

Cyclospora cayetanensis is a globally distributed coccidian protozoal parasite of humans. Infection occurs by ingestion of contaminated water. The incubation period of around 2 to 11 days is followed by diarrhoea and abdominal cramps. The illness is usually self-limiting, but is more severe in immunocompromised patients. Diagnosis is by microscopy or PCR of stool, and treatment, if required, is with cotrimoxazole.

Intestinal nematodes

Adult nematodes in the human gut can cause disease. There are two types:

- hookworms: have a soil stage in which they develop into larvae that then penetrate the host.
- a group of nematodes that survive in the soil merely as eggs, which have to be ingested for their life cycle to continue.

The geographical distribution of hookworms is limited by the larval requirement for warmth and humidity.

Ancylostomiasis (hookworm)

Ancylostomiasis is a leading cause of anaemia in the tropics. The causative organisms are *Ancylostoma duodenale* and *Necator americanus*. The life cycle involves the passage of the hookworm from the soil through the skin via the blood stream to the lungs. The worms ascend the bronchi and are swallowed, with the adult worm inhabiting the duodenum and jejunum. Eggs are passed in faeces, and develop through the larval stage to the filariform infective stage in the soil. Geographic distribution is as follows:
• *A. duodenale*: Far East, Mediterranean coastal regions, Africa. • *N. americanum*: West, East and Central Africa, Central and South America, Far East.

Clinical features
• Cutaneous: allergic dermatitis of the feet at the time of infection. • Pulmonary: paroxysmal cough, blood-stained sputum. • GI: vomiting, epigastric pain, diarrhoea. • Systemic: symptoms of anaemia such as tiredness, malaise, cardiac failure.

Investigations
• Stool sample: ova on microscopy. FOB testing may be positive. • FBC: eosinophilia.

Management

A single dose of albendazole (400 mg) is the treatment of choice. Mebendazole 100 mg twice daily for 3 days is an alternative. Oral iron is effective in anaemic patients.

Strongyloidiasis (threadworm)

Strongyloides stercoralis is a small nematode (2 mm × 0.4 mm). The life cycle involves the passage of the filariform larvae in the soil through the skin to the upper part of the small intestine, where the adult worms live. Eggs hatch in the bowel, and larvae are passed in the faeces. In moist soil, they develop into infective filariform larvae. Autoinfection may lead to chronic disease. It is found in the tropics and subtropics, especially the Far East.

Clinical features

• Cutaneous: itchy rash, urticarial papules and plaques, larva currens (linear urticarial weals on buttocks and abdomen). • GI: diarrhoea, abdominal pain, steatorrhoea, weight loss. • Disseminated infection occurs in the immunosuppressed (e.g. HIV, immunosuppressant treatment), causing abdominal pain, shock, wheeze, cough and neurological symptoms.

Investigations

• Stool sample: microscopy (motile larvae may be seen) and culture. • Jejunal aspirate/string test. • Blood: eosinophilia and antibodies by ELISA.

Management

• Ivermectin (200 µg/kg on two successive days) is the first choice. • Albendazole is an alternative.

Ascaris lumbricoides (roundworm)

This pale yellow nematode is 20 to 35 cm long and causes up to 35% of intestinal obstructions in endemic areas of the tropics. Infection begins with ingestion of mature ova in contaminated food. *Ascaris* larvae hatch in the duodenum, migrate through the lungs, ascend the bronchial tree, are swallowed and mature in the small intestine.

Clinical features

• GI: abdominal pain, severe obstructive complications (particularly at the terminal ileum), intussusception, volvulus, haemorrhagic infarction and perforation. • Hepatobiliary: blockage of the bile or pancreatic duct with worms. • Symptoms attributed to a generalised hypersensitivity reaction caused by tissue migration: pneumonitis, bronchial asthma, urticaria.

Investigations

• Stool sample: adult worms visible; microscopy reveals ova. • FBC: eosinophilia. • Barium studies: occasionally demonstrate worms.

Management

A single dose of albendazole (400 mg) is effective. Alternatives include pyrantel pamoate, ivermectin and mebendazole. Treated patients frequently expel numerous large worms. Intestinal obstruction is treated with nasogastric suction, piperazine and IV fluids, or surgery for complete obstruction.

Enterobius vermicularis (threadworm)

This helminthic infection is common worldwide, especially in children. After the ova are swallowed, the worms develop in the small intestine. Adult worms live in the colon. The adult female lays eggs around the anus, causing intense itching; eggs may be carried on the fingers to the mouth, causing autoinfection.

Clinical features

Intense itch in the perianal or genital area is the most common presenting symptom.

Investigations

Ova may be collected on a strip of adhesive tape applied in the morning to the perianal skin.

Management

• Single dose of mebendazole 100 mg, albendazole 400 mg or piperazine 4 g. Dosing is repeated after 2 weeks to control autoreinfection. • If infection is recurrent, all family members should be treated. • General hygiene measures help to prevent spread: laundering of bedclothes, keeping nails short and clean.

Trichuris trichiura (whipworm)

This is common worldwide with poor hygiene. Infection follows ingestion of ova in contaminated food. Adult worms 3 to 5 cm in length live in the caecum, lower ileum, appendix, colon and anal canal.

Infection is usually asymptomatic; intense infections may cause persistent diarrhoea or rectal prolapse. Diagnosis is by stool microscopy for ova. Treatment involves mebendazole 100 mg twice daily or albendazole for 3 days or 5 to 7 days in heavy infections.

Tissue-dwelling human nematodes

Filarial worms are tissue-dwelling nematodes. The larval stages are inoculated by biting mosquitoes or flies. The larvae develop into adult worms (2–50 cm long), which, after mating, produce millions of microfilariae (170–320 μm long) that migrate in blood or skin, causing a symptomatic immune response. Worms live 10 to 15 years and microfilariae 2 to 3 years. The life cycle is completed when the insect vector ingests microfilariae by biting humans, normally the only host.

Lymphatic filariasis

The causative organisms are Wuchereria bancrofti and Brugia malayi, which have different geographic distributions:
• W. bancrofti: occurs in tropical Africa, coastal areas of North Africa, Asia, Indonesia and northern Australia, the South Pacific islands, the West Indies and North and South America. • B. malayi: affects Indonesia, Borneo, Malaysia, Vietnam, South China, South India and Sri Lanka.

Clinical features

Acute: Filarial lymphangitis presents with fever, pain, tenderness and erythema along the course of inflamed lymphatic vessels. Inflammation of the spermatic cord, epididymitis and orchitis are common. The whole episode lasts a few days but may recur several times a year.

Chronic: Oedema becomes persistent, with regional lymphadenopathy. Progressive enlargement, coarsening, corrugation and fissuring of the skin and subcutaneous tissue develop gradually, causing irreversible 'elephantiasis'. The scrotum may reach an enormous size. Chyluria and chylous effusions are milky and opalescent.

Tropical pulmonary eosinophilia: This may develop when filariae enter pulmonary capillaries, causing a massive allergic response. Mainly seen in India, it presents with cough, wheeze and fever, and may progress to chronic interstitial lung disease.

Investigations

• FBC: massive eosinophilia (higher than other helminthic infections). • Indirect immunofluorescence and ELISA: detects filarial antibodies. • Wet blood film from a nocturnal sample: microfilariae circulate in large numbers at night. • Radiology: calcified filariae may be detected on x-ray.

Management

Diethylcarbamazine (DEC; 6 mg/kg as a single dose) kills microfilariae and adult worms. In the first 24 to 36 hours of therapy, a severe allergic response to dying microfilariae, characterised by fever, headache, nausea, vomiting, arthralgia and prostration, may be seen, and severity is proportional to the filarial load. Antihistamines and oral glucocorticoids may be used to control the symptoms. Chronic lymphoedema should be managed with physiotherapy, tight bandaging and elevation, as well as scrupulous attention to skin care to prevent infection. Surgery is useful in selected cases. DEC can also be used for prophylaxis in endemic areas with a once-yearly dose.

Loiasis

The causative organism is the filaria *Loa*. The adults, 3 to 7 cm × 4 mm, chiefly parasitise the subcutaneous tissue of humans.

Clinical features

The infection is often symptomless. The first sign is usually a Calabar swelling, which is an irritating, tense, localised swelling up to a few centimetres in diameter that develops around an adult worm. The swelling is generally on a limb, and may be particularly painful if near a joint. It usually disappears after a few days, but may persist for 2 or 3 weeks. Other cutaneous signs include urticaria or, rarely, a visible worm wriggling under the skin (especially that of an eyelid) or across the eye under the conjunctiva.

Investigations

• Blood: direct visualisation of microfilariae, eosinophilia. • Immunology: antifilarial antibodies are positive in 95%. • X-rays: may demonstrate a calcified worm.

Management

DEC for 3 weeks is curative, but a febrile reaction to treatment is common, and may require glucocorticoids. Protective clothing and insect repellent prevent inoculation.

Onchocerciasis (river blindness)

The causative organism is *Onchocerca volvulus*; it is transmitted to humans by a bite from the *Simulium* fly. Onchocerciasis is a major cause of blindness in sub-Saharan Africa, Yemen and parts of Central and South America. The worms live for up to 17 years in human tissue. Live microfilariae are poorly immunogenic, but dead ones elicit severe allergic inflammation. Death of microfilariae in the eye may cause blindness.

Clinical features

• May be symptomless for months or years. • Itchy papular urticaria: excoriated papules, patchy hyperpigmentation, thickened, wrinkled skin. • Superficial lymphadenopathy: may become pendulous in the groin. • Firm subcutaneous nodules (onchocercomas): result from fibrosis around adult worms. • Eyes: itch, lacrimation, conjunctivitis, progressing to sclerosing keratitis, 'snowflake' deposits on the cornea, choroidoretinitis and optic neuritis.

Investigations

• Direct microscopy of skin snip/shaving: demonstrates microfilariae. • FBC: eosinophilia. • Slit-lamp–microfilariae in the eye • Filarial antibodies: present in serum in 95% of cases.

Management

Ivermectin (single dose 100–200 µg/kg) kills the microfilariae with minimal toxicity. Dosing is repeated every 3 months to prevent relapses. Prevention measures include the use of protective clothing, population prophylaxis with ivermectin and the use of insecticides to kill the *Simulium* fly.

Dracunculiasis (Guinea worm)

The Guinea worm (*Dracunculus medinensis*) is a tissue-dwelling nematode that is transmitted to humans by the ingestion of the crustacean *Cyclops*, now found only in sub-Saharan Africa. Management is by extraction of the protruding worm (which is over 1 m long) by winding it out gently over several days on a matchstick. The worm must never be broken.

Zoonotic nematodes

Trichinosis (trichinellosis)

Trichinella spiralis is a nematode that parasitises rats and pigs and is transmitted to humans by eating partially cooked, infected pork products. Symptoms result from invasion of intestinal submucosa by ingested larvae, which develop into adult worms, and the secondary invasion of tissues, particularly striated muscle, by fresh larvae produced by these adult worms. Outbreaks may occur wherever pork is eaten.

Clinical features

Light infection may be asymptomatic. Heavy infection causes nausea and diarrhoea 24 to 48 hours after the infected meal. Larval invasion on day 4 to 5 produces fever and oedema of the face, eyelids and conjunctivae. Larval invasion of muscle produces myositis. Larval migration may cause acute myocarditis and encephalitis.

Investigations

• Muscle biopsy: microscopy may demonstrate encysted larvae. • Public health investigations: may reveal a cluster of cases who have eaten infected pork from a common source.

Management

Albendazole (400 mg twice daily for 8–14 days) kills newly formed adult worms. Glucocorticoids are required to counteract the effects of acute inflammation.

Cutaneous larva migrans

Larvae of the dog hookworm (*Ancylostoma caninum*) migrate 2 to 3 cm per day across the skin, causing intense itch and a linear serpiginous track. Treatment is with topical 15% thiabendazole or systemic albendazole.

Trematodes (flukes)

These leaf-shaped worms are parasitic to humans and animals. Their complex life cycles may involve one or more intermediate hosts, often freshwater molluscs.

Schistosomiasis

Schistosomiasis is a major cause of morbidity in the tropics, and is being spread by irrigation schemes. The five species commonly causing humans disease are: *Schistosoma haematobium*, *S. mansoni*, *S. japonicum*, *S. mekongi* and *S. intercalatum*. The life cycle of *Schistosoma* is illustrated in Fig. 5.12. The human is the definitive host, and the freshwater snail is the intermediate host. Infection can be acquired after a brief exposure, such as swimming in freshwater lakes in Africa.

Clinical features

These vary between species and are dependent on the stage of infection. After a symptom-free period of 3 to 5 weeks, the acute presentation (Katayama syndrome) is with fever, urticaria, muscle aches, abdominal pain and cough. Chronic schistosomiasis is caused by egg deposition, months to years after infection. Painless terminal haematuria is commonest symptom with *S. haematobium*. Urinary frequency, infections and renal failure may develop later. *S. mansoni* and *S. japonicum* mainly pass through the wall of the bowel or are carried to the liver. Diarrhoea with mucus and blood is common. A summary of the symptoms of schistosomiasis as they correlate with the stage and type of infection is given in Box 5.20.

Investigations

Blood tests show eosinophilia. Serology (ELISA) aids screening but remains positive after treatment.

    S. haematobium: Dipstick urine testing demonstrates blood and albumin. Microscopy of a centrifuged terminal urine sample shows eggs. USS may demonstrate bladder wall thickening, hydronephrosis and bladder calcification. Cystoscopy reveals 'sandy' patches, bleeding mucosa and later distortion.

5

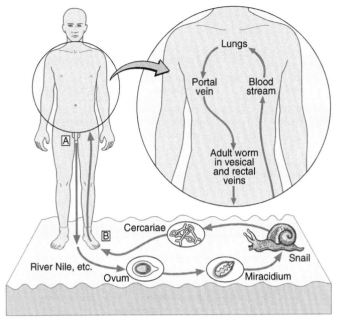

Fig. 5.12 Life cycle of *Schistosoma*. (A) Ova are passed into fresh water in urine and faeces. (B) Cercariae in fresh water penetrate the skin of bathers, infecting a new host.

***S. mansoni* and *S. japonicum*:** Stool microscopy demonstrates the characteristic egg with its lateral spine. Rectal biopsy may demonstrate schistosomes. Sigmoidoscopy may show inflammation or bleeding.

Management
Praziquantel (dose depending on species) is the drug of choice for schistosomiasis, producing parasitological cure in 80% of individuals. Side effects are uncommon but include nausea and abdominal pain. Surgery may be required for ureteric stricture or bladder thickening.

Liver flukes

Liver flukes infect at least 20 million people and remain an important public health problem in endemic areas. They are associated with abdominal pain, hepatomegaly and relapsing cholangitis. *Clonorchis sinensis* and *Opisthorchis felineus* are major causes of bile duct cancer.

Cestodes (tapeworms)

Cestodes are ribbon-shaped worms that inhabit the intestinal tract of humans who have ingested undercooked beef, pork or fish infected

i	**5.20 Clinical pathology of schistosomiasis**		
Stage	Time	*Schistosoma haematobium*	*S. mansoni* and *S. japonicum*
Cercarial penetration	Days	Papular dermatitis at site of penetration	As for *S. haematobium*
Larval migration and maturation	Weeks	Pneumonitis; myositis; hepatitis; fever; 'serum sickness'; eosinophilia; seroconversion	As for *S. haematobium*
Early egg deposition	Months	Cystitis; haematuria; ectopic granulomatous lesions: skin, CNS; immune complex glomerulonephritis	Colitis; granulomatous hepatitis; acute portal hypertension; ectopic lesions as for *S. haematobium*
Late egg deposition	Years	Fibrosis and calcification of ureters, bladder: bacterial infection, calculi, hydronephrosis, carcinoma; pulmonary granulomas and pulmonary hypertension	Colonic polyposis and strictures; periportal fibrosis; portal hypertension; pulmonary features as for *S. haematobium*

with *Taenia saginata*, *T. solium* or *Diphyllobothrium latum*, respectively. Tapeworms cause two distinct patterns of disease: intestinal infection and systemic cysticercosis. Some tapeworms, for example, *T. saginata* and *D. latum*, cause only intestinal infection, whereas *T. solium* can cause intestinal infection or cysticercosis, and *Echinococcus granulosus* causes only systemic infection (hydatid disease).

Intestinal tapeworm

T. solium is common in Central Europe, South Africa, South America and parts of Asia, whereas *T. saginata* occurs worldwide. Adult *T. saginata* worms may be several metres long. Infection is diagnosed by finding ova or segments in the stool and is treated with praziquantel. Prevention depends on efficient meat inspection and thorough cooking of meat.

Cysticercosis

Human cysticercosis is acquired either by ingesting *T. solium* ova on contaminated fingers (faecal–oral route) or by eating undercooked, contaminated pork (Fig. 5.13). The larvae emerge from eggs in the stomach, penetrate the intestinal mucosa and are carried to subcutaneous tissue, skeletal muscles and brain, where they develop and form cysticerci, 0.5 to 1 cm cysts containing the head of a young worm.

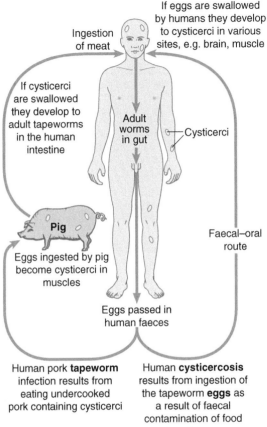

Fig. 5.13 Cysticercosis: life cycle of *Taenia solium*.

Clinical features

There are palpable subcutaneous nodules that may calcify. Infection of the cerebral tissue may cause personality change, epilepsy, hydrocephalus or encephalitis.

Investigations

Biopsy of a subcutaneous nodule may demonstrate cysticerci. CT/MRI will demonstrate cerebral cysts. X-rays of muscles may show calcified cysts. Antibody detection is available for serodiagnosis.

Management and prevention

Albendazole (15 mg/kg daily for at least 8 days) is the drug of choice for parenchymal neurocysticercosis. Praziquantel is another option.

Prednisolone is also given for 14 days. Seizures should be controlled with anticonvulsants.

◼ *Echinococcus granulosus (Taenia echinococcus)* and hydatid disease

Dogs are the definitive hosts of the tiny tapeworm *E. granulosus*; ova produced by the adult worms inhabiting the dog are ingested by intermediate hosts, which include sheep, cattle, camels and humans. The embryo is liberated from the ovum in the small intestine and invades the blood stream, spreading to the liver. The resultant cyst grows very slowly, sometimes intermittently, and may outlive the patient. It may calcify or rupture, giving rise to multiple cysts. The disease is common in the Middle East, North and East Africa, Australia and Argentina. Foci of infection persist in rural Wales and Scotland.

Clinical features
Hydatid disease is typically acquired in childhood; it causes cysts in the liver (75% of cases), lung, bone or brain. Symptoms are slow to develop and are a result of local pressure.

Investigations
USS or CT usually demonstrates the cyst. Serology is positive in 70% to 90% of cases.

Management and prevention
Surgical excision is the treatment of choice, with praziquantel administered peri-operatively to kill protoscolices. Albendazole should also be used, and may be combined effectively with aspiration. Good personal hygiene and animal handling practices, as well as deworming of dogs, can reduce disease prevalence.

Fungal infections

Superficial fungal infections of the skin are described in Chapter 18.

Subcutaneous mycoses

◼ Chromoblastomycosis

Chromoblastomycosis is a tropical fungal disease of the cutaneous and subcutaneous tissue. The usual cause is *Fonsecaea pedrosoi*, and the disease is inoculated by trauma, particularly in those walking barefoot. Lesions may start several months after the injury in the form of a papule, which later turns into an irregular plaque. Later there may be hypertrophy of the tissue, leading to a characteristic cauliflower-like appearance.

Investigations
Biopsy shows pigmented, rounded sclerotic bodies. Culture confirms the aetiological agent.

Management
• Oral itraconazole or terbinafine. • Cryosurgery with liquid nitrogen.

Mycetoma (eumycetoma and actinomycetoma)

Mycetoma is a chronic suppurative infection of the deep soft tissues and bones, occurring mainly in the tropics. The limbs are most commonly affected. It is caused by either the filamentous fungus Eumyces (eumycetoma, 40%) or by aerobic Actinomycetes (60%, actinomycetoma). Both groups produce characteristically coloured grains (microcolonies), the colour depending on the organism.

Clinical features

The causative organism is usually introduced by a thorn, and most commonly affects the foot (Madura foot). Mycetoma begins as a painless swelling at the implantation site, which grows and spreads steadily within the soft tissues, causing further swelling and eventually penetrating bones. Nodules develop under the epidermis and rupture, revealing sinuses through which grains are discharged. Deeper tissue invasion and bone involvement are less rapid and extensive in eumycetoma than in actinomycetoma. There is little pain and usually no fever or lymphadenopathy, but there is progressive disability.

Investigations

Biopsy/aspiration of pus should be sent for microscopy, culture and determination of sensitivity.

Management

• Eumycetes: surgery plus ketoconazole or itraconazole. • Actinomycetes: prolonged antibiotics—usually streptomycin and dapsone. • Surgical amputation may be required in severe cases.

Sporotrichosis

Sporotrichosis is caused by *Sporothrix schenckii*. It presents as a localised subcutaneous nodule at the site of inoculation (often a thorn scratch), which subsequently ulcerates with a pustular discharge (fixed cutaneous). The disease may then spread along the cutaneous lymphatic channels, forming multiple cutaneous nodules that ulcerate and discharge (lymphocutaneous). Pulmonary involvement occurs but is rare.

Investigations

Biopsies should be sent for microscopy and culture.

Management

• Oral itraconazole for cutaneous and lymphocutaneous disease. • Amphotericin B for systemic life-threatening illness.

Systemic mycoses

Aspergillosis

This is primarily respiratory and is described in Chapter 9.

Candidiasis

The species of *Candida* most commonly involved in human disease is *C. albicans*. Other species increasingly implicated are *C. tropicalis*, *C. glabrata* and *C. krusei*. Infection is most common in the immunosuppressed, particularly neutropenic patients, as neutrophils form the body's main defence against *Candida*. The source of infection is usually endogenous, originating in flora in the patient's oropharyngeal and genital areas, commonly producing oropharyngeal or vaginal candidiasis or 'thrush'.

Systemic *Candida* infection may be acute or chronic:

Acute disseminated candidiasis: Usually presents as candidaemia, often in the presence of a central venous catheter. Recent abdominal surgery, antibiotics, total parenteral nutrition and IV drug misuse predispose to candidaemia. Up to 40% have ophthalmic involvement, with 'cotton wool' retinal exudates progressing to vitreous haze and threatening sight.

Chronic disseminated (hepatosplenic) candidiasis: Presents in neutropenic patients as persistent fever despite antibacterial therapy. There is abdominal pain and elevated alkaline phosphatase, and multiple lesions are seen in the liver and spleen on imaging. This infection may last for months despite therapy.

Management

Infection detected on blood culture must be treated aggressively. Indwelling catheters should be removed. Treatments for candidaemia include an echinocandin, amphotericin B, voriconazole and fluconazole.

Cryptococcosis

This is found worldwide and is caused by *Cryptococcus neoformans* and *C. gattii*. The former causes opportunistic infection, most commonly in those with HIV, whereas the latter causes severe disease in immunocompetent hosts. Spread is by inhalation. Disseminated cryptococcal infection mainly affects the immunocompromised. CNS manifestations include meningitis and cryptococcoma. Pulmonary cryptococcus can present as severe pneumonia in the immunocompromised, or as cavitating nodules in patients with lesser immunosuppression.

Diagnosis is by biopsy and/or culture. Treatment is with IV antifungal agents such as amphotericin B. Recovery may be monitored by a fall in antigen titres.

Mild pulmonary disease is treated with fluconazole or resection of nodules.

Other systemic mycoses affecting patients with severe immunosuppression include fusariosis and mucormycosis. Both are rare but serious and require treatment with IV amphotericin B or posaconazole.

Histoplasmosis

Histoplasmosis is caused by *Histoplasma capsulatum* var. *capsulatum* and is found in all parts of the United States, especially in the east central states. A variant, *H. capsulatum* var. *duboisii*, is found in parts of tropical Africa. *H. capsulatum* multiplies in soil enriched by the droppings of birds and bats. Infection is by inhalation of infected dust.

Clinical features

Histoplasma infection is usually asymptomatic or self-limiting. Pulmonary symptoms may include fever, nonproductive cough, pleuritic pain and an influenza-like illness. Erythema nodosum, myalgia and joint pain frequently occur. *H. capsulatum* var. *duboisii* usually spares the lungs, but can cause cutaneous ulcers and destructive bone lesions. On examination, lymphadenopathy, hepatosplenomegaly, rashes and pulmonary crackles may be found.

Investigations

• Biopsy: tissue should be sent for smear, histology and culture. • CXR: may show soft infiltrates, cavitating or calcified nodules and hilar lymphadenopathy. • Antigen or antibody detection in blood.

Management

• IV amphotericin B in severe infection. • Itraconazole for chronic infection.
• Glucocorticoids may be added initially in severe pulmonary disease.

Coccidioidomycosis

This is caused by the airborne organisms *Coccidioides immitis* and *C. posadasii*, and is found in Central and South America. It is acquired by inhalation and is asymptomatic in 60%. In others it affects the lungs, lymph nodes and skin. In immunocompromised patients, adrenal and meningeal spread occurs. Pulmonary coccidioidomycosis has two forms:

Primary coccidioidomycosis: If symptomatic, causes cough, fever, dyspnoea and rashes.

Progressive coccidioidomycosis: Systemic upset and lobar pneumonia; may mimic TB. Diagnosis is by complement fixation and precipitin tests, and treatment is with antifungal azoles, or amphotericin B in severe disease.

Paracoccidioidomycosis

This is caused by *Paracoccidioides brasiliensis* and occurs in South America. Mucocutaneous lesions occur early. It affects the lungs, mucous membranes, skin, lymph nodes and adrenal glands. Treatment is with oral itraconazole.

Blastomycosis

This is caused by *Blastomyces dermatitidis* and occurs in parts of North America and occasionally in Africa. Systemic infection begins in the lungs and mediastinal lymph nodes and resembles pulmonary TB. Bones, skin and the genitourinary tract may also be affected. Treatment is with itraconazole or amphotericin B.

Sexually transmitted bacterial infections

Syphilis

Syphilis is caused by infection, through abrasions in the skin or mucous membranes, with the spirochaete *Treponema pallidum*. In adults the infection is usually sexually acquired; however, transmission by kissing, blood transfusion and percutaneous injury has been reported. Transplacental infection of the fetus can occur.

Primary syphilis: The incubation period is usually between 14 and 28 days, with a range of 9 to 90 days. The primary lesion or chancre develops at the site of infection, usually in the genital area. A dull red macule develops, becomes papular and then erodes to form an indurated, painless ulcer (chancre) with associated inguinal lymphadenopathy. Without treatment, the chancre will resolve within 2 to 6 weeks to leave a thin, atrophic scar.

Secondary syphilis: This occurs 6 to 8 weeks after the development of the chancre when treponemes disseminate to produce a multisystem disease. Constitutional features such as mild fever, malaise and headache are common. Over 75% of patients present with a maculopapular rash on the trunk and limbs that may later involve the palms and soles. Generalised nontender lymphadenopathy is present in more than 50% of patients. Mucosal lesions, known as mucous patches, may affect the genitalia, mouth, pharynx or larynx, and are essentially modified papules, which become eroded. Rarely, confluence produces characteristic 'snail track ulcers' in the mouth.

Tertiary syphilis: This may develop between 3 and 10 years after infection. The characteristic feature is a chronic granulomatous lesion called a gumma, which may be single or multiple and can affect skin, mucosa, bone, muscles or viscera. Resolution of active disease should follow treatment, although some tissue damage may be permanent.

After several years, cardiovascular syphilis, particularly aortitis with aortic incompetence, angina and aneurysm, and neurosyphilis, with meningovascular disease, tabes dorsalis or general paralysis of the insane, may develop.

Congenital syphilis: This is rare where antenatal serological screening is practised. Antisyphilitic treatment in pregnancy treats the fetus, if infected, as well as the mother. Treponemal infection in pregnancy may result in:

• Miscarriage or stillbirth. • A syphilitic baby (a very sick baby with hepatosplenomegaly and a bullous rash). • A baby who develops signs of congenital syphilis (condylomata lata, oral/anal/genital fissures, 'snuffles', lymphadenopathy and hepatosplenomegaly).

Diagnosis is by identification of the organism in smears from lesions, or by testing serum for IgG or IgM treponemal antibodies. Older nonspecific serological tests such as the VDRL can yield false positives in infectious mononucleosis, chickenpox and malaria.

The treatment of choice is penicillin by injection, which sometimes precipitates an acute febrile reaction (Jarich-Herxheimer reaction).

Gonorrhoea

Gonorrhoea is caused by infection with *Neisseria gonorrhoeae*. and may involve columnar epithelium in the lower genital tract, rectum, pharynx and eyes. Transmission is usually the result of vaginal, anal or oral sex. The incubation period is usually 2 to 10 days.

In men, the anterior urethra is commonly infected, causing urethral discharge and dysuria, but symptoms are absent in around 10% of cases.

Epididymo-orchitis may occur. In women, the urethra, para-urethral glands/ducts, Bartholin's glands/ducts or endocervical canal may be infected, but 80% are asymptomatic. Acute PID (see later) is a rare complication. The rectum may also be involved, either because of contamination from a urogenital site or as a result of anal sex.

Gram-negative intracellular diplococci are seen on direct smears from infected sites. Antibiotic resistance complicates treatment. The UK recommendation has changed to intramuscular ceftriaxone 500 mg given with an oral dose of azithromycin 1 g, in the hope that combination therapy will slow down the development of cephalosporin resistance.

Chlamydial infection

Chlamydia is transmitted and presents in a similar way to gonorrhoea.

In men, urethral symptoms are usually mild and occur in less than 50% of cases. Epididymo-orchitis may occur. In women, the cervix and urethra are commonly involved. Infection is asymptomatic in around 80% of women, but may cause vaginal discharge, dysuria, intermenstrual and/or postcoital bleeding. Lower abdominal pain, dyspareunia and intermenstrual bleeding suggest complicating PID. Examination may reveal mucopurulent cervicitis, contact bleeding from the cervix, evidence of PID or no obvious clinical signs. PID, with the risk of tubal damage and subsequent infertility or ectopic pregnancy, is an important long-term complication. Treatment options for chlamydia include a single 1-g oral dose of azithromycin, although PID requires more prolonged treatment.

Sexually transmitted viral infections

Herpes simplex

Genital herpes simplex transmission is usually sexual (vaginal, anal, orogenital or oroanal), but perinatal infection of the neonate may also occur. The manifestations of herpes simplex infection are covered on p. 124.

Human papilloma virus and anogenital warts

Of the many subtypes of HPV, genotypes 6, 11, 16 and 18 most commonly infect the genital tract through sexual transmission.

Genotypes HPV-6 and 11 cause benign anogenital warts. Genotypes such as 16 and 18 are associated with dysplastic conditions and cancers, but not benign warts. Anogenital warts are the result of HPV-driven hyperplasia, and usually develop after an incubation period of between 3 months and 2 years. Local treatment with cryotherapy or podophyllotoxin may help, and condoms offer some protection. Vaccines are highly effective in preventing cervical neoplasia and are in routine use in several countries.

HIV infection

AIDS is caused by HIV-1 and was first recognised in 1981. HIV-2 causes a similar but less aggressive illness occurring mainly in West Africa. AIDS has become the second leading cause of disease worldwide and the leading cause of death in Africa (causing >20% of deaths). Immune deficiency arises from continuous HIV replication leading to virus- and immune-mediated destruction of CD4 lymphocytes.

Global epidemic and regional patterns

In 2015, the WHO estimated that there were 36.7 million people living with HIV/AIDS, 2.1 million new infections and 1.1 million deaths. The epidemiology of HIV has changed with use of combination ART, which reached 17 million people in 2015: AIDS-related deaths have almost halved since 2005, new infections have decreased by 40% since 1997, and the population living with HIV has increased. Regions differ in prevalence, incidence and mode of transmission. In southern Africa, average life expectancy fell below 40 years before the introduction of ART.

HIV is transmitted by sexual contact, by exposure to blood and blood products (e.g. injection drug use, occupational exposure in health-care workers) or to infants of HIV-infected mothers (who may be infected in utero, perinatally or via breastfeeding). Worldwide, the major route of transmission is heterosexual. The risk of contracting HIV after exposure to infected body fluid depends on the integrity of the exposed site, the type and volume of fluid and the level of viraemia in the source. The transmission risk after exposure is given in Box 5.21.

5.21 Risk of HIV transmission after single exposure to an HIV-infected source	
HIV exposure	Approximate risk
Sexual intercourse	
Vaginal: female to male	0.05%
male to female	0.1%
Anal: insertive	0.05%
receptive	0.5%
Oral: insertive	0.005%
receptive	0.01%
Blood exposure	
Transfusion	90%
IV drug user sharing needle	0.67%
Percutaneous needle stick	0.3%
Mucous membrane splash	0.09%
Mother to child	
Vaginal delivery	15%
Breastfeeding (per month)	0.5%

A high proportion of patients with haemophilia had been infected through contaminated blood products by the time HIV antibody screening was adopted in the United States and Europe in 1985. Screening of blood products has virtually eliminated this as a mode of transmission in developed countries; however, the WHO estimates that 5% to 10% of blood transfusions globally are with HIV-infected blood.

Virology and immunology

HIV is an enveloped RNA retrovirus of the lentivirus family. It infects cells bearing the CD4 receptor; these are T-helper lymphocytes, monocyte-macrophages, dendritic cells and microglial cells in the CNS. A small percentage of T-helper lymphocytes enter a postintegration latent phase and represent sanctuary sites from antiretroviral drugs, which only act on replicating virus. This prevents current ART from eradicating HIV. Latently infected CD4 cells also evade CD8 cytotoxic T lymphocytes.

Diagnosis and initial testing

HIV infection is detected by testing for host antibodies; most tests are sensitive to antibodies to both HIV-1 and HIV-2. Global trends are towards more widespread testing, but in the UK testing is still targeted at high-risk groups (Box 5.22). Counselling is essential both before testing and after the result is obtained.

 5.22 Patients who should be offered HIV testing in the UK

Patients attending services for:
  Sexually transmitted infection
  Drug dependency
  Pregnancy termination
  Hepatitis B or C, lymphoma or TB
Patients who:
  Have symptoms suggesting HIV or for which HIV is a possible diagnosis
  Request testing for sexually transmitted infection
  Are from a country/group with high HIV prevalence
  Are men or trans women who have sex with men
  Disclose high-risk sexual practices, for example, 'chemsex'
  Use injected drugs
  Have sexual contacts who are HIV-positive, at high risk of HIV or come from a country
    with high HIV prevalence
New prison inmates

N.B.: Exclude those already known to be HIV positive. In areas of high and extremely high prevalence, testing should be considered at every encounter in primary and secondary care.

Following diagnosis, the CD4 lymphocyte count should be determined. This indicates the degree of immune suppression and is used to guide treatment. Counts between 200 and 500/mm^3 have a low risk of major opportunistic infection; below 200/mm^3 there is a high risk of AIDS-defining conditions. Quantitative PCR of HIV-RNA, known as viral load, is used to monitor the response to ART.

Clinical manifestations of HIV

Primary HIV infection

Primary infection is symptomatic in more than 50% of cases, and usually occurs 2 to 4 weeks after exposure. Many of the clinical manifestations resemble infectious mononucleosis:

- Fever.
- Pharyngitis with lymphadenopathy.
- Myalgia/arthralgia.
- Headache.
- Diarrhoea.

The presence, in addition, of a maculopapular rash or oral and genital ulceration suggests HIV rather than infectious mononucleosis. Lymphopenia with oropharyngeal candidiasis may occur. Symptoms seldom last longer than 2 weeks. In many patients the illness is mild and is only identified by retrospective enquiry.

Diagnosis is made by detecting HIV-RNA in the serum by PCR, as seroconversion to positive anti-HIV antibodies takes 2 to 12 weeks after the development of symptoms. This 'window period' of false negative antibody tests is prolonged if postexposure prophylaxis is used.

The differential diagnosis includes:

- EBV.
- CMV.
- Streptococcal pharyngitis.
- Toxoplasmosis.
- Secondary syphilis.

Asymptomatic infection

This lasts for a variable period, during which the infected individual remains well with no evidence of disease, except for persistent generalised lymphadenopathy (defined as enlarged glands at two extra-inguinal sites at least). Viraemia peaks during this phase, and high viral loads predict a more rapid rate of decline in CD4 count (Fig. 5.14). The median time from infection to development of AIDS in adults is 9 years.

Minor HIV-associated disorders

A wide range of disorders indicating some impairment of cellular immunity occurs in most patients before they develop AIDS. Careful examination of the mouth is important, as oral candidiasis and oral hairy leucoplakia are common conditions that require the initiation of prophylaxis against opportunistic infections, irrespective of the CD4 count.

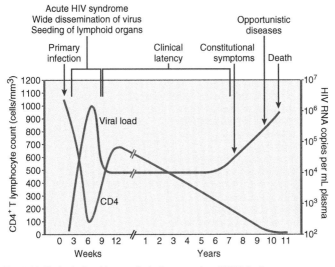

Fig. 5.14 Virological and immunological progression of HIV infection.

AIDS

AIDS is defined by the development of specified opportunistic infections, tumours and other features of advanced HIV (CDC category C or WHO stage 4 disease, Box 5.23).

Presenting problems in HIV infection

The CD4 count is useful in differential diagnosis (Box 5.24). For example, with a pulmonary infiltrate and a CD4 count of 350 cells/mm³, tuberculosis is likely and PJP very unlikely, but if the CD4 count is 50 cells/mm³, both PJP and tuberculosis are likely.

Lymphadenopathy

Lymphadenopathy in HIV can be attributed to asymptomatic infection (see previously), malignancy (Kaposi's sarcoma or lymphoma) or infections, especially TB. Enlarging lymph nodes should undergo needle biopsy for mycobacterial stain and culture and cytology for lymphoma.

Weight loss

HIV wasting syndrome is an AIDS-defining condition comprising 10% weight loss and either chronic diarrhoea or chronic weakness with unexplained fever. Infections, painful oral conditions and depression should be excluded before diagnosis.

5.23 Clinical features of advanced HIV infection (CDC category C/WHO stage 4); AIDS

Candidiasis of oesophagus, trachea, bronchi or lungs
Cervical carcinoma—invasive
Cryptococcosis—extrapulmonary
Cryptosporidiosis, chronic
Cytomegalovirus disease outside liver, spleen and nodes
Herpes simplex chronic ulcers or visceral
HIV encephalopathy or wasting syndrome
Cystoisosporiasis, chronic
Kaposi's sarcoma
Lymphoma (cerebral or B-cell non-Hodgkin's)
Mycobacterial infection, nontuberculous, extrapulmonary or disseminated
Mycosis—disseminated endemic (e.g. coccidioidomycosis, histoplasmosis)
Pneumocystis jirovecii pneumonia
Pneumonia, recurrent bacterial
Progressive multifocal leucoencephalopathy
Toxoplasmosis—cerebral
Tuberculosis
Sepsis, recurrent
Symptomatic HIV-associated nephropathy or cardiomyopathy[a]
Leishmaniasis, atypical disseminated[a]

[a]*World Health Organisation criteria, not Centers for Disease Control and Prevention*

 5.24 Correlations between CD4 count and HIV-associated diseases

<500 cells/mm³

- TB, bacterial pneumonia, herpes zoster, oropharyngeal candidiasis, nontyphoid salmonellosis, Kaposi's sarcoma, non-Hodgkin's lymphoma, HIV-associated idiopathic thrombocytopenic purpura

<200 cells/mm³

- PJP, chronic herpes simplex ulcers, oesophageal candidiasis, *Cystisospora belli* diarrhoea, HIV wasting syndrome, HIV-associated dementia, peripheral neuropathy, endemic mycoses

<100 cells/mm³

- Cerebral toxoplasmosis, cryptococcal meningitis, cryptosporidiosis and microsporidiosis, primary CNS lymphoma, CMV, disseminated MAI, progressive multifocal leucoencephalopathy

Fever

Fever is a very common presenting feature. Nontyphoid *Salmonella* bacteraemia can present with fever without diarrhoea. PUO in HIV should be investigated with abdominal CT, which may reveal lymphadenopathy or splenic microabscesses, suggesting tuberculosis. Bone marrow should be sampled if there are cytopenias. TB or disseminated MAI are common underlying causes of fever.

Mucocutaneous disease

HIV-associated skin diseases include:

Psoriasis and drug rashes: Exacerbated by HIV.

Seborrhoeic dermatitis: Scaly patches in skin folds. Fungal infection contributes.

Herpes simplex: May affect the nasolabial and anogenital regions. Ulcers lasting more than 4 weeks are AIDS-defining.

Herpes zoster: Usually presents with a dermatomal vesicular rash on an erythematous base. In advanced disease it may be multidermatomal, with a high risk of postherpetic neuralgia.

Kaposi's sarcoma: (Fig. 5.15) A lympho-endothelial tumour attributed to sexually transmitted herpesvirus 8. Predominantly affects men, and presents with red-purple papular or nodular mucocutaneous lesions. May spread to lymph nodes, lungs and the GI tract. Chemotherapy is reserved for those who fail to improve on ART.

Bacillary angiomatosis: An infection caused by *Bartonella* bacteria. Causes red-purple skin lesions. May become disseminated with fevers, lymphadenopathy and hepatosplenomegaly.

Oral Candida infection: Very common in HIV, and nearly always caused by *C. albicans*. Treatment is with an oral azole drug.

Oral hairy leucoplakia: Corrugated white plaques running vertically on the side of the tongue; virtually pathognomonic of HIV. It is usually asymptomatic and is attributed to EBV.

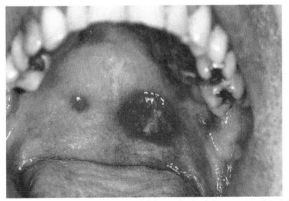

Fig. 5.15 Oral Kaposi's sarcoma. A full examination is important to detect disease that may affect the palate, gums, fauces or tongue.

Gastrointestinal disease

Oesophageal candidiasis: Causes dysphagia. Concomitant oral candidiasis is usual. Systemic fluconazole is usually curative.

Large-bowel diarrhoea: Usually caused by *Campylobacter*, *Shigella* or *Salmonella*. CMV colitis may occur in those with CD4 counts less than 100/mm³.

Small-bowel diarrhoea: Presents with watery diarrhoea and wasting without fever and may be attributed to HIV enteropathy or have an infective cause—typically, cryptosporidiosis, microsporidiosis, cystoisosporiasis or disseminated mycobacterium avium complex.

Hepatobiliary disease

Because of shared risk factors, co-infection of HIV patients with HBV and/or HCV is common, particularly in injection drug users and patients with haemophilia. In both HBV and HCV infection, HIV increases viraemia and also the risk of hepatic fibrosis and hepatoma. During treatment, a flare of hepatitis may be seen with immune recovery.

Hepatitis B: Treatment with anti-HBV drugs is indicated in all those with active HBV replication, hepatitis or fibrosis. HBV co-infection increases the risk of antiretroviral hepatotoxicity.

Hepatitis C: Treatment for HCV should be deferred in patients with CD4 counts less than 200 cells/mm³ until they are stable on ART. Response to anti-HCV therapy is similar to that in HIV-negative patients, but drug interactions with ART are common.

HIV cholangiopathy: A sclerosing cholangitis may occur in patients with severe immune suppression. Co-infection with CMV, cryptosporidiosis and microsporidiosis may be present. ERCP with cautery may be needed, and ART may also improve this condition.

Respiratory disease

Respiratory admissions in HIV patients are most frequently as a result of bacterial pneumonia, PJP (in high-income countries) or TB (in low-income countries).

Pneumocystis jirovecii pneumonia

Clinical features include:
• Progressive dyspnoea. • Dry cough. • Fever. • Exercise-induced desaturation. • Arterial hypoxaemia. • Impaired gas transfer. • Raised LDH (from lung damage). • Pneumothorax.

Auscultation is unremarkable, and the CXR may be normal in early disease (15%–20%), but classically shows perihilar ground-glass infiltrates. Induced sputum is a sensitive diagnostic test. Co-trimoxazole is used for treatment and prophylaxis. Glucocorticoids are useful if there is hypoxia.

Pulmonary tuberculosis

TB is the most common cause of admission in countries with a high TB incidence. The presentation depends on immune function. When the CD4 count is greater than 200 cells/mm^3, disease is more likely to be reactivated, upper-lobe, open cavitary disease. As immunosuppression increases, the clinical pattern changes:

• Disease progresses more rapidly. • X-ray appearances become atypical, with lymphadenopathy or effusions rather than apical cavitation. • Sputum smears are often negative in the absence of cavitation. • Many patients have disseminated disease with miliary shadowing, or infiltrates along with pleural or lymph node disease. TB in HIV responds well to standard short-course therapy (p. 311).

Bacterial infections: Bacterial pneumonia (p. 311) is common in HIV.

Nervous system and eye disease

Cognitive impairment: HIV invades the nervous system early, and meningo-encephalitis may occur at seroconversion. Neuropsychiatric tests may reveal neurocognitive disorders ranging from asymptomatic impairment to dementia. HIV-associated dementia is associated with cerebral atrophy on CT or MRI, but usually responds to ART. Progressive multifocal leucoencephalopathy is a fatal demyelinating disease caused by the JC virus; it presents with stroke-like episodes and cognitive impairment. Vision is often affected. The presence of JC-DNA in CSF is diagnostic. No specific treatment exists, and the prognosis is poor. CMV encephalitis may also cause cognitive impairment, and responds poorly to treatment.

Space-occupying lesions: *Toxoplasma* infection (p. 154) is the most common cause. Cerebral toxoplasmosis is caused by reactivation of residual *Toxoplasma gondii* cysts from past infection. Imaging reveals multiple ring-enhancing space-occupying lesions with surrounding oedema. Diagnosis is by imaging supported by serology. Treatment is with sulfadiazine and pyrimethamine, although co-trimoxazole may also be effective, with improvement in 1 to 2 weeks and shrinkage of lesions in 2 to 4 weeks. Primary CNS lymphomas are high-grade B-cell lymphomas associated with EBV infection. Imaging typically shows a single enhancing periventricular lesion with surrounding oedema. If lumbar puncture can be safely performed, EBV-DNA can be demonstrated by PCR. Treatment is usually palliative, with dexamethasone and symptom relief. The prognosis is poor. Tuberculoma is identified by lesions resembling toxoplasmosis on imaging. CSF shows features of tuberculous meningitis (p. 633).

Stroke: Atherosclerosis is enhanced by HIV and by some antiretroviral drugs. HIV can also cause vasculitis. The result is an increased incidence of stroke in patients with HIV.

Meningitis: *Cryptococcus neoformans* is the most common cause of meningitis in AIDS patients. It presents subacutely with headache, vomiting and decreased level of consciousness. Neck stiffness is often absent (<50%). CSF cryptococcal antigen tests have sensitivity and specificity close to 100%, whereas CSF protein, cell counts and glucose may be normal. Treatment is 2 weeks of amphotericin B followed by fluconazole. Tuberculous meningitis is also common and presents in a similar way to that in patients without HIV.

Peripheral nerve disease: HIV causes axonal degeneration, resulting in a sensorimotor peripheral neuropathy in about one-third of AIDS patients.

Myelopathy and radiculopathy: Myelopathy most commonly results from tuberculous spondylitis. Vacuolar myelopathy causes paraparesis in advanced HIV disease. CMV polyradiculitis causes painful legs, flaccid paraparesis, saddle anaesthesia and sphincter dysfunction. Functional recovery is poor despite ganciclovir treatment.

Retinopathy: CMV retinitis causes painless, progressive visual loss in patients with severe immunosuppression. Haemorrhages and exudates are seen on the retina. Treatment with ganciclovir or valganciclovir may halt progression but does not restore lost vision. The eyes may also be affected by toxoplasmosis or varicella zoster infection. In addition, immune recovery with ART sometimes causes uveitis.

Rheumatological problems

HIV can cause seronegative arthritis resembling rheumatoid arthritis, or it can exacerbate reactive arthritis.

Diffuse infiltrative lymphocytosis syndrome is a benign lymphocytic tissue infiltration that commonly presents with bilateral parotid swelling and lymphadenopathy. Hepatitis, arthritis and polymyositis may occur. Treatment is with glucocorticoids and ART, but the response is variable.

Haematological problems

Normochromic normocytic anaemia and thrombocytopenia are common in advanced HIV. Antiretroviral drugs may cause haematological disorders, for example, zidovudine causes macrocytic anaemia and neutropenia. Immune thrombocytopenia in HIV responds to glucocorticoids or immunoglobulins, together with ART.

Renal disease

HIV-associated nephropathy is an important cause of chronic kidney disease and presents with nephrotic syndrome. Outcomes of renal transplantation on ART are good.

Cardiac disease

HIV-associated cardiomyopathy is a rapidly progressive dilated cardiomyopathy. Tuberculous pericarditis and accelerated coronary atheroma are other HIV-associated cardiac disorders.

Management of HIV

Prevention of opportunistic infections

Effective ART is the best protection, but other protective measures remain important:
• Avoidance of contaminated water and undercooked food. • Condom use. • Avoidance of animal-borne infection (cats). • Malaria vector control in endemic areas. • Co-trimoxazole prophylaxis: protects against pneumocystis, toxoplasmosis and cystoisosporiasis. • Vaccination against

pneumococcus, seasonal influenza and HBV is useful once CD4 counts are greater than 200 cells/mm^3. • Isoniazid may prevent TB in HIV-infected patients with a tuberculin skin test of 5 mm or more.

Antiretroviral therapy

The goals of ART are to:
• Reduce the viral load to an undetectable level for as long as possible. • Improve the CD4 count to greater than 200 cells/mm^3, making severe HIV-related disease unlikely. • Improve quantity and quality of life without unacceptable drug toxicity. • Reduce transmission.

Guidelines recommend starting ART in all people with HIV infection, irrespective of CD4 count or clinical status. Early initiation reduces morbidity, mortality and the risk of transmission. Urgent treatment is rarely necessary, and patient education about lifelong treatment and the need for adherence is the early priority. Adherence is improved by:
• Disclosure of HIV status. • Joining support groups. • Patient-nominated treatment supporters. • Management of coincident depression and substance abuse.

In patients with major opportunistic infections, ART should be started within 2 weeks, except in cryptococcal meningitis, where initiation before 5 weeks increases mortality, and in tuberculosis, where initiation before 8 weeks increases the risk of the immune reconstitution inflammatory syndrome (IRIS). IRIS is characterised by an exaggerated immune response with pronounced inflammatory features and paradoxical deterioration in opportunistic infections.

Commonly used drugs are shown in Box 5.25. Standard starting regimens include dual nucleoside reverse transcriptase inhibitors (NRTIs) combined with a non-NRTI, or a protease or integrase inhibitor.

CD4 counts and viral load are monitored every 6 months. CD4 count rises by 100 to 150 cells/mm^3 in the first year and about 80 cells/mm^3 per year thereafter, provided viral load is suppressed.

Pregnancy, HIV and ART

All pregnant women should be recommended for HIV screening. ART has reduced the risk of mother-to-child transmission of HIV to less than 1%. Caesarean section reduces the risk of transmission, but makes no

5.25 Commonly used antiretroviral drugs	
Classes	**Drugs**
Nucleoside reverse transcriptase inhibitors	Abacavir, emtricitabine, lamivudine, tenofovir, zidovudine
Non-nucleoside reverse transcriptase inhibitors	Efavirenz, rilpivirine
Protease inhibitors	Atazanavir, darunavir, lopinavir
Integrase inhibitors	Raltegravir, dolutegravir, elvitegravir
Chemokine receptor inhibitor	Maraviroc

difference to risk in those on ART. HIV is also transmitted by breastfeeding, but risk can be reduced by treating the infant with ART.

Pre-exposure prophylaxis

PrEP with tenofovir plus emtricitabine reduces the risk of HIV acquisition in people at ongoing high risk. Regular HIV testing should be done during PrEP.

Post-exposure prophylaxis

When risk of infection is deemed to be significant after careful risk assessment, PEP should be given. The first dose should be given as soon as possible, preferably within 6 to 8 hours; after 72 hours, PEP is ineffective. Tenofovir and emtricitabine are usually recommended, with a protease or integrase inhibitor. HIV antibody testing should be repeated at 3 months after exposure.

Clinical biochemistry and metabolic medicine

Between 60% and 70% of all critical decisions taken in regard to patients in health-care systems in developed countries involve a laboratory service or result. This chapter describes disorders whose primary manifestation is in abnormalities of biochemistry laboratory results, or whose underlying pathophysiology involves disturbance in specific biochemical pathways.

Biochemical investigations

Because the blood consists of both intracellular (red cell) and extracellular (plasma) components, it is important to avoid haemolysis of the sample, which causes contamination of the plasma by intracellular elements, particularly potassium. Blood should not be drawn from an arm into which an IV infusion is being given, to avoid contamination by the infused fluid.

A guide to the interpretation of disorders of urea and electrolytes is given in Box 6.1.

Because the kidneys maintain body fluid composition by adjusting urine volume and composition, it is often helpful to obtain a simultaneous sample of urine ('spot' specimen or 24-hour collection) at the time of blood analysis.

Water and electrolyte homeostasis

Total body water (TBW) constitutes around 60% of body weight in men, averaging about 40 L. Approximately 25 L is intracellular fluid (ICF), whereas the remainder is extracellular fluid (ECF). Plasma constitutes a small fraction (some 3 L) of the ECF, whereas the remainder is interstitial fluid that is within the tissues but outside the cells.

The dominant cation in the ICF is potassium, whereas in the ECF it is sodium (Fig. 6.1). Phosphates and negatively charged proteins constitute the major intracellular anions, whereas chloride and bicarbonate dominate the ECF anions. An important difference between the plasma and interstitial ECF is that only plasma contains significant concentrations of protein.

The major force maintaining the difference in cation concentration between the ICF and ECF is the sodium–potassium pump (Na,K ATPase) integral to all cell membranes. Maintenance of these gradients across cell membranes

6.1 How to interpret urea and electrolyte results

Sodium	Largely reflects reciprocal changes in body water
Potassium	May reflect K shifts in and out of cells
	Low: usually excess loss (renal, GI)
	High: usually renal dysfunction
Chloride	Generally changes in parallel with Na
	Low in metabolic alkalosis
	High in some metabolic acidosis
Bicarbonate	Abnormal in acid–base disorders—Box 6.6
Urea	Rises with ↓glomerular filtration rate, ↓renal perfusion, ↓urine flow, catabolic states or high protein intake
Creatinine	Rises with ↓glomerular filtration rate, high muscle mass, some drugs

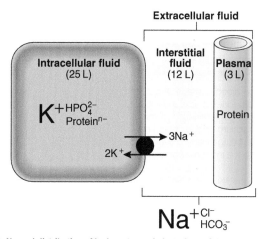

Fig. 6.1 Normal distribution of body water and electrolytes. Schematic representation of volume (*L*, litres) and composition (dominant ionic species only shown) of the intracellular fluid and extracellular fluid in a 70-kg male.

is essential for many cell processes, including the excitability of conducting tissues such as nerve and muscle. The difference in protein content between the plasma and the interstitial fluid compartment is maintained by the protein permeability barrier at the capillary wall. This protein concentration gradient contributes to the balance of forces across the capillary wall that favour fluid retention within the capillaries (the colloid osmotic, or oncotic, pressure of the plasma), maintaining circulating plasma volume.

Presenting problems in sodium and water balance

When the sodium balance is disturbed as a result of imbalance between intake and excretion, any tendency for the plasma sodium concentration to change is usually corrected by the osmotic mechanisms controlling water balance (see later). As a result, disorders in sodium balance present chiefly as altered ECF volume, rather than altered sodium concentration.

Hypovolaemia

Aetiology includes the following factors:

- Inadequate sodium intake
- GI sodium loss: vomiting, diarrhoea, external fistula
- Skin sodium loss: excess sweating, burns
- Renal sodium loss: diuretics, mineralocorticoid deficiency
- Internal sequestration: bowel obstruction, pancreatitis
- Acute blood loss

Clinical features

Symptoms and signs of hypovolaemia are:

• Thirst • Dizziness on standing • Weakness • Low JVP • Postural hypotension • Tachycardia • Dry mouth • Delirium • Weight loss

Investigations

Serum sodium is usually normal in hypovolaemia. The GFR is usually maintained (unless hypovolaemia is very severe or prolonged), but urinary flow is reduced by renal sodium- and water-retaining mechanisms. Serum creatinine, which reflects GFR, is usually normal, but serum urea is typically elevated as a result of low urine flow rate with increased tubular reabsorption of urea. Urine osmolality increases because of increased reabsorption of sodium and water. The urine sodium concentration falls, and sodium excretion may fall to less than 0.1% of the filtered sodium load.

Management

This has two main components:

- Treat the cause where possible, to stop ongoing salt and water losses.
- Replace salt and water deficits, and provide ongoing maintenance requirements by IV infusion when depletion is severe.

  IV fluid therapy. A typical adult requires 2.45 to 3.15 L of water, 105 to 140 mmol of sodium and 70 to 105 mmol of potassium per day. Infusions containing neither sodium nor protein will distribute to the body fluid compartments according to the normal distribution of TBW. For example, only 3/40 of the infused volume of 5% dextrose contributes towards the plasma volume, making it unsuitable for treating hypovolaemia. IV normal saline, on the other hand, is more effective at expanding the ECF, although only about 3/15 of the infused volume contributes to plasma volume.

Studies show no advantage of giving albumin-containing infusions for acute hypovolaemia, and synthetic colloids such as dextrans carry an increased risk of acute kidney injury and mortality in the critically ill. Therefore crystalloids are the treatment of choice for acute hypovolaemia.

Hypervolaemia

Hypervolaemia is the result of excess sodium and water and is rare in patients with normal cardiac and renal function because the kidney has a large capacity to increase sodium and water excretion.

Causes of sodium and water excess in clinical practice include:

- Impaired renal function: primary renal disease.
- Primary hyperaldosteronism: Conn's syndrome.
- Secondary hyperaldosteronism: congestive cardiac failure, cirrhotic liver disease, nephrotic syndrome.

In cardiac failure, cirrhosis and nephrotic syndrome, sodium retention results from circulatory insufficiency caused by the primary disorder (Fig. 6.2). In renal failure, the reduction in GFR impairs sodium and water excretion.

Peripheral oedema is the most common physical sign associated with these conditions, although it is not usually a feature of Conn's syndrome.

Management

The management of hypervolaemia involves:

- Specific treatment directed at the cause, for example, ACE inhibitors in heart failure, glucocorticoids in minimal change nephropathy.
- Restriction of dietary sodium to 50 to 80 mmol/day.
- Diuretics (loop or thiazide).

Water homeostasis

Daily water intake can vary over a wide range, from 500 mL to several litres a day. Although some water is lost through stool, sweat and the respiratory tract, the kidneys are chiefly responsible for adjusting water excretion to balance intake and maintain body fluid osmolality (reference range: 280–296 mmol/kg).

Regulation of total ECF volume is largely achieved through renal control of sodium excretion; however, the kidneys can excrete urine that is hypertonic or hypotonic in relation to plasma to maintain constant plasma osmolality. Failure of this regulation causes abnormalities of plasma sodium concentration, and hence of plasma osmolality. The main consequence of changes in plasma osmolality, especially when rapid, is altered cerebral function. This is because, when extracellular osmolality changes abruptly, water flows rapidly across cell membranes with resultant cell swelling (during hypoosmolality) or shrinkage (during hyperosmolality). Cerebral cell function is very sensitive to such volume changes, particularly during cell swelling, when an increase in intracerebral pressure causes reduced cerebral perfusion.

Hyponatraemia

Hyponatraemia is defined as a serum Na <135 mmol/L and indicates retention of water relative to sodium. It is often asymptomatic but can cause disturbances of cerebral function such as anorexia, nausea, vomiting, delirium, lethargy, seizures and coma. Symptoms are related to the speed of onset of hyponatraemia, rather than the severity.

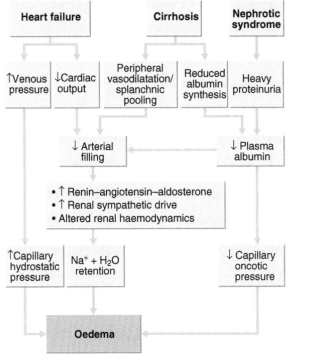

Fig. 6.2 Secondary mechanisms causing sodium excess and oedema in cardiac failure, cirrhosis and nephrotic syndrome. Primary renal retention of Na and water may also contribute to oedema formation when the glomerular filtration rate is significantly reduced.

Its causes are organised according to any associated change in ECF volume:

- *Hypovolaemic* (large Na deficit, relatively smaller water deficit): renal Na loss (diuretics), GI Na loss (vomiting, diarrhoea), skin Na loss (burns)
- *Euvolaemic* (excess body water with normal body sodium): primary polydipsia, syndrome of inappropriate antidiuretic hormone (SIADH; Box 6.2)
- *Hypervolaemic* (sodium retention with relatively greater water retention): heart failure, liver disease or kidney disease

Investigations

Plasma and urine electrolytes and osmolality (Box 6.3) are usually the only tests required to classify the hyponatraemia.

Management

The treatment for hyponatraemia is critically dependent on the rate of development and severity, and on the underlying cause.

6.2 SIADH: causes and diagnosis

Causes

- Tumours, especially small-cell lung cancer
- CNS disorders: stroke, trauma, infection, psychosis
- Pulmonary disorders: pneumonia, TB
- Drugs: anticonvulsants, psychotropics, antidepressants, cytotoxics, oral hypoglycae-mics, opiates
- Idiopathic

Diagnosis

- Low plasma sodium concentration (typically <130 mmol/L)
- Low plasma osmolality (<275 mmol/kg)
- Urine osmolality not minimally low (>100 mmol/kg)
- Urine sodium concentration not minimally low (>30 mmol/L)
- Low-normal plasma urea, creatinine, uric acid
- Exclusion of other causes of hyponatraemia
- Appropriate clinical context (see earlier)

6.3 Urine Na and osmolality in the differential diagnosis of hyponatraemia

Urine Na (mmol/L)	Urine osmolality (mmol/kg)	Possible diagnoses
<30	<100	Primary polydipsia, low intake
<30	>100	Hypovolaemia: vomiting, diarrhoea
		Hypervolaemia: heart failure, cirrhosis
>30	<100	Diuretic action (acute phase)
>30	>100	Hypovolaemia: diuretics, adrenal insufficiency
		Euvolaemia: SIADH

Urine analysis may yield results of indeterminate significance; if so, diagnosis depends on comprehensive clinical assessment.

If hyponatraemia has developed rapidly (<48 hours), with signs of cerebral oedema (patient is obtunded or convulsing), sodium levels should be restored rapidly to normal by infusion of hypertonic (3%) sodium chloride.

Rapid correction of hyponatraemia that has developed slowly (>48 hours) may lead to 'central pontine myelinolysis', which may cause permanent structural and functional cerebral changes, and is generally fatal. The rate of plasma sodium correction in chronic asymptomatic hyponatraemia should not exceed 10 mmol/L/day, and an even slower rate is generally safer.

Treatment should be directed at the underlying cause. For hypovolaemic patients, this will involve controlling sodium loss and giving IV saline if clinically warranted. Patients with euvolaemic hyponatraemia usually respond to fluid restriction in the range of 600 to 1000 mL/day and removal of the precipitating stimulus (e.g. a drug causing SIADH). Oral urea therapy (30–45 g/day) can be beneficial in persistent SIADH.

Hypernatraemia

Hypernatraemia (defined as serum Na >145 mmol/L) reflects inadequate concentration of urine in the face of restricted water intake. Patients with hypernatraemia generally have reduced cerebral function, as well as cerebral dehydration. This triggers thirst and drinking, and if adequate water is obtained, is self-limiting. If adequate water is not obtained, dizziness, delirium, weakness and ultimately coma and death can result.

Management

Treatment of hypernatraemia depends on both the rate of development and the underlying cause.

If there is reason to think that the condition has developed quickly, correction with appropriate volumes of IV hypotonic fluid may be attempted relatively rapidly.

In older, institutionalised patients, however, it is more likely that the disorder has developed slowly, and extreme caution should be exercised in lowering the plasma sodium to avoid the risk of cerebral oedema.

Potassium homeostasis

Potassium is the major intracellular cation (Fig. 6.1), and the steep concentration gradient for potassium across the membranes of excitable cells plays an important part in generating the resting membrane potential and allowing propagation of the action potential, which is crucial to normal functioning of nerve, muscle and cardiac tissues. The kidneys normally excrete 90% of the daily intake of potassium (80–100 mmol). Hypokalaemia may occur when potassium is driven into cells by extracellular alkalosis, insulin, catecholamines or aldosterone. Extracellular acidosis, lack of insulin and insufficiency or blockade of catecholamines or aldosterone can cause hyperkalaemia because of efflux of potassium from cells.

Hypokalaemia

Causes of hypokalaemia include:

- *Redistribution into cells:* alkalosis, insulin excess, β_2-agonists
- *Reduced potassium intake:* dietary, IV therapy
- *Excessive renal loss:*
  - Activation of mineralocorticoid receptor: Conn's or Cushing's syndrome, glucocorticoids, carbenoxolone—all associated with hypertension
  - Diuresis—thiazides, loop, recovery from acute tubular necrosis or obstruction
  - Genetic tubular defects, for example, Bartter's syndrome
  - Renal tubular acidosis—inherited or acquired
- *Excessive GI loss:*
  - Vomiting
  - NG aspiration

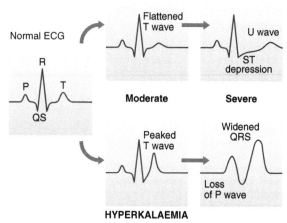

Fig. 6.3 The *ECG* in hypokalaemia and hyperkalaemia.

- Diarrhoea
- Bowel obstruction
- Laxative abuse

Clinical features

Hypokalaemia is asymptomatic if mild (3–3.3 mmol/L). Larger reductions cause:

- Muscular weakness
- Tiredness
- ECG changes (Fig. 6.3), ventricular ectopics or more serious arrhythmias; potentiation of the adverse effects of digoxin
- Functional bowel obstruction caused by paralytic ileus
- Damage to renal tubules (hypokalaemic nephropathy, in prolonged hypokalaemia) and interference with the tubular response to ADH (acquired nephrogenic diabetes insipidus), causing polyuria and polydipsia

Investigations

Measurement of plasma electrolytes, bicarbonate, urine potassium and sometimes calcium and magnesium is usually sufficient to establish the diagnosis.

Plasma renin activity is low in patients with primary hyperaldosteronism (p. 406) and other mineralocorticoid excesses, but high in other causes of hypokalaemia. Urinary potassium is high in renal loss and low with GI loss. Occasionally the cause of hypokalaemia is obscure, especially when the history is incomplete or unreliable and the level of potassium in the urine is inconclusive. Many such cases are associated with metabolic alkalosis, and measurement of urine chloride concentration can then be helpful:

- A low urine chloride level (<30 mmol/L) is characteristic of vomiting (spontaneous or self-induced)
- A chloride level greater than 40 mmol/L suggests diuretic therapy (acute phase) or a tubular disorder

Management

If the problem is redistribution of potassium into cells, reversal of the underlying cause (e.g. correction of alkalosis) may restore plasma potassium without supplements. In most cases, potassium replacement (oral or IV) will be required. The rate of administration depends on the severity of hypokalaemia and the presence of cardiac or neuromuscular complications, but should generally not exceed 10 mmol per hour. If higher rates are needed, the concentration of potassium infused may be increased to 40 mmol/L if a peripheral vein is used, but higher concentrations must be infused into a large 'central' vein with continuous cardiac monitoring.

Hyperkalaemia

Causes of hyperkalaemia include:

- *Artefactual:* haemolysis during or after venepuncture
- *Increased intake:* exogenous (diet, IV therapy)
- *Redistribution from cells:* acidosis, insulin deficiency, β-blockers, severe hyperglycaemia, haemolysis, rhabdomyolysis
- *Reduced urinary excretion:* acute and chronic kidney disease, reduced mineralocorticoid receptor activation (Addison's, ACE inhibitors and ARBs, spironolactone), renin inhibition (NSAIDs), tubulointerstitial disease

Clinical features

Mild to moderate hyperkalaemia (<6.5 mmol/L) is usually asymptomatic. More severe hyperkalaemia can present with progressive weakness, but sometimes there are no symptoms until cardiac arrest occurs. Typical ECG changes are shown in Fig. 6.3. Peaking of the T wave is an early ECG sign but widening of the QRS complex presages a dangerous cardiac arrhythmia.

Investigations

Plasma electrolyte, creatinine and bicarbonate results, together with consideration of the clinical scenario, will usually provide the explanation for hyperkalaemia. Addison's disease should be excluded, unless there is an obvious alternative diagnosis, as described on page 402.

Management

Treatment of hyperkalaemia depends on the severity and rate of development. In the absence of neuromuscular symptoms or ECG changes, reduction of potassium intake and correction of underlying abnormalities may be sufficient. In acute and/or severe hyperkalaemia, more urgent measures must be taken (Box 6.4).

✚ 6.4 Treatment of hyperkalaemia

Mechanism	Therapy
Stabilise cell membrane potential[a]	IV calcium gluconate (10 mL of 10% solution)
Shift K into cells	Inhaled β_2-agonist, e.g. salbutamol
	IV glucose (50 mL of 50% solution) and insulin (5 U Actrapid)
	IV sodium bicarbonate[b]
Remove K from body	IV furosemide and normal saline[c]
	Ion exchange resin (e.g. Resonium) orally or rectally
	Dialysis

[a]If severe hyperkalaemia (K typically >6.5 mmol/L).
[b]If acidosis present.
[c]If adequate residual renal function.

Acid-base homeostasis

The pH of the ECF is maintained within narrow limits by blood and tissue buffers, of which the most important is the bicarbonate buffer (because ECF contains a high concentration of bicarbonate):

$$CO_2 + H_2O \underset{\text{carbonic anhydrase}}{\leftrightarrow} H_2CO_3 \rightleftharpoons H^+ + HCO_3^-$$

Two of the key components of this buffer are under physiological control: CO_2 by the lungs, and bicarbonate by the kidneys. Altered ventilation and renal bicarbonate absorption can correct disturbed blood acidity, but respiratory and renal disease can also cause disorders of acid–base homeostasis.

Patients with disturbances of the acid–base balance may present clinically either with the effects of tissue malfunction as a result of disturbed pH (such as altered cardiac and CNS function), or with secondary changes in respiration as a response to the underlying metabolic change (e.g. Kussmaul respiration during metabolic acidosis). The clinical picture is often dominated by the underlying cause of the acid–base change, such as uncontrolled diabetes or primary lung disease. Frequently, the acid–base disturbances only become evident when the venous plasma bicarbonate concentration is found to be abnormal, or when ABG analysis shows abnormalities in the pH, PCO_2 or bicarbonate.

The common blood gas abnormities in acid–base disturbances are shown in Box 6.5. Interpretation of blood gas results is made easier by blood gas diagrams (e.g. Fig. 6.4), which indicate whether any acidosis or alkalosis is due to acute or chronic respiratory derangements of $PaCO_2$ or to metabolic causes.

In metabolic disturbances, respiratory compensation is almost immediate; that is, the compensatory change in PCO_2 is achieved soon after the onset of the metabolic disturbance. In respiratory disorders, on the

i 6.5 Principal patterns of acid–base disturbance

Disturbance	H⁺	Primary change	Compensatory response
Metabolic acidosis	>40[a]	HCO_3^- <24 mmol/L	PCO_2 <5.33 kPa[b]
Metabolic alkalosis	<40[a]	HCO_3^- >24 mmol/L	PCO_2 >5.33 kPa[b,c]
Respiratory acidosis	>40[a]	PCO_2 >5.33 kPa[b]	HCO_3^- >24 mmol/L
Respiratory alkalosis	<40[a]	PCO_2 <5.33 kPa[b]	HCO_3^- <24 mmol/L

[a]H^+ of 40 nmol/L = pH of 7.40.
[b]PCO_2 of 5.33 kPa = 40 mmHg.
[c]PCO_2 does not rise above 7.33 kPa (55 mmHg) because hypoxia intervenes to drive ventilation.

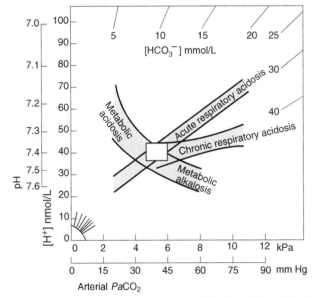

Fig. 6.4 Changes in blood [H⁺], $PaCO_2$ and plasma [HCO_3^-] in acid–base disorders. The shaded rectangle indicates the limits of normal. The bands represent 95% confidence limits of single disturbances in human blood in vivo. The diagonal lines (*top* and *right*) indicate bicarbonate levels. For any measured value of [H⁺], the corresponding value of $PaCO_2$ indicates whether the acidosis or alkalosis is primarily respiratory or metabolic in origin.

other hand, a small initial change in bicarbonate occurs as a result of chemical buffering of CO_2, largely within red blood cells, but further compensatory changes in bicarbonate occur via long-term adjustments in acid secretory capacity by the kidney, requiring days to weeks. When clinically obtained acid–base parameters do not accord with the predicted compensation shown, a mixed acid–base disturbance should be suspected.

Metabolic acidosis

Metabolic acidosis occurs when an acid other than carbonic acid (attributed to CO_2 retention) accumulates in the body, resulting in a fall in the plasma bicarbonate. Causes of metabolic acidosis are classified according to the anion gap, which is the difference between the main measured cations [$Na^+ + K^+$] and the main measured cations [$Cl^- + HCO_3^-$]. This is normally 12 to 16 mmol/L, but increases when an acid accumulates accompanied by a corresponding anion.

Metabolic acidosis with normal anion gap: this occurs either with loss of bicarbonate from the ECF or the result of poisoning. Causes include:
- GI HCO_3^- loss (diarrhoea, small bowel fistula, urinary diversion procedure)
- RTA (urinary loss of HCO_3^- in proximal RTA, impaired tubular acid secretion in distal RTA)
- Therapeutic infusion or poisoning with HCl or NH_4Cl

Metabolic acidosis with increased anion gap
- Diabetic ketoacidosis (accumulation of ketones with hyperglycaemia)
- Lactic acidosis (shock or liver disease)
- Renal failure
- Poisoning (aspirin, methanol, ethylene glycol)

Management

Identify and correct the underlying cause. Because metabolic acidosis is frequently associated with sodium and water depletion, resuscitation with appropriate IV fluids will often be needed. Use of IV bicarbonate in metabolic acidosis is controversial and reserved for severe acidosis.

Metabolic alkalosis

Metabolic alkalosis is characterised by an increase in the plasma bicarbonate concentration and the plasma pH (see Box 6.5). There is a compensatory rise in PCO_2 because of hypoventilation, but this is limited by the need to avoid hypoxia.

Clinically, apart from manifestations of the underlying cause, there may be few symptoms or signs related to alkalosis itself. When the rise in systemic pH is abrupt, plasma ionised calcium falls, and signs of increased neuromuscular irritability, such as tetany, may develop (p. 397).

The causes are classified by the accompanying disturbance of ECF volume:

Hypovolaemic metabolic alkalosis (most common pattern): sustained vomiting—acid-rich fluid is lost from the body, hypokalaemia stimulates renal H^+ excretion. Hypovolaemia leads to secondary hyperaldosteronism, triggering proximal sodium bicarbonate reabsorption and additional acid secretion by the distal tubule.

Normovolaemic (or hypervolaemic) metabolic alkalosis: occurs when both bicarbonate retention and volume expansion are found together. Causes include:

- Conn's syndrome
- Cushing's syndrome
- Glucocorticoids
- Overuse of antacids

Management

Metabolic alkalosis associated with hypovolaemia is treated with IV fluids, specifically isotonic sodium chloride. Replacement of potassium helps correct the hypokalaemia and its consequences in the kidney.

In metabolic alkalosis associated with normal or increased volume, treatment should focus on correcting the underlying cause.

Respiratory acidosis

Respiratory acidosis occurs when there is accumulation of CO_2 owing to type II respiratory failure (p. 311). This results in a rise in the PCO_2, with a compensatory increase in plasma bicarbonate concentration, particularly when the disorder is of long duration and the kidney has fully developed its capacity for increased acid excretion.

The aetiology, clinical features and management of respiratory acidosis are covered in Chapter 9.

Respiratory alkalosis

Respiratory alkalosis develops when there is a period of hyperventilation resulting in a reduction of PCO_2 and increase in plasma pH. If the condition is sustained, renal compensation occurs, such that tubular acid secretion is reduced, and the plasma bicarbonate falls.

This acid–base disturbance is frequently of short duration, as in anxiety states or over-vigorous assisted ventilation. It can be prolonged in the context of pregnancy, pulmonary embolism, chronic liver disease and ingestion of certain drugs that stimulate the brainstem respiratory centre (e.g. salicylates).

Clinical features of hyperventilation are described in Chapter 9. The characteristic perioral and digital tingling occurs because alkalosis promotes the binding of calcium to albumin, causing reduced ionised calcium. In severe cases, Trousseau's sign and Chvostek's sign may be positive, and tetany or seizures may develop (p. 397).

Mixed acid-base disorders

In patients with complex illnesses, it is not uncommon for more than one independent disturbance of acid–base metabolism to be present at the same time. In these situations, the arterial pH will represent the net effect of all primary and compensatory changes. Indeed, the pH may be normal, but the presence of underlying acid–base disturbances can be gauged from concomitant abnormalities in the PCO_2 and bicarbonate concentration (Fig. 6.4).

Calcium homeostasis

This is covered in Chapter 10.

Magnesium homeostasis

Magnesium is mainly an intracellular cation, and is functionally important for many enzymes, including the Na/K ATPase. It can also regulate potassium and calcium channels.

Free plasma magnesium (~70% of the total) is filtered at the glomerulus, with the majority of this reabsorbed in the loop of Henle and tubules. Reabsorption is enhanced by parathyroid hormone (PTH).

Hypomagnesaemia

Causes include:

- Inadequate intake: starvation, parenteral nutrition.
- Excessive losses: GI (vomiting, diarrhoea, fistulae), renal (diuretics, alcohol, acute tubular necrosis).
- Complex formation: acute pancreatitis.

Clinical features

The clinical features of hypomagnesaemia and hypocalcaemia are similar: tetany; arrhythmias, especially torsades de pointes (p. 269); and seizures. Hypomagnesaemia is associated with hypocalcaemia because magnesium is required for normal PTH secretion in response to a fall in serum calcium; also, hypomagnesaemia induces resistance to PTH in bone. Hypomagnesaemia is also associated with hyponatraemia and hypokalaemia, and these may mediate some of the clinical manifestations.

Management

Treat the underlying cause. Oral magnesium is poorly absorbed and may cause diarrhoea. If disease is symptomatic, correct with IV magnesium. If caused by diuretic use, adjunctive use of a potassium-sparing diuretic will also reduce renal magnesium losses.

Hypermagnesaemia

Hypermagnesaemia is much less common than hypomagnesaemia. It may be attributed to:

- Acute kidney injury or chronic kidney disease.
- Adrenocortical insufficiency.
- Increased intake (antacids, laxatives, enemas).

Clinical features

- Bradycardia.
- Hypotension.
- Reduced consciousness.
- Respiratory depression.

Management

- Restrict magnesium intake.
- Optimise renal function.

- Promote renal magnesium excretion with IV hydration and a loop diuretic.
- Administer calcium gluconate IV to reverse overt cardiac effects.
- Prescribe dialysis, if poor renal function is present.

Phosphate homeostasis

Inorganic phosphate is involved in energy metabolism, intracellular signalling and bone/mineral homeostasis. It is freely filtered at the glomerulus, with around 65% reabsorbed in the proximal tubule and a further 10% to 20% reabsorbed in the distal tubules. Proximal reabsorption is reduced by PTH.

Hypophosphataemia

Causes include:

- Redistribution into cells: refeeding after starvation, respiratory alkalosis.
- Inadequate intake or absorption: malabsorption, diarrhoea.
- Increased renal excretion: hyperparathyroidism, volume expansion.

Clinical features
- Impaired function and survival of all blood cell lines.
- Muscle weakness, respiratory failure, congestive cardiac failure, ileus.
- Decreased consciousness, coma.
- Osteomalacia.

Management
Measurement of phosphate, calcium, PTH and 25(OH)D helps to exclude osteomalacia, rickets and primary hyperparathyroidism.

- Oral phosphate supplements.
- IV sodium or potassium phosphate salts: may be used in critical situations, but there is a risk of hypocalcaemia and metastatic calcification.

Hyperphosphataemia

Hyperphosphataemia is most commonly caused by acute kidney injury or chronic kidney disease. Redistribution of phosphate from cells in tumour lysis syndrome is another cause.

Clinical features
These relate to hypocalcaemia and metastatic calcification, especially in chronic renal failure and tertiary hyperparathyroidism, where a high calcium-phosphate product occurs.

Management
- Dietary phosphate restriction and phosphate binders in kidney disease.
- If renal function is normal, volume expansion with normal saline promotes renal phosphate excretion.

Disorders of amino acid metabolism

These usually present in the neonatal period and involve lifelong treatment regimens.

Phenylketonuria

This autosomal recessive condition causes deficiency of phenylalanine hydroxylase. Affected infants accumulate phenylalanine, causing intellectual disability. This can be prevented by neonatal screening and dietary phenylalanine restriction.

Homocystinuria

An autosomal recessive deficiency of cystathionine β-synthase results in the accumulation of homocystine and methionine in the blood. Clinical manifestations include:

- Displacement of the ocular lens
- Intellectual disability, seizures, psychiatric disturbances
- Marfan-like skeleton, with osteoporosis
- Thrombosis of arteries and veins
- Skin hypopigmentation

Treatment involves a methionine-restricted, cystine-supplemented diet and large doses of pyridoxine.

Disorders of carbohydrate metabolism

Diabetes is described in Chapter 11.

Galactosaemia

Galactosaemia is caused by an autosomal recessive mutation in the galactose-1-phosphate uridyl transferase gene. The neonate is unable to metabolise galactose, leading to vomiting or diarrhoea after milk ingestion. Failure to thrive, cataracts and intellectual disability may result. Treatment involves lifelong avoidance of galactose- and lactose-containing foods.

Lipids and lipoprotein metabolism

Lipids are absorbed from the gut or released from the liver. They are transported in the blood as chylomicrons and lipoproteins, which are classified by their density: very low (VLDL), low (LDL), intermediate (IDL) and high density lipoproteins (HDL). VLDL is important in the transport of triglycerides, and LDL and HDL in the transport of cholesterol. High LDL and IDL levels and low HDL levels predict atherosclerosis.

Lipid measurements are usually performed for the following reasons:

- Screening for primary or secondary prevention of cardiovascular disease.
- Investigation of patients with clinical features of lipid disorders.
- Testing of relatives of patients with genetic dyslipidaemia.

Nonfasting measurements of total cholesterol and HDL-C allow estimation of non-HDL cholesterol, but a 12-hour fasting sample is required for TG measurement and calculation of LDL-C.

Following the exclusion of secondary causes (Box 6.6), primary lipid abnormalities may be diagnosed.

---

i 6.6 Causes of secondary hyperlipidaemia

Secondary hypercholesterolaemia

- Hypothyroidism[a]
- Pregnancy[a]
- Cholestatic liver disease[a]
- Drugs (diuretics, ciclosporin, glucocorticoids, androgens, antiretrovirals)[a]
- Nephrotic syndrome
- Anorexia nervosa
- Hyperparathyroidism

Secondary hypertriglyceridaemia

- Type 2 diabetes mellitus
- Chronic kidney disease
- Abdominal obesity
- Excess alcohol
- Hepatocellular disease
- Drugs (β-blockers, retinoids, glucocorticoids, antiretrovirals)

[a]Common causes.

Hypercholesterolaemia

This is usually polygenic and causes raised LDL-C and increased cardiovascular risk. Familial hypercholesterolaemia is a more severe disorder, and is usually autosomal dominant.

Clinical features include:

- Xanthelasma.
- Corneal arcus.
- Tendon xanthomas.

Hypertriglyceridaemia

Hypertriglyceridaemia is most commonly polygenic, but many cases are secondary to alcohol, diabetes or insulin resistance syndrome (p. 425). TGs are raised and HDL-C is low, increasing cardiovascular risk.

Clinical features of severe TG elevation include:

- Lipaemia retinalis.
- Lipaemic blood and plasma.
- Eruptive xanthomas.
- Acute pancreatitis.
- Hepatomegaly.

Mixed hyperlipidaemia

This is usually polygenic with no pathognomonic features.

Management of dyslipidaemia

Risk and benefit should be assessed individually using prediction charts.

Nonpharmacological management

Patients with lipid abnormalities should receive medical advice and, if necessary, dietary counselling to:

- Reduce intake of saturated and transunsaturated fat to less than 7% to 10% of total energy
- Reduce cholesterol intake to less than 250 mg/day
- Replace sources of saturated fat and cholesterol with alternative foods such as lean meat, low-fat dairy products, polyunsaturated spreads and low glycaemic index carbohydrates
- Reduce the consumption of energy-dense foods, such as fats and soft drinks, while increasing activity and exercise to maintain or lose weight
- Increase consumption of cardioprotective and nutrient-dense foods, such as vegetables, unrefined carbohydrates, fish, nuts, pulses, legumes and fruit
- Reduce alcohol intake if excessive or if associated with hypertension, hypertriglyceridaemia or central obesity
- Achieve additional benefits with preferential intake of foods containing lipid-lowering nutrients, such as n-3 fatty acids, dietary fibre and plant sterols

Response to diet appears within 3 to 4 weeks. Hyperlipidaemia in general and hypertriglyceridaemia in particular can be very responsive to these measures. Explanation and encouragement are important to assist patient adherence. Even minor weight loss can substantially reduce cardiovascular risk, especially in centrally obese patients.

All other modifiable cardiovascular risk factors should be assessed and treated. Where possible, intercurrent drug treatments that adversely affect the lipid profile should be replaced.

Pharmacological management

Statins are used to inhibit cholesterol synthesis, and ezetimibe to inhibit cholesterol absorption. Fibrates and fish oil are used to treat hypertriglyceridaemia. Treatment choices are summarised in Fig. 6.5.

Other biochemical disorders

Amyloidosis

Amyloidosis is characterised by the extracellular deposition of insoluble proteins. These deposits consist of amyloid protein fibrils linked to glycosaminoglycans, proteoglycans and serum amyloid P component. The diagnosis should be considered in unexplained nephrotic syndrome, cardiomyopathy and peripheral neuropathy. Amyloid diseases are classified by aetiology and type of protein deposited:

- *Reactive (AA) amyloidosis:* increased production of serum amyloid A owing to chronic infection (e.g. TB, bronchiectasis) or inflammation (e.g. RA). Some 90% of patients have proteinuria.
- *Light chain (AL) amyloidosis:* increased production of monoclonal light chains owing to monoclonal gammopathies (myeloma, plasmacytoma).

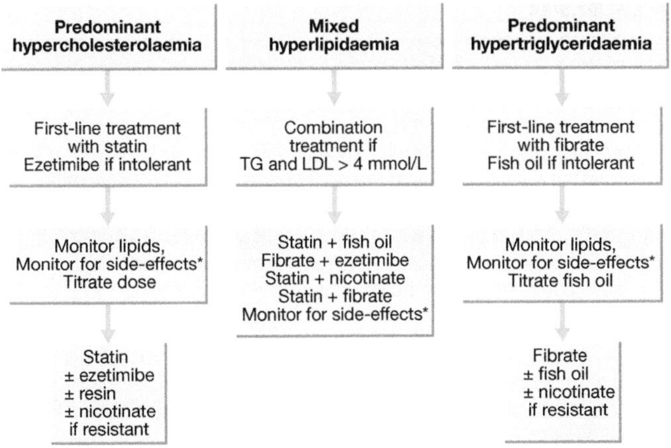

Predominant hypercholesterolaemia	Mixed hyperlipidaemia	Predominant hypertriglyceridaemia
First-line treatment with statin Ezetimibe if intolerant	Combination treatment if TG and LDL > 4 mmol/L	First-line treatment with fibrate Fish oil if intolerant
Monitor lipids, Monitor for side-effects* Titrate dose	Statin + fish oil Fibrate + ezetimibe Statin + nicotinate Statin + fibrate Monitor for side-effects*	Monitor lipids, Monitor for side-effects* Titrate fish oil
Statin ± ezetimibe ± resin ± nicotinate if resistant		Fibrate ± fish oil ± nicotinate if resistant

Fig. 6.5 Flow chart for drug treatment of hyperlipidaemia. *Interrupt treatment if the creatine kinase level is more than 5 to 10 times normal, if it is elevated with muscle symptoms or if the alanine aminotransferase level is more than 2 to 3 times normal.

Clinical features include restrictive cardiomyopathy, neuropathy and macroglossia (pathognomonic). Prognosis is poor.

- *Dialysis-associated (Aβ2M) amyloidosis:* Accumulation of β_2-microglobulin as a result of renal failure. Presents 5 to 10 years after starting dialysis, with carpal tunnel syndrome, arthropathy and pathological fractures owing to amyloid bone cysts.

Investigations

Biopsy of an affected organ, rectum or subcutaneous fat, when stained with Congo red dye, shows the pathognomonic apple-green birefringence of amyloid deposits under polarised light. Quantitative scintigraphy with radiolabelled SAP determines distribution of amyloid deposits.

Management

The aims of treatment are to support affected organs and, in acquired amyloidosis, to prevent further amyloid deposition through treatment of the primary cause. Liver transplantation may provide definitive treatment in selected patients with hereditary amyloidosis.

The porphyrias

These are rare disorders caused by inherited enzyme deficiencies of the haem biosynthetic pathway. They are divided into hepatic or erythropoietic, depending on the major site of excess porphyrin production. Inheritance is dominant with low penetrance, and environmental factors influence expression.

Clinical features

Two patterns are recognised:

- *Photosensitive skin manifestations:* pain, erythema, bullae, erosions, hirsutism and hyperpigmentation are characteristic of the most common form of porphyria, PCT.
- *Acute neurological syndrome:* presents with acute abdominal pain and autonomic dysfunction (tachycardia, hypertension and constipation), and is characteristic of AIP.

Attacks are often provoked by drugs such as anticonvulsants, sulfonamides, oestrogen and progesterone (oral contraceptive pill); alcohol; and even fasting. In some cases, no precipitant can be identified.

Investigations

Measure porphyrins, their precursors and metabolites in blood, urine and faeces. It is now possible to measure some of the affected enzymes. Identification of the underlying gene mutations has made family testing possible for some variants.

Management

With neurovisceral attacks, patients should avoid any known precipitants of acute porphyria. IV glucose can terminate acute attacks through a reduction in δ-aminolaevulinic acid synthetase activity. For photosensitive manifestations, the primary goal is to avoid sun exposure and skin trauma. Barrier sun creams containing zinc or titanium oxide are the most effective products.

Nephrology and urology

This chapter describes the disorders of the kidneys and urinary tract that are commonly encountered in routine practice, as well as giving an overview of the highly specialised field of renal replacement therapy. Disorders of renal tubular function, which may cause alterations in electrolyte and acid–base balance, are described in Chapter 6.

Measurement of renal function

The key measurement of renal function, glomerular filtration rate (GFR), is normally assessed using the serum level of endogenously produced creatinine, using a formula that allows for sex, age and ethnicity, for example:

$$\text{eGFR} = 175 \times (\text{creatinine in } \mu\text{mol/L}/88.4)^{-1.154} \times (\text{age in yrs})^{-0.203} \times (0.742 \text{ if female}) \times (1.21 \text{ if black})$$

(To convert creatinine in mg/dL to µmol/L, multiply by 88.4.)

Presenting problems in renal and urinary tract disease

Oliguria/anuria

Daily urine volumes less than 400 mL are termed oliguria. Anuria is defined as less than 100 mL urine passed per day. Impaired GFR does not always cause oliguria; a high solute load or tubular dysfunction may produce normal or high urine volumes. A low measured urine volume is a consequence of reduced production, obstruction to urine flow or both. Patients should be assessed for signs of dehydration or hypotension, and for signs of urinary obstruction (enlarged bladder). Catheterisation relieves distal obstruction and allows monitoring of urine flow rate. USS reveals the site of obstruction.

Clinical examination of the kidney and urinary tract

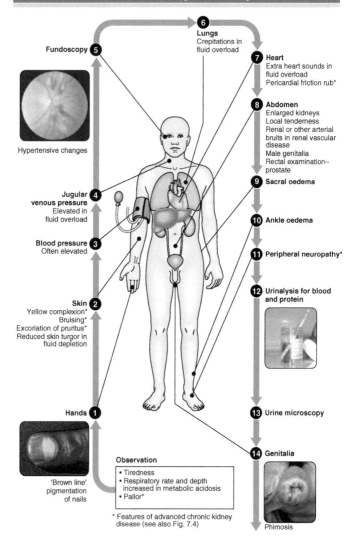

6 Lungs
Crepitations in fluid overload

Fundoscopy 5

Hypertensive changes

7 Heart
Extra heart sounds in fluid overload
Pericardial friction rub*

8 Abdomen
Enlarged kidneys
Local tenderness
Renal or other arterial bruits in renal vascular disease
Male genitalia
Rectal examination– prostate

9 Sacral oedema

Jugular 4 venous pressure
Elevated in fluid overload

Blood pressure 3
Often elevated

10 Ankle oedema

11 Peripheral neuropathy*

Skin 2
Yellow complexion*
Bruising*
Excoriation of pruritus*
Reduced skin turgor in fluid depletion

12 Urinalysis for blood and protein

Hands 1

'Brown line' pigmentation of nails

13 Urine microscopy

14 Genitalia

Observation
- Tiredness
- Respiratory rate and depth increased in metabolic acidosis
- Pallor*

* Features of advanced chronic kidney disease (see also Fig. 7.4)

Phimosis

i	**7.1 Interpretation of dipstick-positive haematuria**	
Dipstick test positive	**Urine microscopy**	**Suggested cause**
Haematuria	White blood cells	Infection
	Abnormal epithelial cells	Tumour
	Red cell casts, dysmorphic RBC	Glomerular bleeding
Haemoglobinuria	No red cells	Intravascular haemolysis
Myoglobinuria	No red cells	Rhabdomyolysis

Haematuria

This indicates bleeding anywhere within the urinary tract and may be visible (macroscopic) or only detectable on urinalysis (microscopic). Macroscopic haematuria is most commonly caused by tumours, urine infection and stones. Causes of dipstick-positive haematuria are shown in Box 7.1. Investigations and management of haematuria are outlined in Fig. 7.1.

Nephritic syndrome

This means the presence of haematuria together with hypertension, oliguria, fluid retention and impaired renal function. It is typical of rapidly progressive glomerulonephritis and warrants urgent investigation.

Proteinuria

Moderate amounts of low molecular weight proteins pass through the GBM, but are reabsorbed by tubular cells, so that less than 150 mg/day appears in the urine. Quantification and interpretation of proteinuria are covered in Box 7.2.

Proteinuria is usually asymptomatic and detected on urinalysis. It can occur transiently after exercise, during fever, in heart failure and with UTI. 'Orthostatic proteinuria', with positive daytime samples and negative morning samples, is usually benign.

Moderately elevated albuminuria (formerly known as microalbuminuria) is abnormal, and may indicate early glomerular disease. Patients with diabetes should be screened for this, as ACE inhibitors can prevent loss of renal function. Persistently elevated levels are associated with atherosclerosis and cardiovascular mortality.

Overt (dipstick-positive) proteinuria often indicates glomerular damage, and should be quantified (protein:creatinine ratio, PCR) and investigated. Nephrotic syndrome features heavy proteinuria (>3.5 g/24 hours; PCR >350 mg/mmol), hypoalbuminaemia and oedema. Stimulation of the renin–angiotensin system leads to renal sodium retention. Hypercholesterolaemia and hypercoagulability are other features. Infection is common as a result of urinary loss of immunoglobulins. Management includes treating the underlying renal disease, plus supportive therapy with diuretics, low-sodium diet, statins, prophylactic anticoagulation and vaccination against infection.

Investigation of proteinuria is summarised in Fig. 7.2.

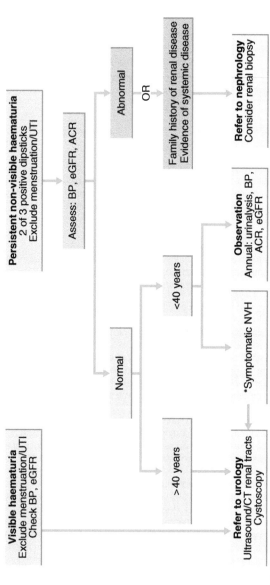

Fig. 7.1 Investigation of haematuria. *Symptomatic: voiding symptoms including hesitancy, frequency, urgency, dysuria. *ACR*, Albumin:creatinine ratio; *BP*, blood pressure; *GFR*, glomerular filtration rate; *NVH*, nonvisible haematuria; *UTI*, urinary tract infection.

	7.2 Quantification and interpretation of proteinuria		
ACR	**PCR**	**Dipstick results**	**Significance**
<3.5 female <2.5 male	<25	–	Normal
3.5–30	25–50	–	Moderately elevated albuminuria
30–70	50–100	+ to ++	Dipstick-positive
70–300	100–350	++ to +++	Glomerular disease more likely Equivalent to >1 g/24 hrs
>300	>350	+++ to ++++	Nephrotic; always glomerular disease, equivalent to >3.5 g/24 hrs

ACR, Urinary albumin (mg/L)/urine creatinine (mmol/L); PCR, urine protein (mg/L)/urine creatinine (mmol/L).

Oedema

Oedema is an excessive accumulation of fluid within the interstitial space.

Investigations

The cause of oedema (Box 7.3) is usually apparent from the history and examination of the cardiovascular system and abdomen, combined with measurement of renal and liver function, urinary protein and serum albumin. Where ascites or pleural effusion in isolation is causing diagnostic difficulty, aspiration of fluid with measurement of protein and glucose, and microscopy for cells, will usually clarify the diagnosis (p. 316).

Management

Mild fluid retention will respond to a diuretic such as a thiazide or low-dose loop diuretic. Restrict sodium (and sometimes fluid) in resistant cases. In nephrotic syndrome, renal failure and severe cardiac failure, very large doses of diuretics, sometimes in combination, may be required. Specific causes (e.g. venous thrombosis) should be treated.

Hypertension

Hypertension is a very common feature of renal disease. As the GFR declines, hypertension becomes increasingly common, regardless of the renal diagnosis. Hypertension also identifies a population at risk of developing CKD (and associated cardiovascular risk), so hypertensive patients should have renal function checked annually. Management is discussed on p. 78.

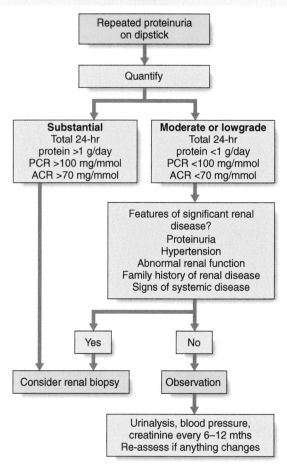

Fig. 7.2 Investigation of proteinuria. *ACR*, Albumin:creatinine ratio; *PCR*, protein:creatinine ratio.

Loin pain

Dull ache in the loin is often musculoskeletal in origin, but may be caused by renal stone, renal tumour, acute pyelonephritis or obstruction of the renal pelvis. Acute loin pain radiating to the groin ('renal colic'), together with haematuria, is typical of ureteric obstruction, most commonly caused by calculi (p. 241).

Dysuria

Dysuria refers to painful urination, often with suprapubic pain, frequency and a feeling of incomplete emptying. The cause is usually UTI (p. 236),

7.3 Causes of oedema	
Increased extracellular fluid	Heart failure, renal failure, liver disease
High local venous pressure	Deep vein thrombosis, pregnancy, pelvic tumour
Low plasma oncotic pressure	Nephrotic syndrome, liver failure, malabsorption
Increased capillary permeability	Infection, sepsis, calcium channel blockers
Lymphatic obstruction	Infection (filariasis), malignancy, radiation injury

7.4 Causes of polyuria

- Excess fluid intake
- Osmotic: hyperglycaemia, hypercalcaemia
- Cranial diabetes insipidus
- Nephrogenic diabetes insipidus:
  Lithium, diuretics
  Interstitial nephritis
  Hypokalaemia, hypercalcaemia

but sexually transmitted diseases and bladder stone may also present with dysuria.

Frequency

Frequency describes micturition more often than a patient's expectations. It may be a consequence of polyuria, when urine volume is normal or high, but is also found in patients with dysuria or prostatic disease when urine volume is normal.

Polyuria

Causes of an inappropriately high urine volume (>3 L/day) are shown in Box 7.4. Assessment involves measuring U&Es, calcium, glucose, albumin and fluid intake and output.

Nocturia

Waking up at night to void urine may be a consequence of polyuria but may also result from fluid intake or diuretic use in the late evening. Nocturia also occurs in CKD, and in prostatic enlargement where it is associated with poor stream, hesitancy, incomplete bladder emptying, terminal dribbling and urinary frequency.

Urinary incontinence

Urinary incontinence is defined as any involuntary leakage of urine. Urinary tract pathology causing incontinence is described later. It may also occur

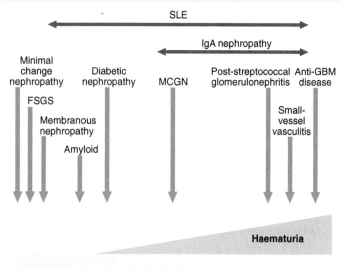

Fig. 7.3 Spectrum of glomerular diseases. *FSGS*, Focal segmental glomerulosclerosis; *GBM*, glomerular basement membrane; *IgA*, immunoglobulin A; *MCGN*, mesangiocapillary glomerulonephritis; *SLE*, systemic lupus erythematosus; *PCR*, protein:creatinine ratio = urine protein (mg/L)/urine creatinine (mmol/L).

with a normal urinary tract, for example, in association with dementia or poor mobility, or transiently during an acute illness or hospitalisation, especially in older people. Diuretics, alcohol and caffeine may worsen incontinence. Investigation is described on p. 245.

Glomerular diseases

Glomerular diseases may cause acute and CKD, and may follow a number of insults: immunological injury (glomerulonephritis), inherited abnormality (e.g. Alport's syndrome), metabolic stress (e.g. diabetes mellitus), deposition of abnormal proteins (e.g. amyloid) or other direct glomerular injury. The response of the glomerulus to injury varies according to the nature of the insult (Fig. 7.3). At one extreme, specific podocyte injury, or structural alteration of the glomerulus affecting podocyte function (e.g. by scarring or deposition of matrix or other material), causes proteinuria and nephrotic syndrome. At the other end of the spectrum, inflammation leads to cell damage and proliferation, causing breakage of the GBM and blood leakage into the urine. In its extreme form, with acute sodium retention and hypertension, this is referred to as nephritic syndrome.

Glomerulonephritis

Glomerulonephritis means 'inflammation of glomeruli', although inflammation is not apparent in all varieties. Most types of glomerulonephritis are immunologically mediated, and several respond to immunosuppressive drugs. Classifications of glomerulonephritis are largely histopathological.

Diseases presenting with nephrotic syndrome

Minimal change nephropathy

Minimal change disease occurs at all ages, but accounts for nephrotic syndrome (PCR >300 mg/mmol, hypoalbuminaemia [< 30 g/L], oedema and fluid retention) in most children and about one-quarter of adults. It is caused by reversible dysfunction of podocytes. It typically remits with high-dose glucocorticoid therapy (1 mg/kg prednisolone for 6 weeks). Some patients who respond incompletely or relapse frequently need maintenance glucocorticoids, cytotoxic therapy or other agents. Minimal change disease does not progress to CKD but can present with problems related to nephrotic syndrome and complications of treatment.

Focal segmental glomerulosclerosis

Primary FSGS can occur at any age and presents with massive proteinuria and nephrotic syndrome. It is particularly common in people of West African descent who carry an apolipoprotein L1 gene variant predicting increased risk of FSGS. Histology shows sclerosis affecting segments of the glomeruli, with positive immunofluorescence staining for C3 and IgM. Because disease is focal, abnormal glomeruli may be missed on small renal biopsies.

Primary FSGS may respond to high-dose glucocorticoid therapy (0.5–2.0 mg/kg/day), but the response is rarely rapid or complete. Ciclosporin and mycophenylate have also been used to uncertain effect. Progression to CKD is common in patients who do not respond to glucocorticoids, and the disease frequently recurs after renal transplantation, sometimes immediately.

FSGS can also be secondary to HIV infection, morbid obesity, hypertension or haemolytic uraemic syndrome. Secondary FSGS presents with the same histology as primary FSGS, but with less proteinuria. Management involves ACE inhibitors and treating the cause.

Membranous nephropathy

This is the most common cause of nephrotic syndrome in adults. It is usually caused by autoantibodies to surface antigens on podocytes. Some cases are associated with known causes (malignancy, hepatitis B, lupus) but most are idiopathic. Of this group, approximately one-third remit spontaneously, one-third remain nephrotic and one-third develop progressive CKD. Short-term glucocorticoids and cyclophosphamide may improve both the nephrotic syndrome and the long-term prognosis. However, because of the toxicity of these regimens, most nephrologists reserve such treatment for those with severe nephrotic syndrome or deteriorating renal function.

Diseases presenting with mild nephritic syndrome

IgA nephropathy and Henoch–Schönlein purpura

IgA nephropathy is the most common glomerulonephritis, and presents in many ways. Haematuria is the earliest sign (nonvisible haematuria is universal), and hypertension is also common. Proteinuria occurs later. There may be progressive loss of renal function leading to end stage renal disease (ESRD). Some young adults develop acute self-limiting exacerbations, often with visible haematuria, associated with minor respiratory infections.

Management of IgA nephropathy involves control of BP with ACE inhibitors and high-dose glucocorticoids if there is progressive renal disease.

In children, and occasionally in adults, systemic vasculitis occurs in response to an infectious trigger and is called Henoch–Schönlein purpura. A characteristic petechial rash (cutaneous vasculitis, typically affecting the buttocks and lower legs), abdominal pain (GI vasculitis) and arthralgia usually dominate the clinical picture, with mild glomerulonephritis indicated by haematuria. Renal biopsy shows mesangial IgA deposition, indistinguishable from acute IgA nephropathy. Treatment is supportive, and the prognosis is good.

Mesangiocapillary glomerulonephritis

MCGN is characterised by increased mesangial cellularity, with thickening of glomerular capillary walls. It presents with proteinuria and haematuria. There are two main subtypes:

- Deposition of immunoglobulins within the glomeruli; associated with chronic infections, autoimmune diseases and monoclonal gammopathy
- Deposition of complement; associated with inherited or acquired abnormalities in the complement pathway

Management of MCGN with immunoglobulin deposits consists of treatment of the underlying disease and the use of immunosuppressive drugs. There is no proven treatment for MCGN with complement deposition, although eculizumab shows promise.

Diseases presenting with rapidly progressive glomerulonephritis

Rapidly progressive glomerulonephritis causes rapid loss of renal function over days to weeks. Renal biopsy shows crescentic lesions often associated with necrotising lesions within the glomerulus. Causes include:

- Postinfectious glomerulonephritis.
- Anti-GBM disease.
- Small-vessel vasculitides (p. 628).
- SLE (p. 622).
- IgA and other nephropathies (occasionally).

Antiglomerular basement membrane disease

This is a rare autoimmune condition in which specific anti-GBM antibodies damage the basement membrane in glomeruli and pulmonary capillaries, leading to renal impairment and lung haemorrhage (Goodpasture's disease). Management includes plasma exchange, glucocorticoids and immunosuppressants.

Infection-related glomerulonephritis

Bacterial infections, usually subacute (e.g. bacterial endocarditis), may cause a variety of histological patterns of glomerulonephritis, but usually with extensive immunoglobulin deposition and complement consumption.

Postinfectious glomerulonephritis is most common following infection with certain strains of streptococcus (poststreptococcal nephritis) but can occur after other infections. It is more common in children than adults but is now rare in the developed world. It presents around 10 days after throat infection or longer after skin infection. An acute nephritis of varying severity occurs, with sodium retention, hypertension and oedema. Tests show a reduced GFR, proteinuria, haematuria, reduced urine volume, low serum C3 and C4 and evidence of streptococcal infection (positive antistreptolysin O test). Treatment is supportive, with control of blood pressure and fluid overload, as well as salt restriction, diuretics and dialysis if required. Antibiotics are unnecessary, as the renal disease occurs after the infection has subsided. The prognosis is good, with recovery of renal function typical even in those requiring dialysis therapy.

Tubulo-interstitial diseases

These diseases affect renal tubules and the surrounding interstitium. The clinical presentation is with tubular dysfunction and electrolyte abnormalities, moderate proteinuria and varying degrees of renal impairment.

Acute interstitial nephritis

AIN may be caused by allergic drug reactions (e.g. to proton pump inhibitors, NSAIDs), autoimmune nephritis, infections (e.g. pyelonephritis, TB) or toxins (e.g. mushrooms or myeloma light chains). Clinical presentation is with nonoliguric renal impairment or an eosinophilic reaction with fever and rash.

Investigations

Renal biopsies show intense inflammation surrounding tubules and blood vessels and invading tubules, with occasional eosinophils (especially in drug-induced disease). The degree of chronic inflammation in a biopsy is a useful predictor of long-term renal function. Eosinophiluria may be present, but it is not a good discriminator for AIN.

Management

Remove/treat the cause. High-dose glucocorticoids may accelerate recovery and prevent long-term scarring.

Chronic interstitial nephritis

Known causes of CIN are shown in Box 7.5; however, it is often diagnosed late with no apparent cause.

> ### 7.5 Causes of chronic interstitial nephritis
>
> - Any cause of acute interstitial nephritis
> - Glomerulonephritis
> - Immune/inflammatory (sarcoid, Sjögren's, SLE, transplant rejection)
> - Toxic (mushrooms, Balkan nephropathy, lead)
> - Drugs (ciclosporin, tacrolimus, tenofovir, lithium, analgesics)
> - Infection (severe pyelonephritis)
> - Congenital/developmental (reflux, sickle cell nephropathy)
> - Metabolic and systemic diseases (hypokalaemia, hyperoxaluria)

Clinical features, investigations and management

Most patients present in adult life with moderate CKD, hypertension and small kidneys. Because of tubular dysfunction, electrolyte abnormalities (e.g. hyperkalaemia, acidosis) may be severe. Urinalysis is nonspecific.

Management is supportive, with correction of acidosis and hyperkalaemia and renal replacement therapy if required.

Papillary necrosis

The renal papillae may become necrotic when their vascular supply is impaired by diabetes, sickle-cell disease or long-term NSAIDs. Some patients are asymptomatic, but others present with renal colic and renal impairment when the necrosed papillae cause ureteric obstruction. Urinalysis frequently shows haematuria and sterile pyuria. Diagnosis is by CT urography or IV pyelography. Management is by relieving any obstruction and avoiding precipitating drugs.

Genetic renal diseases

Alport's syndrome is an uncommon X-linked condition in which abnormal collagen deposition at basement membranes results in haematuria, progressive renal failure and sensorineural deafness. ACE inhibitors slow but do not prevent loss of function, and many patients require RRT.

Nephrotic syndrome with an FSGS pattern on biopsy may be inherited through several autosomal dominant and recessive gene defects.

Isolated defects of tubular function

An increasing number of disorders (e.g. renal glycosuria and cystinuria) are now known to be caused by specific defects of transporter molecules in renal tubular cells.

The term *Fanconi syndrome* is used to describe generalised proximal tubular dysfunction. This presents with low blood phosphate and uric acid, glycosuria, aminoaciduria and proximal renal tubular acidosis. Renal tubular acidosis describes the common endpoint of a variety of diseases affecting distal (classical or type 1) or proximal (type 2) renal tubular function. They cause metabolic acidosis with a normal anion gap (p. 198).

Cystic kidney diseases

Adult polycystic kidney disease

PKD is common condition (prevalence ~1:1000) and is inherited as an autosomal dominant trait. Small cysts lined by tubular epithelium develop from infancy or childhood and enlarge slowly and irregularly. Surrounding normal kidney tissue is progressively damaged, and as renal function declines, the kidneys become grossly enlarged. *PKD1* gene mutations account for 85% of cases, and *PKD2* for around 15%. ESRD occurs in around 50% of patients with *PKD1* mutations, with a mean age of onset of 52 years of age, as well as in a minority of patients with *PKD2* mutations with a mean age of onset of 69 years of age. Between 5% and 10% of patients on renal replacement therapy (RRT) have PKD.

Clinical features
See Box 7.6.

Investigations and screening
These are based on family history, clinical examination and USS. USS demonstrates cysts in around 95% of affected patients aged older than 20 years of age, but may not detect smaller cysts in younger patients. Genetic diagnosis is possible, but not routinely used. Screening for intracranial aneurysms is not generally indicated but can be done using MRI in those with a family history of subarachnoid haemorrhage.

Management
Good BP control is important because of cardiovascular morbidity and mortality, but there is no evidence that this retards the loss of renal function in PKD. The vasopressin V2 receptor antagonist tolvaptan may retard kidney volume increase and slow the rate of GFR decline. Patients with PKD are usually good candidates for dialysis and transplantation. Sometimes the kidneys are so large that one or both have to be removed to make space for a renal transplant.

7.6 Adult PKD: common clinical features

- Asymptomatic until later life
- Vague discomfort in loin or abdomen caused by increasing mass of renal tissue
- One or both kidneys palpable, with nodular surface
- Acute loin pain or renal colic caused by haemorrhage into a cyst
- Hypertension gradually develops over age 20 years
- Haematuria (with little or no proteinuria)
- Urinary tract or cyst infections
- Gradual-onset renal failure
- Associated features:
  Hepatic cysts (30%)
  Berry aneurysms of the cerebral vasculature
  Mitral and aortic regurgitation (common but rarely severe)
  Colonic diverticula
  Abdominal wall hernias

Other cystic diseases

Renal cysts and diabetes syndrome are caused by a genetic mutation with a renal phenotype varying from cysts to a tubulo-interstitial pattern of injury or congenital absence of a kidney.

Tuberous sclerosis (p. 772) may cause renal angiomyolipomas and cysts, occasionally resulting in CKD.

Von Hippel–Lindau syndrome (p. 697) is associated with multiple renal cysts, renal adenomas and renal adenocarcinoma. Other features include CNS haemangioblastomas, pancreatic cystadenomas and adrenal phaeochromocytoma.

Acquired cystic disease can develop in patients with a very long history of renal failure, so it is not an inherited cystic disease. It is associated with increased erythropoietin production and sometimes with the development of renal cell carcinoma.

Renal vascular diseases

Diseases that affect renal blood vessels may cause renal ischaemia, leading to acute or chronic renal failure or secondary hypertension. The rising prevalence of atherosclerosis and diabetes in ageing populations has made renal vascular disease an important cause of ESRD.

Renal artery stenosis

Atherosclerosis is the most common cause of renal artery stenosis, occurring in up to 4% of older patients with widespread arterial disease. In patients younger than 50 years of age, fibromuscular dysplasia is a more likely cause of renal artery stenosis. This is an uncommon congenital disorder of unknown cause; it affects the media ('medial fibroplasia'), which narrows the artery but rarely leads to total occlusion. It most commonly presents with hypertension in patients aged 15 to 30 years of age and presents in women more frequently than men.

Clinical features

- **Hypertension:** This is driven by activation of the renin–angiotensin system in response to renal ischaemia. In atherosclerotic renal artery disease, there is usually evidence of arterial disease elsewhere, particularly in the legs. Factors that predict renovascular disease are shown in Box 7.7.

7.7 Renal artery stenosis

Renal artery stenosis is more likely if:
- Hypertension is severe, *or* of recent onset *or* difficult to control
- Kidneys are asymmetrical in size
- Flash pulmonary oedema occurs repeatedly
- There is peripheral vascular disease of lower limbs
- Renal function has deteriorated on ACE inhibitors

- **Deterioration of renal function on ACE inhibitors:** When renal perfusion pressure drops, the renin–angiotensin–aldosterone system is activated, and angiotensin-mediated glomerular efferent arteriolar vasoconstriction maintains glomerular filtration pressure. ACE inhibitors or ARBs block this physiological response. A drop in GFR (or a >30% rise in creatinine) on ACE inhibitors raises the possibility of renal artery stenosis.
- **Flash pulmonary oedema:** Repeated episodes of acute pulmonary oedema associated with severe hypertension, without other obvious cause (e.g. myocardial infarction) in patients with normal or mildly impaired renal and cardiac function, can indicate renal artery stenosis.
- **Renal impairment:** This may be the presenting feature in bilateral renal artery stenosis.

Investigations

Imaging of the renal arteries with CT or MRI angiography should confirm the diagnosis. USS may reveal asymmetry of kidney size. Biochemistry may show impaired renal function and elevated plasma renin, sometimes with hypokalaemia because of hyperaldosteronism.

Management

First-line management is with antihypertensives supplemented by statins and low-dose aspirin in those with atherosclerotic disease. Interventions to correct vessel narrowing should be considered in all patients aged younger than 40 years, those with hypertension that is hard to control medically, those with deteriorating renal function and those with episodes of 'flash' pulmonary oedema. Angioplasty with stenting is of proven value in fibromuscular dysplasia, but the results are less certain in atherosclerotic disease. Risks include renal infarction and failure to improve as a result of distal small-vessel disease.

Acute renal infarction

Sudden occlusion of the renal arteries usually presents as acute loin pain with nonvisible haematuria, but pain is occasionally absent. Severe hypertension is common but not universal. LDH and CRP are commonly raised. Infarction may be caused by renal artery thrombosis or by thromboemboli from a distant source, which may cause occlusion in branch arteries with multiple parenchymal infarcts, visible on CT scanning. Bilateral infarction or infarction of a single functioning kidney results in AKI with anuria. Patients with bilateral occlusion usually have widespread vascular disease, and may show evidence of aortic occlusion, with absent femoral pulses and reduced leg perfusion.

Management is largely supportive and includes anticoagulation for an identified source of thromboemboli. It is sometimes possible to restore renal blood flow and function by stenting an acutely blocked main renal artery.

Diseases of small intrarenal vessels

A number of conditions are associated with acute damage and occlusion of small blood vessels (arterioles and capillaries) in the kidney (Box 7.8). They may be associated with similar changes elsewhere in the body. A common feature of these syndromes is microangiopathic haemolytic anaemia, in which fragmented red cells can be seen on a blood film as a consequence of damage during passage through the abnormal vessels.

> **7.8 Thrombotic microangiopathies associated with acute renal damage**
>
> **Primary thrombotic microangiopathies**
>
> * Haemolytic uraemic syndrome—Shiga toxin, complement-mediated and drug-induced
> * Thrombotic thrombocytopenic purpura
>
> **Thrombotic microangiopathy associated with systemic disorders**
>
> * Disseminated intravascular coagulation
> * Malignancy—breast, prostate, lung, pancreas and GI
> * Systemic sclerosis
> * Preeclampsia
> * Malignant hypertension

Small-vessel vasculitis

Renal small-vessel vasculitis usually presents with a glomerulonephritis (see p. 223).

Renal involvement in systemic disorders

Diabetes mellitus

Patients with diabetes advance steadily from moderately elevated albuminuria to dipstick-positive proteinuria, then to hypertension and progressive renal failure. Few require diagnostic renal biopsy, but atypical features should raise suspicion of an alternative condition.

ACE inhibitors and ARBs slow progression, as described on p. 455. In some patients, proteinuria may be eradicated and progression halted, even if renal function is abnormal.

Multiple myeloma

In myeloma, malignant plasma cells produce a paraprotein, often a monoclonal light chain (p. 581). These paraproteins may cause AKI, tubular injury, amyloidosis and proteinuria. Hypercalcaemia may also occur as a result of bony metastases.

Hepatic–renal disease

Severe hepatic dysfunction may cause a type of renal failure, hepatorenal syndrome (p. 519). Patients with liver disease can also develop AKI in response to bleeding, diuretics and infection.

Sarcoidosis

The most common renal manifestation of sarcoidosis is hypercalcaemia from 1-α-vitamin D formation in granulomas. Less commonly, it causes a granulomatous interstitial nephritis.

Systemic vasculitis

Small-vessel vasculitis

This causes a focal inflammatory glomerulonephritis, often with crescentic changes. It may be a kidney-limited disorder with rapidly deteriorating renal function, or may be associated with a systemic illness with acute phase response, weight loss and arthralgia; in some patients it causes pulmonary haemorrhage, which can be life threatening.

The most important cause is ANCA-positive vasculitis (p. 628), of which two subtypes occur: microscopic polyangiitis, and granulomatosis with polyangiitis (formerly known as Wegener's granulomatosis). Both may present with glomerulonephritis and pulmonary haemorrhage with constitutional symptoms. Antibodies are nonspecific, so biopsy is often required.

Treatment of small-vessel vasculitis is with glucocorticoids, cyclophosphamide and biological agents such as rituximab. Plasma exchange offers additional benefit in patients with progressive renal damage who are not responding to drugs.

Medium- to large-vessel vasculitis (e.g. polyarteritis nodosa) does not cause glomerulonephritis, but can cause hypertension, renal infarction or haematuria.

Systemic sclerosis

Renal complications of systemic sclerosis occur most frequently in the diffuse cutaneous systemic sclerosis form of the disease. Intrarenal vasospasm causes severe hypertension, microangiopathic features and progressive oliguric renal failure. Treatment is with ACE inhibitors and RRT.

Systemic lupus erythematosus

Subclinical renal involvement, with nonvisible haematuria and proteinuria but minimally impaired or normal renal function, is common in SLE. Usually this is caused by glomerular disease, although interstitial nephritis may also occur in overlap syndromes (e.g. mixed connective tissue disease, Sjögren's syndrome). SLE can produce almost any glomerular histology, and clinical features range from florid, rapidly progressive glomerulonephritis to nephrotic syndrome. High-dose glucocorticoids and cyclophosphamide reduce the risk of ESRD in lupus nephritis.

Sickle-cell nephropathy

Improved survival of patients with sickle-cell disease (p. 571) means that a larger proportion live to develop chronic complications of microvascular occlusion.

Clinical features

Damage to the medullary vasa recta causes loss of urine-concentrating ability with polyuria. Distal renal tubular acidosis with hyperkalaemia is typical. Papillary necrosis also occurs. A minority of patients develop ESRD.

Acute kidney injury

AKI refers to a sudden and often reversible loss of renal function that develops over a period of days or weeks. There are many possible causes (Fig. 7.4), and AKI is frequently multifactorial.

Clinical features

Early recognition and intervention are important in AKI; all emergency admissions to hospital should have renal function checked and should undergo assessment of risk for developing AKI. This includes detecting coexisting diabetes, vascular and liver disease, which increase risk, and recording drugs (e.g. ACE inhibitors, NSAIDs) that may impair renal function. If a high serum creatinine is found, establish (ideally using prior renal function measurements) whether this is acute, acute-on-chronic or a sign of chronic kidney disease (CKD) (see Fig. 7.5). Clinical features and pertinent investigations for the different causes of AKI are shown in Box 7.9.

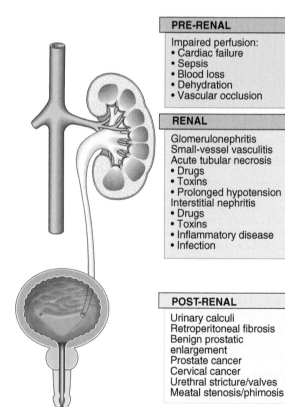

PRE-RENAL

Impaired perfusion:
• Cardiac failure
• Sepsis
• Blood loss
• Dehydration
• Vascular occlusion

RENAL

Glomerulonephritis
Small-vessel vasculitis
Acute tubular necrosis
• Drugs
• Toxins
• Prolonged hypotension
Interstitial nephritis
• Drugs
• Toxins
• Inflammatory disease
• Infection

POST-RENAL

Urinary calculi
Retroperitoneal fibrosis
Benign prostatic enlargement
Prostate cancer
Cervical cancer
Urethral stricture/valves
Meatal stenosis/phimosis

Fig. 7.4 Causes of acute kidney injury.

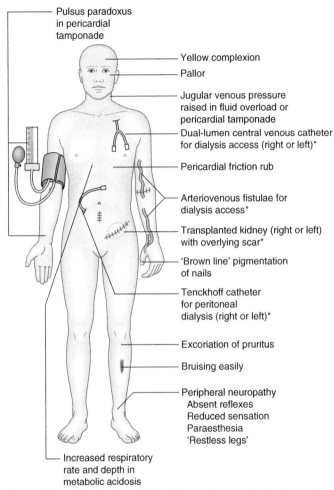

Fig. 7.5 Physical signs in chronic kidney disease. *Features of renal replacement therapy.

Prerenal AKI: Patients with prerenal AKI are typically hypotensive and tachycardic, with signs of hypovolaemia including postural hypotension (>20/10 mmHg decrease from lying to standing). Patients with sepsis may have peripheral vasodilatation and yet have relative under-filling of the arterial tree and renal vasoconstriction, leading to AKI with ATN. Although the cause of renal hypoperfusion may be obvious, concealed blood loss may occur

i 7.9 Categorising AKI by history, examination and investigations

Type of AKI	History	Examination	Investigations
Prerenal	Volume depletion Drugs Liver disease Cardiac failure	Low BP (postural drop), Tachycardia, Weightloss, Dry mouth, ↑ skin turgor, JVP not visible	Urine Na <20mmol/L High urea:creatinine ratio Urinalysis bland
Renal			
ATN	Prolonged prerenal state Sepsis Toxic:drugs Other (rhabdomyolysis, snake bite, mushrooms)	Vital signs Fluid assessment Limbs (compartment syndrome)	Urine Na >40 mmol/L Dense granular ('muddy brown') casts Creatine kinase
Glomeru-lar	Rash, weight loss, arthralgia Chest symptoms IV drug use	Hypertension Oedema Purpuric rash, uveitis, arthritis	Proteinuria, haematuria, Red cell casts, dysmorphic red cells, ANCA, anti-GBM, ANA, C3, C4, Hepatitis, HIV, Renal biopsy
Tubulo-interstitial	Interstitial nephritis: drugs Sarcoidosis Tubular obstruction: 1.Myeloma 2.Crystal nephropathy: Drugs, Oxalate, Urate	Fever, rash	Leucocyturia Eosinophiluria Eosinophilia White cell casts Minimal proteinuria Paraprotein Calcium Urine for crystals Serum urate Urine oxalate
Vascular	Flank pain, trauma Anticoagulation Recent angiography Nephrotic syndrome (renal vein thrombosis) Systemic sclerosis Diarrhoea (HUS)	BP Fundoscopy Livedo reticularis Sclerodactyly	Haematuria C3, C4 Doppler renal ultrasound CT angiography Platelets, haemolytic screen, lactate dehydrogenase

Continued

7.9 Categorising AKI by history, examination and investigations—cont'd

Type of AKI	History	Examination	Investigations
Postrenal	Prostate cancer history Neurogenic bladder Cervical carcinoma Retroperitoneal fibrosis Bladder outlet symptoms	Rectal examination (prostate and anal tone) Distended bladder Pelvic mass	Urinalysis normal or haematuria Renal ultrasound (hydronephrosis) Isotope renogram if ultrasound inconclusive

7.10 Management of AKI

- Assess fluid status to determine fluid prescription:
  Hypovolaemic: optimise systemic haemodynamic status with fluid challenge and inotropes if necessary
  Euvolaemic: match fluid intake to urine output plus 500 mL for insensible losses
  Fluid-overloaded: prescribe loop diuretics (high dose often required); if unsatisfactory response, prescribe dialysis
- Give calcium resonium to stabilise myocardium and glucose + insulin to correct hyperkalaemia if K^+ >6.5 mmol/L (p. 195) until dialysis or restoration of renal function allows adequate potassium excretion
- Consider sodium bicarbonate (100 mmol) to correct acidosis if H^+ is >100 nmol/L (pH <7.0)
- Discontinue any nephrotoxic drugs, and reduce doses of other drugs according to level of renal function
- Ensure adequate nutrition
- Consider PPIs to reduce the risk of upper gastrointestinal bleeding
- Screen for infections and treat if present
- If obstructed, drain lower or upper urinary tract as necessary

following trauma (e.g. pelvic fractures) or into a pregnant uterus. Also, large intravascular volumes may be lost with injuries, burns, severe inflammatory skin diseases or sepsis. Finally, prerenal AKI may occur without hypotension in those taking NSAIDs or ACE inhibitors.

Renal and postrenal AKI: Factors that can differentiate the causes of renal and postrenal AKI are summarised in Box 7.9. Patients should be examined clinically and by USS for bladder enlargement and hydronephrosis.

Management

Management common to all forms of AKI is summarised in Box 7.10.

Haemodynamic status: If hypovolaemia is present, it should be corrected by replacement of intravenous fluid or blood; excessive volume should be avoided because it can provoke pulmonary oedema. Balanced crystalloid solutions, such as Plasma-Lyte, Hartmann's or Ringer's lactate, may be preferable to isotonic saline (0.9% NaCl) to avoid hyperchloraemic acidosis. Critically ill patients may require inotropes to restore blood pressure, but trials do not support the use of low-dose dopamine.

Metabolic derangements: Hyperkalaemia greater than 6.5 mmol/L should be treated immediately to prevent arrhythmias. Restoration of blood volume will usually correct acidosis, but severe acidosis may be treated with sodium bicarbonate if volume status allows. Dilutional hyponatraemia may occur if the patient has drunk freely despite oliguria or has received intravenous dextrose. Hypocalcaemia is common, but rarely requires treatment. Serum phosphate levels are usually high.

Cardiopulmonary complications: Pulmonary oedema may be caused by administration of excessive fluid relative to urine output and by increased pulmonary capillary permeability. If urine output cannot be rapidly restored, dialysis may be required to remove excess fluid. Temporary respiratory support may also be necessary.

Nutrition: Parenteral or enteral tube feeding may be needed in hypercatabolic patients. Feed should include sufficient energy and adequate protein, although high protein intake should be avoided.

Infection: Patients with AKI are at risk of intercurrent infection, and prompt diagnosis and treatment are essential.

Medications: Drugs known to cause kidney injury and any nonessential drugs should be stopped. Vasoactive medications (e.g. NSAIDs and ACE inhibitors) should be discontinued because they may prolong AKI. H_2-receptor antagonists or PPIs should be given to prevent GI bleeding. Remaining essential treatments should have the doses adjusted if necessary.

Renal tract obstruction: Relieving obstruction in postrenal AKI may involve catheterisation for bladder outflow obstruction, or a ureteric stent or percutaneous nephrostomy for ureteric obstruction.

Renal replacement therapy: If uraemia and hyperkalaemia fail to respond to the previously mentioned measures, a period of renal replacement therapy may be required. The two main options for AKI are haemodialysis or high-volume haemofiltration. Both carry risks, including haemodynamic instability and infected catheters, so careful assessment of individual cases is required. Peritoneal dialysis can be used if haemodialysis is unavailable.

Recovery from AKI:

A gradual return of urine output and a steady improvement in biochemistry accompany recovery. Some patients, primarily those with ATN or those in whom chronic urinary obstruction has been relieved, develop a 'diuretic phase'. Sufficient fluid to replace the urine output should be given. After a few days, urine volume falls to normal as the concentrating mechanisms recover. During the diuretic phase, supplements of sodium, chloride, potassium and phosphate may be necessary to compensate for increased urinary losses.

Chronic kidney disease

CKD refers to an irreversible deterioration in renal function that classically develops over a period of years. Initially, it is manifest only as a biochemical abnormality. Eventually, loss of the excretory, metabolic and endocrine functions of the kidney leads to the clinical symptoms and signs of renal failure, which are referred to as uraemia. The stages of CKD are defined in Box 7.11. When death is likely without renal replacement therapy (stage 5 CKD), it is called end stage renal disease (ESRD).

CKD may be caused by any condition that damages the normal function of the kidney. Common causes are shown in Box 7.12.

Clinical features

The typical presentation is for a raised urea and creatinine to be found incidentally during routine blood tests, often when screening high-risk patients, such as those with diabetes or hypertension. Most patients are asymptomatic until their GFR falls below 30 mL/min/1.73 m^2, and some remain

	7.11 Stages of CKD			
Stage[a]	GFR definition[b]	Description	Prevalence	Clinical presentation
1	Kidney damage[c] with normal or high (>90)	Normal function	3.5%	Asymptomatic
2	Kidney damage and GFR 60–89	Mild CKD	3.9%	Asymptomatic
3A	GFR 45–59	Mild to moderate CKD	7.6% (3A and 3B)	Usually asymptomatic
3B	GFR 30–44	Moderate to severe CKD		Anaemia in some 3B patients Most are nonprogressive or progress very slowly
4	GFR 15–29	Severe CKD	0.4%	Symptoms start at GFR <20 Electrolyte problems likely as GFR falls
5	GFR <15 or on dialysis	Kidney failure	0.1%	Significant symptoms and complications Dialysis usually initiated at GFR <10

[a]Stages defined by the US National Kidney Foundation Kidney Disease Quality Outcomes Initiative 2002.
[b]Two GFRs 3 months apart are required to assign a stage. GFR values in mL/min/1.73 m^2.
[c]Pathological abnormalities or markers of damage, including urine test or imaging abnormalities.

7.12 Causes of CKD	
Diabetes mellitus	20%–40%
Interstitial diseases	20%–30%
Glomerular diseases	10%–20%
Hypertension	5%–20%
Systemic inflammatory diseases	5%–10%
Renovascular disease	5%
Congenital and inherited	5%
Unknown	5%–20%

asymptomatic with much lower GFR values than this. An early symptom is nocturia, caused by the loss of concentrating ability and increased osmotic load per nephron, but this is nonspecific. When the GFR falls below 15–20 mL/min/1.73 m^2, symptoms and signs are common, and can affect almost all body systems (Fig. 7.5). They typically include tiredness or breathlessness, which may be related to renal anaemia or fluid overload. With further deterioration in renal function, patients may suffer pruritus, anorexia, weight loss, nausea, vomiting and hiccups. In very advanced renal failure, respiration may be particularly deep (Kussmaul breathing) as a result of metabolic acidosis, and patients may develop muscular twitching, fits, drowsiness and coma.

Investigations

Initial screening tests for CKD are summarised in Box 7.13. The aims are to:
• Exclude AKI. • Identify the underlying cause. • Address reversible factors that are making renal function worse, for example, hypertension, urinary tract obstruction or infection and nephrotoxic medications. • Screen for complications such as osteodystrophy or anaemia. • Screen for cardiovascular risk factors.

Management

This is aimed at preventing further renal damage, managing and limiting metabolic and cardiovascular complications and preparing for RRT if required.

Monitoring of renal function: The rate of change in renal function varies between patients and over time. Renal function should therefore be monitored every 6 months in patients with stage 3 CKD, but more frequently in deteriorating patients and those with stage 4 or 5 CKD. A plot of GFR against time can reveal treatment effects and unexpected declines and help to plan when RRT will be required.

Reduction of rate of progression: Slowing the rate of progression of CKD may reduce complications and delay symptom onset and the need for RRT. The primary cause should be treated where possible; tight blood pressure control is important in CKD regardless of cause, and reducing proteinuria is a key target in those with glomerular disease.

i 7.13 Suggested investigations in CKD	
Initial tests	**Interpretation**
Urea and creatinine	Compare with prior values
Urinalysis and quantification of proteinuria	Haematuria and proteinuria suggest glomerular disease and need for biopsy. Proteinuria: risk of progressive CKD requiring preventive ACE inhibitors or ARBs
Electrolytes	To identify hyperkalaemia and acidosis
Calcium, phosphate, PTH and 25(OH)D	Assessment of renal osteodystrophy
Albumin	Low albumin: consider malnutrition, inflammation, nephrotic syndrome
FBC ($\pm$ Fe, ferritin, folate, B_{12})	If anaemic, exclude common nonrenal explanations, then manage as renal anaemia
Lipids, glucose, $\pm$ HbA$_{1c}$	Cardiovascular risk high in CKD: treat risk factors aggressively
Renal ultrasound	If obstructive urinary symptoms, persistent haematuria, family history of PKD or progressive CKD. Small kidneys suggest chronicity. Asymmetric renal size suggests renovascular or developmental disease
Hepatitis and HIV serology	If dialysis or transplant is planned. Hepatitis B vaccination recommended if seronegative
Other tests	Consider relevant tests from Box 7.10, especially if cause is unknown

7

Antihypertensive therapy: Lowering BP slows the rate of decline of renal function in CKD, with associated reductions in the risk of heart failure, stroke and peripheral vascular disease. No threshold for this benefit has been identified, and any reduction appears beneficial. The suggested target BP is 130/80 mmHg for patients with CKD and moderate albuminuria, and 125/75 mmHg for those with CKD and heavy proteinuria (PCR >100 mg/mmol). Achieving these targets requires multiple drugs and good adherence to treatment.

Reduction of proteinuria: The degree of proteinuria is clearly related to the rate of progression of renal disease, and reducing proteinuria slows progression. ACE inhibitors and ARBs reduce proteinuria and retard progression of CKD, as well as reducing cardiovascular events and all-cause mortality. They may produce an initial reduction in GFR, but can be continued, provided the reduction is not greater than 25% or progressive.

Treatment of complications:

Fluid and electrolyte balance: Urea is a product of protein degradation and accumulates in patients with CKD. All patients with stage 4 or 5 CKD

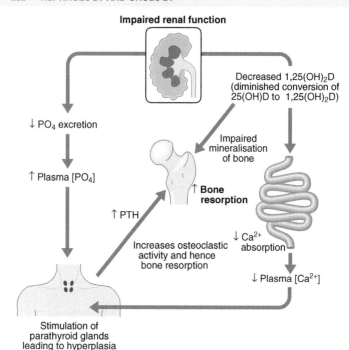

Impaired renal function

↓ PO₄ excretion

↑ Plasma [PO₄]

Decreased 1,25(OH)₂D
(diminished conversion of
25(OH)D to 1,25(OH)₂D)

Impaired
mineralisation
of bone

↑ **Bone
resorption**

↑ PTH

Increases osteoclastic
activity and hence
bone resorption

↓ Ca²⁺
absorption

↓ Plasma [Ca²⁺]

Stimulation of
parathyroid glands
leading to hyperplasia

Fig. 7.6 Pathogenesis of renal osteodystrophy. The net result of decreased 1,25(OH)₂ cholecalciferol levels and increased parathyroid hormone (PTH) levels in the presence of high [PO₄] is bone that exhibits increased osteoclastic activity and increased osteoid content as a consequence of decreased mineralisation.

should be advised to avoid excessive protein consumption. Severe protein restriction is not recommended, however, as it may lead to malnutrition.

Potassium often accumulates in patients with advanced CKD, who should be advised to reduce daily potassium intake to below 70 mmol. The inability of the failing kidney to excrete sodium and water loads commonly leads to their accumulation, which may manifest as oedema and exacerbate hypertension. Patients with fluid overload should be recommended a low-sodium diet (<100 mmol/24 hours) and in severe cases fluid intake should also be restricted. Correction of acidosis using sodium bicarbonate supplements to keep plasma bicarbonate greater than 22 mmol/L may be beneficial.

Renal bone disease: The pathogenesis of renal bone disease is summarised in Fig. 7.6. Hypocalcaemia is corrected by giving 1α-hydroxylated synthetic analogues of vitamin D, adjusting the dose to avoid hypercalcaemia and to reduce PTH levels to between two and four times normal. This will usually prevent or control osteomalacia. Hyperphosphataemia is controlled by dietary restriction of high-phosphate foods (milk, cheese, eggs) and the use of phosphate-binding drugs with food. These agents form insoluble complexes with dietary phosphate and prevent its absorption (e.g. calcium carbonate). Secondary hyperparathyroidism is usually controlled by these measures but, in severe bone disease with autonomous parathyroid function, parathyroidectomy may become necessary.

Anaemia: Recombinant human erythropoietin is effective in correcting the anaemia associated with CKD. The target haemoglobin level is between 100 and 120 g/L. Complications of treatment include hypertension and thrombosis. Erythropoietin is less effective in the presence of iron deficiency, active inflammation or malignancy. These factors should be sought and, if possible, corrected before treatment.

Cardiovascular risk: Patients with CKD are at increased cardiovascular risk and should be encouraged to exercise, maintain a healthy weight and avoid smoking. Hypercholesterolaemia and raised triglycerides are common in CKD. Control of dyslipidaemia with statins may slow disease progression.

Preparing for RRT: When patients are known to have progressive CKD and are under regular clinic review, preparation for RRT should begin at least 12 months before the predicted start date. This involves psychological and social support, assessment of home circumstances and discussion about choice of treatment between haemodialysis, peritoneal dialysis and referral for renal transplantation.

Renal replacement therapy

RRT may be required temporarily for AKI or permanently for CKD. In the UK the median age at which patients start dialysis is 65 years, and 24% of patients have CKD resulting from diabetic nephropathy. The aim is to start RRT when symptoms of CKD have appeared but before serious complications develop. Although this varies between patients, it typically occurs when the eGFR approaches 10 mL/min/1.73 m^2.

Prognosis or the need for RRT depend on age and comorbidity. Young patients without extrarenal disease can lead normal active lives on RRT, but those aged 30 to 34 years have a 25 times higher mortality than age-matched controls. The aim of RRT is to replace the excretory functions of the kidney, and to maintain normal fluid and electrolyte balance. Options include haemodialysis, haemofiltration, peritoneal dialysis and transplantation (Fig. 7.7). The major side effects of dialysis (Box 7.14) relate to haemodynamic disturbance caused by fluid removal or the extracorporeal circulation of blood, and reactions between blood and components of the dialysis system (bioincompatibility).

Conservative treatment

In older patients with stage 5 CKD and multiple comorbidities, conservative symptomatic treatment is viewed increasingly as a positive choice. Survival may be similar to those undergoing RRT, and patients are spared hospitalisation and invasive procedures. Patients are offered full medical, psychological and social support to optimise and sustain existing renal function for as long as possible, and appropriate palliative care in the terminal phases of disease. Many patients enjoy a good quality of life for

A: Haemodialysis

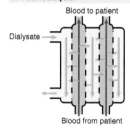

B: Haemofiltration

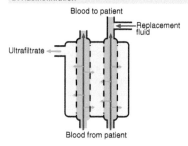

C: Peritoneal dialysis

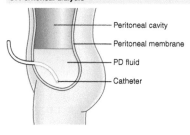

- Peritoneal cavity
- Peritoneal membrane
- PD fluid
- Catheter

D: Transplantation

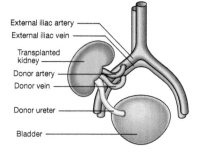

- External iliac artery
- External iliac vein
- Transplanted kidney
- Donor artery
- Donor vein
- Donor ureter
- Bladder

Fig. 7.7 Options for renal replacement therapy. A In haemodialysis, there is diffusion of solutes from blood to dialysate across a semi-permeable membrane down a concentration gradient. **B** In haemofiltration, both water and solutes are filtered across a semi-permeable membrane by a pressure gradient. Replacement fluid is added to the filtered blood before it is returned to the patient. **C** In peritoneal dialysis, fluid is introduced into the abdominal cavity using a catheter. Solutes diffuse from blood across the peritoneal membrane into the fluid down a concentration gradient. **D** In transplantation, the blood supply of the transplanted kidney is anastomosed to the internal iliac vessels, and the ureter to the bladder. The transplanted kidney replaces all the functions of the failed kidneys.

7.14 Problems with haemodialysis

- Hypotension during dialysis
- Cardiac arrhythmias
- Haemorrhage
- Air embolism
- Dialyser hypersensitivity
- Emergencies between treatments (pulmonary oedema, sepsis)

several years. It is also appropriate to discontinue dialysis, with the consent of the patient, and to offer conservative therapy and palliative care when quality of life on dialysis is poor.

Haemodialysis

Haemodialysis (Fig. 7.7A) is the most common form of RRT used for ESRD and is also used in AKI. Vascular access must be gained using either a central venous catheter or an arteriovenous shunt. The composition of the dialysate can be varied to achieve the desired solute flows, and the pressure can be varied to remove water from the circulation if required. Anticoagulation with heparin during dialysis is standard practice. Haemodialysis for CKD may be performed at home or hospital, and typically takes 3 to 5 hours three times weekly. Complications are shown in Box 7.14.

Haemofiltration

Haemofiltration (Fig. 7.7B) is principally used for AKI. It may be either intermittent or continuous, and allows control of intravascular volume by adjustment of the rate of fluid replacement.

Peritoneal dialysis

Peritoneal dialysis (Fig. 7.7C) is used principally for CKD and is useful in children and in adults with residual renal function. In CAPD, 2 L of sterile isotonic dialysis fluid is introduced into and left in the abdomen for 4 to 6 hours. Automated peritoneal dialysis is similar but fluid exchanges are performed by a pump overnight, reducing the daily treatment burden. Complications are summarised in Box 7.15.

Renal transplantation

Renal transplantation (Fig. 7.7D) offers the best chance of long-term survival in patients with ESRD. It can restore normal kidney function and correct all the metabolic abnormalities of CKD. All patients should be considered for transplantation unless there are contraindications. Active malignancy, vasculitis, cardiovascular disease and a high risk of recurrence of renal disease (generally glomerulonephritides) are common contraindications to transplantation.

> **7.15 Problems with continuous ambulatory peritoneal dialysis**
>
> • Peritonitis
> • Catheter exit site infection
> • Ultrafiltration failure
> • Peritoneal membrane failure
> • Sclerosing peritonitis

Kidney grafts may be taken from a deceased donor or a living donor. The matching of a donor to a specific recipient is strongly influenced by immunological factors, as graft rejection is the major cause of failure of the transplant. ABO (blood group) compatibility between donor and recipient is essential, and the degree of matching for MHC antigens—particularly HLA–DR—influences the incidence of rejection. Tests should be performed for antibodies against HLA antigens and antibodies that can bind to donor lymphocytes; both predict early rejection. Some ABO- and HLA-incompatible transplants are now possible with pretransplant plasma exchange or immunosuppression, but the preparation required restricts this to live donor transplants. Paired exchanges, in which a donor–recipient pair who are incompatible, either in blood group or HLA, are computer-matched with another pair to overcome the mismatch, are used increasingly to increase the number of successful transplants.

Once the graft begins to function, normal or near-normal biochemistry is usually achieved within a few days. Complications after transplant are summarised in Box 7.16.

Management after transplantation

All transplant patients require regular lifelong clinic follow-up to monitor renal function and immunosuppression. Common immunosuppressive regimens combine prednisolone with ciclosporin or tacrolimus, together with azathioprine or mycophenolate mofetil. Treatment is associated with an increased incidence of infection, particularly opportunistic infections such as cytomegalovirus and *Pneumocystis jirovecii*. There is also an increased risk of malignancy, especially of the skin. Lymphomas are rare, but may occur early, and are often related to infection with herpes viruses, especially Epstein-Barr virus.

In the UK, the prognosis for transplants from cadaver donors is 96% patient and 93% graft survival at 1 year, and 88% patient and 84% graft survival at 5 years. Even better results follow living donor transplantation (91% graft survival at 5 years).

Drugs and the kidney

The kidney is susceptible to damage because of concentration of drugs and metabolites during excretion. Specific examples are shown in Box 7.17.

Urinary tract infection

UTI is the term used to describe acute urethritis and cystitis caused by bacteria. It is the most common bacterial infection managed in general

i	7.16 Common causes of renal allograft dysfunction

Time post transplant	Cause
Hours to days	Renal artery/vein thrombosis Ureteric leak Delayed graft function Hyperacute rejection
Weeks	Acute rejection (esp. <3 months; later if insufficient immunosuppression)
Months	BK virus nephropathy Renal artery stenosis
Years	Chronic allograft injury (often antibody-mediated)

Any time	Tacrolimus/ciclosporin toxicity
	Sepsis
	Recurrence of disease:
	    Early (FSGS/MCGN)
	    Later (IgA nephropathy/membranous glomerulonephritis)

i	7.17 Drug-induced renal dysfunction: examples and mechanisms

Drug or toxin	Comments
Haemodynamic	
NSAIDs	↓renal blood flow by inhibition of prostaglandin synthesis
ACE inhibitors	↓efferent glomerular arteriolar tone. Toxic in renal artery stenosis/other renal hypoperfusion
Radiographic contrast media	May cause intense vasoconstriction, among other toxic effects
Acute tubular necrosis	
Aminoglycosides, amphotericin	Direct tubular toxicity but haemodynamic factors probably contribute
Paracetamol	± serious hepatotoxicity
Radiographic contrast media	May precipitate in tubules. Furosemide is a co-factor
Loss of tubular/collecting duct function	
Lithium, cisplatin Aminoglycosides, amphotericin	Loss of concentrating ability. Occurs at lower exposures than those that cause acute tubular necrosis

Continued

ℹ️ 7.17 Drug-induced renal dysfunction: examples and mechanisms—cont'd	
Drug or toxin	**Comments**
Glomerulonephritis (immune-mediated)	
Penicillamine, gold	Membranous nephropathy
Penicillamine	Crescentic or focal necrotising glomerulonephritis in association with ANCA-positive small-vessel vasculitis
NSAIDs	Minimal change nephropathy
Interstitial nephritis (immune-mediated)	
NSAIDs, penicillins, PPIs	Acute interstitial nephritis
Interstitial nephritis (toxicity)	
Lithium	Acute toxicity
Ciclosporin, tacrolimus	The major problem with these drugs
Tubular obstruction (crystal formation)	
Aciclovir	Drug crystallises in tubules
Chemotherapy	Uric acid crystals form as a consequence of tumour lysis
Nephrocalcinosis	
Bowel-cleansing agents	Ca, PO_4 precipitation—mild but sometimes irreversible damage
Retroperitoneal fibrosis	
Methysergide, practolol	No longer used in the UK. Idiopathic form is more common

medical practice, and accounts for 1% to 3% of consultations. The prevalence in women is 3% at age 20 years, rising by 1% per decade thereafter.

Clinical features

Typical features of cystitis and urethritis include:

• Abrupt onset of frequency and urgency of micturition. • Burning pain in the urethra during micturition (dysuria). • Suprapubic pain during and after voiding. • Intense desire to pass more urine after micturition caused by spasm of the inflamed bladder wall (strangury). • Cloudy urine with an unpleasant odour. • Nonvisible or visible haematuria.

Systemic symptoms are usually slight or absent. However, infection in the lower urinary tract can spread; prominent systemic symptoms with fever, rigors and loin pain suggest acute pyelonephritis and may be an indication for hospitalisation.

The differential diagnosis includes urethritis resulting from an STI (p. 174) or reactive arthritis.

Investigations

An approach to investigation is shown in Box 7.18. Investigation should be used selectively, most commonly in children, men and those with recurrent infections. Typical organisms causing UTI in the community include:
• *Escherichia coli* derived from the GI tract (~75% of infections). • *Proteus.*
• *Pseudomonas* spp. • Streptococci. • *Staphylococcus epidermidis.*

In hospital, *E. coli* still predominates, but *Klebsiella* and streptococci are more common. Certain strains of *E. coli* have a particular propensity to invade the urinary tract.

Management

Antibiotics are recommended in all cases of proven UTI. If urine culture has been performed, treatment may be started while awaiting the result. Treatment for 3 days is the norm and is less likely to induce alterations in bowel flora than more prolonged therapy. Trimethoprim is the usual choice for initial treatment; however, 10% to 40% of organisms causing UTI are resistant, the lower rates being seen in community-based practice. Nitrofurantoin, ciprofloxacin and cefalexin are also generally effective. High fluid intake and urinary alkalinising agents are often recommended but are not evidence-based.

Persistent or recurrent UTI

Treatment failure with persistence of organisms on repeat culture suggests an underlying cause such as:
• Incomplete bladder emptying (prostatic disease, neurological problems).
• Foreign body (catheter, stone). • Failure of host defences (diabetes, postmenopausal atrophic urethritis).

7.18 Investigation of patients with UTI

All patients

- Dipstick[a] for nitrite, leucocyte esterase and glucose
- Microscopy/cytometry of urine for white blood cells, organisms
- Urine culture

Infants, children and anyone with fever or complicated infection

- Full blood count; urea, electrolytes, creatinine
- Blood cultures

Pyelonephritis: men; children; women with recurrent infections

- Renal tract ultrasound or CT
- Pelvic examination in women, rectal examination in men

Continuing haematuria or other suspicion of bladder lesion

- Cystoscopy

[a]May substitute for microscopy and culture in uncomplicated infection.

Reinfection with a different organism, or with the same organism after an interval, may also occur. In women, recurrent infections are common, and further investigation is only justified if infections are severe or frequent (>2 per year).

If the cause cannot be removed, suppressive antibiotic therapy can be used to prevent recurrence and reduce the risk of septicaemia and renal damage. Regular urine culture and a regimen of two or three antibiotics in sequence, rotating every 6 months, are used to reduce the emergence of resistant organisms. Other simple measures to prevent recurrence include:
• Fluid intake greater than 2 L per day. • Regular complete bladder emptying. • Good personal hygiene. • Emptying of bladder before and after sexual intercourse. • Cranberry juice.

Asymptomatic bacteriuria

This is defined as greater than 10^5/mL organisms in the urine of apparently healthy asymptomatic patients. There is no evidence that this condition causes renal scarring in adults who are not pregnant and have a normal urinary tract, and in general, treatment is not indicated. Up to 30% of patients will develop symptomatic infection within 1 year.

Acute pyelonephritis

The kidneys are infected in a minority of patients with lower UTI by ascending infection from the bladder. Rarely, bacteraemia leads to complications, including renal or perinephric abscesses, and papillary necrosis.

Clinical features

• Acute onset of pain in one or both loins, which may radiate to the iliac fossae and suprapubic area. • Lumbar tenderness and guarding. • Dysuria caused by associated cystitis in 30%. • Fever with rigors, vomiting and hypotension.

In papillary necrosis, fragments of papillary tissue are passed per urethra and can be identified histologically. They may cause ureteric obstruction and, if bilateral or in a single kidney, may lead to AKI. Predisposing factors include diabetes mellitus, chronic urinary obstruction, analgesic nephropathy and sickle-cell disease.

Investigations and management

In addition to the investigations for UTI, renal tract USS or CT excludes a perinephric collection and obstruction as a predisposing factor. Adequate fluid intake must be ensured, IV if necessary by Cefalexin 1 g four times daily for 14 days, with ciprofloxacin 500 mg twice daily for 7 days is first-line treatment. Severe cases require initial IV therapy with a cephalosporin, quinolone or gentamicin.

Tuberculosis

TB of the kidney and urinary tract results from haematogenous spread of infection from elsewhere in the body.

Clinical features

• Bladder symptoms (frequency, dysuria), haematuria, malaise, fever, night sweats, loin pain. • CKD as a result of urinary tract obstruction or destruction of renal tissue. • Renal calcification and ureteric strictures are typical.

Investigations and management

Urine reveals neutrophils but is negative on routine culture. Early-morning urine cultures should be sent to identify tubercle bacilli. Perform cystoscopy if there is bladder involvement. Radiology of urinary tract and CXR are mandatory. Standard anti-TB chemotherapy (p. 339) is effective. Surgical relief of obstruction and nephrectomy are sometimes necessary for severe infection.

Reflux nephropathy

This chronic interstitial nephritis is associated with vesico-ureteric reflux in early life and with the appearance of scars in the kidney.

Clinical features

Usually the renal scarring and renal/ureteric dilatation are asymptomatic. Presentation may be at any age, with hypertension, proteinuria or features of CKD. Frequency, dysuria and lumbar back pain may be present; however, there may be no history of UTIs. There is an increased prevalence of urinary calculi.

Investigations

• Radionuclide scans: sensitive to detect reflux. • Serial CT/MRI: may be useful to assess progression. • USS: will exclude significant obstruction but is not helpful in identifying renal scarring. • Urinalysis shows leucocytes and proteinuria (usually <1 g/24 hours).

Management and prognosis

Treat infection; if recurrent, use prophylactic therapy. Nephrectomy is indicated if infection recurs in an abnormal kidney with minimal function. Hypertension is occasionally cured by the removal of a diseased kidney when disease is unilateral. Otherwise, surgery is rarely indicated, as most childhood reflux disappears spontaneously. Children and adults with small or unilateral renal scars have a good prognosis, provided renal growth is normal. Severe reflux may be managed by ureteric reimplantation or subtrigonal injection of Teflon or polysaccharide beneath the ureteric orifice.

Urolithiasis

The incidence of renal stones varies in frequency around the world, probably as a consequence of dietary and environmental factors, but genetic factors may also contribute. In Europe, 75% of renal stones contain calcium oxalate or phoshpate, around 15% contain magnesium ammonium phosphate, and small numbers of pure cystine or uric acid stones are found. In developing countries, bladder stones are common, particularly in children. In developed countries, the incidence of childhood bladder stones is low; renal stones in adults are more common. Staghorn calculi fill

7.19 Predisposing factors for kidney stones

Environmental and dietary

- Low urine volumes: high ambient temperatures, low fluid intake
- Diet: high protein, high sodium, low calcium
- High sodium excretion
- High oxalate or urate excretion
- Low citrate excretion

Acquired causes

- Hypercalcaemia of any cause (p. 395)
- Ileal disease or resection (increases oxalate absorption and urinary excretion)
- Renal tubular acidosis type I (distal, p. 218)

Congenital and inherited causes

- Familial hypercalciuria
- Medullary sponge kidney
- Cystinuria
- Renal tubular acidosis type I (distal)
- Primary hyperoxaluria

the whole renal pelvis and branch into the calyces; they are usually associated with infection and composed largely of struvite. Several risk factors for renal stone formation are known (Box 7.19); however, in developed countries, most calculi occur in healthy young men with no clear predisposing cause.

Clinical features

Most renal stones are asymptomatic. Ureteric obstruction by stone causes these typical symptoms:

• Renal colic: sudden pain in the loin, radiating to the groin, testis or labium, in the L1 distribution. • Pain escalates to a peak in a few minutes; the patient tries unsuccessfully to obtain relief by changing position. • Pallor, sweating, restlessness and often vomiting. • Frequency, dysuria and haematuria. • Intense pain usually subsides within 2 hours, but may continue for hours or days. It is usually constant during attacks, although slight fluctuations in severity may occur. A dull, persistent loin ache may follow.

Similar symptoms may occur with ureteric obstruction by papillary necrosis, clot or tumour.

Investigations

• Urinalysis: shows red cells. • AXR: around 90% of stones are radio-opaque. • CT of the kidneys, ureters and bladder is superior to AXR because it can also show nonopaque stones. • USS may show stones and dilatation of the renal pelvis above an obstruction and saves the patient radiation exposure.

Patients with a first renal stone should have a minimum set of investigations (Box 7.20); more detailed investigation is reserved for those with recurrent or multiple stones, or complicated or unexpected presentations.

	7.20 Investigations for renal stones		
Sample	**Test**	**First stone**	**Recurrent stone**
Stone	Chemical—most valuable test if stone can be recovered		✓
Blood	Calcium	✓	✓
	Phosphate	✓	✓
	Uric acid	✓	✓
	U&Es	✓	✓
	Bicarbonate	✓	✓
	PTH—only if serum calcium or urine calcium excretion high		(✓)
Urine	Dipstick test for protein, blood, glucose	✓	✓
	Amino acids		✓
24-hour urine	Urea		✓
	Creatinine clearance		✓
	Sodium		✓
	Calcium		✓
	Oxalate		✓
	Uric acid		✓

Because most stones pass spontaneously, urine should be sieved for a few days after an episode of colic to collect the calculus for analysis.

Management

• Powerful analgesia, for example, diclofenac (100 mg) orally or by suppository, morphine (10–20 mg) or pethidine (100 mg) IM. • Antiemetics are often required.

Around 90% of stones less than 4 mm in diameter pass spontaneously, but only 10% of stones of greater than 6 mm do, and these may require active intervention. Immediate action is required if there is anuria or infection in the stagnant urine proximal to the stone (pyonephrosis). Stones that do not pass spontaneously need to be removed surgically, using ureteroscopy and stone fragmentation by laser, or percutaneous nephrolithotomy and fragmentation with an ultrasonic disaggregator. Alternatively, stones can be fragmented by extracorporeal shock wave lithotripsy, in which externally generated shock waves are focused on the stone, fragmenting it into pieces that can be easily passed.

Measures to prevent recurrent stone formation depend on the results of investigations (Box 7.20) and include dietary modifications, adequate fluid intake and diuretics.

Diseases of the collecting system and ureters

Congenital abnormalities

These include single kidneys, duplex kidneys with two ureters and obstruction at the pelviureteric junction. The latter causes hydronephrosis in children and can be treated by laparoscopic pyeloplasty.

Medullary sponge kidney is a congenital disorder in which malformation of the papillary collecting ducts leads to the formation of medullary cysts. Patients present as adults with renal stones, but the prognosis is good. Diagnosis is by USS, CT or intravenous urography (IVU).

Retroperitoneal fibrosis

Fibrosis of retroperitoneal connective tissue may compress and obstruct the ureters.

Causes include idiopathic (most commonly), drugs, radiation, aortic aneurysm or malignancy. Presentation is with symptoms of ureteric obstruction. Investigations show high ESR/CRP; CT or IVU shows obstruction and medial deviation of ureters. Immediate treatment is usually by ureteric stenting. The idiopathic type responds to glucocorticoids; surgical ureterolysis is necessary if there is no response.

Tumours of the kidney and urinary tract

Renal cell cancer

This is by far the most common malignant tumour of the kidney in adults, with a prevalence of 16 cases per 100 000 individuals. It is twice as common in males as in females. The peak incidence is between 65 and 75 years of age, and it is uncommon before 40 years of age. Spread may be local, lymphatic or blood-borne (usually to lungs, bone or brain).

Clinical features

• 50% of cases are asymptomatic and discovered incidentally. • If symptomatic: haematuria (60%), loin pain (40%), abdominal mass (25%), or PUO. • Systemic effects include fever, raised ESR and coagulopathy. • Tumour may secrete ectopic hormones, for example, EPO, PTH, renin. The effects of these disappear when the tumour is removed.

Investigations

• USS: allows differentiation between solid tumour and simple renal cysts. • CT abdomen/chest: for staging. • USS- or CT-guided biopsy: avoids nephrectomy for benign disease.

Management and prognosis

Radical nephrectomy should be performed whenever possible (even in the presence of metastases, which may regress after surgery). Partial nephrectomy is appropriate if the tumour is smaller than 4 cm in diameter. Renal cell cancer is resistant to radiotherapy and most chemotherapy, but some benefit has been seen in recent years with tyrosine kinase inhibitors and mTOR inhibitors. If the tumour is confined to the kidney, 5-year survival is 75%. This falls to only 5% when there are distant metastases.

Urothelial tumours

These usually have a transitional cell origin, and can affect the renal pelvis, ureter, bladder (most commonly) or urethra. They are 3 to 4 times more common in men than women, and are rare under the age of 40 years. Risk factors include smoking and exposure to aromatic amines, aniline dyes and aldehydes.

Tumour appearance ranges from a delicate papillary structure, which usually indicates good prognosis, to a solid ulcerating mass, which usually signifies aggressive disease.

Clinical features and investigations

Over 80% of patients present with painless, visible haematuria (see p. 209). Obstructive symptoms may also occur. Examination is generally unhelpful. Cystoscopy is mandatory for suspected bladder cancer. CT urogram or IVU demonstrates lesions in the upper urinary tract. Tumour staging is by chest/abdomen/pelvis CT.

Management and prognosis

Superficial tumours are treated by transurethral surgery and/or intravesical chemotherapy; cystectomy is rarely required. Regular cystoscopy is needed to detect recurrence. Carcinoma *in situ* responds well to intravesical BCG treatment. Invasive bladder tumours are generally treated with radical cystectomy and urinary diversion. Overall, 5-year survival for patients with muscle-invasive bladder cancer is 50% to 70%.

Urinary incontinence

Stress incontinence

Leakage occurs because passive bladder pressure exceeds the urethral pressure, because of either poor pelvic floor support or a weak urethral sphincter, most often both. This is very common in women, especially following childbirth. It is rare in men, in whom it usually follows prostate surgery. It presents with incontinence during coughing, sneezing or exertion. In women, perineal inspection may reveal leakage of urine with coughs.

Urge incontinence

Leakage usually occurs when detrusor over-activity produces an increased bladder pressure that overcomes the urethral sphincter. Urgency with or without incontinence may also be driven by a hypersensitive bladder resulting from UTI or bladder stone. Detrusor over-activity may be neurogenic (in spina bifida or multiple sclerosis) or idiopathic. The incidence of urge incontinence increases with age and is also seen in men with lower urinary tract obstruction; it most often remits after the obstruction is relieved.

Continual incontinence

This is suggestive of a vesicovaginal or ureterovaginal fistula, often complicating previous surgery or radiotherapy.

Overflow incontinence

This occurs when the bladder becomes chronically over-distended. It is most common in men with benign prostatic hyperplasia or bladder neck obstruction but may occur in either sex as a result of detrusor muscle failure (atonic bladder). This may be idiopathic, but more commonly results from pelvic nerve damage from surgery (e.g. hysterectomy or rectal excision), trauma or infection, or from compression of the cauda equina from disc prolapse, trauma or tumour.

Postmicturition dribble

This is very common in men, even in the relatively young. It is caused by a small amount of urine becoming trapped in the U-bend of the bulbar urethra, which leaks out when the patient moves. It is more pronounced if associated with a urethral diverticulum or urethral stricture. It may occur in females with a urethral diverticulum and may mimic stress incontinence.

Clinical assessment and investigations

A voiding diary is used to record the pattern of micturition, including the measured volume voided, frequency of voiding, precipitating factors and associated features, for example, urgency. Cognitive function and mobility are assessed. Neurological assessment reveals disorders such as MS that may affect the nervous supply of the bladder. Perineal sensation and anal sphincter tone should be examined because the same sacral nerve roots also supply the bladder and urethral sphincter. The lumbar spine should be inspected for features of spina bifida occulta. Rectal examination is needed to assess the prostate in men and to exclude faecal impaction. Urinalysis and culture should be performed in all patients. An assessment of postmicturition volume should be made, either by postmicturition USS or by catheterisation. Urine flow rates and full urodynamic assessment may also be helpful in selected cases.

Management includes weight reduction in obesity, physiotherapy for women with stress incontinence, anticholinergic medication for urge incontinence and surgery for fistulae.

Prostatic disease

Benign prostatic enlargement

From 40 years of age, the prostate increases in volume by 2.4 cm^3 per year on average. Approximately 50% of men aged over 80 years will have lower urinary tract symptoms associated with BPE. Benign prostatic hyperplasia is the accompanying histological abnormality.

Clinical features

There is hesitancy, urinary frequency and urgency, poor urine flow and a sensation of incomplete emptying. Presentation may be with acute urinary retention, often precipitated by alcohol, constipation or prostatic infection.

The painful distended bladder requires emergency catheter drainage. Chronic urinary retention involves a painless distended bladder that may lead to dilatation of the ureters and kidneys, with eventual renal failure. These patients may develop acute-on-chronic retention.

Investigations

• Symptom scoring systems: allow baseline values to be established and further deterioration/improvement to be assessed. • Urine flow meter readings. • Prostate volume assessment (PR and transrectal ultrasound) • Urodynamic studies. • Renal function and renal ultrasound.

Management

Medical treatment (α-adrenoceptor blockers, e.g. tamsulosin; 5α-reductase inhibitors, e.g. finasteride alone or in combination) may relieve obstruction. TURP or enucleation by holmium laser is effective; open prostatectomy is rarely needed unless the prostate is very large.

Prostate cancer

Prostatic cancer is common in northern Europe and the United States, but rare in China and Japan. In the UK the prevalence is 105 per 100 000 individuals. It rarely occurs before the age of 50 years and has a mean age at presentation of 70 years.

Almost all prostate cancers are adenocarcinomas. Metastatic spread to pelvic lymph nodes occurs early, and metastases to bone, mainly the lumbar spine and pelvis, are common.

Clinical features

Patients are either asymptomatic or have urinary symptoms indistinguishable from BPE. Symptoms and signs owing to metastases are much less common, and include back pain, weight loss, anaemia and obstruction of the ureters. The prostate may feel nodular and hard on digital rectal examination, with loss of the central sulcus (although up to 45% of tumours are impalpable).

Investigations

• PSA: a good tumour marker — 40% of patients with a serum PSA greater than 4.0 ng/mL will have prostate cancer on biopsy. Screening programmes remain unproven, however, as the pickup rate is low. • Transrectal ultrasound-guided needle biopsy: to confirm diagnosis. • Ultrasound of urinary tract and U&Es. • If diagnosis is confirmed: pelvic MRI and isotope bone scans are useful for staging, although high levels of serum PSA (>100 ng/mL) almost always indicate distant bone metastases. • PSA: most useful for monitoring response to treatment and disease progression.

Management and prognosis

Tumours confined to the prostate are potentially curable by either radical prostatectomy, radical radiotherapy or brachytherapy (implantation of radioactive particles), and these options should be considered in all patients with a life expectancy greater than 10 years. A small focus of tumour found incidentally at TURP does not significantly alter life expectancy, and only requires follow-up.

Approximately half of men with prostate cancer will have metastatic disease at the time of diagnosis. Prostatic cancer is sensitive to hormonal influences; androgen depletion, either by orchidectomy or, more commonly, by androgen-suppressing drugs, leads to a high initial response rate in locally advanced or metastatic prostate cancer; androgen receptor blockers, such as bicalutamide or cyproterone acetate, may also prevent tumour cell growth. A small proportion of patients fail to respond to endocrine treatment. More respond initially but experience disease progression after a year or two. Radiotherapy is useful for localised bone pain.

The 10-year survival of patients with focal prostate carcinoma is 95%, but if metastases are present this falls to 10%.

Testicular tumours

These uncommon tumours occur mainly in men between 20 and 40 years of age; 85% are either seminomas or teratomas. Seminomas are relatively low grade but may metastasise to the lungs. Teratomas may contain differentiated bone, cartilage or other tissue. Testicular tumours may secrete α-fetoprotein or β-human chorionic gonadotrophin.

Presentation is with a testicular lump, which should be imaged by ultrasound. CT of the chest, abdomen and pelvis is required for staging. Treatment is by orchidectomy with radiotherapy and/or chemotherapy for metastases.

Erectile dysfunction

Erectile disfunction is most commonly caused by psychological, vascular or neuropathic factors. With the exception of diabetes mellitus, endocrine causes are uncommon and are characterised by simultaneous loss of libido. If the patient has erections on wakening in the morning, vascular and neuropathic causes are much less likely, and a psychological cause should be suspected.

Cardiology

Cardiovascular disease is the most frequent cause of adult death in the Western world. Although the incidence of ischaemic heart disease is declining in many developed countries, it is rising in Eastern Europe and Asia. Valvular heart disease is also common, but although rheumatic fever still predominates in the Indian subcontinent and Africa, calcific aortic valve disease is now the most common problem in developed countries. Prompt recognition of the development of heart disease is limited by two factors. Firstly, patients often remain asymptomatic despite the presence of advanced disease, and secondly, the diversity of symptoms attributable to heart disease is limited, and so different conditions frequently present similarly.

Presenting problems in cardiovascular disease

A close relationship between symptoms and exercise is a hallmark of cardiovascular disease. The NYHA functional classification is often used to grade disability (Box 8.1).

Chest pain on exertion

The many noncardiac causes of chest pain are covered in Chapter 4. This section covers exertional chest pain, which is typical of coronary artery disease.

A careful history is crucial in determining whether chest pain is cardiac. The reproducibility and predictability of the relationship between exertion and chest pain are the most important features. The duration is also

i 8.1 NYHA functional classification

Class I	No limitation during ordinary activity
Class II	Slight limitation during ordinary activity
Class III	Marked limitation of normal activities without symptoms at rest
Class IV	Unable to undertake physical activity without symptoms; symptoms may be present at rest

Clinical examination of the cardiovascular system

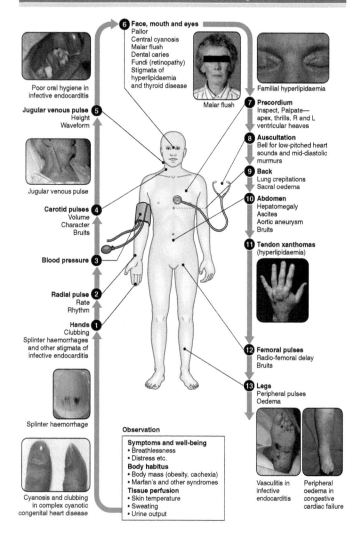

6 Face, mouth and eyes
Pallor
Central cyanosis
Malar flush
Dental caries
Fundi (retinopathy)
Stigmata of hyperlipidaemia and thyroid disease

Poor oral hygiene in infective endocarditis

Malar flush

Familial hyperlipidaemia

5 Jugular venous pulse
Height
Waveform

Jugular venous pulse

7 Precordium
Inspect, Palpate—apex, thrills, R and L ventricular heaves

8 Auscultation
Bell for low-pitched heart sounds and mid-diastolic murmurs

9 Back
Lung crepitations
Sacral oedema

4 Carotid pulses
Volume
Character
Bruits

10 Abdomen
Hepatomegaly
Ascites
Aortic aneurysm
Bruits

3 Blood pressure

11 Tendon xanthomas
(hyperlipidaemia)

2 Radial pulse
Rate
Rhythm

1 Hands
Clubbing
Splinter haemorrhages and other stigmata of infective endocarditis

12 Femoral pulses
Radio-femoral delay
Bruits

13 Legs
Peripheral pulses
Oedema

Splinter haemorrhage

Observation

Symptoms and well-being
• Breathlessness
• Distress etc.
Body habitus
• Body mass (obesity, cachexia)
• Marfan's and other syndromes
Tissue perfusion
• Skin temperature
• Sweating
• Urine output

Cyanosis and clubbing in complex cyanotic congenital heart disease

Vasculitis in infective endocarditis

Peripheral oedema in congestive cardiac failure

important; recent-onset angina indicates greater risk than long-standing and unchanged symptoms. Examination is often normal, but may reveal risk factors such as xanthelasma indicating hyperlipidaemia. Signs of anaemia or thyrotoxicosis may be identified, both of which can exacerbate angina. Cardiovascular examination may reveal left ventricular dysfunction or cardiac murmurs in patients with aortic valve disease and hypertrophic cardiomyopathy. Evidence of arterial disease, such as bruits and loss of peripheral pulses, may also be observed.

Investigations

Blood count, fasting glucose, lipids, thyroid function tests and a 12-lead ECG are the basic investigations. An exercise ECG may identify high-risk patients requiring further investigation, but false-negative and false-positive results can occur. Patients with chest pain suggestive of coronary disease but with a normal exercise ECG should undergo CT coronary angiography. If a murmur is found, echocardiography should be performed to exclude valve disease or hypertrophic cardiomyopathy.

Severe prolonged chest pain

Severe prolonged cardiac chest pain may represent acute myocardial infarction or unstable angina (p. 279)—the acute coronary syndromes.

Clinical assessment

Acute coronary syndrome is often preceded by stable angina, but unheralded severe chest pain at rest can be the first presentation of coronary disease. History and examination may reveal pallor or sweating caused by accompanying autonomic disturbance, arrhythmia, hypotension or heart failure. Patients with symptoms suggesting acute coronary syndrome require hospital admission and urgent investigation.

Investigations

Initial triage is by 12-lead ECG and serum troponin I or T. Acute coronary syndrome is suggested by ST elevation or depression and elevated troponin I or T, indicating myocardial damage.

If the diagnosis remains unclear, repeat ECGs are useful, particularly if recorded during pain. If baseline plasma troponin is normal, repeat measurements should be made 6 to 12 hours after the onset of symptoms or after admission. New ECG changes or elevated troponin confirm the diagnosis of an acute coronary syndrome. If the pain settles, there are no new ECG changes and troponin remains normal, the patient can be discharged, but further investigations may still be indicated (p. 284).

The differential diagnosis and management of acute coronary syndrome are described in more detail on pp. 279 and 282.

Breathlessness

Cardiac causes of breathlessness include arrhythmias, heart failure, acute coronary syndrome, valvular disease, cardiomyopathy and constrictive pericarditis, all discussed later. The differential diagnosis however, includes many noncardiac causes, and is discussed on pp. 61 and 311.

Syncope

This refers to loss of consciousness caused by reduced cerebral perfusion, and is covered on p. 63.

Palpitation

Palpitation is a term used to describe a variety of sensations, including an erratic, fast, slow or forceful heartbeat.

Clinical assessment

Take a detailed history (Box 8.2) and ask the patient to tap out the heartbeat on the table.

Recurrent but short-lived bouts of an irregular heartbeat, such as dropped or missed beats, are usually because of atrial or ventricular extrasystoles. Attacks of a pounding, forceful, fast heartbeat are a common manifestation of anxiety, but may also occur in anaemia, pregnancy and thyrotoxicosis. Discrete bouts of a very rapid (>120/min) heartbeat suggest a paroxysmal arrhythmia. Atrial fibrillation typically presents with a completely irregular tachycardia.

Investigation and management

An ECG during an attack of palpitation (ambulatory monitoring or patient-activated recorder) is necessary to establish a definitive diagnosis. Most cases are attributed to an awareness of the normal heartbeat, sinus tachycardia or benign extrasystoles, in which case an explanation and reassurance will often suffice. Palpitation associated with syncope should be investigated without delay. Arrhythmia management is described on pp. 262-263.

Cardiac arrest

Cardiac arrest describes the sudden, complete loss of cardiac output as a result of asystole, catastrophic arrhythmia or loss of mechanical contraction (pulseless electrical activity). The patient is unconscious and pulseless. Coronary disease is the commonest cause, but valvular disease, cardiomyopathy, drugs and electrolyte abnormalities can all cause catastrophic arrhythmias. Death is inevitable without prompt effective treatment.

 8.2 How to evaluate palpitation

- Is the palpitation continuous or intermittent?
- Is the heart beat regular or irregular?
- What is the approximate heart rate?
- Do symptoms occur in discrete attacks?
  - Is the onset abrupt? How do attacks terminate?
- Are there any associated symptoms?
  - Chest pain, lightheadedness, polyuria (a feature of supraventricular tachycardia, p. 266)?
- Are there any precipitating factors, e.g. exercise, alcohol?
- Is there a history of structural heart disease, e.g. coronary artery disease, valvular heart disease?

Clinical assessment and management

Basic life support: The ABCDE approach to management should be followed: restoration of the **A**irway; rescue **B**reathing ('mouth-to-mouth'); maintenance of **C**irculation using chest compressions; **D**isability (assessment of neurological status); and **E**xposure (removal of clothes to enable defibrillation, auscultation, assessment for rash, injuries, etc.).

Chest compression–only ('hands-only') cardiopulmonary resuscitation is simpler to teach and do, and is now advocated for members of the public.

Advanced life support: Advanced life support (Fig. 8.1) aims to restore normal cardiac rhythm by defibrillation when the cause of arrest is tachyarrhythmia, or to restore cardiac output by correcting other reversible causes of cardiac arrest. The initial priority is to assess the cardiac rhythm using a defibrillator or monitor. Treatment is based on the ECG findings.

Ventricular fibrillation (VF) (Fig. 8.2) or pulseless ventricular tachycardia (VT) should be treated with immediate 150 J defibrillation, then a further 2 minutes of CPR, because cardiac output rarely resumes immediately after successful defibrillation. After 2 minutes, if there is still no pulse, a further shock (150–200 J) should be given. Thereafter, additional shocks are given every 2 minutes after each cycle of CPR. Adrenaline (epinephrine, 1 mg IV) should be given every 3 to 5 minutes, and intravenous amiodarone should be considered, especially if VF or VT recurs after successful defibrillation.

VF of low amplitude, or 'fine VF', may mimic asystole. If asystole cannot be confidently diagnosed, the patient should be defibrillated. If the observed ECG rhythm would be expected to produce a cardiac output, 'pulseless electrical activity' is present. This should be treated by continuing CPR and adrenaline (epinephrine) administration while seeking reversible causes. Asystole should be treated similarly, with the additional support of atropine and sometimes external or transvenous pacing in an attempt to generate an electrical rhythm. The main reversible causes of cardiac arrest are listed in Fig. 8.1.

The chain of survival: Survival is most likely if all the key elements of resuscitation happen rapidly: that is the arrest is witnessed, basic life support is administered immediately by a trained individual, and the emergency services deliver defibrillation and advanced life support within a few minutes. Training in life support is essential and should be maintained by regular refresher courses. In recent years, public-access automated defibrillators have been introduced in places of high population density, particularly where congestion may delay the emergency services.

Survivors of cardiac arrest: Patients who survive a cardiac arrest caused by acute MI have a similar prognosis to those recovering from an uncomplicated infarct. Those with reversible causes, such as exercise-induced ischaemia or aortic stenosis, should have the cause treated. Survivors of VT or VF arrest in whom no reversible cause can be identified may be at risk of another episode, and should be considered for an implantable cardiac defibrillator (p. 275) and antiarrhythmic drugs. In these patients, the risk is reduced by treatment of heart failure with β-adrenoceptor antagonists and ACE inhibitors, and by coronary revascularisation.

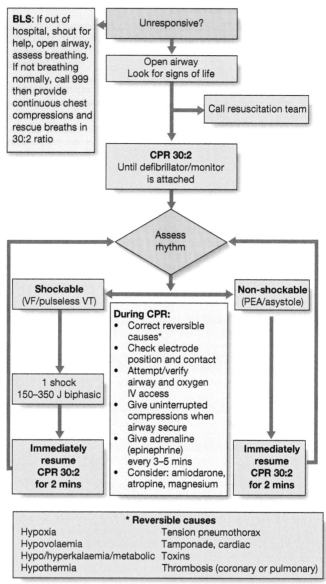

BLS: If out of hospital, shout for help, open airway, assess breathing. If not breathing normally, call 999 then provide continuous chest compressions and rescue breaths in 30:2 ratio

Unresponsive?

Open airway
Look for signs of life

Call resuscitation team

CPR 30:2
Until defibrillator/monitor is attached

Assess rhythm

Shockable
(VF/pulseless VT)

Non-shockable
(PEA/asystole)

During CPR:
- Correct reversible causes*
- Check electrode position and contact
- Attempt/verify airway and oxygen IV access
- Give uninterrupted compressions when airway secure
- Give adrenaline (epinephrine) every 3–5 mins
- Consider: amiodarone, atropine, magnesium

1 shock
150–350 J biphasic

Immediately resume CPR 30:2 for 2 mins

Immediately resume CPR 30:2 for 2 mins

* Reversible causes	
Hypoxia	Tension pneumothorax
Hypovolaemia	Tamponade, cardiac
Hypo/hyperkalaemia/metabolic	Toxins
Hypothermia	Thrombosis (coronary or pulmonary)

Fig. 8.1 Algorithm for basic and adult advanced life support. For further information see www.resus.org.uk. *BLS*, Basic life support; *CPR*, cardiopulmonary resuscitation; *PEA*, pulseless electrical activity; *VF*, ventricular fibrillation; *VT*, pulseless ventricular tachycardia.

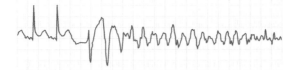

Fig. 8.2 VF. A bizarre chaotic rhythm, initiated in this case by two ectopic beats in rapid succession.

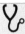 **8.3 How to assess heart murmurs**

When does it occur?

- Time the murmur using heart sounds, carotid pulse and apex beat. Is it systolic or diastolic?
- Does the murmur extend throughout systole or diastole, or is it confined to a shorter part of the cardiac cycle?

How loud is it? (intensity)

- Grade 1 Very soft (only audible in ideal conditions)
- Grade 2 Soft
- Grade 3 Moderate
- Grade 4 Loud with associated thrill
- Grade 5 Very loud
- Grade 6 Heard without stethoscope

N.B. Diastolic murmurs are rarely louder than grade 4.

Where is it heard best? (location)

- Listen over the apex and base of the heart, including the aortic and pulmonary areas

Where does it radiate?

- Evaluate radiation to the neck, axilla or back

What does it sound like? (pitch and quality)

- Pitch is determined by flow (high pitch indicates high-velocity flow)
- Is the intensity constant or variable?

Abnormal heart sounds and murmurs

The first clinical manifestation of heart disease may be the incidental discovery of an abnormal sound on auscultation. Clinical evaluation (Box 8.3) is helpful, but an echocardiogram is often necessary to confirm the nature of an abnormal heart sound or murmur. Some added sounds are physiological but may also occur in pathological conditions; for example, a third sound is common in young people and in pregnancy, but is also a feature of heart failure. Similarly, an ejection systolic murmur may occur in hyperdynamic states (e.g. anaemia, pregnancy) but also in aortic stenosis. Benign murmurs do not occur in diastole, and systolic murmurs that radiate or are associated with a thrill are almost always pathological. Valvular heart disease is covered on p. 295.

Systolic murmurs: Ejection systolic murmurs occur in ventricular outflow obstruction and have a mid-systolic crescendo–decrescendo pattern. Pansystolic murmurs occur with mitral or tricuspid regurgitation and ventricular septal defect and have constant intensity from the first to beyond the second heart sound.

Diastolic murmurs: Soft, low-pitched mid-diastolic murmurs occur with turbulent flow across stenotic mitral or tricuspid valves, and are best heard with the stethoscope bell. Early diastolic murmurs accompany aortic or pulmonary regurgitation, and have a decrescendo, soft, blowing quality best heard with the diaphragm of the stethoscope.

Heart failure

Heart failure describes the state that develops when the heart cannot maintain an adequate cardiac output or can do so only at the expense of elevated filling pressures. Initially it causes mainly exertional symptoms, but advanced heart failure may cause symptoms at rest.

Left-sided heart failure: This causes a reduction in LV output and an increase in the left atrial or pulmonary venous pressure. An acute increase in left atrial pressure may cause pulmonary oedema; a more gradual increase leads to reflex pulmonary vasoconstriction and pulmonary hypertension.

Right-sided heart failure: This causes a reduction in RV output and an increase in right atrial pressure. The common causes are chronic lung disease and pulmonary embolism.

Biventricular heart failure: This may develop because disease affects both ventricles (e.g. dilated cardiomyopathy), or because left heart failure leads to chronic elevation of left atrial pressure, pulmonary hypertension and right heart failure.

Epidemiology

Heart failure mainly affects older patients, the prevalence rising from around 1% in those aged 50 to 59 years to more than 10% of those aged 80 to 89 years. The prognosis is poor; around 50% of patients with severe heart failure caused by LV dysfunction die within 2 years, either from pump failure or ventricular arrhythmias. Ischaemic heart disease is the most common cause, but most forms of heart disease can cause heart failure (Box 8.4).

Pathophysiology

Cardiac output is determined by preload, afterload and myocardial contractility (Fig. 8.3). Ventricular dysfunction can occur because of impaired systolic contraction or abnormal diastolic relaxation because of a stiff, noncompliant ventricle (usually caused by left ventricular hypertrophy). Systolic and diastolic dysfunction often coexist, particularly in coronary artery disease. Falling cardiac output activates the SNS, causing vasoconstriction, and the RAAS, causing sodium and water retention mediated by

i 8.4 Mechanisms of heart failure

Cause	Examples
Reduced ventricular contractility	MI (segmental dysfunction) Myocarditis/cardiomyopathy (global dysfunction)
Ventricular outflow obstruction (pressure overload)	Hypertension, aortic stenosis (left heart failure) Pulmonary hypertension, pulmonary valve stenosis (right heart failure)
Ventricular inflow obstruction	Mitral stenosis, tricuspid stenosis
Ventricular volume overload	LV volume overload (e.g. mitral or aortic regurgitation) Ventricular septal defect RV volume overload (e.g. atrial septal defect)
Arrhythmia	Atrial fibrillation Complete heart block Tachycardia-induced cardiomyopathy
Diastolic dysfunction	Constrictive pericarditis Restrictive cardiomyopathy LV hypertrophy and fibrosis Cardiac tamponade

8

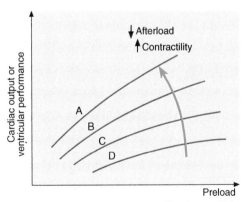

Fig. 8.3 Starling's Law. Normal (A), mild (B), moderate (C) and severe (D) heart failure. Ventricular performance is related to the degree of myocardial stretching. An increase in preload (end-diastolic volume, end-diastolic pressure, filling pressure or atrial pressure) will therefore enhance function; however, overstretching causes marked deterioration. In heart failure, the curve moves to the right and becomes flatter. An increase in myocardial contractility or a reduction in afterload will shift the curve upwards and to the left (green arrow).

angiotensin II, aldosterone, endothelin-1 and antidiuretic hormone. This leads to a vicious cycle of increased afterload and preload.

Although sympathetic activation initially sustains cardiac output through increased contractility and HR, prolonged activation causes cardiac myocyte apoptosis, hypertrophy and focal myocardial necrosis, and predisposes to arrhythmias. Natriuretic peptides are released from the dilated atria and compensate for the sodium-conserving effect of aldosterone, but this mechanism is overwhelmed in heart failure. Pulmonary and peripheral oedema develop, compounded by impairment of renal perfusion and secondary hyperaldosteronism.

High output failure: Heart failure can occur in the absence of heart disease if there is an excessively high cardiac output, for example, with large arteriovenous shunts or thyrotoxicosis.

Clinical features: Heart failure can develop acutely as with MI, or gradually as in valvular disease. 'Compensated heart failure' describes a patient with gradually impaired cardiac function in whom adaptive changes have prevented overt heart failure. An infection or arrhythmia may precipitate acute heart failure in such patients.

Acute left heart failure: This usually presents with sudden-onset dyspnoea at rest with acute respiratory distress, orthopnoea and prostration. A precipitant (e.g. acute MI) may be apparent from the history. The patient appears agitated, pale and clammy. The peripheries are cool to the touch, the pulse is rapid, and the JVP is usually elevated. The apex is not displaced, as there has been no time for ventricular dilatation. Auscultation may reveal a triple 'gallop' rhythm, a systolic murmur if there is mitral regurgitation or septal rupture and crepitations at the lung bases. Acute-on-chronic heart failure will have additional features of long-standing heart failure (see later). Potential precipitants (e.g. arrhythmia, changes in medication, intercurrent infective illness) should be identified.

Chronic heart failure: This commonly follows a relapsing and remitting course, with periods of stability interrupted by episodes of decompensation. A low cardiac output causes fatigue, listlessness and a poor effort tolerance; the peripheries are cold, and BP is low. Pulmonary oedema as a result of left heart failure may present with breathlessness, orthopnoea, paroxysmal nocturnal dyspnoea and pulmonary crepitations. Right heart failure produces a high JVP, with hepatic congestion and dependent peripheral oedema. In ambulant patients the oedema affects the ankles, whereas in bed-bound patients it collects around the thighs and sacrum.

Chronic heart may cause additional complications:

- *Weight loss* (cardiac cachexia) as a result of anorexia and impaired absorption because of GI congestion.
- *Renal failure* from poor renal perfusion as a result of a low cardiac output — exacerbated by diuretics, ACE inhibitors and angiotensin receptor blockers.
- *Hypokalaemia* caused by diuretics and hyperaldosteronism.
- *Hyperkalaemia* caused by the effects of drugs (particularly ACE inhibitors given with spironolactone) and renal dysfunction.

- *Hyponatraemia* caused by diuretic therapy or inappropriate water retention because of high ADH secretion—a poor prognostic sign.
- *Thromboembolism*—either DVT with pulmonary embolism or systemic emboli from cardiac thrombus in atrial fibrillation or complicating MI.
- *Atrial and ventricular arrhythmias* may be related to electrolyte changes (e.g. hypokalaemia, hypomagnesaemia), underlying cardiac disease and accompanying sympathetic activation. Sudden death occurs in up to 50% of patients, probably caused by VF.

Investigations

• CXR: may reveal cardiomegaly, and shows characteristic changes in pulmonary oedema (Fig. 8.4), including distension of upper lobe pulmonary veins, Kerley B lines (horizontal lines near the costal margin indicating interstitial oedema), hazy hilar opacification (alveolar oedema) and pleural effusions. • Echocardiography: consider in all patients with heart failure to determine the aetiology (e.g. valvular disease, regional wall motion defect in MI) and assess LV impairment. • ECG: may reveal LV hypertrophy, evidence of previous MI. • U&Es, LFTs, TFTs and FBC: may identify some of the associated causes and complications listed previously. • Brain natriuretic peptide (BNP): elevated in heart failure and is a prognostic marker, as well as being useful in differentiating heart failure from other causes of breathlessness or peripheral oedema.

Management of acute pulmonary oedema

This is summarised in Box 8.5. For severe or unresponsive patients, treatment of cardiogenic shock is covered on p. 84.

Management of chronic heart failure

General measures

The aim of treatment is to improve cardiac function by increasing contractility, optimising preload or decreasing afterload and controlling cardiac rate and rhythm. In addition to treating the underlying cause, both nondrug and drug therapies are important.

Nondrug measures include:
• Effective education about heart failure. • Maintenance of nutritional status.
• Smoking cessation. • Avoidance of excessive salt or alcohol intake.
• Regular moderate exercise. • Vaccinations for influenza and pneumococcus.

Drug treatment

Drugs that reduce preload are indicated if there is pulmonary or systemic venous congestion. Drugs that reduce after load and increase contractility are useful if cardiac output is low.

Diuretics: Promote sodium and water excretion, reducing plasma volume and preload, thereby improving pulmonary and systemic venous congestion. In some patients with severe chronic heart failure, IV loop diuretics or combination therapy with a loop and thiazide diuretic may be required. Aldosterone receptor antagonists such as spironolactone are potassium-sparing diuretics that improve long-term outcome in patients with severe heart failure and those with heart failure following MI.

ACE inhibitors: Interrupt the vicious circle of neurohormonal activation in chronic heart failure, preventing salt and water retention, peripheral

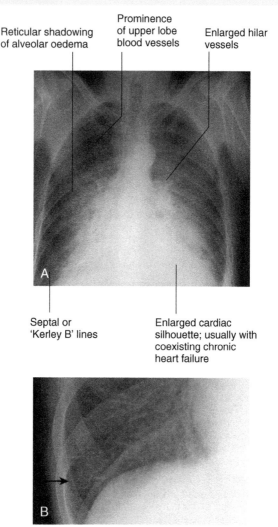

Reticular shadowing of alveolar oedema

Prominence of upper lobe blood vessels

Enlarged hilar vessels

Septal or 'Kerley B' lines

Enlarged cardiac silhouette; usually with coexisting chronic heart failure

Fig. 8.4 Radiological features of heart failure. (A) CXR of a patient with pulmonary oedema. (B) Enlargement of lung base showing septal or 'Kerley B' lines (arrow).

vasoconstriction, and sympathetic nervous system activation. They improve effort tolerance and mortality in moderate to severe heart failure and following MI. They may cause hypotension and renal impairment, especially in hypovolaemic and elderly patients, and should therefore be started cautiously.

ARBs: Produce haemodynamic and mortality benefits similar to those of ACE inhibitors, and are a useful alternative for patients intolerant of ACE inhibitors.

8.5 Management of acute pulmonary oedema

Action	Effect
Sit the patient up	Reduces preload
Give high-flow oxygen	Corrects hypoxia
Ensure CPAP of 5–10 mmHg by tight-fitting mask	Reduces preload and pulmonary capillary hydraulic gradient
Administer nitrates:[a] IV glyceryl trinitrate (10–200 μg/min) Buccal glyceryl trinitrate 2–5 mg	Reduces preload and afterload
Administer a loop diuretic: Furosemide (50–100 mg IV)	Combats fluid overload

[a]The dose of nitrate should be titrated upwards every 10 minutes until there is an improvement or systolic blood pressure is less than 110 mmHg.

Neprilysin inhibitors: Sacubitril inhibits breakdown of the endogenous diuretics ANP and BNP. Combined with the ARB valsartan (sacubitril–valsartan), it improves symptoms and mortality compared with ACE treatment, and is now recommended for resistant heart failure.

Vasodilators: Valuable in chronic heart failure when ACE inhibitors or ARBs are contraindicated. Venodilators (e.g. nitrates) and arterial dilators (e.g. hydralazine) may be used, but may cause hypotension.

β-Blockers: Help to counteract the adverse effects of sympathetic stimulation in chronic heart failure and reduce the risk of arrhythmias and sudden death. They must be introduced gradually to avoid precipitating acute-on-chronic failure, but when used appropriately have been shown to increase ejection fraction, improve symptoms and reduce mortality.

Ivabradine: Acts on the SA node to reduce HR. It reduces mortality and admissions in moderate to severe LV dysfunction, and is useful if β-blockers are not tolerated or not effective.

Digoxin: Can be used for rate control in heart failure with AF. It may reduce episodes of hospitalisation in patients with severe heart failure, but has no effect on long-term survival.

Amiodarone: Useful for controlling arrhythmias in patients with poor LV function because it has little negative inotropic effect.

Nondrug therapies

Implantable cardiac defibrillators (p. 275): Reduce the risk of sudden death in selected patients with chronic heart failure, particularly those with symptomatic ventricular arrhythmia.

Cardiac resynchronisation therapy (p. 275): Restores the normal contraction pattern of the left ventricle, which may be dysynchronous in patients with impaired LV function and left bundle branch block.

Coronary revascularisation: Bypass grafting or percutaneous coronary intervention may improve function in areas of 'hibernating' myocardium with inadequate blood supply, and can be used to treat carefully selected patients with heart failure and coronary artery disease.

Cardiac transplantation: An established and successful form of treatment for patients with intractable heart failure. Coronary artery disease and dilated cardiomyopathy are the most common indications. The use of transplantation is limited by the availability of donor hearts, and so is generally reserved for young patients with severe symptoms. Serious complications include rejection, infection (because of immunosuppressive therapy) and accelerated atherosclerosis.

Ventricular assist devices: Have been employed as a bridge to cardiac transplantation, and more recently as potential long-term therapy. They assist cardiac output by using a roller, centrifugal or pulsatile pump. There is currently a high rate of complication (e.g. haemorrhage, systemic embolism, infection).

Cardiac arrhythmias

Arrhythmias are generally classified as either tachycardias (HR >100/min) or bradycardias (HR <60/min). There are two main mechanisms of tachycardia:

Increased automaticity: Repeated spontaneous depolarisation of an ectopic focus, often in response to catecholamines.

Re-entry: This occurs when there are two alternative pathways with different conducting properties (e.g. a normal and an ischaemic area). In sinus rhythm, each impulse passes down both pathways before entering a common distal pathway. If the refractory periods of the paths differ, a premature impulse may travel down one pathway, then retrogradely up the alternative pathway, establishing a closed loop or re-entry circuit and initiating a tachycardia.

'Supraventricular' (sinus, atrial or junctional) arrhythmias usually produce narrow QRS complexes because the ventricles are depolarised via normal pathways. Ventricular arrhythmias cause broad, bizarre QRS complexes because the ventricles are activated in an abnormal sequence.

Clinical features
Tachycardias can cause palpitation, dizziness, syncope, chest pain or breathlessness, and trigger heart failure or even sudden death. Bradycardias cause fatigue and syncope.

Investigations
A 12-lead ECG will be diagnostic in many cases. If arrhythmias are intermittent, the rhythm should be recorded using an ambulatory ECG or a patient-activated ECG.

Management
This depends on the rhythm.

Sinus arrhythmia: Refers to the normal increase in HR during inspiration and slowing during expiration. It is mediated by the parasympathetic nerves, and may be pronounced in young patients.

Sinus bradycardia: May occur in healthy people at rest, especially athletes. Pathological causes include MI, raised intracranial pressure, hypothermia, hypothyroidism, cholestatic jaundice and drug therapy (e.g. β-blockers, verapamil, digoxin). Asymptomatic sinus bradycardia requires no treatment; symptomatic patients may require IV atropine or a pacemaker.

Sinus tachycardia: Usually because of an increase in sympathetic activity with exercise, emotion or pregnancy. Pathological causes include anaemia, fever, thyrotoxicosis, phaeochromocytoma, cardiac failure, shock and drug therapy (e.g. inhaled β-agonists).

Sick sinus syndrome

Sick sinus syndrome results from degeneration of the sinus node, and is more common in the elderly. It typically presents with palpitation, dizzy spells or syncope, because of intermittent tachycardia, bradycardia or pauses with no atrial or ventricular activity (sinus arrest or sinoatrial block). A permanent pacemaker may benefit patients with symptomatic bradycardias, but is not indicated in asymptomatic patients.

Atrial arrhythmias

Atrial ectopic beats (extrasystoles): Usually cause no symptoms, but can give the sensation of a missed beat or abnormally strong beat. The ECG shows a premature but otherwise normal QRS complex; the preceding P wave has a different morphology because the atria activate from an abnormal site. Treatment is rarely necessary.

Atrial tachycardia: Produces a narrow-complex tachycardia with abnormal P-wave morphology caused by increased atrial automaticity, sinoatrial disease or digoxin toxicity. It may respond to β-blockers, which reduce automaticity, or class I or III antiarrhythmic drugs (Box 8.9). Catheter ablation may be useful for recurrent tachycardias.

Atrial flutter: Results from a large re-entry circuit in the right atrium. The atrial rate is around 300/min, but associated 2:1, 3:1 or 4:1 AV block usually produces a ventricular HR of 150, 100 or 75/min. The ECG shows saw-tooth flutter waves. With regular 2:1 AV block, these may be buried in the QRST complexes, but can be revealed by transiently increasing the AV block through carotid sinus massage (Fig. 8.5) or IV adenosine. Digoxin, β-blockers or verapamil can limit the ventricular rate, but electrical or chemical cardioversion using amiodarone or flecainide is often

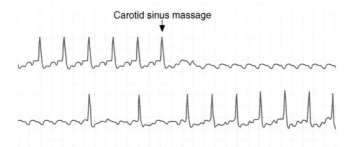

Carotid sinus massage

Fig. 8.5 Atrial flutter with 2:1 block: flutter waves revealed by carotid sinus massage.

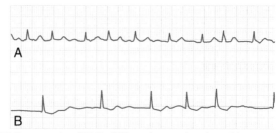

Fig. 8.6 Two examples of AF. The QRS complexes are irregular, and there are no P waves. (A) There is usually a fast ventricular rate, often between 120 and 160/min, at the onset of AF. (B) In chronic AF the ventricular rate may be much slower as a result of the effects of medication and AV nodal fatigue.

preferable. β-Blockers or amiodarone may be used to prevent recurrent atrial flutter, but catheter ablation is now the treatment of choice for patients with persistent symptoms. Anticoagulants are used to manage thrombotic risk around cardioversion as for atrial fibrillation (see below).

Atrial fibrillation

AF is the most common sustained cardiac arrhythmia, and its prevalence rises with age. The atria beat rapidly, but in an uncoordinated and ineffective manner. The ventricles are activated irregularly at a rate determined by conduction through the AV node, giving rise to an 'irregularly irregular' pulse. The ECG (Fig. 8.6) shows normal but irregularly spaced QRS complexes with absent P waves.

AF can be classified as:
• Paroxysmal (intermittent, self-terminating episodes). • Persistent (prolonged episodes that can be terminated by electrical or chemical cardioversion). • Permanent.

Paroxysmal AF often becomes permanent, with progression of underlying disease and electrical and structural remodeling of the atria. Common causes are shown in Box 8.6; however, many patients have 'lone atrial fibrillation', where no underlying cause is identified.

Clinical features

AF is occasionally asymptomatic, but typically presents with palpitation, breathlessness and fatigue. It may provoke angina in patients with coronary disease or cardiac failure in those with poor ventricular function or valve disease. Asymptomatic AF may present with embolic stroke in the elderly.

Investigation and management

All patients should have an ECG, echocardiogram and TFTs.

Paroxysmal AF: When AF complicates an acute illness (e.g. chest infection), treatment of the primary disorder usually restores sinus rhythm. Occasional attacks of paroxysmal AF do not necessarily need treatment. For repeated symptomatic episodes, β-blockers can be used to reduce the

8.6 Common causes of atrial fibrillation

- Coronary artery disease (including acute MI)
- Valvular heart disease, especially rheumatic mitral valve disease
- Hypertension
- Sinoatrial disease
- Hyperthyroidism
- Alcohol
- Cardiomyopathy
- Congenital heart disease
- Chest infection
- Pulmonary embolism
- Pericardial disease
- Idiopathic (lone AF)

8

ectopics that initiate AF, and are the usual first-line therapy, especially in patients with associated ischaemic heart disease, hypertension or cardiac failure. Flecainide, along with β-blockers, prevents episodes, but should be avoided in coronary disease or LV dysfunction. Amiodarone is also effective, but side effects restrict use. Digoxin and verapamil limit rate in AF but do not prevent episodes. Catheter ablation is useful in drug-resistant cases.

Persistent AF: *Rhythm control*—Successful restoration of sinus rhythm is most likely if AF has been present for less than 3 months and the patient is young and has no structural heart disease. Immediate cardioversion is indicated within 48 hours of onset. In stable patients without structural heart disease, IV flecainide is usually effective; amiodarone by central venous catheter is used in those with structural heart disease, and DC cardioversion is used if drugs fail. Beyond 48 hours, the ventricular rate should be controlled and cardioversion deferred until more than 4 weeks of oral anticoagulation. Prophylactic amiodarone may help to reduce recurrence, and catheter ablation may help in resistant cases.

Rate control—If sinus rhythm cannot be restored, β-blockers and rate-limiting calcium antagonists (e.g. verapamil) are more effective than digoxin at controlling HR during exercise. In exceptional cases, AF can be treated by inducing complete heart block with catheter ablation after first implanting a permanent pacemaker.

Thromboprophylaxis

Left atrial dilatation and loss of contraction may lead to thrombus formation, predisposing patients to stroke and systemic embolism. Patients undergoing cardioversion require temporary anticoagulation with warfarin (INR target 2.0–3.0) or direct-acting oral anticoagulant drugs, which should be started 4 weeks before and maintained for 3 months after successful cardioversion.

In chronic AF, the risk of stroke is balanced against the risk of bleeding complicating anticoagulation. Patients with underlying mitral valve disease should always be anticoagulated; in others, clinical scores (Box 8.7) are

i	8.7 CHA_2DS_2-VAS_c stroke risk score for nonvalvular atrial fibrillation	
	Parameter	**Score**
C	Congestive heart failure	1 point
H	Hypertension history	1 point
A_2	Age ≥75 years	2 points
D	Diabetes mellitus	1 point
S_2	Previous stroke or TIA	2 points
V	Vascular disease	1 point
A	Age 65–74 years	1 point
S_c	Sex category female	1 point
	Maximum total score	9 points

Annual stroke risk
0 points = 0% (no prophylaxis required)
1 point = 1.3% (oral anticoagulant recommended–males only)
2+ points = > 2.2% (oral anticoagulant recommended)

European Society of Cardiology Clinical Practice Guidelines: Atrial Fibrillation (Management of) 2010 and Focused Update (2012). Eur Heart J 2012; 33:2719–2747.

used to assess stroke risk. Risk is weakly related to frequency and duration of AF episodes, so guidelines do not distinguish between paroxysmal, persistent and permanent AF.

Directly acting oral anticoagulants (e.g. apixaban, dabigatran) are at least as effective as warfarin at preventing thrombotic stroke and have a lower risk of intracranial haemorrhage. They also do not require monitoring and have fewer drug interactions. Comorbid conditions (e.g. frequent falls) and drug interactions must be considered before anticoagulation is recommended.

Supraventricular tachycardia

This term describes a group of narrow-complex tachycardias (Fig. 8.7) caused by atrial re-entry circuits or abnormal atria foci, including AVNRT and AVRT (see later).

Atrioventricular nodal re-entrant tachycardia

AVNRT is attributed to re-entry in the right atrium and AV node, and tends to occur in structurally normal hearts. It produces episodes of regular tachycardia, with a rate of 120 to 240/min lasting from a few seconds to many hours.

The patient experiences a rapid, forceful, regular heartbeat and may feel faint or breathless. Polyuria may occur. The ECG usually shows a regular tachycardia with normal QRS complexes, but occasionally there is rate-dependent bundle branch block.

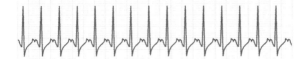

Fig. 8.7 Supraventricular tachycardia. The rate is 180/min, and the QRS complexes are normal.

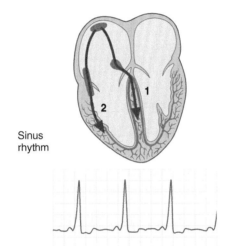

Sinus
rhythm

Fig. 8.8 Wolff–Parkinson–White syndrome. A strip of accessory conducting tissue allows electricity to bypass the AV node and spread from atria to ventricles without delay. When ventricular activation occurs through the AV node (1), the ECG is normal; however, when it occurs through the accessory pathway (2), a very short PR interval and a broad QRS complex are seen. In sinus rhythm, ventricular activation occurs by both paths, causing the characteristic short PR and slurring of the upstroke of the QRS complex (delta wave). The proportion of activation occurring via the accessory pathway may vary; therefore, at times, the ECG can look normal.

Management

Attacks may be terminated by carotid sinus pressure or Valsalva manœuvre, but if not, IV adenosine or verapamil will usually restore sinus rhythm. If there is severe haemodynamic compromise, the tachycardia should be terminated by DC cardioversion (p. 273). For recurrent attacks, catheter ablation (p. 275) is the most effective therapy, and is preferable to long-term medication with β-blockers or verapamil.

Atrioventricular re-entrant tachycardia

In this condition an abnormal band of rapidly conducting tissue ('accessory pathway') connects the atria and ventricles (Fig. 8.8). In 50% of cases, premature ventricular activation via the pathway produces a short PR interval and a 'slurred' upstroke of the QRS complex, called a delta wave. As the AV node and accessory pathway have different conduction speeds and refractory periods, a re-entry circuit can develop, causing tachycardia. When associated with symptoms, this is known as Wolff–Parkinson–White syndrome. The ECG during tachycardia is indistinguishable from that of AVNRT.

Management

Carotid sinus pressure, Valsalva manœuvre or IV adenosine can terminate the tachycardia. If AF occurs, it may produce a dangerously rapid ventricular rate (because the accessory pathway lacks the rate-limiting properties of the AV node) causing syncope. This is treated with emergency DC cardioversion. Catheter ablation (p. 275) of the accessory pathway is first-line treatment in symptomatic patients, and is nearly always curative. Prophylactic flecainide or propafenone can be used, but long-term medication cannot be justified, as ablation is safer and more effective. Digoxin and verapamil shorten the refractory period of the accessory pathway and must be avoided.

Ventricular premature beats

VPBs occur frequently in healthy people at rest, disappearing on exercise. They also occur in subclinical coronary artery disease, cardiomyopathy or following an MI. Most patients are asymptomatic, but some feel irregular or missed beats. The pulse reveals weak or missed beats because VPBs have a low stroke volume. The ECG shows broad and bizarre QRS complexes as depolarization propagates outside the conducting system.

Treatment (β-blockers) is only necessary in highly symptomatic cases. Frequent VPBs in patients with heart failure or those who have survived the acute phase of MI are associated with an adverse prognosis. Treatment should be directed at the underlying cause.

Ventricular tachycardia

VT usually occurs in patients with coronary heart disease or cardiomyopathies, and may cause haemodynamic compromise or degenerate into VF (Fig. 8.4). The ECG shows tachycardia with broad, abnormal QRS complexes and a rate greater than 120/min (Fig. 8.9). VT is by far the most common cause of a broad-complex tachycardia, but may be difficult to distinguish from supraventricular tachycardia with bundle branch block or Wolff–Parkinson–White syndrome. When there is doubt, it is safer to manage the problem as VT.

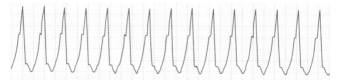

Fig. 8.9 VT: rhythm strip. Typical broad, bizarre QRS complexes with a rate of 160/min.

Management

Prompt DC cardioversion is required if systolic BP is less than 90 mmHg, but if VT is well tolerated, then IV amiodarone may be tried. Hypokalaemia, hypomagnesaemia, acidosis and hypoxaemia must be corrected. β-Blockers and/or amiodarone may be effective for subsequent prophylaxis. Class Ic anti-arrhythmic drugs should be avoided because they can provoke dangerous arrhythmia. An implantable cardiac defibrillator is recommended in patients with poor LV function, or those with refractory VT causing haemodynamic compromise. VT occasionally occurs in patients with otherwise healthy hearts; in such cases prognosis is good and catheter ablation can be curative.

Torsades de pointes

This form of VT complicates a prolonged QT interval, which may be congenital or secondary to drugs (e.g. class Ia, Ic and III antiarrhythmics, macrolide antibiotics, tricyclic antidepressants, phenothiazines) or electrolyte disturbance ($\downarrow Ca^{2+}$, $\downarrow Mg^{2+}$, $\downarrow K^+$). The ECG shows rapid broad complexes that seem to twist around the baseline as the QRS axis changes. It is typically nonsustained but may degenerate into VF. The ECG in sinus rhythm shows a prolonged QT interval (>0.44 seconds in men, >0.46 seconds in women when corrected to a HR of 60/min).

Management

IV magnesium should be given in all cases. Atrial pacing or IV isoprenaline shortens the QT interval by increasing HR. Otherwise, treatment is directed at the underlying cause. Patients with congenital long QT syndrome often require an implantable cardiac defibrillator.

Atrioventricular block

This usually indicates disease affecting the AV node. Block may be intermittent and only apparent when tachycardias stress the conducting tissue.

First-degree AV block

AV conduction is delayed, producing a prolonged PR interval (>0.20 seconds). It rarely causes symptoms.

Second-degree AV block

Here, dropped beats occur because some atrial impulses fail to conduct to the ventricles.

Mobitz type I block ('Wenckebach's phenomenon'): There is progressive lengthening of the PR intervals, culminating in a dropped beat. The cycle then repeats itself. It is sometimes observed at rest or during sleep in athletic young adults with high vagal tone.

Mobitz type II block: The PR interval of conducted impulses remains constant, but some P waves are not conducted. It is usually caused by disease of the His–Purkinje system, and carries a risk of asystole. In 2:1 AV block (Fig. 8.10), alternate P waves are conducted, so it is impossible to distinguish between Mobitz type I and type II block.

Third-degree AV block

AV conduction fails completely, the atria and ventricles beat independently (AV dissociation, Fig. 8.11) and ventricular activity is maintained by an

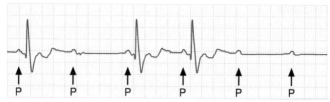

Fig. 8.10 Second-degree atrioventricular block (Mobitz type II). The PR interval of conducted beats is normal, but some P waves are not conducted. The constant PR interval distinguishes this from Wenckebach's phenomenon.

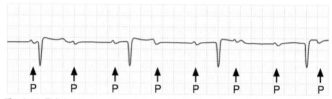

Fig. 8.11 Third-degree atrioventricular block. There is complete dissociation of atrial and ventricular complexes. The atrial rate is 80/min, and the ventricular rate is 38/min

escape rhythm arising in the AV node or bundle of His (narrow QRS) or the distal Purkinje tissues (broad QRS). Distal escape rhythms are slower and less reliable. The pulse is slow, regular and unresponsive to exercise. Cannon waves may be visible in the neck, and the intensity of the first heart sound varies because of loss of AV synchrony.

Clinical features

The typical presentation is with recurrent sudden loss of consciousness, typically without warning ('Stokes–Adams' attacks). Anoxic seizures (because of cerebral ischaemia) may occur if asystole is prolonged. There is pallor and a death-like appearance during the attack, but when the heart starts beating again there is a characteristic flush. In contrast to epilepsy, recovery is rapid.

Management

Acute inferior MI is often complicated by transient AV block because the right coronary artery supplies the AV node. There is usually a reliable escape rhythm, and if the patient remains well, no treatment is required. Symptomatic second-degree or third-degree block may respond to IV atropine or, if this fails, a temporary pacemaker. In most cases the AV block resolves within 7 to 10 days.

Second- or third-degree AV block complicating acute anterior MI indicates extensive ventricular damage involving both bundle branches, and carries a poor prognosis. Asystole may ensue, and a temporary pacemaker

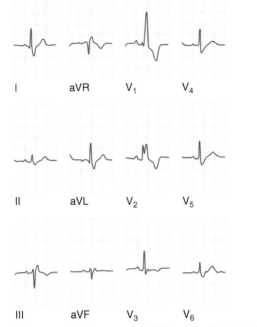

Fig. 8.12 RBBB. Note the wide QRS complexes with 'M'-shaped configuration in leads V_1 and V_2 and a wide S wave in lead I.

should be inserted promptly. If the patient presents with asystole, IV atropine (3 mg) or IV isoprenaline (2 mg in 500 mL 5% dextrose, infused at 10–60 mL/hour) may help to maintain the circulation until a temporary pacing electrode can be inserted.

Patients with symptomatic bradyarrhythmias associated with AV block should receive a permanent pacemaker. Asymptomatic first-degree or Mobitz type I second-degree AV block does not require treatment, but a permanent pacemaker is usually indicated in patients with asymptomatic Mobitz type II second-degree or third-degree heart block on prognostic grounds.

Bundle branch block

Interruption of the right or left branch of the conducting system delays activation of the corresponding ventricle, broadens the QRS complex (≥0.12 seconds) and produces characteristic alterations in QRS morphology (Figs. 8.12 and 8.13). RBBB can be a normal variant, but LBBB usually signifies important underlying heart disease (Box 8.8).

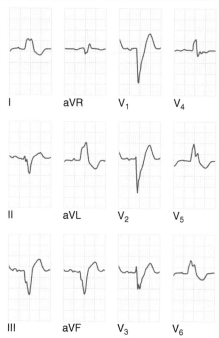

Fig. 8.13 LBBB. Note the wide QRS complexes with the loss of the Q wave or septal vector in lead I and 'M'-shaped QRS complexes in V_5 and V_6.

---

i   **8.8 Common causes of bundle branch block**

Right

- Normal variant
- RV hypertrophy or strain, e.g. PE
- Congenital heart disease, e.g. atrial septal defect
- CAD

Left

- CAD
- Aortic valve disease
- Hypertension
- Cardiomyopathy

Antiarrhythmic drugs

The major classes of antiarrhythmic drugs and their side effects are summarised in Box 8.9.

Nonpharmacological treatment of arrhythmias

Electrical cardioversion

This is useful for terminating rhythms such as AF or VT. The shock interrupts the arrhythmia and produces a brief asystole, followed by the resumption of sinus rhythm. Cardioversion is usually carried out electively under general anaesthesia. The shock is delivered immediately after the R wave, because a shock applied during the T wave may provoke VF. High-energy shocks may cause chest wall pain postprocedure, so it is usual to begin with a shock of 50 J, proceeding to larger shocks if necessary.

Defibrillation

Defibrillators deliver a high-energy DC shock via two large paddles coated with conducting jelly or a gel pad, positioned over the upper right sternal edge and the apex. They are used in the management of cardiac arrest because of VF or VT. Modern units deliver a biphasic shock, during which the shock polarity is reversed mid-shock, reducing the energy required to depolarise the heart. In VF and other emergencies, the energy of the first and second shocks should be 150 J and thereafter up to 200 J.

Temporary pacemakers

Transvenous pacing: Delivered by positioning a pacing electrode at the apex of the right ventricle via the internal jugular, subclavian or femoral vein using fluoroscopic imaging. The electrode is connected to an external pacemaker that delivers an adjustable electrical impulse if the HR falls below a set rate. Temporary pacing may be indicated in the management of transient heart block or of other causes of transient bradycardia (e.g. drug overdose), or as a prelude to permanent pacing. Complications include pneumothorax, brachial plexus or subclavian artery injury, infection or sepsis (usually *Staphylococcus aureus*) and pericarditis.

Transcutaneous pacing: Administered by delivering an electrical stimulus sufficient to induce cardiac contraction through two adhesive gel pad electrodes placed externally over the apex and upper right sternal edge. It is easy and quick to set up, but causes significant discomfort.

Permanent pacemakers

These use the same principles, but the pulse generator is implanted under the skin. Electrodes can be placed in the right ventricular apex, the right atrial appendage or both (dual-chamber). Atrial pacing may be appropriate for patients with sinoatrial disease without AV block. In dual-chamber pacing, the atrial electrode can be used to detect spontaneous atrial activity and trigger ventricular pacing, thereby preserving AV synchrony and allowing the ventricular rate to increase together with the atrial rate during exercise, leading to improved exercise tolerance. A code is used to signify the pacing mode (Box 8.10). Most dual-chamber pacemakers are programmed to DDD mode. Rate-responsive pacemakers trigger a rise in HR in response to

| i | 8.9 Classification, use and side effects of antiarrhythmic drugs |

Drug	Main uses	Route	Important side effects
Class 1: Membrane stabilizing agents			
Disopyramide	Atrial and ventricular tachyarrhythmias	IV, oral	Myocardial depression
Lidocaine	Ventricular tachycardia and fibrillation	IV	Convulsions
Mexilitine	Atrial and ventricular tachyarrhythmias	IV, oral	Myocardial depression
Flecainide	Atrial and ventricular tachyarrhythmias	IV, oral	Myocardial depression
Class II: Beta adrenoceptor antagonists			
Atenolol	Treatment and prevention of SVT and AF, prevention of VPBs and exercise induced VT	IV, oral	Myocardial depression, bronchospasm, cold peripheries
Bisoprolol		oral	
Metoprolol		IV, oral	
Class III: Drugs prolonging action potential			
Amiodarone	Atrial and ventricular tachyarrhythmias	IV, oral	Thyroid, lung toxicity
Dronedarone	Paroxysmal atrial fibrillation	oral	Renal, liver toxicity
Sotalol[a]	AF, rarely ventricular arrhythmias	IV, oral	Torsades de pointes
Class IV: Slow calcium channel blockers			
Verapamil	Treatment of SVT, control of AF	IV, oral	Myocardial depression
Other			
Atropine	Treatment of vagal bradycardia	IV	Dry mouth, poor vision
Adenosine	Identification/treatment of SVT	IV	Flushing, dyspnea
Digoxin	Treatment of SVT, rate control in AF	IV, oral	GI upset, arrhythmias

[a]Sotalol also has class II β-blocker activity

movement or increased respiratory rate and are used in patients unable to raise their HR during exercise. Complications of permanent pacing include:

Early: pneumothorax, cardiac tamponade, lead displacement, infection.
Late: infection, erosion of the generator or lead, lead fracture because of mechanical fatigue.

8.10 International generic pacemaker code

Chamber paced	Chamber sensed	Response to sensing
O = none	O = none	O = none
A = atrium	A = atrium	T = triggered
V = ventricle	V = ventricle	I = inhibited
D = both	D = both	D = both

8.11 Key indications for implantable cardiac defibrillator therapy

Primary prevention

- After MI, if LV ejection fraction <30%
- Mild to moderate symptomatic heart failure, on optimal drug therapy, with LV ejection fraction <35%
- Selected inherited conditions e.g. long QT syndrome, cardiomyopathy

Secondary prevention

- Survivors of VF or VT cardiac arrest not attributed to transient or reversible cause
- VT with haemodynamic compromise or significant LV impairment (LV ejection fraction <35%)

Implantable cardiac defibrillators

In addition to the functions of a permanent pacemaker, ICDs sense rhythm and deliver current through leads implanted in the heart via the subclavian or cephalic vein. They automatically sense and terminate life-threatening ventricular arrhythmias. These devices can treat ventricular tachyarrhythmias using overdrive pacing, synchronised cardioversion or defibrillation. ICD implantation is subject to similar complications as pacemaker implantation (see earlier). Indications for ICDs are shown in Box 8.11.

Cardiac resynchronisation therapy

CRT is a useful treatment for selected patients with LBBB, which causes uncoordinated LV contraction, exacerbating heart failure. CRT systems pace the septum through an RV lead and the epicardial surface of the LV using a lead placed via the coronary sinus into an epicardial vein. Simultaneous septal and epicardial pacing resynchronise LV contraction, improving heart failure and mortality in selected patients.

Catheter ablation therapy

This is the treatment of choice for many patients with AVNRT, AV re-entrant tachycardias and atrial flutter, and is useful for some patients with AF or ventricular arrhythmias. A series of catheter electrodes are inserted into the heart via the venous system and used to record the activation sequence of the heart in sinus rhythm, during tachycardia and after pacing manœuvres. Once the arrhythmia focus or circuit is identified, a catheter is used to ablate the culprit tissue using radiofrequency current or cryoablation. Serious complications are rare (<1%), but include complete heart block requiring pacemaker implantation, and cardiac tamponade. Successful ablation spares the patient long-term drug treatment.

Coronary artery disease

CAD is the most common cause of angina and acute coronary syndrome and the most common cause of death worldwide. In the UK, 1 in 3 men and 1 in 4 women die from CAD.

Disease of the coronary arteries is almost always caused by atherosclerosis and its complications, particularly thrombosis. Atherosclerosis is a progressive inflammatory disorder of the arterial wall, characterised by focal lipid-rich deposits of atheroma that remain clinically silent until they become large enough to impair arterial perfusion or until disruption of the lesion results in thrombotic occlusion or embolisation of the vessel. Several risk factors have been identified:

Age and sex: Age is the most powerful independent risk factor for athero-sclerosis. Premenopausal women have lower rates of disease than men, but thereafter risk is similar. Hormone replacement therapy has no role in prevention of atherosclerosis, however.

Genetics: A positive family history is common in patients with early-onset disease (age <50 in men and <55 in women). A monozygotic twin of a case has an eightfold risk and a dizygotic twin a fourfold risk of dying from CAD, because of shared genetics, environment and lifestyle. Other risk factors, such as hypertension, hyperlipidaemia and diabetes, have polygenic inheritance.

Smoking: The most important modifiable risk factor, smoking is strongly related to CAD.

Hypertension: The incidence of atherosclerosis increases as BP (systolic and diastolic) rises. Antihypertensive therapy reduces cardiovascular mortality and stroke.

Hypercholesterolaemia: Risk rises with serum cholesterol concentration. Lowering serum total and LDL cholesterol reduces the risk of cardiovascular events.

Diabetes mellitus: This is a potent risk factor for atherosclerosis, and is often associated with diffuse disease. Insulin resistance (normal glucose homeostasis with high levels of insulin) is also a risk factor for CAD.

Lifestyle factors: Alcohol excess is associated with hypertension and cerebrovascular disease. Physical inactivity and obesity are independent risk factors for atherosclerosis; regular exercise appears to have a protective effect. Diets deficient in fresh fruit, vegetables and polyunsaturated fatty acids are associated with an increased risk of cardiovascular disease.

Social deprivation: This is an independent risk factor for cardiovascular disease. Guidelines recommend lower treatment thresholds for socially deprived patients.

Management

Primary prevention: This aims to prevent atherosclerosis in healthy individuals with elevated risk. Public health measures are used to actively discourage risk factors such as obesity and smoking. In addition, scoring systems can identify high-risk individuals for treatment.

Secondary prevention: This means treating patients who already have disease, to prevent subsequent events. Following an event such as an MI, patients are usually receptive to lifestyle advice, such as diet and smoking cessation. Additional interventions are discussed below.

Angina pectoris

Angina pectoris is the symptom complex occurring when an imbalance between myocardial oxygen supply and demand causes transient myocardial ischaemia. Atherosclerosis is by far the most common cause of angina; however, it can also occur with aortic valve disease, hypertrophic cardiomyopathy, vasculitis or aortitis. Angina may accompany coronary vasospasm, and when accompanied by transient ST elevation, this is termed *Prinzmetal's angina*.

Angina on effort with myocardial ischaemia on stress testing but with normal coronary angiography is known as syndrome X. This disorder is poorly understood, but carries a good prognosis.

Clinical features

The history is the most important factor in making the diagnosis (p. 1). Stable angina is characterised by central chest pain, discomfort or breathlessness that is precipitated by exertion or other stress, and is promptly relieved by rest. Examination is frequently negative, but may reveal evidence of:
• Aortic stenosis (an occasional cause of angina). • Risk factors (e.g. hypertension, diabetes; check fundi). • LV dysfunction (e.g. cardiomegaly). • Other arterial disease (e.g. carotid bruits, peripheral vascular disease). • Conditions that exacerbate angina (e.g. anaemia, thyrotoxicosis).

Investigations

Symptoms are a poor guide to the extent of CAD, so stress testing and noninvasive imaging are advisable in patients who are potential candidates for revascularisation.

Exercise ECG: performed using a standard treadmill or bicycle ergometer protocol is the first-line investigation. Horizontal or down-sloping ST segment depression of 1 mm or more is indicative of ischaemia; up-sloping ST depression is less specific. Exercise testing is of value in identifying high-risk individuals with severe coronary disease, but false negatives and positives do occur, the predictive accuracy is lower in women and not all patients can exercise to the required level.

Myocardial perfusion scanning: is helpful if suspicion of CAD is high but the exercise test is equivocal, uninterpretable (e.g. LBBB) or cannot be done. A perfusion defect present during stress but not at rest indicates reversible myocardial ischaemia; a persistent defect suggests previous MI.

CT coronary arteriography: is used increasingly to investigate patients with suspected CAD. It can clarify the diagnosis and (if negative or showing only mild disease) can avoid the need for cardiac catheterisation.

Coronary angiography: provides detailed anatomical information about the extent of CAD. It is usually performed when coronary bypass surgery or percutaneous coronary intervention are being considered.

Management

This should begin with a careful explanation of the problem and a discussion of the lifestyle and medical interventions that can relieve symptoms and improve prognosis. Management then involves:

- Assessment of extent and severity of CAD.
- Identification and control of risk factors (see earlier).
- Symptom control using medication.
- Identification of high-risk patients for treatment to improve life expectancy.

All patients with angina secondary to CAD should receive low-dose (75 mg) aspirin (or clopidogrel 75 mg daily if aspirin causes dyspepsia), continued indefinitely because it reduces the risk of MI. Similarly, all patients should be prescribed a statin, even if cholesterol is normal.

Antianginal drug therapy

The goal is control of angina with minimum side effects and the simplest possible drug regimen. Five groups of drug are used, but there is little evidence that one group is more effective than another. It is conventional to start with glyceryl trinitrate and a β-blocker, adding a calcium channel antagonist or a long-acting nitrate if needed. If two drugs fail to control symptoms, revascularisation should be considered.

Nitrates: Sublingual GTN spray (400 μg) is used for acute attacks and as prophylaxis before exercise. GTN patches have a longer effect. Isosorbide dinitrate or mononitrate can be given by mouth. Headache is a common side effect.

β-Blockers: These limit myocardial oxygen demand by reducing HR, BP and myocardial contractility, but may provoke bronchospasm in asthmatic patients. Cardioselective preparations such as bisoprolol (5–15 mg daily) are widely used.

Calcium channel antagonists: These lower myocardial oxygen demand by reducing BP and myocardial contractility. Nifedipine and amlodipine may cause a reflex tachycardia, so are often combined with a β-blocker. Verapamil and diltiazem can be used as monotherapy. All can aggravate heart failure and cause peripheral oedema and dizziness.

Potassium channel activators: Nicorandil acts as an arterial and venous vasodilator, and has the advantage that it does not exhibit the tolerance seen with nitrates.

I_f channel antagonist: Ivabradine induces bradycardia by modulating ion channels in the sinus node. It does not inhibit contractility or exacerbate heart failure.

Nonpharmacological treatments

Percutaneous coronary intervention: involves passing a fine guidewire across a coronary stenosis under radiographic control and using it to position a balloon, which is then inflated to dilate the stenosis. This can be combined with deployment of a coronary stent, which is metallic 'scaffolding' impregnated with antiproliferative drugs, used to dilate and maintain a stenosed vessel. PCI is an effective symptomatic treatment, but does not improve survival in patients with chronic stable angina. It is mainly used in single- or two-vessel disease, and can also be used to dilate stenosed bypass grafts. The main acute complication is vessel occlusion by thrombus or dissection, which may lead to myocardial damage (2%–5%) requiring stenting or emergency CABG. The main long-term complication is restenosis. Stenting substantially reduces the risk of restenosis, probably because it allows more complete dilatation. Antiproliferative drug-eluting stents can reduce this risk even further. Adjunctive therapy with a potent platelet inhibitor such as the P2Y12 receptor antagonists (clopidogrel, prasugrel or ticagrelor) in combination with aspirin and heparin improves the outcome following PCI.

Coronary artery bypass grafting: The internal mammary arteries, radial arteries or reversed segments of saphenous vein can be used to bypass coronary artery stenoses, usually under cardiopulmonary bypass. The operative mortality is ~1.5%, but higher in elderly patients and those with poor LV function or significant comorbidity (e.g. renal failure). There is a 1% to 5% risk of perioperative stroke. Approximately 90% of patients are free of angina 1 year after surgery, but less than 60% of patients are asymptomatic 5 years or more after CABG. Arterial grafts have much better long-term patency rates than vein grafts. Long-term aspirin or clopidogrel improves graft patency, whereas intensive lipid-lowering therapy slows progression of disease in the native coronary arteries and grafts. Persistent smokers are twice as likely to die in the 10 years following surgery compared with those who give up at surgery. CABG improves survival in patients with left main stem coronary stenosis and those with symptomatic three-vessel coronary disease; the benefit is greatest in those with impaired LV function or positive stress testing before surgery.

Acute coronary syndrome

This term encompasses unstable angina and MI. Unstable angina refers to new-onset or rapidly worsening (crescendo) angina, and angina on minimal exertion or at rest without myocardial damage. In MI there is evidence of myocardial necrosis in a clinical setting of acute myocardial ischaemia. Criteria for diagnosing an MI are a rise in cardiac biomarker values (e.g. cardiac troponin), to more than the 99th centile and at least one of the following:

1. Symptoms of ischaemia
2. New/presumed new significant ST–T changes or new LBBB
3. Development of pathological Q waves
4. New loss of viable myocardium or new regional wall motion abnormality on imaging
5. Identification of an intracoronary thrombus by angiography or postmortem

Acute coronary syndrome may present de novo or against a background of chronic stable angina. The underlying pathophysiology is usually a fissured atheromatous plaque with adherent thrombus formation.

Clinical features

The cardinal symptom is severe and prolonged angina-like pain occurring at rest. Other symptoms include:

• Breathlessness. • Vomiting because of vagal stimulation, particularly in inferior MI. • Syncope or sudden death because of arrhythmia.

MI may occasionally be painless, especially in diabetic or elderly patients.

Complications of acute coronary syndromes

Arrhythmias: Arrhythmias are common with acute coronary syndrome, but often transient. The risks can be minimised by pain relief, rest and correction of hypokalaemia. VF occurs in 5% to 10% of hospitalised patients. The prognosis of patients defibrillated for VF in the first 48 hours is identical to that of patients without VF. Ventricular arrhythmias during convalescence signify poor ventricular function, and selected patients may benefit from ICDs (p. 275). AF is common and only requires cardioversion if it causes tachycardia with hypotension, otherwise digoxin or a β-blocker are usually given. Anticoagulation is required if AF persists.

Bradycardia does not require treatment unless there is hypotension, in which case atropine (0.6–1.2 mg IV) is given. Inferior MI may cause AV block, which often resolves following reperfusion. If there is compromise because of second- or third-degree AV block, or block complicating anterior MI, a temporary pacemaker is required.

Recurrent angina: Patients who develop recurrent angina following acute coronary syndrome are at high risk and should be considered for coronary angiography and urgent revascularisation. Angiography is also indicated in all those who have had successful thrombolysis, to treat residual stenosis.

Patients with dynamic ECG changes and ongoing pain should be treated with intravenous glycoprotein IIb/IIIa receptor antagonists.

Acute heart failure: Acute heart failure usually reflects extensive myocardial damage and carries a poor prognosis. The management of heart failure is discussed on p. 259.

Pericarditis: This complicates infarction and is particularly common on the second and third days. A distinct new pain develops, which is often positional or exacerbated by inspiration. A pericardial rub may be heard. Opiate analgesics are preferred over NSAIDs and glucocorticoids because the latter may increase the risk of aneurysm and myocardial rupture.

Dressler's syndrome: This is an autoimmune disorder that occurs weeks to months after the infarct, and is characterised by persistent fever, pericarditis and pleurisy. Severe symptoms may require treatment with an NSAID or glucocorticoids.

Papillary muscle rupture: This causes acute pulmonary oedema and shock with a pansystolic murmur because of the sudden onset of severe mitral regurgitation. Emergency mitral valve replacement may be necessary.

Ventricular septum rupture: Usually presents with sudden haemodynamic deterioration accompanied by a new, loud pansystolic murmur. It may be difficult to distinguish from acute mitral regurgitation, but tends to cause right heart failure rather than pulmonary oedema. Doppler echocardiography will confirm the diagnosis. Without prompt surgery, the condition is usually fatal.

Ventricular rupture: Leads to cardiac tamponade and is usually fatal.

Other recognised peri-infarct complications

These include:
• Systemic embolism from a cardiac thrombus. • Development of a ventricular aneurysm.

Investigations

ECG: This is the most important investigation in the assessment of acute chest pain, and guides initial therapy. It shows a characteristic series of changes in MI (Fig. 8.14):

The earliest change is ST elevation followed by diminution in the size of the R wave, and development of a Q wave (indicating full-thickness infarction). Subsequently, the T wave becomes inverted, and this change persists after the ST segment has returned to normal. ECG changes are best seen in the leads that 'face' the infarcted area. With anteroseptal infarction, abnormalities are found in one or more leads from V_1 to V_4. Anterolateral infarction produces changes from V_4 to V_6, in aVL and lead I. Inferior infarction is best shown in leads II, III and aVF. Infarction of the posterior wall of the left ventricle does not cause ST elevation or Q waves in the standard leads, but can be diagnosed by the presence of reciprocal changes (ST depression and a tall R wave in leads V_1–V_4).

In non-ST segment elevation acute coronary syndrome, partial or minor coronary occlusion causes unstable angina or subendocardial MI (termed NSTEMI). The ECG shows ST depression and T-wave changes.

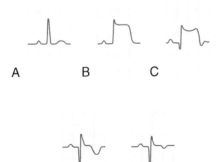

A   B   C

D   E

Fig. 8.14 The serial evolution of ECG changes in full-thickness myocardial infarction.
(A) Normal ECG complex. (B) (Minutes) Acute ST elevation. (C) (Hours) Progressive loss of the R wave, developing Q wave, resolution of the ST elevation and terminal T-wave inversion. (D) (Days) Deep Q wave and T-wave inversion. (E) (Weeks or months) Old or established infarct pattern; the Q wave tends to persist, but the T-wave changes become less marked.

Occasionally, new-onset LBBB is the only ECG change with infarction.

Patients with ST elevation or new LBBB block require immediate reperfusion therapy. Patients with unstable angina or NSTEMI have a high risk of progression to STEMI or death.

Cardiac biomarkers: Serial measurements of serum troponin should be taken. In unstable angina, there is no rise in troponin, and the diagnosis is made from the history and ECG. In contrast, MI causes a rise in plasma troponin T and I concentrations and other cardiac muscle enzymes (Fig. 8.15). Troponins T and I increase within 3 to 6 hours, peak at about 36 hours and remain elevated for up to 2 weeks.

ECG: This is useful for assessing ventricular function and for detecting complications such as mural thrombus, cardiac rupture, ventricular septal defect, mitral regurgitation and pericardial effusion.

Coronary angiography: Angiography with a view to revascularisation should be considered in patients at moderate or high risk, including those with: • failure to settle on medical therapy • extensive ECG changes • elevated plasma troponin • severe preexisting stable angina

Other investigations: A CXR may reveal pulmonary oedema or cardiomegaly. Lipids should be measured within 24 hours as cholesterol falls following infarction.

Management

Urgent hospital admission is required, as appropriate medical therapy reduces the risk of death and recurrent ischaemia by at least 60%. Initial therapy is summarised in Fig. 8.16.

Clinical risk stratification using defined scores (e.g. the GRACE score; Box 8.12) should be used to select patients for early coronary angiography or early mobilisation and discharge.

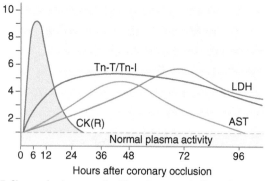

Fig. 8.15 Changes in plasma cardiac biomarker concentrations after myocardial infarction. Creatine kinase (CK) and troponins T (TnT) and I (Tn I) are the first to rise, followed by aspartate aminotransferase (AST) and then lactate (hydroxybutyrate) dehydrogenase (LDH). In patients treated with reperfusion therapy, a rapid rise in plasma creatine kinase (curve CK [R]) occurs, because of a washout effect.

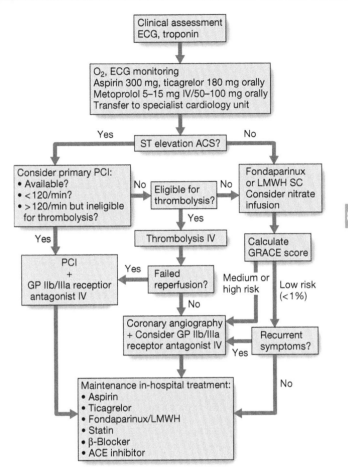

Fig. 8.16 Summary of treatment for acute coronary syndrome. *PCI*, Percutaneous coronary intervention: *GP*, glycoprotein: *LMWH*, low molecular weight heparin.

Analgesia: This is essential to relieve distress, and also to lower adrenergic drive and susceptibility to arrhythmias. IV opiates with an appropriate antiemetic (e.g. metoclopramide) should be titrated until the patient is comfortable.

Reperfusion therapy: Immediate reperfusion therapy is indicated when the ECG shows new bundle branch block or characteristic ST segment elevation of more than 1 mm in the limb leads or 2 mm in the chest leads. PCI is the treatment of choice for those presenting within 12 hours of symptom onset (Fig. 8.16). If PCI cannot be performed within 120 minutes, and thrombolysis is contraindicated, the procedure should

i	**8.12 Risk stratification in acute coronary syndrome: GRACE score**		
Clinical feature	Points range		
Heart failure score (Killip class)	No failure: 0	to	Cardiogenic shock: 59
Systolic BP (mmHg)	≥200: 0	to	≤80: 58
Heart rate	≤50: 0	to	≥200: 46
Age (years)	≤30: 0	to	≥90: 100
Serum creatinine (μmol/L)	0–34: 1	to	≥353: 28
Cardiac arrest at admission	39		
ST-segment deviation	28		
Elevated cardiac enzyme levels	14		
The first five factors score points according to defined ranges (see SIGN Guideline 93; Feb 2007; pp. 42 (annex 1) and 47 (annex 4): http://www.sign.ac.uk/guidelines/fulltext/93/. Sum of points predicts in-hospital death: 0.2% for points ≤60, rising to 52% for points totalling >240			

be performed as soon as possible. Patients should be considered for PCI within 24 hours, even after spontaneous reperfusion or thrombolysis. PCI restores coronary patency in more than 95% of patients, with more than 95% 1-year survival and marked reductions in heart failure and recurrent MI. Successful PCI also leads to rapid pain relief, resolution of acute ST elevation and occasional transient arrhythmias. PCI confers no immediate mortality benefit in patients with non-ST segment elevation acute coronary syndrome.

Thrombolysis: If primary PCI cannot be achieved in a timely manner (see Fig. 8.16), thrombolysis should be administered. The survival advantage following thrombolysis is significant, but less than for primary PCI. The benefit is greatest within the first 12 hours, and especially the first 2 hours. Tenecteplase and reteplase, analogues of human tissue plasminogen activator, are given as an IV bolus, assisting emergency treatment including in the prehospital setting. The major hazard of thrombolysis is bleeding. Cerebral haemorrhage causes four extra strokes per 1000 patients treated, and the incidence of other major bleeds is between 0.5% and 1%. Thrombolysis should therefore be withheld if there is a risk of serious bleeding (Box 8.13). PCI should be considered if thrombolysis is contraindicated but there is evidence of cardiogenic shock, and also within 24 hours of successful thrombolysis, to prevent recurrent infarction and improve outcome.

Antithrombotic therapy: Antiplatelet therapy with oral aspirin (300 mg initially, then 75 mg long term) improves survival (25% reduction in mortality). A P2Y12 receptor antagonist such as ticagrelor (180 mg, then 90 mg twice daily) should be given with the aspirin for up to 12 months. Patients intolerant of aspirin should receive clopidogrel (300 mg, then 75 mg daily).

> **i** **8.13 Relative contraindications to thrombolytic therapy (potential candidates for primary percutaneous coronary intervention)**
>
> - Active internal bleeding
> - Previous subarachnoid or intracerebral haemorrhage
> - Uncontrolled hypertension
> - Recent surgery (within 1 month)
> - Recent trauma (including traumatic resuscitation)
> - High probability of active peptic ulcer
> - Pregnancy

Glycoprotein IIb/IIIa receptor antagonists (e.g. tirofiban) block platelet aggregation and are given IV to high-risk patients with acute coronary syndromes undergoing PCI.

Anticoagulation: This reduces thromboembolic complications and reinfarction. Fondaparinux (2.5 mg SC daily) has the best safety and efficacy profile, but LMWH is a useful alternative. Anticoagulation should be continued for 8 days or until hospital discharge.

Antianginal therapy: Sublingual GTN (300–500 µg) is valuable first aid in unstable angina, and IV nitrates are useful for the treatment of LV failure and for recurrent or persistent ischaemic pain. Intravenous β-blockers (atenolol or metoprolol) relieve pain, reduce arrhythmias and improve short-term mortality in patients who present within 12 hours of the onset of symptoms, but should be avoided if there is heart failure, hypotension or bradycardia. Nifedipine or amlodipine can be added to the β-blocker if there is persistent chest discomfort. Long-term oral β-blockers reduce mortality by around 25% in survivors of MI.

Renin–angiotensin blockade: Long-term ACE inhibitors (e.g. enalapril 10 mg twice daily or ramipril 2.5–5 mg daily) counteract ventricular remodelling, prevent heart failure, improve survival and reduce recurrent MI and rehospitalisation. Patients with heart failure benefit most, but they should be considered in all patients with acute coronary syndrome. ACE inhibitors may exacerbate hypotension, in which case ARBs (e.g. candesartan) may be better tolerated.

Mineralocorticoid receptor antagonists: Patients with acute MI complicated by heart failure and LV dysfunction, and either pulmonary oedema or diabetes, further benefit from eplerenone (25–50 mg daily) or spironolactone (25–50 mg daily).

Lipid lowering therapy: All patients should receive therapy with HMG CoA reductase enzyme inhibitors (statins) after acute coronary syndrome, irrespective of serum cholesterol. Patients with serum LDL cholesterol concentrations greater than 3.2 mmol/L (~120 mg/dL) benefit from more intensive therapy, such as atorvastatin (80 mg daily). Ezetimibe, fibrates and anion exchange resins may be used in cases resistant to statins alone.

Smoking cessation: Giving up smoking is the single most effective thing a patient can do after acute coronary syndrome, as cessation halves mortality at 5 years. Cessation success rates are improved by supportive advice and pharmacological therapy.

Diet and exercise: Maintaining an ideal weight, eating a Mediterranean-style diet, taking regular exercise, and controlling hypertension and diabetes mellitus all improve the long-term outlook.

Rehabilitation

When there are no complications, the patient can mobilise on the second day, return home in 2 to 3 days and gradually increase activity, aiming to return to work in 4 weeks. Most patients may resume driving after 1 to 4 weeks, but drivers of trucks and buses usually require special assessment. Emotional problems such as anxiety and depression are common, and must be recognised and dealt with accordingly. Formal rehabilitation programmes, based on graded exercise protocols with individual and group counselling, are often very successful.

Prognosis

In almost one-quarter of cases of MI, death occurs within a few minutes without medical care. Half of deaths occur within 24 hours of the onset of symptoms, and around 40% of all affected patients die within the first month. Of those who survive an acute attack, more than 80% live for a further year, around 75% for 5 years and 50% for 10 years. Early death is usually caused by an arrhythmia but, later on, the outcome is determined by the extent of myocardial damage. Unfavourable features include poor LV function, AV block and persistent ventricular arrhythmias. The prognosis is worse for anterior than for inferior infarcts.

Peripheral arterial disease

Around 20% of UK adults aged 55 to 75 years have PAD, but only one-quarter have symptoms, usually intermittent claudication. Almost all PAD is because of atherosclerosis, and it shares the same risk factors as CAD. Some 5% to 10% of patients with PAD have diabetes, but this increases to 30% to 40% in those with severe limb ischaemia. The mechanism of PAD in diabetes is atheroma of medium to large arteries, so diabetes is not a contraindication to lower limb revascularisation.

Clinical features

Symptomatic PAD affects the legs eight times more commonly than the arms. Several vessels may be affected in a variable and asymmetric manner. Box 8.14 lists the clinical signs of chronic PAD.

Intermittent claudication: IC is the most common presentation of PAD and refers to ischaemic pain in the leg muscles. It is usually felt in the calf (superficial femoral artery disease) but may occur in the thigh or buttock (iliac artery disease). Typically, the pain comes on after a reasonably constant distance and resolves rapidly on stopping.

---

i **8.14 Examination findings in chronic lower limb ischaemia**

- Pulses—diminished or absent
- Bruits—denote turbulent flow but bear no relationship to the severity of the underlying disease
- Reduced skin temperature
- Pallor on elevation and rubor on dependency (Buerger's sign)
- Superficial veins that fill sluggishly and empty ('gutter') upon minimal elevation
- Muscle wasting
- Skin and nails—dry, thin and brittle
- Loss of hair

✚ **8.15 Symptoms and signs of ALI**

Symptoms/signs	Comment
Pain Pallor Pulselessness }	May be absent in complete acute ischaemia, and can be present in chronic ischaemia
Perishing cold	Unreliable, as the ischaemic limb takes on the ambient temperature
Paraesthesia Paralysis }	Important features of impending irreversible ischaemia

Critical limb ischaemia: CLI is defined as rest pain requiring opiate analgesia and/or ulceration or gangrene, present for more than 2 weeks, in the presence of an ankle BP less than 50 mmHg. Rest pain with ankle pressures greater than 50 mmHg is known as subcritical limb ischaemia (SCLI). Severe limb ischaemia (SLI) comprises both CLI and SCLI. Whereas IC is usually because of single-segment plaque, SLI is always because of multilevel disease. Patients are at risk of losing their limb (or life) in a matter of weeks or months without surgical bypass or endovascular revascularisation, but treatment is difficult because most are elderly with significant multisystem comorbidity and extensive disease.

Acute limb ischaemia: This is most frequently caused by acute thrombotic occlusion of a preexisting arterial stenosis or thromboembolism (often secondary to AF). The typical presentation is with the so-called 'Ps of acute ischaemia' (Box 8.15). Pain on squeezing the calf indicates muscle infarction and impending irreversible ischaemia. All suspected acutely ischaemic limbs must be discussed immediately with a vascular surgeon. If there are no contraindications, an IV bolus of heparin (3000–5000 U) should be given to limit thrombus propagation and protect the collateral circulation. Distinguishing thrombosis from embolism is frequently difficult. Evidence of chronic lower limb ischaemia (e.g. previous IC symptoms, bruits, diminished contralateral pulses) favours thrombosis, whereas sudden onset and the presence of AF favour embolism.

ALI because of thrombosis can often be treated medically with IV heparin (target APTT 2.0–3.0), antiplatelet agents, high-dose statins, IV fluids and oxygen. ALI because of embolus (no collateral circulation) normally results in extensive tissue necrosis within 6 hours unless the limb is revascularised. Irreversible ischaemia mandates early amputation or palliative therapy.

Investigations

The ankle–brachial pressure index (ABPI, the ratio between the systolic ankle and brachial blood pressures) is over 1.0 in health. In IC, the ABPI is typically 0.5 to 0.9, and in CLI usually less than 0.5. Further investigation with duplex ultrasonography, MRI or contrast CT is used to define the sites of involvement. Intra-arterial digital subtraction angiography is reserved for those undergoing endovascular revascularisation. Other investigations should include a full blood count to exclude anaemia and thrombocythaemia, as well as measurement of lipids and blood glucose.

Management

Medical management consists of smoking cessation, exercise, antiplatelet therapy (aspirin or clopidogrel), statins and treatment of coexisting diabetes, hypertension or polycythaemia. Vorapaxar, an inhibitor of platelet activation, has recently been licensed in combination with either aspirin or clopidogrel in patients with PAD. The peripheral vasodilator cilostazol may improve walking distance in patients who fail to respond to usual therapy. Angioplasty, stenting, endarterectomy or bypass is usually considered in patients who remain severely disabled by symptoms despite 6 months of medical therapy. Subclavian artery disease is usually treated by angioplasty and stenting.

Buerger's disease–thrombangitis obliterans

This inflammatory obliterative arterial disease usually affects male smokers aged 20 to 30 years, causing claudication and finger pain, with absent wrist and ankle pulses. Smoking cessation is essential, and sympathectomy and prostaglandin infusions may help.

Raynauld's syndrome

This disorder affects 5% to 10% of young women aged 15 to 30 years in temperate climates. It is usually benign, so the patient should be reassured and advised to avoid cold. More severe Raynauld's syndrome with digital ulceration occurs with connective tissue disease (p. 770).

Diseases of the aorta

Aortic aneurysms

An aortic aneurysm is an abnormal dilatation of the aortic lumen. Abdominal aortic aneurysms (AAAs) affect men three times more commonly than women, and occur in about 5% of men over the age of 60 years.

The most common cause of aortic aneurysm is atherosclerosis, for which the risk factors are described earlier (p. 276). Additional genetic factors cause aortic aneurysm to run in families. Marfan's syndrome (p. 290) is a rare cause.

Clinical features

The clinical presentation depends on the site of the aneurysm. Thoracic aneurysms may typically present with acute severe chest pain, but other features, including aortic regurgitation, stridor, hoarseness and superior vena cava syndrome, may occur. Erosion into the oesophagus or bronchus may present with massive bleeding.

AAAs can present in a number of ways, including central abdominal or back pain, lower limb thromboemboli and compression of the duodenum or IVC. The usual age is 65 to 75 years for elective presentations and 75 to 85 years for emergency presentations. Many AAAs are asymptomatic and found incidentally or on screening.

Investigation

Ultrasound establishes the diagnosis and is used to monitor asymptomatic AAAs; elective repair is considered if the diameter exceeds 5.5 cm. CT and MRI scanning are used to assess thoracic aneurysms and to plan surgical intervention.

Management

All symptomatic AAAs should be considered for repair, not least because pain often predates rupture. Distal embolisation is a strong indication for repair. Rupture of an AAA produces severe abdominal pain with hypovolaemic shock, and is rapidly fatal. Operative mortality for ruptured AAA is around 50%, but survivors have a good prognosis. Endovascular repair using a stent-graft introduced through the femoral artery is used increasingly to replace open surgery.

Aortic dissection

A breach in the intima of the aortic wall allows arterial blood to enter the media, which is then split into two layers, creating a 'false lumen' alongside the existing or 'true lumen'. Aortic dissection is classified into type A and type B, involving or sparing the ascending aorta, respectively. Aortic atherosclerosis and hypertension are common aetiological factors, but other predisposing conditions include thoracic aortic aneurysm, aortic coarctation, previous aortic surgery, Marfan's syndrome, trauma and pregnancy.

Clinical features

The patient typically presents with sudden-onset, severe, 'tearing' anterior chest pain or interscapular back pain, often associated with collapse. Occlusion of aortic branches may cause stroke, MI or paraplegia, as well as asymmetry of the brachial, carotid or femoral pulses.

Investigation

CT and MRI are the investigations of choice. The CXR may show broadening of the upper mediastinum and distortion of the aortic 'knuckle', but these findings are absent in 10% of cases. Transoesophageal echocardiography is useful; transthoracic echocardiography shows only 3 to 4 cm of the ascending aorta.

Management

Early mortality of acute dissection is 1% to 5% per hour. Initial management comprises pain control and IV labetalol (target systolic BP <120 mmHg). Endoluminal repair with fenestration of the intimal flap or insertion of a stent-graft may be effective.

Marfan's syndrome

This is a rare autosomal dominant connective tissue disorder that is associated with a high risk of aortic aneurysm and dissection.

Clinical features

Aortic and mitral regurgitation, skin laxity, joint hypermobility, long arms, legs and fingers (arachnodactyly), scoliosis, pectus excavatum, high-arched palate, lens dislocation retinal detachment and pneumothorax.

Investigations

The clinical diagnosis is confirmed by genetic testing. Patients should undergo serial echocardiography of the aortic root; if dilatation is observed, elective surgery should be considered.

Management

β-Blockers reduce the risk of aortic dilatation and should be given to all patients. Activities associated with increases in cardiac output are best avoided. Surgery to replace the aortic root can be performed in patients with progressive aortic dilatation.

Hypertension

The risk of cardiovascular diseases such as stroke and CAD is closely related to BP; however, there is no specific cut-off above which the risk of cardiovascular risk suddenly increases. The diagnosis of hypertension is made when BP rises above a specific threshold where the risk of cardiovascular complications and benefits of treatment outweigh the costs and side effects of therapy. The British Hypertension Society defines hypertension as a BP greater than 140/90 mmHg.

In more than 95% of cases, no specific underlying cause of hypertension can be found, and such patients are said to have essential hypertension. Important predisposing factors for essential hypertension include:
• Age. • Ethnicity (higher incidence in African Americans and Japanese). • Genetic factors. • High salt intake. • Alcohol excess. • Obesity. • Lack of exercise. • Impaired intrauterine growth.

In around 5% of cases, hypertension results from a specific underlying disorder (secondary hypertension). Causes include:

	8.16 Hypertensive retinopathy
Grade 1	Arteriolar thickening, tortuosity and increased reflectiveness ('silver wiring')
Grade 2	Grade 1 plus constriction of veins at arterial crossings ('arterio-venous nipping')
Grade 3	Grade 2 plus evidence of retinal ischaemia (flame-shaped or blot haemorrhages and 'cotton wool' exudates)
Grade 4	Grade 3 plus papilloedema

• Renal disease (renal vascular disease, glomerulonephritis, polycystic kidney disease; see Chapter 7). • Endocrine disorders (phaeochromocytoma, Cushing's syndrome, Conn's syndrome, acromegaly, thyrotoxicosis, congenital adrenal hyperplasia; see Chapter 10). • Pregnancy. • Drugs (corticosteroids, oestrogen-containing oral contraceptive pill, anabolic steroids). • Coarctation of the aorta.

Clinical features

Hypertension is usually asymptomatic until discovered at a routine examination or when a complication arises. A BP check is therefore advisable every 5 years in adults older than 40 years to detect occult hypertension. The history may reveal familial hypertension, lifestyle factors (exercise, salt intake, smoking, alcohol intake) and potential drug causes. Examination may reveal radio-femoral delay (coarctation of the aorta), enlarged kidneys (polycystic kidney disease), abdominal bruits (renal artery stenosis) or features of Cushing's syndrome. More commonly, there may be evidence of risk factors such as central obesity or hyperlipidaemia, or of complications such as LV hypertrophy (LV heave, fourth heart sound), aortic aneurysm, stroke or retinopathy (Box 8.16).

Investigations

Antihypertensive therapy is commonly lifelong, so it is vital that the BP readings on which the diagnosis is based are accurate. Measurements should be made to the nearest 2 mmHg, sitting with the arm supported, using an appropriately sized cuff and repeated after 5 minutes' rest if initial values are high. Sphygmomanometry, particularly when performed by a doctor, can cause a transient rise in BP ('white coat' hypertension). A series of automated ambulatory BP measurements obtained over 24 hours or longer provides a better profile than a limited number of clinic readings. Home self-measurement is an alternative that is less well established. Ambulatory or home measurements may be particularly helpful in patients with unusually labile or refractory BP, those with symptomatic hypotension and those in whom white coat hypertension is suspected.

All hypertensive patients should also be investigated by urinalysis for blood, protein and glucose, U&Es, blood glucose, serum lipids, thyroid function and 12-lead ECG. Additional investigations are appropriate in selected patients to identify target organ damage (e.g. echocardiography) or potential causes of secondary hypertension (e.g. renal USS, urinary catecholamines).

Management

The objective of antihypertensive therapy is to reduce the incidence of adverse cardiovascular events. The relative benefit of BP reduction (~30% reduction in risk of stroke and 20% reduction in risk of CAD) is similar in all patient groups, so the absolute benefit of treatment is greatest in those at highest risk. Decisions on treatment should therefore be guided by an overall assessment of cardiovascular risk. In practice this is best calculated using risk-prediction charts (Fig. 8.18). The British Hypertension Society management guidelines are summarised in (Box 8.17).

The following lifestyle measures can not only lower BP but also reduce cardiovascular risk:

• Correcting obesity. • Reducing alcohol intake. • Restricting salt intake. • Engaging in regular physical exercise. • Increasing consumption of fruit and vegetables.

Drug therapy

Thiazides: The antihypertensive action of thiazides is incompletely understood, and may take up to a month to take effect. The daily dose of bendroflumethiazide is 2.5 mg.

ACE inhibitors: ACE inhibitors (e.g. lisinopril 10–40 mg daily) are effective, but can precipitate renal failure in patients with renal impairment or renal artery stenosis. U&E should be checked before and 1 to 2 weeks into therapy. Side effects include first-dose hypotension, cough, rash, hyperkalaemia and renal dysfunction.

Angiotensin receptor blockers: ARBs (e.g. irbesartan 150–300 mg daily) have similar efficacy to ACE inhibitors but do not cause cough and are better tolerated.

Calcium channel antagonists: Amlodipine (5–10 mg daily) and nifedipine (30–90 mg daily) are particularly useful in older people. Side effects include flushing, palpitations and fluid retention.

β-Blockers: These are not first-line antihypertensive therapy, except in patients with a second indication such as angina. Atenolol (50–100 mg daily) and bisoprolol (5–10 mg daily) are β_1-selective and less likely than nonselective agents to cause the side effects of poor circulation and bronchospasm.

Combined β- and α-blockers: Labetalol (200 mg–2.4 g daily in divided doses) can be used as an infusion in accelerated hypertension (see below).

Other vasodilators: These include α_1-adrenoceptor antagonists (e.g. doxazosin 1–16 mg daily) and vascular smooth muscle relaxants (e.g. hydralazine 25–100 mg twice daily). Side effects include first-dose and postural hypotension, headache, tachycardia and fluid retention.

Combination therapy is often required to achieve adequate control, and a recommended treatment algorithm is shown in Fig. 8.19. However, comorbid conditions may have an important influence on initial drug selection (e.g. a β-blocker might be the most appropriate treatment for a patient with angina, but should be avoided in asthma).

Accelerated hypertension

This rare complication of hypertension is characterised by rapidly progressive end-organ damage, including retinopathy, renal dysfunction and

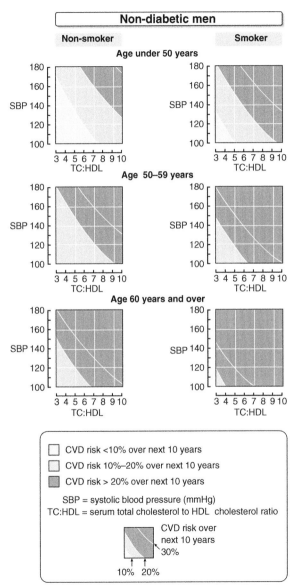

Fig. 8.17 Example of cardiovascular risk prediction chart for nondiabetic men.
Cardiovascular risk is predicted from the patient's age, sex, smoking habit, BP and
cholesterol ratio.

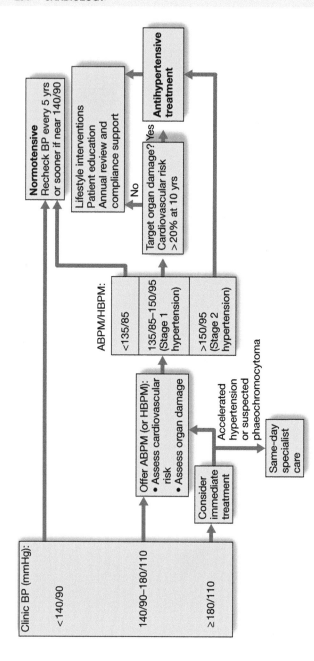

Fig. 8.18 Management of hypertension: British Hypertension Society guidelines. Consider specialist referral for stage 1 hypertension in those aged younger than 40 years. *ABPM*, Ambulatory blood pressure monitoring; *HBPM*, home blood pressure monitoring.

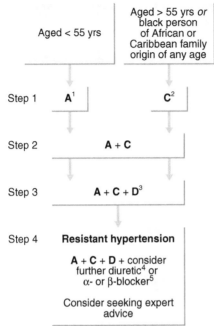

Fig. 8.19 Antihypertensive drug combinations. [1]A = ACE inhibitor or ARB. [2]C = calcium channel blocker (CCB); consider thiazide if CCB not tolerated or in heart failure. [3]D = thiazide. [4]Low-dose spironolactone or higher-dose thiazide. [5]Consider an α- or β-blocker if further diuretics are not tolerated, contraindicated or ineffective. *CCB,* Calcium channel blocker.

encephalopathy. Sudden lowering of BP may compromise perfusion, leading to cerebral, coronary or renal insufficiency. A controlled reduction to around 150/90 mmHg over 24 to 48 hours using oral agents is ideal. Where necessary, IV labetalol, GTN and sodium nitroprusside are effective alternatives, but require careful supervision.

Diseases of the heart valves

A diseased valve may be narrowed (stenosed), or it may fail to close adequately, and thus permit regurgitation of blood. Sudden valve failure can occur with aortic dissection, traumatic rupture, endocarditis or papillary muscle rupture complicating MI. Valve disease may also be congenital or acquired through rheumatic carditis, syphilitic aortitis, ventricular dilatation in heart failure or senile degeneration.

Acute rheumatic fever

This usually affects children or young adults. It is now rare in Western Europe and North America, but remains endemic in the Indian subcontinent,

Africa and South America. It is triggered by an immune-mediated delayed response to infection with specific strains of group A streptococci that have antigens that cross-react with cardiac myosin and sarcolemmal membrane protein. Antibodies produced against the streptococcal antigens mediate inflammation in the endocardium, myocardium and pericardium, as well as the joints and skin.

Clinical features

ARF typically follows 2 to 3 weeks after an episode of streptococcal pharyngitis, and presents with fever, anorexia, lethargy and joint pains. The diagnosis is based on the revised Jones criteria (Box 8.17). Carditis may involve the endocardium, myocardium and pericardium to varying degrees, and manifests as breathlessness (heart failure or pericardial effusion), palpitations or chest pain (pericarditis). Other features include tachycardia, cardiac enlargement, new murmurs (especially mitral regurgitation) or a soft mid-diastolic murmur because of mitral valvulitis (Carey Coombs murmur).

Acute, painful, asymmetric and migratory arthritis of the large joints (knees, ankles, elbows, wrists) is the most common major manifestation.

Erythema marginatum appears as red macules, which fade in the centre but remain red at the edges; they occur mainly on the trunk and proximal extremities, but not the face. Subcutaneous nodules are small, firm, painless and best felt over extensor surfaces of bone or tendons. They usually appear more than 3 weeks after the onset of other manifestations.

 8.17 Jones criteria for the diagnosis of rheumatic fever

Major manifestations

- Carditis
- Polyarthritis
- Chorea
- Erythema marginatum
- Subcutaneous nodules

Minor manifestations

- Fever
- Arthralgia
- Previous rheumatic fever
- Raised ESR or CRP
- Leucocytosis
- First-degree AV block

Notes

- Diagnosis depends on two or more major manifestations, or one major and two or more minor manifestations PLUS supporting evidence of preceding streptococcal infection: recent scarlet fever, raised ASO or other streptococcal antibody titre, positive throat culture
- Evidence of recent streptococcal infection is particularly important if there is only one major manifestation

Sydenham's chorea (St. Vitus' dance) is a late (>3 months) neurological manifestation characterised by emotional lability and purposeless involuntary choreiform movements of the hands, feet or face; spontaneous recovery usually occurs within a few months.

Investigations

Raised WCC, ESR and CRP indicate systemic inflammation, and are useful for monitoring the disease. Throat swabs are often negative because infection has already resolved. ASO titre indicates preceding streptococcal infection—either rising titres or high titres (children >300 U, adults >200 U). ECG (AV block, pericarditis) and echocardiography (cardiac dilatation, valve abnormalities) may reveal evidence of carditis.

Management

Benzathine benzylpenicillin (1.2 million U IM once) or oral phenoxymethyl-penicillin (250 mg four times daily for 10 days) should be given to eliminate residual streptococcal infection. Bed rest lessens joint pain and reduces cardiac workload. Cardiac failure should be treated. High-dose aspirin (60–100 mg/kg up to 8 g per day) usually relieves arthritic pain, and a response within 24 hours helps to confirm the diagnosis. Prednisolone 1 to 2 mg/kg per day produces more rapid symptomatic relief, and is indicated for carditis or severe arthritis until the ESR returns to normal. Patients are susceptible to further attacks of rheumatic fever if subsequent streptococcal infection occurs, and long-term prophylaxis with penicillin should be given, usually until the age of 21 years.

Chronic rheumatic heart disease

This is characterised by progressive valve fibrosis, and develops in at least half of those affected by rheumatic fever with carditis. Some episodes of rheumatic fever may pass unrecognised, and a positive history is only found in about half of patients. The mitral valve is affected in more than 90% of cases, with the aortic valve the next most frequently involved.

Mitral stenosis

Mitral stenosis is almost always rheumatic in origin. The valve orifice is slowly diminished by progressive fibrosis, leaflet calcification and fusion of the cusps and subvalvular apparatus. Restricted blood flow from left atrium to ventricle causes a rise in left atrial pressure, leading to pulmonary venous congestion and breathlessness, whereas low cardiac output may cause fatigue. Patients usually remain asymptomatic until the mitral valve area is less than 2 cm^2 (normal = 5 cm^2). AF occurs frequently because of progressive left atrial dilatation, and the onset of AF often causes rapid decompensation with pulmonary oedema because ventricular filling depends on left atrial contraction. Exercise and pregnancy also increase left atrial pressure and cause decompensation. More gradual rises in left atrial pressure cause pulmonary hypertension, RV hypertrophy and dilatation, tricuspid regurgitation and right heart failure.

Clinical features

Effort-related dyspnoea is usually the dominant symptom and produces a gradual reduction in exercise tolerance over many years, culminating in dyspnoea at rest. Acute pulmonary oedema or pulmonary hypertension may cause haemoptysis. On examination, the patient is usually in AF, and a malar flush may be apparent. Thromboembolism is a common complication, especially in patients with AF. The apex beat is characteristically tapping in nature. On auscultation there may be a loud first heart sound, an opening snap and a low-pitched mid-diastolic murmur. An elevated JVP, RV heave, loud pulmonary component of the second heart sound and features of tricuspid regurgitation all signify the presence of pulmonary hypertension.

Investigations

• Doppler echocardiography provides the definitive evaluation of mitral stenosis, allowing estimation of valve area, pressure gradient across the valve and pulmonary artery pressure. • ECG may show bifid P waves (P mitrale) because of left atrial hypertrophy, or AF. • CXR may show an enlarged left atrium and features of pulmonary congestion.

Management

Medical management consists of diuretics for pulmonary congestion, digoxin, β-blockers or calcium antagonists for rate limitation, plus anticoagulants if there is AF. For persistent symptoms or pulmonary hypertension, valvuloplasty, valvotomy or valve replacement are indicated. Balloon valvuloplasty or valvotomy are useful in noncalcific pure stenosis; valve replacement is needed for calcific disease or stenosis with regurgitation.

Mitral regurgitation

Causes of mitral regurgitation are shown in Box 8.18. Chronic mitral regurgitation causes gradual dilatation of the LA with little increase in pressure; progressive LV dilatation occurs because of chronic volume overload. Acute mitral regurgitation causes a rapid rise in left atrial pressure, resulting in pulmonary oedema.

Mitral valve prolapse: A common cause of mild mitral regurgitation, this arises from congenital anomalies or degenerative myxomatous changes, and rarely as a feature of Marfan's syndrome. In mild cases, the valve remains competent but bulges back into the atrium during systole, causing a midsystolic click but no murmur. If the valve becomes regurgitant, the click is followed by a late systolic murmur. Sudden deterioration may occur if the chordae tendinae rupture. The condition is associated with a variety of benign arrhythmias, atypical chest pain and a very small risk of embolic stroke or transient ischaemic attack. Nevertheless, the long-term prognosis is good.

8.18 Causes of mitral regurgitation

- Mitral valve prolapse
- Dilatation of the LV and mitral valve ring (e.g. coronary artery disease, cardiomyopathy)
- Damage to valve cusps and chordae (e.g. rheumatic heart disease, endocarditis)
- Ischaemia or infarction of papillary muscle
- Myocardial infarction

Clinical features

Chronic mitral regurgitation typically causes progressive exertional dyspnoea and fatigue, whereas sudden-onset mitral regurgitation usually presents with acute pulmonary oedema. The regurgitant jet causes an apical pan-systolic murmur that radiates to the axilla. The first heart sound is quiet, and there may be a third heart sound. The apex beat feels hyperdynamic and is usually displaced to the left, indicating LV dilatation. Signs of AF, pulmonary venous congestion and pulmonary hypertension may be present.

Investigations

Doppler echocardiography reveals chamber dimensions, LV function, the severity of regurgitation and structural abnormalities of the valve. ECG commonly shows AF. Cardiac catheterisation is indicated if surgery is being considered. The severity of regurgitation can be assessed by left ventriculography and by the size of the v (systolic) waves in the left atrial or pulmonary artery wedge pressure trace.

Management

Medical treatment includes diuretics and afterload reduction with vasodilators (e.g. ACE inhibitors). AF requires digoxin and anticoagulation. Regular review is important to detect worsening symptoms, progressive cardiac enlargement and LV impairment, as these are all indications for surgical intervention. Mitral valve repair is now the treatment of choice for severe mitral regurgitation, even in asymptomatic patients, because early repair prevents irreversible left ventricular damage. Acute severe mitral regurgitation necessitates emergency valve replacement or repair.

Aortic stenosis

The three common causes of aortic stenosis are:
• Rheumatic fever (usually associated with mitral valve disease). • Calcification of a congenitally bicuspid valve. • In the elderly, senile degenerative aortic stenosis.

Cardiac output is initially maintained, but the left ventricle becomes increasingly hypertrophied. Eventually it can no longer overcome the outflow tract obstruction and heart failure develops. Patients with aortic stenosis typically remain asymptomatic for many years but deteriorate rapidly when symptoms develop.

Clinical features

Mild to moderate aortic stenosis is usually asymptomatic, but may be detected incidentally on routine examination. The three cardinal symptoms are angina, syncope and breathlessness.
• Angina: arises because of the increased oxygen demands of the hypertrophied LV working against the high-pressure outflow tract obstruction (or coexisting CAD). • Syncope: usually occurs on exertion when cardiac output fails to rise to meet demand because of severe outflow obstruction, causing a fall in BP. • Exertional breathlessness: suggests cardiac decompensation as a consequence of chronic excessive pressure overload.

The characteristic clinical signs are:
• Harsh ejection systolic murmur radiating to the neck (often with a thrill).
• Soft second heart sound. • Slow-rising carotid pulse. • Narrow pulse pressure. • Thrusting but undisplaced apex beat.

Investigations

• Doppler echocardiography is the key investigation. It demonstrates restricted opening and any structural abnormalities, and permits calculation of the systolic pressure gradient. • The ECG: usually shows features of LV hypertrophy, often with down-sloping ST segments and T inversion ('strain pattern'), but can be normal despite severe stenosis. • CT or MRI to assess calcification. • Cardiac catheterisation: is usually necessary to assess the coronary arteries before surgery.

Management

Patients with asymptomatic aortic stenosis have a good prognosis with conservative management, but should be kept under review, as the development of angina, syncope or heart failure are indications for prompt surgery. Old age is not a contraindication to valve replacement, and results are very good, even for those in their eighties. This is especially true for transcatheter aortic valve implantation (TAVI). Balloon valvuloplasty is useful in congenital stenosis but not in calcific stenosis.

Aortic regurgitation

This condition may be caused by disease of the aortic valve cusps (e.g. rheumatic fever, infective endocarditis) or dilatation of the aortic root (e.g. ankylosing spondylitis, Marfan's syndrome, aortic dissection or aneurysm). The LV dilates and hypertrophies to compensate for the regurgitation, producing a large increase in stroke volume. As disease progresses, LV end-diastolic pressure rises, and pulmonary oedema develops.

Clinical features

In mild to moderate aortic regurgitation, patients are frequently asymptomatic, but may experience an awareness of the heartbeat because of the increased stroke volume. Exertional dyspnoea is the dominant symptom in more severe disease. The pulse is typically of large volume and collapsing in nature, the pulse pressure is wide and the apex beat is heaving and displaced laterally. The characteristic soft early diastolic murmur is usually best heard to the left of the sternum with the patient leaning forward, with the breath held in expiration. A systolic murmur because of the increased stroke volume is common. In acute severe regurgitation (e.g. perforation of aortic cusp in endocarditis) there may be no time for compensatory LV hypertrophy and dilatation to develop, and the features of heart failure may predominate.

Investigations

• Doppler echocardiography: confirms the diagnosis and may show a dilated, hyperdynamic left ventricle. • Cardiac catheterisation and aortography: can also be helpful in assessing the severity of regurgitation, aortic dilatation and the presence of coexisting coronary artery disease. • MRI is useful in assessing aortic dilatation if this is suspected on CXR or echocardiography.

Management

Underlying conditions, such as endocarditis and syphilis, should be treated. Replacement of the aortic valve (and aortic root, if dilated) is indicated in symptomatic regurgitation. Asymptomatic patients should also be followed up annually to detect the development of symptoms or increasing ventricular size on echocardiography; if the end-systolic dimension increases to 55 mm or more, then aortic valve replacement should be undertaken. Systolic BP should be controlled with vasodilating drugs such as nifedipine or ACE inhibitors.

Tricuspid stenosis

This is uncommon, usually rheumatic in origin and almost always associated with mitral and aortic valve disease. It may cause signs and symptoms of right heart failure.

Tricuspid regurgitation

This is common and most frequently secondary to RV dilatation caused by pulmonary hypertension or MI. It may also be caused by endocarditis (especially in IV drug-users), rheumatic fever or carcinoid syndrome. Symptoms result from reduced forward flow (tiredness) and venous congestion (oedema, hepatic enlargement). The most prominent sign is a large systolic *v* wave in the JVP. Other features include a pansystolic murmur at the left sternal edge and a pulsatile liver. Tricuspid regurgitation caused by RV dilatation often improves when the cause of RV overload is corrected, for example, diuretic and vasodilator therapy in congestive cardiac failure.

Pulmonary stenosis

This can occur in the carcinoid syndrome but is usually congenital, when it may be isolated or associated with other abnormalities, such as tetralogy of Fallot (p. 305). On examination there is an ejection systolic murmur, loudest at the left upper sternum and radiating towards the left shoulder. Mild to moderate pulmonary stenosis is nonprogressive and does not require treatment. Severe pulmonary stenosis (gradient >50 mmHg) is treated by percutaneous balloon valvuloplasty or, if this is not available, surgical valvotomy.

Pulmonary regurgitation

Rarely an isolated phenomenon and usually associated with pulmonary artery dilatation caused by pulmonary hypertension of any cause.

Prosthetic valves

Diseased valves can be replaced with mechanical or biological prostheses. Common mechanical prostheses include ball and cage, tilting disc and tilting bi-leaflet valves. All generate audible clicks and require long-term anticoagulation to prevent thromboembolism. Pig or allograft valves are the commonest biological valves. They generate normal heart sounds and do not require anticoagulation.

Infective endocarditis

Infective endocarditis is caused by microbial infection of a heart valve (native or prosthetic) or the lining of a cardiac chamber or blood vessel. It typically occurs at sites of preexisting endocardial damage, although infection with particularly virulent organisms (e.g. *Staphylococcus aureus*) can cause endocarditis in a previously normal heart. Areas of endocardial damage caused by a high-pressure jet of blood (e.g. VSD, mitral regurgitation, aortic regurgitation) are particularly vulnerable. When the infection is established, vegetations composed of organisms, fibrin and platelets grow and may break away as emboli. Adjacent tissues are destroyed, abscesses may form and valve regurgitation may develop through cusp perforation, distortion or rupture of chordae. Extracardiac manifestations, such as vasculitis and skin lesions, are caused by emboli or immune complex deposition.

Microbiology

S. aureus is the commonest cause of acute endocarditis, originating from skin infections, abscesses or vascular access sites such as intravenous lines or intravenous drug use. *Streptococcus viridans* (from the upper respiratory tract or gums) and enterococci (from the gut or urinary tract) may enter the blood stream, and are common causes of subacute endocarditis. *S. epidermidis*, a normal skin commensal, is the most common organism in endocarditis, complicating cardiac surgery. Rarer causes include the Gram-negative HACEK-group organisms (*Haemophilus* spp., *Actinobacillus actinomycetemcomitans*, *Cardiobacterium hominis*, *Eikenella* spp. and *Kingella kingae*). *Coxiella burnetii* (Q fever) and *Brucella* cause occasional cases in patients exposed to farm animals. Yeasts and fungi may be responsible in immunocompromised patients.

Clinical features

Subacute endocarditis: Should be suspected when a patient with congenital or valvular heart disease develops a persistent fever, unusual tiredness, night sweats, weight loss or new signs of valve dysfunction. Other features include embolic stroke, petechial rash, splinter haemorrhages, nonvisible haematuria and splenomegaly. Osler's nodes (painful swellings at the fingertips) are rare, and finger clubbing is a late sign.

Acute endocarditis: Usually presents as a severe febrile illness with prominent and changing heart murmurs and petechiae. Clinical stigmata of chronic endocarditis are usually absent, but embolic events (e.g. cerebral) are common, and cardiac or renal failure may develop rapidly.

Postoperative endocarditis: This presents as unexplained fever in a patient who has had heart valve surgery. The pattern may resemble subacute or acute endocarditis, depending on the virulence of the organism. Morbidity and mortality are high, and revision surgery is often required.

Investigations

Diagnosis is based on the modified Duke criteria (Box 8.19). Blood culture is the key investigation to identify the causative organism and guide antibiotic therapy; 3 to 6 sets should be taken, using scrupulous aseptic technique, before commencing therapy. Echocardiography allows detection of vegetations and abscess formation, as well as assessment of valve damage. Transoesophageal echo has a higher sensitivity than transthoracic echo for detecting vegetations (90% vs. 65%), and is particularly valuable for investigating patients with prosthetic heart valves. Failure to detect vegetations does not exclude the diagnosis. A normochromic, normocytic

8.19 Diagnosis of infective endocarditis (modified Duke's criteria)

Major criteria

- Positive blood culture: typical organism from two cultures; persistent positive blood cultures taken >12 hours apart; three or more positive cultures taken over >1 hour
- Endocardial involvement: positive echocardiographic findings of vegetations; new valvular regurgitation

Minor criteria

- Predisposing valvular or cardiac abnormality
- IV drug misuse
- Pyrexia ≥38°C
- Embolic phenomenon
- Vasculitic phenomenon
- Blood cultures suggestive—organism grown but not achieving major criteria
- Suggestive echocardiographic findings

Definite endocarditis: two major, or one major and three minor, or five minor
Possible endocarditis: one major and one minor, or three minor

8

anaemia and elevated WCC, ESR and CRP are common. CRP is superior to ESR for monitoring progress. Nonvisible haematuria is usually present. ECG may show the development of AV block (caused by abscess formation). CXR may show evidence of cardiac failure.

Management

Any source of infection (e.g. dental abscess) should be removed immediately. Empirical antibiotic therapy is with vancomycin (1 g IV twice daily) and gentamicin (1 mg/kg IV twice daily) if the presentation is acute, or with amoxicillin (2 g IV six times daily) with or without gentamicin if subacute. Subsequent antibiotic treatment is guided by culture results and is usually continued for 4 weeks. Indications for surgery (debridement of infected material, valve replacement) include heart failure, abscess formation, failure of antibiotic therapy and large vegetations on left-sided heart valves (high risk of systemic emboli).

Prevention

Until recently, antibiotic prophylaxis was given routinely to people at risk of infective endocarditis undergoing interventional procedures. However, as the link between episodes of infective endocarditis and interventional procedures has not been demonstrated, antibiotic prophylaxis is no longer offered routinely.

Congenital heart disease

This usually presents in childhood, but defects such as atrial septal defect may be asymptomatic until adulthood or discovered incidentally on routine examination or CXR. Defects that were previously fatal in childhood can now be corrected or mitigated, so prolonged survival is the norm. Such patients may re-present as adults with arrhythmia or heart failure.

Persistent ductus arteriosus

During fetal life, most of the blood from the pulmonary artery passes through the ductus arteriosus into the aorta. Normally, the ductus closes soon after birth but in this anomaly it fails to do so. Because the pressure in the aorta is higher than that in the pulmonary artery, there will be a continuous left to right shunt.

Usually there is no disability in infancy, but cardiac failure may eventually ensue, dyspnoea being the first symptom. A continuous 'machinery' murmur is heard, maximal in the second left intercostal space below the clavicle. Closure of the patent ductus is usually performed by catheterisation using an implantable occlusive device in early childhood.

Coarctation of the aorta

This condition is associated with other abnormalities, including bicuspid aortic valve and cerebral 'berry' aneurysms. It is an important cause of cardiac failure in the newborn, but is often asymptomatic in older children or adults. Headaches may occur from hypertension proximal to the coarctation, and occasionally leg weakness or cramps from decreased distal circulation. The BP is raised in the upper body but normal or low in the legs, with weak, delayed femoral pulses. A systolic murmur is heard posteriorly, over the coarctation. CXR may show an altered contour of the aorta and notching of the under-surfaces of the ribs from collaterals. MRI is the investigation of choice. Surgical correction is advisable in all but the mildest cases. If this is done sufficiently early, persistent hypertension can be avoided, but patients repaired in late childhood or adult life often remain hypertensive. Recurrence of stenosis may be managed by balloon dilatation and stenting, which can also be used as the primary treatment in some cases.

Atrial septal defect

This common congenital defect results in shunting of blood from left to right atrium, and then to the RV and pulmonary arteries. As a result, there is gradual enlargement of the right side of the heart and of the pulmonary arteries.

The condition is frequently asymptomatic but may cause dyspnoea, cardiac failure or arrhythmias, for example, AF. Characteristic physical signs include wide, fixed splitting of the second heart sound and a systolic flow murmur over the pulmonary valve. Echocardiography can directly demonstrate the defect, and may show RV dilatation or hypertrophy. The CXR typically shows enlargement of the heart and the pulmonary artery, as well as pulmonary plethora. The ECG usually shows incomplete RBBB. The defect is often first detected when a CXR or ECG is carried out for incidental reasons. Atrial septal defects in which pulmonary flow is increased by 50% above systemic flow should be closed either surgically or by catheter implantation of a closure device.

Ventricular septal defect

This is the most common congenital cardiac defect; it may be isolated or part of complex congenital heart disease. Flow from the high-pressure

LV to the low-pressure RV produces a pansystolic murmur, best heard at the left sternal edge but radiating all over the precordium. VSD may present as cardiac failure in infants, as a murmur with minimal haemodynamic disturbance in older children or adults, or rarely as Eisenmenger's syndrome (see later). Doppler echocardiography helps to identify small, haemodynamically insignificant VSDs that are likely to close spontaneously. With larger defects, the CXR shows pulmonary plethora, and the ECG shows bilateral ventricular hypertrophy. Small VSDs require no treatment. Larger VSDs should be followed with serial ECG and echo. Surgical repair is indicated for those with cardiac failure or developing pulmonary hypertension.

Eisenmenger's syndrome

Persistently raised pulmonary flow (e.g. with left to right shunting) leads to increased pulmonary resistance and pulmonary hypertension. In severe pulmonary hypertension, a left to right shunt may reverse, resulting in right to left shunting and marked cyanosis (Eisenmenger's syndrome). Patients with Eisenmenger's syndrome are at particular risk from changes in afterload that exacerbate right to left shunting, for example, vasodilatation, anaesthesia, pregnancy.

Tetralogy of Fallot

This is the most common cause of cyanotic disease in childhood and comprises:
• Right ventricular outflow obstruction (usually subvalvular). • Right ventricular hypertrophy. • Ventricular septal defect. • Aorta overriding the septum.

Cyanosis is usual, but may be absent in the newborn, until RV pressure rises to above LV pressure. The subvalvular obstruction may increase suddenly after feeding or crying, causing apnoea and unconsciousness ('Fallot's spells'). In older children, Fallot's spells are uncommon, but cyanosis increases as rising RV pressure causes increasing right to left shunting across the VSD, together with stunted growth, clubbing and polycythaemia. A loud ejection systolic murmur is heard in the pulmonary area. Investigation is by echocardiography, which is diagnostic. ECG shows RV hypertrophy, and CXR a 'boot-shaped' heart. Definitive management is by surgical relief of the outflow obstruction and closure of the VSD, and the prognosis is good following childhood surgery.

Adult congenital heart disease

Many patients who would not previously have survived childhood now do so following corrective surgery. These adult survivors may develop problems; for example, those with transposition of the great arteries corrected by 'Mustard' repair, in which blood is redirected at the atrial level, leaving the RV supplying the aorta, may develop right ventricular failure in adulthood. Adults with repaired ventricular defects may develop ventricular arrhythmias as a result of postoperative scarring, and may require an implantable defibrillator. All such patients require careful follow-up through adult life in specialist clinics.

Diseases of the myocardium

Myocarditis

This is an acute inflammatory condition of the myocardium, caused by infection, autoimmune disease (e.g. lupus) or toxins (e.g. cocaine). Viral infection is the most common cause, particularly Coxsackie and influenza viruses A and B. Other causes include Lyme disease (p. 131), Chagas' disease (p. 153) and acute rheumatic fever.

Four presentations occur:

- **Fulminant myocarditis:** follows a viral illness, causing severe heart failure or cardiogenic shock.
- **Acute myocarditis:** presents more gradually with heart failure; can lead to dilated cardiomyopathy.
- **Chronic active myocarditis:** rare, with chronic myocardial inflammation.
- **Chronic persistent myocarditis:** can cause chest pain and arrhythmia, sometimes without ventricular dysfunction.

Echocardiography may reveal LV dysfunction, which is sometimes regional (focal myocarditis). MRI may show diagnostic patterns of inflammation. Troponins and CK are elevated in proportion to the extent of damage.

In most patients, treatment is supportive and the prognosis is good; however, death may occur because of ventricular arrhythmia or rapidly progressive heart failure. Some forms of myocarditis (e.g. Chagas' disease) may lead to chronic low-grade myocarditis or dilated cardiomyopathy. Treatment for cardiac failure or arrhythmias may be required, and intense physical exertion should be avoided. Transplantation is occasionally required.

Dilated cardiomyopathy

This condition is characterised by dilatation and impaired contraction of the LV and often the RV. The causes include:
• Alcohol. • Inherited mutations of cytoskeletal proteins. • X-linked muscular dystrophies. • Autoimmune reactions to viral myocarditis.

Most patients present with heart failure. Arrhythmia, thromboembolism and sudden death may occur at any stage, and chest pain also occurs. The differential diagnosis includes CAD, and dilated cardiomyopathy should only be diagnosed when this has been excluded.

Echocardiography and MRI are useful investigations. Treatment is aimed at controlling heart failure and preventing arrhythmias. The prognosis is variable, and cardiac transplantation may be required.

Hypertrophic cardiomyopathy

This is the most common form of cardiomyopathy, and is characterised by elaborate LV hypertrophy with malalignment of the myocardial fibres. The hypertrophy may be generalised or confined largely to the interventricular septum. Heart failure develops because the stiff, noncompliant ventricles impede diastolic filling. Septal hypertrophy may also cause dynamic LV outflow tract obstruction (hypertrophic obstructive cardiomyopathy). The condition is a genetic disorder with autosomal dominant transmission, a high degree of penetrance and variable expression.

Effort-related symptoms (angina and breathlessness), arrhythmia and sudden death (mainly from ventricular arrhythmias) are the dominant clinical problems. Signs are similar to those of aortic stenosis, except that in hypertrophic cardiomyopathy the character of the arterial pulse is jerky. Echocardiography is usually diagnostic. The ECG is abnormal and may show LV hypertrophy or deep T-wave inversion.

β-Blockers, rate-limiting calcium antagonists and disopyramide can relieve symptoms and prevent syncopal attacks. Arrhythmias often respond to amiodarone, but no drug is definitely known to improve prognosis. Outflow tract obstruction can be improved by partial surgical resection or by iatrogenic infarction of the basal septum using a catheter-delivered alcohol solution. An ICD should be considered in patients with risk factors for sudden death, including previous syncope or ventricular arrhythmias or severe hypertrophy.

Restrictive cardiomyopathy

In this rare condition, ventricular filling is impaired because the ventricles are 'stiff'. This leads to high atrial pressures with atrial hypertrophy, dilatation and later AF. Amyloidosis is the most common cause in the UK.

Diagnosis can be difficult, and requires Doppler echocardiography, CT or MRI, and endomyocardial biopsy. Treatment is symptomatic, but the prognosis is poor and transplantation may be indicated.

Other diseases affecting the myocardium are listed in Box 8.20.

  8.20 Specific diseases of heart muscle

Infections

- Viral, e.g. Coxsackie A and B, influenza, HIV
- Bacterial, e.g. diphtheria, *Borrelia burgdorferi*
- Protozoal, e.g. trypanosomiasis

Endocrine and metabolic disorders

- e.g. diabetes, hypo- and hyperthyroidism, acromegaly, carcinoid syndrome, phaeochromocytoma, inherited storage diseases

Connective tissue diseases

- e.g. systemic sclerosis, systemic lupus erythematosus, polyarteritis nodosa

Infiltrative disorders

- e.g. haemochromatosis, haemosiderosis, sarcoidosis, amyloidosis

Toxins

- e.g. doxorubicin, alcohol, cocaine, irradiation

Neuromuscular disorders

- e.g. dystrophia myotonica, Friedreich's ataxia, X-linked muscular dystrophies

Cardiac tumours

Primary cardiac tumours are rare, but metastases can affect the heart and mediastinum. Most primary tumours are benign (75%), and of these, the majority are left atrial polypoid myxomas. Treatment is by surgical excision.

Diseases of the pericardium

Acute pericarditis

This may be attributed to infection (viral, bacterial, TB), immunological reaction (e.g. post-MI, connective tissue disorder), trauma, uraemia or neoplasm. Pericarditis and myocarditis often coexist, and all forms of pericarditis may produce a pericardial effusion (see later).

Clinical features

The characteristic pain of pericarditis is retrosternal, radiates to the shoulders and neck and is aggravated by deep breathing and movement. A low-grade fever is common. A pericardial friction rub is heard; this is a high-pitched, superficial scratching or crunching noise produced by movement of the inflamed pericardium, and is diagnostic of pericarditis.

Investigations

The ECG shows widespread ST elevation with upward concavity over the affected area. PR interval depression is a very sensitive indicator of acute pericarditis.

Management

The pain is usually relieved by aspirin, but a more potent antiinflammatory agent, such as indometacin, may be required. Glucocorticoids may suppress symptoms, but there is no evidence that they accelerate cure. Viral pericarditis usually resolves in a few days or weeks.

Pericardial effusion

This refers to accumulation of fluid within the pericardial sac and often accompanies pericarditis. Cardiac tamponade describes acute heart failure caused by compression of the heart by a large or rapidly developing effusion.

Typical physical findings include hypotension, a markedly raised JVP that rises paradoxically with inspiration, pulsus paradoxus (exaggerated fall in BP during inspiration) and muffled heart sounds. Echocardiography confirms the diagnosis and helps identify the optimum site for aspiration of fluid. The QRS voltages on the ECG are often reduced in the presence of a large effusion. CXR may show an increase in the size of the cardiac shadow, which may have a globular appearance if the effusion is large. The patient usually responds promptly to percutaneous pericardiocentesis or surgical drainage; the latter is safer in cardiac rupture and aortic dissection. Tuberculous pericarditis causes effusion, is diagnosed on periocardiocentesis and responds to antituberculous therapy and glucocorticoids.

Chronic constrictive pericarditis

Constrictive pericarditis is caused by progressive thickening, fibrosis and calcification of the pericardium. In effect, the heart is encased in a solid shell and cannot fill properly. It often follows tuberculous pericarditis, but can also complicate haemopericardium, viral pericarditis, rheumatoid arthritis and purulent pericarditis.

The symptoms and signs of systemic venous congestion are the hallmarks of constrictive pericarditis. AF is common, and there is often dramatic ascites and hepatomegaly. Breathlessness is not prominent because the lungs are seldom congested. The condition should be suspected in any patient with unexplained right heart failure and a small heart. A CXR showing pericardial calcification and echocardiography often help to establish the diagnosis, although it may be difficult to distinguish from restrictive cardiomyopathy.

Management

Surgical resection of the diseased pericardium can lead to a dramatic improvement, but carries a high morbidity and produces disappointing results in up to 50% of patients.

Respiratory medicine

Respiratory diseases are responsible for much morbidity and avoidable mortality, with TB, pandemic influenza and pneumonia the most important in world health terms. Increasing prevalence of allergy, asthma and COPD, together with a rise in worldwide smoking rates, contributes to a high burden of chronic disease. Despite improved detection and treatment, the outlook for lung cancer remains poor.

Presenting problems in respiratory disease

Cough

Cough is the most common respiratory symptom, and the underlying cause is often clear from other clinical features, particularly in more serious disease. Common causes of acute or transient cough are:
• Viral lower respiratory tract infection. • Postnasal drip (rhinitis/sinusitis). • Foreign body aspiration. • Laryngitis or pharyngitis. • Pneumonia. • Congestive heart failure. • Pulmonary embolism.

Chronic cough presents more of a challenge, especially if physical examination, CXR and lung function are normal. In this context, consider:
• Postnasal drip. • Cough-variant asthma. • Gastro-oesophageal reflux with aspiration. • Drug-induced cough (ACE inhibitors). • Bordetella pertussis infection. • Interstitial disease.

Although most patients with lung cancer have an abnormal CXR on presentation, fibreoptic bronchoscopy and thoracic CT are advisable for unexplained cough of recent onset in adults (especially smokers) because these may reveal a small endobronchial tumour, unexpected foreign body or early interstitial lung disease.

Breathlessness (dyspnoea)

Breathlessness or dyspnoea can be defined as the feeling of an uncomfortable need to breathe. It is unusual among sensations in having no defined receptors, no localised representation in the brain and multiple causes both in health (e.g. exercise) and in diseases of the lungs, heart or muscles.

Clinical examination of the respiratory system

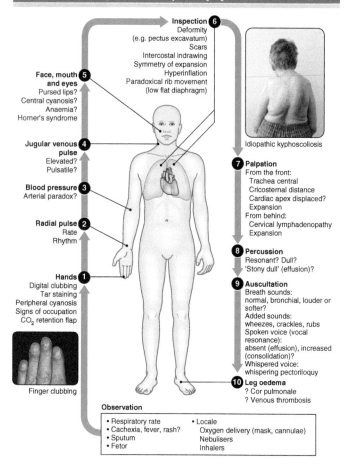

Inspection 6
Deformity
(e.g. pectus excavatum)
Scars
Intercostal indrawing
Symmetry of expansion
Hyperinflation
Paradoxical rib movement
(low flat diaphragm)

Idiopathic kyphoscoliosis

Face, mouth and eyes 5
Pursed lips?
Central cyanosis?
Anaemia?
Horner's syndrome

Jugular venous 4 pulse
Elevated?
Pulsatile?

Blood pressure 3
Arterial paradox?

Radial pulse 2
Rate
Rhythm

Hands 1
Digital clubbing
Tar staining
Peripheral cyanosis
Signs of occupation
CO_2 retention flap

Finger clubbing

7 Palpation
From the front:
Trachea central
Cricosternal distance
Cardiac apex displaced?
Expansion
From behind:
Cervical lymphadenopathy
Expansion

8 Percussion
Resonant? Dull?
'Stony dull' (effusion)?

9 Auscultation
Breath sounds:
normal, bronchial, louder or softer?
Added sounds:
wheezes, crackles, rubs
Spoken voice (vocal resonance):
absent (effusion), increased (consolidation)?
Whispered voice:
whispering pectoriloquy

10 Leg oedema
? Cor pulmonale
? Venous thrombosis

Observation
- Respiratory rate
- Cachexia, fever, rash?
- Sputum
- Fetor
- Locale
  Oxygen delivery (mask, cannulae)
  Nebulisers
  Inhalers

Chronic exertional breathlessness

The cause of breathlessness is often apparent from a careful clinical history. Key questions include:

How is your breathing at rest and overnight?

In COPD, there is a fixed, structural limit to maximum ventilation, and progressive hyperinflation during exercise. Breathlessness occurs on exertion, and not usually at rest or overnight. In contrast, patients with significant asthma are often woken overnight by breathlessness with chest tightness and wheeze.

Orthopnoea is common in COPD, as well as in heart disease, because airflow obstruction is made worse by cranial displacement of the diaphragm by the abdominal contents when recumbent, so patients often sleep propped up. Orthopnoea is therefore not a useful symptom for distinguishing respiratory and cardiac dyspnoea.

How much can you do on a good day?

The approximate distance the patient can walk on the level should be documented, along with capacity to climb inclines or stairs. Variability within and between days is characteristic of asthma; in mild asthma, the patient may have days with no symptoms. Gradual, progressive exercise limitation over years, with consistent disability day to day, is typical of COPD. In suspected asthma, variability should be documented using a peak flow diary.

Relentless progressive breathlessness, present also at rest, often with a dry cough, suggests interstitial disease. Impaired left ventricular function can also cause chronic exertional breathlessness, cough and wheeze. A history of angina, hypertension or MI suggests a cardiac cause. This may be confirmed by a displaced apex beat, raised JVP and peripheral oedema (although these may occur in hypoxic lung disease with fluid retention). The CXR may show cardiomegaly, and an ECG and echocardiogram may reveal left ventricular disease. Measurement of ABGs may help, as, in the absence of an intracardiac shunt or pulmonary oedema, the PaO_2 in cardiac disease is normal and the $PaCO_2$ is low or normal.

Did you have breathing problems in childhood or at school?

When present, a history of childhood wheeze increases the likelihood of asthma, although this history may be absent in late-onset asthma. A history of atopic allergy also increases the likelihood of asthma.

Do you have other symptoms with your breathlessness?

Digital or perioral paraesthesiae and a feeling that 'I cannot get a deep enough breath in' are typical of psychogenic hyperventilation, but this cannot be diagnosed until other potential causes are excluded. Additional symptoms of hyperventilation include lightheadedness, central chest discomfort or carpopedal spasm because of respiratory alkalosis. These alarming symptoms may provoke further anxiety, exacerbating hyperventilation. Psychogenic breathlessness rarely disturbs sleep, frequently occurs at rest, may be provoked by stress and may even be relieved by exercise. ABGs show normal PO_2, low PCO_2 and alkalosis.

Pleuritic chest pain in a patient with chronic breathlessness, particularly if it occurs in more than one site over time, suggests pulmonary thromboembolism. This occasionally presents as chronic breathlessness with no other specific features and should always be considered before diagnosing psychogenic hyperventilation.

Morning headache is an important symptom in patients with breathlessness, as it may indicate carbon dioxide retention and respiratory failure. This occurs particularly in patients with musculoskeletal disease impairing ventilation (e.g. kyphoscoliosis or muscular dystrophy).

Acute severe breathlessness

This is one of the most common and dramatic medical emergencies. Although respiratory causes are common, it can result from cardiac disease, metabolic disease or poisoning causing acidosis or from psychogenic causes. The approach to patients with acute severe breathlessness is covered on p. 61.

Chest pain

Chest pain can result from cardiac, respiratory, oesophageal or musculoskeletal disorders. The approach to this common symptom is covered on p. 58.

Finger clubbing

Painless swelling of the soft tissues of the terminal phalanges causes increased longitudinal and lateral convexity of the nail (Fig. 9.1). The antero-posterior diameter of the finger at the nail bed exceeds that at the distal interphalangeal joint, and the normal angle between the proximal nail and the adjoining skin is lost. Clubbing is usually symmetrical (unless the cause is unilateral, e.g. arteriovenous shunts for dialysis), and commonly also involves the toes. It is sometimes congenital, but in more than 90% of patients it indicates a serious underlying disorder. The most common underlying causes are suppurative or malignant lung disease, but a variety of other conditions can cause clubbing:

- Thoracic (80%): TB, bronchiectasis, empyema, lung cancer, pulmonary fibrosis
- Cardiovascular: Cyanotic congenital heart disease, infective endocarditis
- Gastrointestinal: Cirrhosis, inflammatory bowel disease
- Other: Thyroid acropachy
- Congenital (10%)

Clubbing may recede if the cause resolves, for example, following lung transplantation for bronchiectasis in cystic fibrosis.

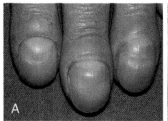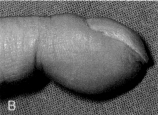

Fig. 9.1 Finger clubbing.

Haemoptysis

Coughing up any amount of blood is an alarming symptom, and nearly always brings the patient to the doctor.

A clear history should be taken to establish that it is true haemoptysis and not haematemesis, gum bleeding or nosebleed. Haemoptysis must always be assumed to have a serious cause until proven otherwise. A history of repeated small haemoptyses, or blood-streaking of sputum, is highly suggestive of lung cancer. Fever, night sweats and weight loss suggest TB. Pneumococcal pneumonia is often the cause of 'rusty'-coloured sputum, but can cause frank haemoptysis, as can all the pneumonic infections that lead to suppuration or abscess formation. Bronchiectasis and aspergilloma can cause catastrophic haemoptysis, and in these patients there may be a history of previous TB or pneumonia in early life. Pulmonary thromboembolism is a common cause of haemoptysis and should always be considered. Many episodes of haemoptysis are unexplained, even after full investigation, most likely resulting from simple bronchial infection.

Investigations and management

In severe acute haemoptysis, the patient should be nursed upright (or on the side of bleeding, if known). Oxygen and haemodynamic resuscitation should be given. Infusions of the antifibrinolytic agent tranexamic acid or the vasopressin precursor terlipressin may limit bleeding, but evidence of efficacy is limited. Bronchial arteriography with embolisation or thoracic surgery may be required to control bleeding.

In the vast majority of cases, however, haemoptysis is not life threatening, and it is possible to follow a logical sequence of investigations including CXR, FBC, clotting screen, bronchoscopy and CTPA to find the cause.

The 'incidental' pulmonary nodule

A pulmonary nodule is defined as a rounded focal opacity on imaging less than 3 cm in diameter, surrounded by aerated lung. The increased use of CT has led to an epidemic of 'incidental' pulmonary nodules; however, these cannot be dismissed as harmless until an early infective or malignant condition is excluded or stability over at least 2 years has been demonstrated.

The list of potential causes of pulmonary nodules is extensive, and most are benign (Box 9.1). Features on CT consistent with a benign lesion include diameter smaller than 5 mm or volume less than $80 mm^3$; diffuse, central, laminated or popcorn calcification; or the presence of macroscopic fat. In addition, perifissural lymph nodes and subpleural nodules with a lentiform or triangular shape do not require any further investigation.

For the remainder, appropriate management depends on both the nodule's appearance and the clinical context, and computer prediction models can clarify risk.

Pulmonary nodules are invariably inaccessible by bronchoscope and, with the exception of pulmonary infection (e.g. tuberculosis), the yield from blind washings is low, although this may improve with advances in endobronchial imaging. Depending on site, size and patient fitness, percutaneous needle

9.1 Causes of pulmonary nodules

Common

- Lung cancer
- Single metastasis
- Localised pneumonia
- Lung abscess
- Tuberculoma
- Pulmonary infarct

Uncommon

- Benign tumours
- Lymphoma
- Arteriovenous malformation
- Hydatid cyst
- Pulmonary haematoma
- Bronchogenic cyst
- Rheumatoid nodule
- Pulmonary sequestration
- Granulomatosis with polyangiitis
- Aspergilloma (usually with surrounding air crescent)

biopsy under ultrasound or CT guidance may be possible. The risk of pneumothorax is approximately 15%, and around 7% require intercostal drainage. Where suspicion of malignancy remains high despite indeterminate investigations, surgical resection may be appropriate, as surgery remains the best chance of curing lung cancer.

PET scanning is useful for nodules of 1 cm or more in diameter. High metabolic activity is strongly suggestive of malignancy, whereas a 'cold' nodule suggests benign disease. However, PET can yield false positives in regions with high endemic rates of infectious or granulomatous disease.

If the nodule is small and inaccessible, interval CT scanning may be employed. A repeat CT at 3 months will reliably detect growth in larger nodules and may also demonstrate resolution. Further interval scans may be needed, depending on the clinical context.

In cases where the probability of cancer is low, the benefits of interval scanning must be balanced against the risk of false-positive findings causing unnecessary patient anxiety and radiation exposure.

Pleural effusion

The accumulation of fluid within the pleural space is termed pleural effusion. Accumulations of frank pus (empyema) or blood (haemothorax) represent separate conditions. Pleural fluid accumulates due either to increased hydrostatic pressure or decreased osmotic pressure ('transudative effusion', as seen in cardiac, liver or renal failure), or to increased microvascular permeability caused by disease of the pleural surface itself, or injury in the adjacent lung ('exudative effusion'). Some causes of pleural effusion are shown in Box 9.2.

Symptoms and signs of pleurisy often precede the development of an effusion, especially in patients with underlying pneumonia, pulmonary infarction or connective tissue disease. However, the onset may be insidious. Breathlessness is often the only symptom related to the effusion, and its severity depends on the size and rate of accumulation.

Investigations

Radiology: The classical appearance of pleural fluid on CXR is that of a curved shadow at the lung base, blunting the costophrenic angle and ascending towards the axilla. Fluid appears to track up the lateral chest wall. In fact, fluid surrounds the whole lung at this level, but casts a radiological shadow only where the x-ray beam passes tangentially through the fluid against the lateral chest wall. Around 200 mL of fluid is required to be detectable on a PA CXR, but smaller effusions can be identified by USS or CT. Previous scarring or adhesions in the pleural space can cause localised effusions. USS is more accurate than plain CXR for determining the volume of pleural fluid and may reveal floating debris, indicating an exudate. The presence of septation suggests an evolving empyema or resolving haemothorax. CT displays pleural abnormalities more readily than either plain radiography or USS and may distinguish benign from malignant pleural disease.

Pleural aspiration and biopsy: In some conditions (e.g. left ventricular failure) it should not be necessary to sample fluid unless atypical features are present. In most other circumstances, diagnostic aspiration is indicated. Pleural aspiration reveals the colour and texture of fluid and on appearance alone may immediately suggest an empyema or chylothorax. The presence

---

9.2 Causes of pleural effusion

Common

- Pneumonia ('para-pneumonic effusion')
- TB
- Pulmonary infarction
- Malignant disease
- Cardiac failure
- Subdiaphragmatic disease (subphrenic abscess, pancreatitis)

Uncommon

- Hypoproteinaemia (nephrotic syndrome, liver failure)
- Connective tissue diseases (systemic lupus erythematosus, rheumatoid arthritis)
- Post-MI syndrome
- Acute rheumatic fever
- Meigs' syndrome (ovarian tumour + pleural effusion)
- Myxoedema
- Uraemia
- Asbestos-related benign pleural effusion

of blood is consistent with pulmonary infarction or malignancy but may represent a traumatic tap. Biochemical analysis allows classification into transudate and exudate (Box 9.3), and Gram stain and culture may reveal infection. The predominant cell type provides useful information, and cytological examination is essential. A low pH suggests infection, but may also be seen in rheumatoid arthritis, ruptured oesophagus or advanced malignancy. USS- or CT-guided pleural biopsy provides tissue for pathological and microbiological analysis. If results are inconclusive, video-assisted thoracoscopy allows the operator to visualise the pleura and guide the biopsy directly.

Management

Therapeutic aspiration may be required to palliate breathlessness but removing more than 1.5 L in one episode is inadvisable because this can cause re-expansion pulmonary oedema. An effusion should never be drained to dryness before establishing a diagnosis, as further biopsy may be precluded until further fluid accumulates. Treatment of the underlying cause—for example, heart failure, pneumonia, pulmonary embolism or subphrenic abscess—will often be followed by resolution of the effusion. The management of pleural effusion in association with pneumonia, TB and malignancy is dealt with later.

Empyema

Empyema means pus in the pleural space. The pus may be as thin as serous fluid or so thick that it is impossible to aspirate, even through a wide-bore needle. Microscopically, neutrophils are present in large numbers. The causative organism may or may not be isolated from the pus. An empyema may involve the whole pleural space or only part of it ('loculated' or 'encysted' empyema) and is usually unilateral. Empyema is always secondary to infection in a neighbouring structure, usually the lung (bacterial pneumonias and TB). Over 40% of patients with community-acquired pneumonia develop an associated pleural effusion ('para-pneumonic' effusion), and around 15% of these become secondarily infected, often where there is a delay in diagnosis or treatment.

Clinical features

• Persistence or recurrence of pyrexia in pulmonary infections, despite the administration of a suitable antibiotic. • Rigors, sweating, malaise and weight loss. • Pleural pain, breathlessness, cough, sputum (copious

9.3 Light's criteria for distinguishing pleural transudate from exudate

Pleural fluid is an exudate if one or more of the following criteria are met:
• Pleural fluid protein : serum protein ratio >0.5
• Pleural fluid LDH : serum LDH ratio >0.6
• Pleural fluid LDH greater than two-thirds of the upper limit of normal serum LDH

amounts if empyema ruptures into a bronchus–bronchopleural fistula).
• Clinical signs of a pleural effusion.

Investigations

• Blood tests: reveal a polymorphonuclear leucocytosis and high CRP.
• CXR: demonstrates a pleural effusion, which often appears loculated against the chest wall ('D-shaped opacity'). When air is present in addition to pus (pyopneumothorax), a horizontal 'fluid level' marks the air/liquid interface. • USS shows the position of the fluid, the extent of pleural thickening and whether fluid is in a single collection or multiloculated by fibrin and debris. • CT: can be useful in assessing the underlying lung parenchyma and patency of the major bronchi. • USS-guided aspiration of pus: confirms the presence of an empyema; the pus is frequently sterile when antibiotics have already been given.

The distinction between tuberculous and nontuberculous disease can be difficult, and often requires pleural histology and culture and/or a nucleic acid amplification test.

Management

When the patient is acutely ill and the pus is thin, a large intercostal tube should be inserted for drainage of the pleural space. If the aspirate reveals turbid fluid or frank pus, or if loculations are seen on USS, the tube should be put on suction (-5 to -10 cmH_2O) and flushed regularly with 20 mL normal saline. An antibiotic directed against the organism causing the empyema should be given for 2 to 4 weeks. Intrapleural fibrinolytic therapy is of no benefit. If the pleural fluid is difficult to drain (when the pus is thick or loculated), surgery is required to clear the empyema cavity. Surgical 'decortication' of the lung may be required if thickening of the visceral pleura is preventing re-expansion of the lung. Surgery is also needed if a bronchopleural fistula develops.

Respiratory failure

The term 'respiratory failure' is used when pulmonary gas exchange fails to maintain normal arterial oxygen and carbon dioxide levels. Its classification into type I and type II relates to the absence or presence of hypercapnia (raised $PaCO_2$). The main causes are shown in Box 9.4.

Acute respiratory failure

Management

Prompt diagnosis and management of the underlying cause are crucial. In type I respiratory failure, high concentrations of oxygen (40%–60% by mask) will usually relieve hypoxia, but occasionally CPAP or mechanical ventilation may be needed.

Acute type II respiratory failure is an emergency. It is useful to distinguish between patients with high ventilatory drive who cannot move sufficient air, and those with reduced or inadequate respiratory effort. In the former, particularly if inspiratory stridor is present, acute upper airway obstruction (e.g. foreign body inhalation or laryngeal obstruction) must be considered,

	9.4 Respiratory failure: underlying causes and blood gas abnormalities			
	Type I		**Type II**	
	Hypoxia (PaO_2 <8.0 kPa [60 mmHg])		Hypoxia (PaO_2 <8.0 kPa [60 mmHg])	
	Normal or low $PaCO_2$ (<6 kPa [45 mmHg])		Raised $PaCO_2$ (>6 kPa [45 mmHg])	
	Acute	**Chronic**	**Acute**	**Chronic**
H^+	→	→	↑	→ or ↑
Bicarbonate	→	→	→	↑
Causes	Acute asthma Pulmonary oedema Pneumonia Lobar collapse Pneumothorax Pulmonary embolus ARDS	COPD Lung fibrosis Lymphangitic carcinomatosis Right-to-left shunts	Acute severe asthma Acute exacerbation of COPD Upper airway obstruction Acute neuropathies/paralysis Narcotic drugs Primary alveolar hypoventilation Flail chest injury	COPD Sleep apnoea Kyphoscoliosis Myopathies/ muscular dystrophy Ankylosing spondylitis

as the Heimlich manoeuvre, immediate intubation or tracheostomy may be life saving.

More commonly, the problem is severe COPD or asthma, or ARDS (see Chapter 4). High-concentration (e.g. 60%) oxygen should be administered with monitoring of ABGs. Patients with asthma or COPD should be treated with nebulised salbutamol 2.5 mg with oxygen, repeated until bronchospasm is relieved. Failure to respond to initial treatment, declining conscious level and worsening respiratory acidosis (H^+ >50 nmol/L [pH <7.3]), $PaCO_2$ >6.6 kPa [50 mmHg]) on blood gases are all indications that supported ventilation is required (see Chapter 4).

Patients with acute type II respiratory failure with reduced drive or conscious level may be suffering from sedative poisoning, CO_2 narcosis or a primary failure of neurological drive (e.g. following intracerebral haemorrhage or head injury). History from a witness may be invaluable, and reversal of sedatives using antagonists occasionally helps, but should not delay intubation and supported mechanical ventilation in appropriate cases.

Chronic and 'acute on chronic' type II respiratory failure

In severe COPD or neuromuscular disease, $PaCO_2$ may be persistently raised, but renal retention of bicarbonate corrects arterial pH to normal. This 'compensated' pattern may be disturbed by further acute illness, such as an exacerbation of COPD, causing 'acute on chronic' respiratory failure, with acidaemia and respiratory distress followed by drowsiness and coma. These patients have lost their chemosensitivity to elevated $PaCO_2$, and depend on hypoxia for respiratory drive; they may therefore develop dangerous respiratory depression if given high concentrations of oxygen.

The aims of treatment in acute on chronic type II respiratory failure are to achieve a safe PaO_2 (>7.0 kPa [52 mmHg]) without increasing $PaCO_2$ and acidosis.

Conscious patients with adequate respiratory drive may benefit from NIV, which has been shown to reduce the need for intubation and to shorten hospital stay. Patients who are drowsy and have low respiratory drive require an urgent decision regarding intubation and ventilation. Important factors to consider include patient and family wishes, presence of a potentially remediable precipitating condition, prior functional capacity and quality of life.

Respiratory stimulant drugs, such as doxapram, have been superseded by intubation and mechanical ventilation in patients with CO_2 narcosis.

Home ventilation for chronic respiratory failure

Some patients with chronic respiratory failure because of spinal deformity, neuromuscular disease or advanced lung disease, for example, cystic fibrosis, benefit from home NIV. In these conditions, morning headache (caused by elevated $PaCO_2$) and fatigue may occur, but the diagnosis may also be revealed by sleep studies or morning blood gas analysis. Overnight home-based NIV is often sufficient to restore the daytime PCO_2 to normal, and to relieve fatigue and headache. In advanced disease, daytime NIV may also be required.

Lung transplantation

This is an established treatment for carefully selected patients with advanced lung disease unresponsive to medical treatment. Single-lung transplantation may be used for selected patients with advanced emphysema or lung fibrosis. It is contraindicated in patients with chronic bilateral pulmonary infection, such as cystic fibrosis, because immunosuppression makes the transplanted lung vulnerable to cross-infection; for these conditions, bilateral lung transplantation is the standard procedure. Heart–lung transplantation is still occasionally needed for patients with advanced congenital heart disease such as Eisenmenger's syndrome and is preferred by some surgeons for the treatment of primary pulmonary hypertension unresponsive to medical therapy.

The prognosis following lung transplantation is improving steadily. Modern immunosuppressive drugs yield over 50% 10-year survival in some UK centres. Chronic rejection with obliterative bronchiolitis continues to afflict some recipients, however.

The major factor limiting the availability of lung transplantation is the shortage of donor lungs. To improve organ availability, techniques to recondition the lungs in vitro after removal from the donor are being developed.

Obstructive pulmonary diseases

Asthma

Asthma is characterised by chronic airway inflammation and increased airway hyper-responsiveness leading to wheeze, cough, chest tightness and dyspnoea. Airflow obstruction in asthma is variable over time and reversible with treatment. As asthma affects all age groups, it is one of the most important long-term respiratory conditions in terms of global years lived with disability.

The relationship between atopy (the propensity to produce IgE in response to allergens) and asthma is well established. Common allergens include house dust mites, cats, dogs, cockroaches and fungi. Allergy is also implicated in some cases of occupational asthma (p. 353).

Aspirin can cause asthma through the production of cysteinyl leukotrienes. In exercise-induced asthma, hyperventilation results in water and heat loss from the airway lining fluid, triggering mediator release.

In persistent asthma, there is a chronic influx of inflammatory cells interacting with airway structural cells, and the secretion of cytokines, chemokines and growth factors. Induced sputum samples demonstrate that, although eosinophils usually dominate, neutrophilic inflammation predominates in some patients, whereas, in others, scant inflammation is observed: so-called 'pauci-granulocytic' asthma.

With increasing severity and chronicity of asthma, airway remodelling may occur, with fibrosis and fixed narrowing of the airways and a reduced bronchodilator response.

Clinical features

Typical symptoms include recurrent episodes of wheezing, chest tightness, breathlessness and cough. In mild intermittent asthma, patients may be asymptomatic between exacerbations. In persistent asthma, the pattern is one of chronic wheeze and breathlessness.

Symptoms may be precipitated by:
• Exercise. • Cold weather. • Allergen exposure (e.g. pets, occupational).
• Viral respiratory tract infections. • Drugs (β-blockers, aspirin and NSAIDs).

There is diurnal variation in symptoms (worse in early morning); sleep is often disturbed by cough and wheeze.

Investigations

A combination of history, examination, pulmonary function and other tests are used to define the probability of asthma in an individual.

Pulmonary function test may show:
• An increase in FEV_1 of 12% or more and at least 200 mL following bronchodilator/trial of glucocorticoids. • More than 20% diurnal variation on 3 or more days in a week for 2 weeks on PEF diary. • A decrease in FEV_1 of 15% or more after 6 minutes of exercise.

In patients with normal FEV_1, bronchial challenge testing (e.g. with mannitol) is a sensitive, although not specific, way to demonstrate airway hyperreactivity.

The diagnosis is supported by evidence of atopy on skin-prick tests, raised total and allergen-specific IgE, an exhaled nitric oxide level (a surrogate of eosinophilic airway inflammation) of 40 or more parts per billion in a glucocorticoid-naïve adult or a peripheral blood eosinophilia.

The CXR is usually normal, but lobar collapse is seen with mucus plugging of a large bronchus, and fleeting shadows with bronchiectasis on CT suggest allergic bronchopulmonary aspergillosis (p. 330).

Management

The goal of asthma therapy is to maintain complete control:
• No daytime symptoms. • No limitation of activities. • No nocturnal symptoms/wakening. • No need for 'rescue' medication. • Normal lung function.
• No exacerbations.

Patients who have symptoms requiring rescue medication more than twice a week have partial control, and those with more than 3 of the previously mentioned features in any week are termed uncontrolled.

Patient education: Patients should be taught about the importance of key symptoms (e.g. nocturnal waking), different types of medication and the use of PEF to guide management. Written action plans may be helpful.

Avoidance of aggravating factors: Asthma control may be improved by reducing exposure to antigens, for example, household pets. In occupational asthma, removal from the offending agent may lead to cure. Many patients are sensitised to several antigens, making avoidance almost impossible. Patients should be advised not to smoke.

Pharmacological treatment

The choice of inhaler device should be based on patient preference and observed competence in its use.

Step 1—Occasional use of inhaled short-acting β_2-adrenoreceptor agonist bronchodilators: This is used for patients with mild intermittent asthma (symptoms less than once a week for 3 months and less than two nocturnal episodes per month). Patients often underestimate the severity of asthma.

Step 2—Regular preventer therapy: Regular ICSs are used for any patient who has experienced an exacerbation in the last 2 years, uses inhaled β_2-agonists three or more times per week, reports symptoms three or more times per week or is awakened by asthma 1 night per week.

Step 3—Add-on therapy: The addition of LABAs to ICSs has been demonstrated to improve asthma control and reduce exacerbations compared with increased doses of ICS alone. Leukotriene receptor antagonists (e.g. montelukast 10 mg daily) are a less effective add-on therapy.

Step 4—Poor control on a moderate dose of inhaled glucocorticoid and add-on therapy: The ICS dose may be increased to 2000 µg BDP or equivalent daily. A nasal glucocorticoid should be used if upper airway symptoms are prominent. Consider trials of leukotriene receptor antagonists, long acting antimuscarinic agents, theophyllines or slow-release β_2-agonists, and stop if ineffective.

Step 5—Continuous or frequent use of oral glucocorticoids: Prednisolone should be prescribed in the lowest dose necessary to control symptoms. Patients receiving more than three or four courses per year or long-term glucocorticoids (>3 months) are at risk of systemic side effects. Osteoporosis should be prevented using bisphosphonates. In atopic patients, omalizumab, a monoclonal anti-IgE antibody, may help to limit glucocorticoid dose and improve symptoms. Mepolizumab should be considered in eosinophil-mediated disease.

Step-down therapy: Once asthma control is established, inhaled (or oral) glucocorticoid dose should be titrated to the lowest dose at which effective control of asthma is maintained.

Exacerbations of asthma

Asthma exacerbations are characterised by increased symptoms, deterioration in PEF and an increase in airway inflammation. They may be precipitated by infections (most commonly viral), moulds (*Alternaria* and *Cladosporium*), pollen (particularly following thunderstorms) and peaks of air pollution. Most attacks are characterised by a gradual deterioration over several hours to days, but some occur with little or no warning: so-called brittle asthma.

Management of mild to moderate exacerbations

Doubling the dose of ICS does not prevent an impending exacerbation. Short courses of 'rescue' oral glucocorticoids (prednisolone 30–60 mg daily) are often required where there are worsening symptoms (morning symptoms persisting until midday, nocturnal wakening or diminishing response to bronchodilator) and a fall of PEF to less than 60% of best recording. Tapering of the dose is not necessary unless given for more than 3 weeks.

Management of acute severe asthma

This is covered in Box 9.5 and Fig. 9.2.

 9.5 Immediate assessment of acute severe asthma

Acute severe asthma

- PEF 33% to 50% predicted (<200 L/min)
- HR ≥110/min
- Respiratory rate ≥25 per minute
- Inability to complete sentences in one breath

Life-threatening features

- PEF <33% predicted (<100 L/min)
- SpO_2 <92% or PaO_2 <8 kPa (60 mmHg), especially on oxygen
- Normal or raised $PaCO_2$
- Silent chest/feeble respiratory effort
- Bradycardia or arrhythmias
- Cyanosis
- Hypotension
- Exhaustion, delirium or Coma

Near-fatal asthma

- ↑$PaCO_2$ and/or requiring mechanical ventilation with raised inflation pressures

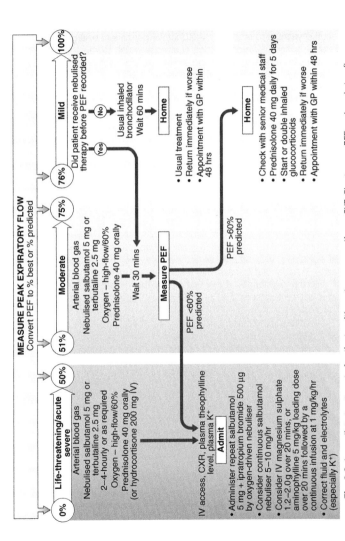

MEASURE PEAK EXPIRATORY FLOW
Convert PEF to % best or % predicted

| 0% | 50% | 51% | 75% | 76% | 100% |

Life-threatening/acute severe

Arterial blood gas
Nebulised salbutamol 5 mg or terbutaline 2.5 mg 2–4-hourly or as required
Oxygen – high-flow/60%
Prednisolone 40 mg orally (or hydrocortisone 200 mg IV)

Moderate

Arterial blood gas
Nebulised salbutamol 5 mg or terbutaline 2.5 mg
Oxygen – high-flow/60%
Prednisolone 40 mg orally

Mild

Did patient receive nebulised therapy before PEF recorded?

No

Usual inhaled bronchodilator
Wait 60 mins

Home

- Usual treatment
- Return immediately if worse
- Appointment with GP within 48 hrs

Yes

Wait 30 mins

Measure PEF

PEF <60% predicted

PEF >60% predicted

Home

- Check with senior medical staff
- Prednisolone 40 mg daily for 5 days
- Start or double inhaled glucocorticoids
- Return immediately if worse
- Appointment with GP within 48 hrs

Admit

IV access, CXR, plasma theophylline level, plasma K^+

- Administer repeat salbutamol 5 mg + ipratropium bromide 500 μg by oxygen-driven nebuliser
- Consider continuous salbutamol nebuliser 5–10 mg/hr
- Consider IV magnesium sulphate 1.2–2.0 g over 20 mins, or aminophylline 5 mg/kg loading dose over 20 mins followed by a continuous infusion at 1 mg/kg/hr
- Correct fluid and electrolytes (especially K^+)

Fig. 9.2 Immediate treatment of patients with acute severe asthma. *CXR*, Chest x-ray; *PEF*, peak expiratory flow.

Chronic obstructive pulmonary disease

COPD is a preventable and treatable disease characterised by persistent progressive airflow limitation associated with chronic inflammation in response to noxious particles or gases. Related diagnoses include chronic bronchitis (cough and sputum for at least 3 consecutive months, in 2 consecutive years) and emphysema (abnormal permanent enlargement of the distal air spaces, with destruction of alveolar walls). Extrapulmonary manifestations include weight loss and skeletal muscle dysfunction, and COPD is associated with cardiovascular disease, cerebrovascular disease, the metabolic syndrome, osteoporosis and depression.

The prevalence of COPD is related to the prevalence of risk factors in the community, particularly tobacco smoking, coal dust exposure and biomass fuel smoke. It has significant social and economic consequences. It is predicted that, by 2030, COPD will be the seventh leading cause of disability and fourth most common cause of death. Not all smokers develop COPD, indicating variable individual susceptibility to smoke, and COPD is unusual in smokers of less than 10 pack years (1 pack year = 20 cigarettes/day for 1 year).

Clinical features

COPD should be suspected in any patient over the age of 40 years with persistent cough and sputum and/or breathlessness. The level of breathlessness should be quantified (e.g. MRC dyspnoea scale, Box 9.6). Physical signs (Fig. 9.3) indicate severe disease, and may be absent in mild cases. In advanced disease with respiratory failure there may be oedema or morning headaches (hypercapnia). Neither finger clubbing nor haemoptysis are typical of COPD — these should trigger a search for underlying malignancy.

Two classical phenotypes have been described, although in practice they often overlap:
• 'Pink puffers': thin and breathless, and maintain a normal $PaCO_2$. • 'Blue bloaters': develop hypercapnia, oedema and secondary polycythaemia.

Investigations

CXR may reveal hyperinflation, bullae or other complications of smoking (lung cancer). FBC may demonstrate polycythaemia. The α_1-antitrypsin level should be checked in younger patients with emphysema.

Assessment of severity has traditionally been based on post–bronchodilator spirometry (% of predicted value; e.g. UK NICE guidelines):

Stage 1 (mild)—FEV_1 greater than 80%, FEV_1/FVC less than 0.7 plus symptoms;
Stage II (moderate)—FEV_1 50% to 79%, FEV_1/FVC less than 0.7;
Stage III (severe)—FEV_1 30% to 49%, FEV_1/FVC less than 0.7;
Stage IV (very severe)—FEV_1 <30%, FEV_1/FVC less than 0.7.

More recent severity assessments also recognise that the impact of COPD on individuals includes the limitations in activity that they experience and whether they suffer frequent exacerbations.

Lung volume measurements are used to quantify hyperinflation. Carbon monoxide transfer factor is reduced in emphysema. Exercise tests provide

i	**9.6 Modified MRC dyspnoea scale**
Grade	Degree of breathlessness related to activities
0	No breathlessness except with strenuous exercise
1	Breathlessness when hurrying on the level or walking up a slight hill
2	Walks slower than contemporaries on level ground because of breathlessness, or has to stop for breath when walking at own pace
3	Stops for breath after walking around 100 m or after a few minutes on level ground
4	Too breathless to leave the house, or breathless when dressing or undressing

Chronic obstructive pulmonary disease

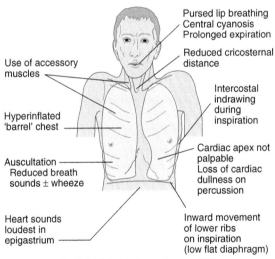

Fig. 9.3 Clinical features of severe COPD.

an objective assessment of exercise tolerance. Pulse oximetry may prompt referral for a domiciliary oxygen assessment if less than 93%.

CT scanning is increasingly used for the detection, characterisation and quantification of emphysema.

Management

This focuses on improving breathlessness, reducing the frequency and severity of exacerbations and improving health status and prognosis.

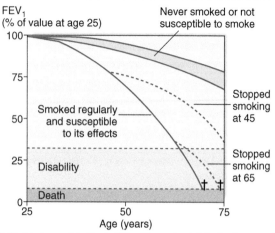

Fig. 9.4 Model of annual decline in FEV$_1$ with accelerated decline in suscepti-ble smokers. When smoking is stopped, subsequent loss is similar to that in healthy nonsmokers.

Reduce exposure to smoke: Always offer the patient help to stop smok-ing, combining pharmacotherapy with an appropriate programme of support. Cessation is proven to decelerate the decline in FEV$_1$ (Fig. 9.4). Smokeless alternatives to biofuels should be promoted wherever possible.

Bronchodilators: Short-acting bronchodilators are given for mild dis-ease (β_2-agonist or anticholinergic). Longer-acting bronchodilators are more appropriate for patients with moderate to severe disease. Select a device that the patient can use effectively.

Significant improvements in breathlessness may be reported despite minimal changes in FEV$_1$, probably reflecting reduced dynamic hyperinfla-tion on exercise. Oral theophylline preparations may be used in patients unable to use inhalers but are limited by side effects. Selective phosphodi-esterase inhibitors are under appraisal.

Combined inhaled glucocorticoids and bronchodilators: The fixed combination of an inhaled glucocorticoid and a LABA improves lung function, reduces the frequency and severity of exacerbations and improves quality of life. These advantages may be accompanied by an increased risk of pneu-monia, particularly in the elderly. LABA/inhaled glucocorticoid combinations are frequently given with a LAMA. LAMAs should be used with caution in patients with significant heart disease or a history of urinary retention.

Oral glucocorticoids: are useful during exacerbations, but maintenance therapy contributes to osteoporosis and impaired muscle function and should be avoided.

Pulmonary rehabilitation: Encourage exercise. Multidisciplinary pro-grammes (usually 6–12 weeks' duration) incorporating physical training, education and nutritional counselling reduce symptoms, improve health status and enhance confidence.

Oxygen therapy: LTOT improves survival in selected patients with COPD and hypoxia (PaO_2 <7.3 kPa [55 mmHg]). A minimum of 15 hours/day is recommended, keeping PaO_2 greater than 8 kPa (60 mmHg) or SaO_2 greater than 90%. Ambulatory oxygen should be considered in patients who desaturate on exercise and show objective improved exercise capacity and/or dyspnoea with oxygen. Short-burst oxygen therapy is of no benefit and should be avoided.

Surgical intervention: In highly selected patients, lung volume reduction surgery (removing nonfunctioning emphysematous lung tissue) reduces hyperinflation and decreases work of breathing. Bullectomy is occasionally performed for large bullae that compress surrounding lung tissue. Lung transplantation may benefit selected patients.

Other measures: Give pneumococcal vaccination and annual influenza vaccination; treat depression and cachexia. Morphine can usefully palliate breathlessness in advanced disease.

Prognosis in COPD is inversely related to age and directly related to FEV_1. Poor prognostic indicators include weight loss and pulmonary hypertension.

Acute exacerbations of COPD

These are characterised by an increase in symptoms and deterioration in lung function. They are more common in severe disease, and may be caused by bacteria, viruses or a change in air quality. Respiratory failure and/or fluid retention may be present. Many patients can be managed at home with the use of increased bronchodilators, a short course of oral glucocorticoids and, if appropriate, antibiotics. Cyanosis, peripheral oedema or altered conscious level should prompt hospital referral.

Oxygen therapy: High concentrations of oxygen may cause respiratory depression and worsening acidosis (p. 320). Controlled oxygen at 24% or 28% should be used, aiming for PaO_2 higher than 8 kPa (60 mmHg) (or SaO_2 >90%) without worsening acidosis.

Bronchodilators: Nebulised short-acting β_2-agonists and anticholinergics are used. The oxygen content of the driving gas should be reduced if there is respiratory depression.

Glucocorticoids: Oral prednisolone (usually 30 mg for 5–10 days) reduces symptoms, improves lung function and shortens hospital stay. Prophylaxis against osteoporosis should be considered if frequent courses are needed.

Antibiotics: These are recommended for an increase in sputum purulence, sputum volume or breathlessness. An aminopenicillin, a tetracycline or a macrolide should be used. Co-amoxiclav is only required where β-lactamase-producing organisms are locally prevalent.

Ventilatory support: In patients with persistent tachypnoea and respiratory acidosis (H^+ ≥45 nmol/L [pH <7.35]), NIV is associated with reduced need for intubation and reduced mortality. Consider intubation and ventilation where there is a reversible cause for deterioration (e.g. pneumonia); the evidence for NIV with pneumonia is much weaker.

Additional therapy: Diuretics should be administered if peripheral oedema has developed. Evidence for IV aminophylline is limited, and there is a risk of arrhythmias and drug interactions. The respiratory stimulant doxapram has been superseded by NIV.

Bronchiectasis

Bronchiectasis means abnormal dilatation of the bronchi because of chronic airway inflammation and infection. It is usually acquired, but may result from an underlying genetic or congenital defect of airway defences (Box 9.7).

Clinical features

• Chronic cough with purulent sputum. • Haemoptysis. • Weight loss and general debility. • Pleuritic pain. • Halitosis.

Acute exacerbations may cause fever and increase these symptoms. Examination reveals coarse crackles caused by sputum in bronchiectatic spaces. Diminished breath sounds may indicate lobar collapse. Bronchial breathing because of scarring may be heard in advanced disease.

Investigations

Sputum: Testing may reveal common respiratory pathogens. As disease progresses, *Pseudomonas aeruginosa, Staphylococcus aureus*, fungi such as *Aspergillus* and various mycobacteria may be seen. Cultures assist appropriate antibiotic selection.

Radiology: CXR may be normal in mild disease. In advanced disease, thickened airway walls, cystic bronchiectatic spaces and areas of pneumonic consolidation or collapse may be seen. CT is much more sensitive and shows dilated airways with thickened walls.

Assessment of ciliary function: Saccharin test or nasal biopsy may be used.

Management and prognosis

In patients with airflow obstruction, inhaled bronchodilators and glucocorticoids may enhance airway patency.

Physiotherapy: Patients should perform regular daily physiotherapy to keep the dilated bronchi empty of secretions. Deep breathing followed by forced expiratory manoeuvres ('active cycle of breathing' technique), and devices that generate positive expiratory pressure (PEP mask or flutter valve) can assist with sputum clearance.

BOX 9.7 Causes of bronchiectasis

Congenital

- Cystic fibrosis
- Primary ciliary dyskinesia
- Kartagener's syndrome (sinusitis and transposition of the viscera)
- Primary hypogammaglobulinaemia

Acquired

- Pneumonia (complicating whooping cough or measles)
- Inhaled foreign body
- Suppurative pneumonia
- Pulmonary TB
- Allergic bronchopulmonary aspergillosis complicating asthma
- Bronchial tumours

Antibiotics: In most patients with bronchiectasis, the same antibiotics are used as in COPD, although higher doses and longer courses are needed. In patients colonised with staphylococci and Gram-negative bacilli, especially *Pseudomonas* spp., antibiotic therapy should be guided by microbiology results.

Surgical treatment: Surgery is only indicated in a few cases where bronchiectasis is unilateral and confined to a single lobe/segment on CT.

The disease is progressive when associated with ciliary dysfunction and cystic fibrosis, and eventually causes respiratory failure. In other patients, the prognosis can be good with regular physiotherapy and judicious use of antibiotics. Bronchiectasis may be prevented by prophylaxis or treatment of common causes, for example, measles, whooping cough, TB.

Cystic fibrosis

CF is the most common lethal genetic disease in Caucasians, affecting 1 in 2500 births. It is caused by mutations of a gene (on chromosome 7) coding for a chloride channel—*CFTR*. The carrier rate of CF mutations is 1 in 25, and inheritance is autosomal recessive. The most common mutation is *ΔF508,* but more than 2000 mutations have been identified. The genetic defect causes increased sodium and chloride in sweat, and depletion of airway lining fluid, leading to chronic bacterial infection in the airways. The gut epithelium, pancreas, liver and reproductive tract are also affected. Neonatal screening for CF is now routine in the United Kingdom. The diagnosis is confirmed by genetic testing and sweat electrolyte measurements.

Clinical features

The lungs are normal at birth, but bronchiectasis develops in childhood. *S. aureus* is the most common childhood organism; however, in adulthood, increasing numbers are colonised with *P. aeruginosa* and other Gram-negative pathogens. Recurrent infective exacerbations cause progressive lung damage, resulting ultimately in death from respiratory failure. Other clinical manifestations of the gene defect include intestinal obstruction, exocrine pancreatic insufficiency with malabsorption, diabetes and hepatic cirrhosis. Men with CF are infertile because of failure of development of the vas deferens.

Management and prognosis

Regular chest physiotherapy is recommended. For exacerbations, *S. aureus* infection is often managed with oral antibiotics; IV treatment is usually needed for *Pseudomonas* spp. Resistant strains of *P. aeruginosa*, *Stenotrophomonas maltophilia* and *Burkholderia cepacia* are a major problem. *Aspergillus* and nontuberculous mycobacteria are also frequently found (may be benign 'colonisers'). Nebulised antibiotic therapy (colistin or tobramycin) is used to suppress chronic *Pseudomonas* infection. Nebulised recombinant human DNase liquefies sputum, reduces exacerbations and improves pulmonary function in some patients. Regular macrolides (e.g. azithromycin) reduce exacerbations and improve lung function in patients with *Pseudomonas* colonisation. In advanced disease, home oxygen and

NIV may be necessary to treat respiratory failure. Ultimately, lung transplantation can produce dramatic improvements but is limited by donor organ availability.

Treatment of nonrespiratory manifestations of CF: Malabsorption is treated with oral pancreatic enzymes and vitamin supplements. Increased calorie requirements of CF patients are met by supplemental feeding, including nasogastric or gastrostomy tube feeding if required. Diabetes eventually appears in around 25% of patients, and often requires insulin. Osteoporosis should be sought and treated.

The prognosis of CF has improved greatly in recent decades, mainly because of better nutrition and treatment of bronchial sepsis. The median survival of patients with CF in the United Kingdom is over 45 years.

Novel oral treatments designed to improve ion channel function, for example, ivacaftor, are beginning to show clinical benefits that are likely to further improve prognosis in coming years.

Infections of the respiratory system

Upper respiratory tract infections

Acute coryza (common cold): Sneezing, blocked nose with watery discharge. The cause is usually a rhinovirus, but it may be complicated by lower respiratory tract infection, sinusitis, acute laryngitis or otitis media. Antibiotics are not necessary in uncomplicated coryza.

Acute bronchitis and tracheitis: Often follow acute coryza. Cough is productive of mucoid/mucopurulent sputum. Patients have pyrexia, chest tightness, wheeze and breathlessness. Tracheitis causes pain on coughing. Disease is usually self-limiting, but may lead to bronchopneumonia or an exacerbation of COPD/asthma.

Bordetella pertussis: The cause of whooping cough; an important source of upper respiratory tract infection. It is highly contagious and is notifiable in the United Kingdom. Vaccination confers protection and is usually offered in infancy, but efficacy wanes in adult life. Adults usually experience mild coryza, but some develop paroxysms of coughing that can persist for up to 100 days. The diagnosis may be confirmed by PCR from a nasopharyngeal swab or serological testing. If recognised early, macrolide antibiotics may ameliorate the course.

Rhinosinusitis: Typically causes nasal congestion, blockage or discharge, and may be accompanied by facial pain or loss of smell. Examination reveals erythematous swollen nasal mucosa with pus. Nasal polyps should be sought, and dental infection excluded. Treatment with topical glucocorticoids, nasal decongestants and regular nasal douching are usually sufficient, and, although bacterial infection is often present, antibiotics are only indicated if symptoms persist for more than 5 days. Persistent or recurrent episodes should prompt a referral to an ear, nose and throat specialist.

Influenza: Discussed on p. 120.

Pneumonia

Pneumonia is defined as an acute respiratory illness associated with recently developed segmental, lobar or multilobar radiological shadowing. It is classified as community-acquired pneumonia, hospital-acquired (nosocomial) pneumonia or pneumonia occurring in immunocompromised hosts. 'Lobar pneumonia' is a radiological and pathological term referring to homogeneous consolidation of one or more lobes, often with pleural inflammation; bronchopneumonia refers to more patchy alveolar consolidation with bronchial and bronchiolar inflammation, often affecting both lower lobes.

Community-acquired pneumonia

In the United Kingdom, 5 to 11/1000 adults contract CAP each year. The incidence is higher in the very young and the elderly. Some 20% of childhood deaths worldwide are attributed to pneumonia. Most patients may be safely managed at home, but hospital admission is necessary in 20% to 40%. In hospital, death rates are typically 5% to 10%, rising to 50% in severe illness. The most common organism is *Streptococcus pneumoniae*. *Haemophilus influenzae* should be considered in elderly patients, whereas *Mycoplasma* and *Chlamydia pneumoniae* are more often seen in the young. Recent influenza may predispose to *S. aureus* pneumonia (although most postinfluenza pneumonia is caused by *S. pneumoniae*). Rarer causes of severe pneumonia include *Legionella* (from infected warm water—ask about foreign travel) and psittacosis (from birds infected with *Chlamydia psittaci*). Recent foreign travel also increases the chances of pneumonia because of rarer causes, for example, MERS-coronavirus (Middle East), *Burkholderia pseudomallei* (SE Asia and northern Australia) and endemic fungal infection (North, Central or South America).

Clinical features

Illness begins acutely with fever, rigors and shivering. Cough, initially dry, later yields mucopurulent sputum, although rust-coloured sputum is characteristic of *S. pneumoniae* infection. Anorexia and headache are also common, as is pleuritic chest pain, which may be the presenting feature. Haemoptysis occasionally occurs. Examination may reveal crepitations or bronchial breathing, suggesting underlying consolidation.

The differential diagnosis of pneumonia includes malignancy, pulmonary infarct, pulmonary eosnophilia and cryptogenic organizing pneumonia.

Investigations

Blood: Very high ($>20 \times 10^9$/L) or low ($<4 \times 10^9$/L) white cell count: marker of severity. Neutrophils greater than 15×10^9/L: suggests bacterial aetiology. Haemolytic anaemia: occasional complication of *Mycoplasma*.

U&Es: Urea greater than 7 mmol/L (~20 mg/dL) or hyponatraemia: marker of severity.

Liver function tests: Hypoalbuminaemia: marker of severity.

ESR/CRP: Nonspecifically elevated.

Blood culture: Bacteraemia: marker of severity.

Cold agglutinins: Positive in 50% of patients with *Mycoplasma*.

ABGs: In severe cases or if SaO_2 is less than 93% to detect respiratory failure.

Sputum: Gram stain, culture and antimicrobial sensitivity testing.

Oropharynx swab: PCR for *Mycoplasma* and other atypical pathogens.

Urine: Pneumococcal and/or *Legionella* antigen.

CXR: Lobar pneumonia (Fig. 9.5)—homogeneous consolidation of affected lobe with air bronchogram. Bronchopneumonia—patchy and segmental shadowing. Multilobar shadowing, cavitation and abscesses suggest *S. aureus.*

Pleural fluid: Always aspirate and culture when significant size, preferably with ultrasound guidance.

Management

A disease severity scoring system (Fig. 9.6) helps to guide antibiotic and admission policies.

High concentrations (>35%) of oxygen (preferably humidified) should be administered to all patients with tachypnoea, hypoxaemia, hypotension or acidosis, aiming to keep PaO_2 at 8 kPa or higher (60 mmHg) or SaO_2 at 92% or higher (except in hypercapnia associated with COPD). IV fluids are given in severe disease, and in elderly or vomiting patients. Give antibiotics (Box 9.8) ideally after taking blood cultures, but do not delay treatment in severe pneumonia. Consider analgesia for pleural pain, and physiotherapy if cough is suppressed, for example, because of pain. Refer to ICU for consideration of CPAP or intubation if there is: a CURB score of 4 to 5 and the patient is failing to respond to treatment; persistent hypoxia despite high inspired O_2; progressive hypercapnia; severe acidosis; shock; or depressed conscious level.

Complications

• Parapneumonic effusion. • Empyema. • Lobar collapse. • Thromboembolic disease. • Pneumothorax. • Lung abscess (*S. aureus*). • Renal failure, ARDS, multiorgan failure. • Ectopic abscess formation (*S. aureus*). • Hepatitis, pericarditis, myocarditis, meningoencephalitis. • Pyrexia attributed to drug hypersensitivity.

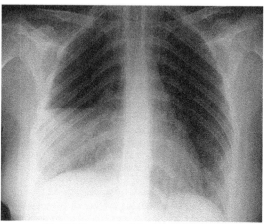

Fig. 9.5 Pneumonia of the right middle lobe.

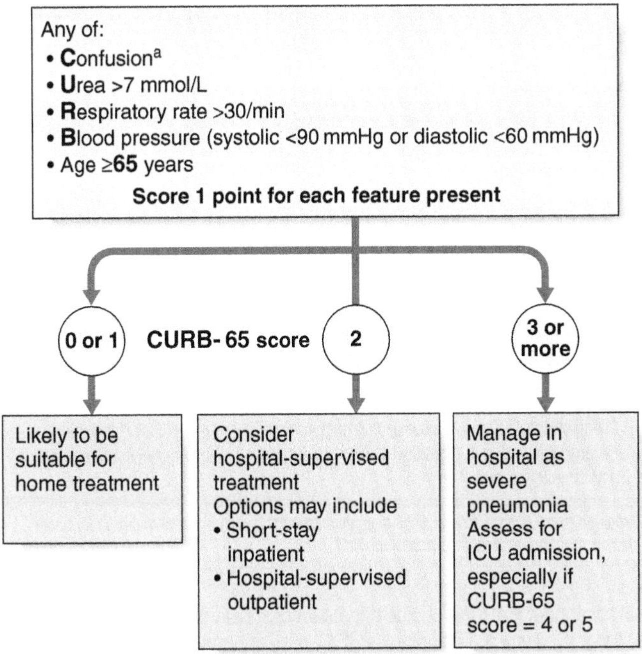

Any of:
- **C**onfusion[a]
- **U**rea >7 mmol/L
- **R**espiratory rate >30/min
- **B**lood pressure (systolic <90 mmHg or diastolic <60 mmHg)
- Age ≥**65** years

Score 1 point for each feature present

(0 or 1) **CURB- 65 score** (2) (3 or more)

| Likely to be suitable for home treatment | Consider hospital-supervised treatment Options may include • Short-stay inpatient • Hospital-supervised outpatient | Manage in hospital as severe pneumonia Assess for ICU admission, especially if CURB-65 score = 4 or 5 |

Fig. 9.6 Hospital CURB-65. [a]Defined as an abbreviated mental test score of 8 or less, or new disorientation in person, place or time. (A urea of 7 mmol/L ≅ 20 mg/dL.)

Follow-up and prevention

Improvement in the CXR typically lags behind clinical recovery. Review should be arranged at around 6 weeks, and a CXR obtained if there are persistent symptoms, physical signs or reasons to suspect underlying malignancy.

Influenza vaccination and pneumococcal vaccination are recommended for selected high-risk patients.

Hospital-acquired pneumonia

HAP is defined as a new episode of pneumonia occurring at least 2 days after admission to hospital. Risk factors for HAP include reduced immune defences (e.g. glucocorticoid treatment, diabetes, malignancy), reduced cough reflex (e.g. postoperative) and bulbar or vocal cord palsy, for example, in stroke. Aspiration because of reduced conscious level, vomiting, dysphagia, reflux or nasogastric intubation also predisposes, as do dental, sinus or abdominal sepsis.

Management and prognosis

Patients who have received no previous antibiotics can be treated with co-amoxiclav or cefuroxime. If the individual has received a course of recent antibiotics, then piperacillin/tazobactam or a third-generation cephalosporin should be considered.

> ### 9.8 Antibiotic treatment for community-acquired pneumonia
>
> **Uncomplicated CAP**
>
> - Amoxicillin 500 mg three times daily orally for 7 to 10 days
> - If penicillin allergy, clarithromycin 500 mg twice daily *or* erythromycin 500 mg four times daily
>
> **If *Staphylococcus* is cultured or suspected**
>
> - Flucloxacillin 1 to 2 g IV four times daily *plus*
> - Clarithromycin 500 mg IV twice daily
>
> **If *Mycoplasma* or *Legionella* is suspected**
>
> - Clarithromycin 500 mg twice daily *or* erythromycin 500 mg four times daily *plus*
> - Rifampicin 600 mg IV twice daily in severe cases
>
> **Severe CAP**
>
> - Clarithromycin 500 mg IV twice daily *or* erythromycin 500 mg–1 g IV four times daily *plus*
> - Co-amoxiclav 1.2 g IV three times daily *or* ceftriaxone 1–2 g IV daily *or* cefuroxime 1.5 g IV three times daily
>
> *(Modified from British Thoracic Society guidelines-https://www.brit-thoracic.org.uk/quality-improvement/guidelines/pneumonia-adults/.)*

In late-onset HAP, the choice of antibiotics must cover the Gram-negative bacteria, *S. aureus* (including MRSA) and anaerobes. Antipseudomonal cover may be provided by meropenem or a third-generation cephalosporin combined with an aminoglycoside. MRSA cover may be provided using vancomycin or linezolid. The choice of agents is most appropriately guided by local patterns of microbiology and antibiotic resistance. It is usual to commence broad-based cover, discontinuing less appropriate antibiotics as culture results become available.

The mortality from HAP is high (~30%). Prevention involves scrupulous hand washing and disinfection of the clinical environment and limiting the use of proton pump inhibitors.

Suppurative and aspiration pneumonia (including pulmonary abscess)

In suppurative pneumonia there is destruction of the lung parenchyma by the inflammatory process. Microabscess formation is a characteristic histological feature of suppurative pneumonia; the term 'pulmonary abscess' refers to large localised collections of pus. Organisms include *S. aureus* and *Klebsiella pneumoniae*. Suppurative pneumonia may be produced by primary infection, inhalation of septic material from the oropharynx or haematogenous spread (e.g. in IV drug abusers). Bacterial infection of a pulmonary infarct or of a collapsed lobe may also produce suppurative pneumonia or lung abscess.

CXR characteristically demonstrates a dense opacity with cavitation and/or a fluid level. Treatment is with amoxicillin with metronidazole, modified as required on culture results. Prolonged treatment for 4 to 6 weeks may be required for abscesses.

Pneumonia in the immunocompromised patient

Pulmonary infection is common in patients receiving immunosuppressive drugs and in diseases causing defects of cellular or humoral immune mechanisms. Most infections are caused by the same common pathogens that cause CAP. Gram-negative bacteria, especially *P. aeruginosa*, are more of a problem than Gram-positive organisms, however, and unusual organisms or those normally considered to be nonpathogenic may become 'opportunistic' pathogens. More than one organism may be present.

Clinical features and investigations

Patients may have nonspecific symptoms, and the onset tends to be less rapid in those with opportunistic organisms such as *Pneumocystis jirovecii* and mycobacterial infections. In *P. jirovecii* pneumonia, cough and breathlessness can precede the CXR abnormality by several days. At presentation the patient is usually pyrexial and hypoxic with normal breath sounds. Induced sputum may yield a diagnosis, and HRCT may reveal cavitation, aspergilloma or the typical bilateral airspace opacities of *Pneumocystis*. Bronchoscopy is useful if safe but often too risky.

Management

Whenever possible, treatment should be directed against an identified organism. Frequently, the cause is not known, and broad-spectrum antibiotic therapy is required (e.g. a third-generation cephalosporin, or a quinolone, + an antistaphylococcal antibiotic, or an antipseudomonal penicillin + an aminoglycoside); treatment is thereafter tailored according to the results of investigations and the clinical response. The investigation and management of *P. jirovecii* infection is described above.

Tuberculosis

TB is caused by infection with *Mycobacterium Tuberculosis* (MTB), which is part of a complex of organisms that also includes *M. bovis* (reservoir cattle) and *M. africanum* (reservoir human).

Incidence of TB in the United Kingdom is slowly falling; however, worldwide, 9.6 million new cases were recorded in 2014, the majority in the poorest nations, who struggle to cover the costs of management and control programmes. In the same year, 1.5 million men, women and children died of TB, and TB continues to rank alongside HIV as a leading cause of death worldwide.

MTB is spread by the inhalation of aerosolised droplet nuclei from other infected patients. At the site of infection, a mass of granulomas forms around an area of caseation, creating the primary lung lesion, a 'Ghon focus'. The combination of a primary lesion and regional lymph node involvement is termed the 'primary complex of Ranke'. If the bacilli spread (either by lymph or blood) before immunity is established, secondary foci may arise in other organs, including lymph nodes, serous membranes, meninges, bones, liver, kidneys and lungs. These foci resolve once an immune response is mounted and the organisms gradually lose viability. However, 'latent bacilli' may persist for years, and can still be detected by tuberculin skin testing or an IGRA. Factors predisposing to TB are summarised in Box 9.9.

9.9 Factors increasing the risk of TB

Patient-related

- Age (children > young adults < elderly)
- First-generation immigrants from high-prevalence countries
- Close contacts of smear-positive patients; worse in overcrowding, e.g. prisons, dormitories
- CXR evidence of self-healed TB
- Primary infection <1 year previously.
- Tobacco use

Associated diseases

- Immunosuppression: HIV, anti-TNF) therapy, high-dose glucocorticoids, cytotoxic agents
- Malignancy (especially lymphoma and leukaemia)
- Type 1 diabetes mellitus
- Chronic kidney disease
- Silicosis
- GI disease with malnutrition (gastrectomy, bypass, pancreatic cancer, malabsorption)
- Deficiency of vitamin D or A
- Recent measles in children

Clinical features

Primary pulmonary TB: This refers to infection of a previously uninfected (tuberculin-negative) individual. A few patients develop a self-limiting febrile illness, but clinical disease occurs only if there is a hypersensitivity reaction or progressive infection. Progressive primary disease may appear during the initial illness or after a latent period of weeks or months.

Miliary TB: Blood-borne dissemination causes miliary TB, which may present acutely or subacutely with 2 to 3 weeks of fever, night sweats, anorexia, weight loss and dry cough. Hepatosplenomegaly may be present, and headache may indicate coexistent tuberculous meningitis. Auscultation is frequently normal, although with more advanced disease widespread crackles occur. Fundoscopy may show choroidal tubercles. CXR demonstrates fine, 1- to 2-mm lesions ('millet seed') distributed throughout the lungs. Anaemia and leucopenia may be present.

Post-primary pulmonary TB: This is the most frequent form of postprimary disease. Onset occurs insidiously over several weeks. Systemic symptoms include fever, night sweats, malaise and loss of appetite and weight, and are accompanied by cough, often with haemoptysis. CXR typically shows an ill-defined opacity situated in one of the upper lobes. As disease progresses, consolidation, collapse and cavitation may develop. A miliary pattern or cavitation suggests active disease.

Extrapulmonary TB (Box 9.10): This accounts for around 20% of cases in HIV-negative individuals, and is more common in HIV-positive individuals. Cervical or mediastinal lymphadenitis is the most common extrapulmonary

i 9.10	**Extrapulmonary manifestations of TB**
Neurological	Tuberculous meningitis, hydrocephalus, tuberculoma, cord compression, cranial nerve palsy
Abdominal	Abdominal mass, psoas abscess, mesenteric adenitis, intestinal obstruction, ascites, anorectal ulceration
Cardiovascular	Pericardial effusion, constrictive pericarditis
Musculoskeletal	Spinal TB with chronic back pain and kyphosis, monoarthritis
Urogenital	Haematuria/dysuria, female infertility, epididymitis
General	Weight loss, fever, night sweats, lymphadenopathy

presentation. Meningeal disease represents the most important form of CNS TB, as it is rapidly fatal if unrecognised and untreated.

Investigations

Typical CXR appearances are shown in Fig. 9.7. Tuberculosis is usually confirmed by direct microscopy (Ziehl–Neelsen or auramine staining) and culture of sputum, bronchial washings or samples from other infected sites. Between 5000 and 10000 acid-fast bacilli must be present for sputum to be smear-positive, whereas only 10 to 100 viable organisms are required for culture-positivity. The slow growth of MTB on solid and liquid culture media has prompted the development of nucleic acid amplification tests (NAATs) which can detect MTB (and rifampicin resistance) in less than 2 hours. Although specific to MTB, NAATs are not sufficiently sensitive to replace culture. With increasing prevalence of drug resistant TB, molecular tests of drug sensitivity are increasingly important.

Chemotherapy

Standard therapy involves 6 months' treatment with isoniazid and rifampicin, supplemented in the first 2 months with pyrazinamide and ethambutol. Fixed-dose tablets combining two or three drugs are preferred. Treatment should be commenced immediately in any patient who is smear-positive or smear-negative but with typical CXR changes and no response to standard antibiotics. Six months of therapy is appropriate for pulmonary TB and most extrapulmonary TB; however, 12 months of therapy is recommended for meningeal TB, including spinal TB with spinal cord involvement—in these cases, ethambutol may be replaced by streptomycin. Pyridoxine should be prescribed in pregnant women and malnourished patients to reduce the risk of peripheral neuropathy with isoniazid. Where drug resistance is not anticipated, patients can be assumed to be noninfectious after 2 weeks of therapy.

Regular monitoring of LFTs is important, as several antituberculous drugs are potentially hepatotoxic. Glucocorticoids reduce inflammation and limit tissue damage and are currently recommended when treating pericardial or meningeal disease, and in children with endobronchial disease. They may also be of benefit in pleural effusion, ureteric TB and severe pulmonary TB.

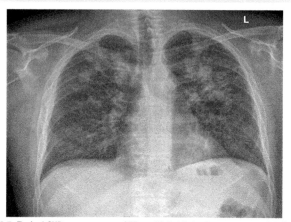

Fig. 9.7 Typical CXR appearances of TB: multiple bilateral upper-zone soft infiltrates with cavitation.

Control and prevention

Detection of latent TB: Latent TB carries a lifetime risk of developing disease of 5% to 15%, with most cases occurring in the first 5 years. It can be detected from the immune response (IGRA test).

Contact tracing allows identification of an index case, other persons infected by the index case and close contacts who should receive BCG vaccination or chemotherapy. Approximately 10% to 20% of close contacts of smear-positive patients and 2% to 5% of those with smear-negative, culture-positive disease have evidence of TB infection. An otherwise asymptomatic contact with a positive tuberculin skin test or IGRA but a normal CXR may be treated with chemoprophylaxis (e.g. rifampicin and isoniazid for 3 months) to prevent progression to clinical disease. Chemoprophylaxis should be offered to adults up to the age of 65. It should also be considered for HIV-infected close contacts of a patient with smear-positive disease. Tuberculin skin testing may be falsely positive in BCG-vaccinated patients and those exposed to nontuberculous mycobacteria. False-negative skin tests occur with immunosuppression or overwhelming infection. These limitations may be overcome by employing IGRAs that are specific to MTB.

Directly observed therapy: Poor adherence to therapy causes prolonged illness, risk of relapse and drug resistance. DOT involves the supervised administration of therapy three times weekly. In the United Kingdom, it is recommended for at-risk groups, including homeless people, alcohol or drug users, patients with serious mental illness and those with a history of nonadherence.

TB and HIV/AIDS

The close links between HIV and TB, particularly in sub-Saharan Africa, are a major challenge. Programmes that link detection and treatment of

TB with detection and treatment of HIV are important, and all patients with TB should be tested for HIV. Mortality is high, and TB is a leading cause of death in HIV patients.

Drug-resistant TB

Globally, 3.3% of new TB cases and 20% of previously treated cases have multi-drug resistant TB (MDR-TB), 9.7% of whom have extremely drug resistant TB (XDR-TB). Cure is possible, but prolonged treatment with less effective, more toxic and more expensive therapies is necessary.

Vaccines

BCG is a live attenuated vaccine used to stimulate protective immunity. It prevents disseminated disease in children, but efficacy in adults is inconsistent. Vaccination policies vary worldwide; in the United Kingdom, vaccination is recommended for infants in high-prevalence communities, health-care workers and selected contacts.

Prognosis

Cure should be anticipated in the majority of patients. There is a small (<5%) risk of relapse, and most recurrences occur within 5 months. Without treatment, a patient with smear-positive TB will remain infectious for around 2 years; in 1 year, 25% of untreated cases will die.

Opportunistic mycobacterial infection

Other species of environmental mycobacteria may colonise damaged lungs or cause disease. They are low-grade pathogens, found most commonly in immunocompromised patients or scarred lungs (e.g. cystic fibrosis). *M. kansasii*, *M. avium* complex (MAC), *M. malmoense*, *M. abscessus* and *M. xenopi* may cause nodular or cavitating lung disease. These organisms are not communicable (except for *M. abscessus* in cystic fibrosis), but they can be multi-resistant, and prolonged treatment is needed if disease occurs.

Respiratory diseases caused by fungi

Allergic bronchopulmonary aspergillosis

ABPA is a hypersensitivity reaction to *Aspergillus fumigatus*. The diagnosis may be suggested by pulmonary infiltrates on routine CXRs of patients with asthma or cystic fibrosis. A persistent vigorous inflammatory response leads to bronchiectasis.

Investigations

• Proximal bronchiectasis on CT. • High serum total IgE and *Aspergillus*-specific IgE. • Elevated *A. fumigatus* precipitins in serum. • Blood eosinophilia. • *A. fumigatus* in sputum.

Management

• Low-dose regular prednisolone (7.5–10 mg daily) suppresses disease. • Itraconazole may be used as a steroid-sparing agent. • Anti-IgE monoclonal antibodies may be helpful in resistant cases.

Chronic pulmonary aspergillosis

This encompasses simple aspergilloma and a range of rare cavitary, fibrosing and semi-invasive conditions, which are hard to diagnose and require prolonged systemic antifungal treatment.

Simple aspergilloma

Aspergillus colonises cavities left by diseases such as TB. CXR and CT reveal an irregular cavity containing a fungal ball, blood tests show elevated precipitins/IgG to *A. fumigatus,* and sputum examination demonstrates *A. fumigatus.*

Aspergillomas are often asymptomatic, but they can cause lethargy, weight loss and recurrent haemoptysis, which may be life threatening.

Asymptomatic cases do not require treatment, but haemoptysis should be controlled by surgery, or tranexamic acid and bronchial artery embolisation if surgery is not possible.

Invasive pulmonary aspergillosis

This serious condition usually occurs in neutropenic patients immunocompromised by either drugs or disease. It should be suspected when such patients develop a severe suppurative pneumonia that has not responded to antibiotics. Demonstration of abundant fungal elements in sputum helps diagnosis. Mortality is high, but treatment with antifungal agents such as voriconazole, amphotericin or caspofungin may be successful.

Tumours of the bronchus and lung

Lung cancer is the most common cause of cancer death worldwide, accounting for 1.59 million deaths per year. Smoking is thought to be directly responsible for at least 90% of lung carcinomas, the risk being directly proportional to the amount smoked and the tar content of cigarettes. Risk falls slowly after smoking cessation but remains above the risk in nonsmokers for many years. Smoking rates and lung cancer incidence are falling in the developed world but rising in developing countries. Exposure to naturally occurring radon is another known risk. The incidence of lung cancer is slightly higher in urban than in rural dwellers; this may reflect differences in atmospheric pollution (including tobacco smoke) or occupation, because a number of industrial materials (e.g. asbestos and silica) are associated with lung cancer.

Lung cancer

This tumour arises from the bronchial epithelium or mucous glands. The common cell types are adenocarcinoma (35%–40%), squamous (25%–30%), small cell (15%) and large cell (10%–15%). Lung cancer presents in many different ways. If the tumour arises in a large bronchus, symptoms arise early, but tumours originating in a peripheral bronchus can grow large without producing symptoms. Peripheral squamous tumours may cavitate. Local spread may occur into the mediastinum and invade or compress the pericardium, oesophagus, superior vena cava, trachea or phrenic or left recurrent laryngeal nerves. Lymphatic spread to supraclavicular and mediastinal lymph nodes is also frequently observed. Blood-borne metastases most commonly affect liver, bone, brain, adrenals and skin. Even a small primary tumour may cause widespread metastatic deposits; this is a particular characteristic of small cell lung cancers.

Clinical features

Cough: This is the most common early symptom.

Haemoptysis: This occurs especially with central tumours.

Bronchial obstruction: Complete obstruction causes collapse of a lobe or lung, with breathlessness, mediastinal displacement, dullness to percussion and reduced breath sounds. Partial obstruction may cause unilateral monophonic wheeze that fails to clear with coughing, and may also impair the drainage of secretions, causing pneumonia or lung abscess. Persistent pneumonia in a smoker suggests an underlying lung cancer. Stridor (a harsh inspiratory noise) occurs when the trachea or larynx is narrowed by tumour or nodes.

Breathlessness: Cancer may present with breathlessness by causing collapse, pneumonia or pleural effusion, or by compressing a phrenic nerve and leading to diaphragmatic paralysis.

Pain and nerve entrapment: Pleural pain may indicate malignant pleural invasion or distal infection. Apical lung cancer may cause Horner's syndrome (ipsilateral partial ptosis, enophthalmos, miosis and hypohidrosis of the face; p. 792) attributed to involvement of the sympathetic nerves in the neck. Pancoast's syndrome (pain in the inner aspect of the arm, with weakness or wasting in the hand) indicates involvement of the brachial plexus by an apical tumour.

Mediastinal spread: Involvement of the oesophagus may cause dysphagia. Pericardial involvement may lead to arrhythmia or effusion. Superior vena cava obstruction by malignant nodes causes suffusion and swelling of the neck and face, conjunctival oedema, headache and dilated veins on the chest wall. Involvement of the left recurrent laryngeal nerve by tumours at the left hilum causes voice alteration and a 'bovine' cough. Enlarged supraclavicular lymph nodes may be palpable.

Metastatic spread: This may lead to focal neurological defects, epileptic seizures, personality change, jaundice, bone pain or skin nodules. Lassitude, anorexia and weight loss usually indicate metastatic spread.

Finger clubbing: This is often seen (p. 314).

Hypertrophic pulmonary osteoarthropathy: This is a painful periostitis of the distal forearm and leg, most often associated with bronchial carcinoma.

Nonmetastatic extrapulmonary effects: These are described in Box 9.11.

Investigations

The main aims of investigation are to:
• Confirm the diagnosis. • Establish the histological cell type. • Define the extent of the disease.

Common CXR features of bronchial carcinoma are illustrated in Fig. 9.8.

Biopsy and histopathology: Central lung tumours can be biopsied at bronchoscopy, and EBUS sampling of mediastinal and hilar nodes can

> **i** **9.11 Nonmetastatic extrapulmonary manifestations of bronchial carcinoma**
>
> - Hyponatraemia (inappropriate ADH secretion)
> - Ectopic ACTH secretion
> - Hypercalcaemia (PTH-related peptide secretion)
> - Myasthenia (Lambert–Eaton syndrome)
> - Digital clubbing
> - Hypertrophic pulmonary osteoarthropathy
> - Polymyositis and dermatomyositis
> - Carcinoid syndrome
> - Gynaecomastia
> - Polyneuropathy
> - Myelopathy
> - Cerebellar degeneration
> - Nephrotic syndrome
> - Eosinophilia

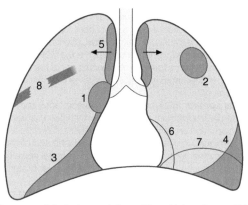

Fig. 9.8 Common radiological presentations of bronchial carcinoma. (1) Hilar mass. (2) Peripheral opacity. (3) Lung, lobe or segmental collapse. (4) Pleural effusion. (5) Broadening of mediastinum. (6) Enlarged cardiac shadow. (7) Elevation of hemidiaphragm. (8) Rib destruction.

facilitate staging at the same procedure. For peripheral tumours, biopsy is performed by percutaneous needle biopsy under CT or USS guidance. There is a small risk of pneumothorax, which may preclude the procedure if there is extensive COPD. In patients with pleural effusions, pleural aspiration and biopsy is the preferred investigation. Thoracoscopy increases yield by allowing biopsies under direct vision. In patients with metastatic disease, the diagnosis can be confirmed by needle aspiration or biopsy of affected lymph nodes, skin lesions, liver or bone marrow.

Staging to guide treatment: Small-cell lung cancer metastasises early, and this normally precludes surgery. In patients with nonsmall cell cancer, CT staging to detect local or distant spread is required to plan treatment. Upper mediastinal or hilar lymph nodes may be sampled using endobronchial ultrasound (EBUS) or mediastinoscopy. Lower mediastinal nodes can be sampled through the oesophageal wall using endoscopic USS. Combined CT and PET is used increasingly to detect metastases. Head CT, radionuclide bone scanning, liver USS and bone marrow biopsy are reserved for patients with clinical or biochemical evidence of spread to these sites. Staging data are used to determine management and prognosis (Fig. 9.9). Physiological testing is also required to assess the patient's fitness for aggressive treatment.

Management and prognosis

Surgical resection carries the best hope of long-term survival, but some patients treated with radical radiotherapy and chemotherapy also achieve prolonged remission or cure. In more than 75% of cases, treatment aimed at cure is not possible or is inappropriate because of extensive spread or comorbidity; these patients receive palliative treatment and best supportive care.

Surgical treatment: Accurate preoperative staging, coupled with improvements in surgical and postoperative care, now offers 5-year survival rates of over 75% in stage I disease and 55% in stage II disease.

Radiotherapy: Patients treated for limited stage disease with radical radiotherapy can also achieve prolonged remission or cure. Radiotherapy is, however, used mainly to palliate complications such as large airway obstruction, superior vena cava obstruction, recurrent haemoptysis and pain from chest wall invasion or skeletal metastases.

Chemotherapy: In small cell carcinoma, chemotherapy with radiotherapy can increase median survival from 3 months to well over a year. Chemotherapy is generally less effective in nonsmall cell lung cancers, although platinum-based regimens offer 30% response rates and a modest increase in survival. Mutation-targeted chemotherapy is used in selected cases.

Malignant pleural effusions should be treated by drainage and pleurodesis if the patient is symptomatic.

The best outcomes are obtained when lung cancer is managed in specialist centres by multidisciplinary teams including oncologists, thoracic surgeons, respiratory physicians and specialist nurses. Effective communication, pain relief and attention to nutrition are important.

Overall, the prognosis in bronchial carcinoma is very poor, with around 70% of patients dying within 1 year of diagnosis and less than 8% of patients surviving 5 years after diagnosis.

Secondary tumours of the lung

The most common tumours that metastasise to the lung are those of the breast, kidney, uterus, ovary, testes and thyroid, often with multiple deposits. Lymphatic infiltration (lymphangitis) may develop in patients with carcinoma of the breast, stomach, bowel, pancreas or bronchus. This grave condition causes severe and rapidly progressive breathlessness associated with marked hypoxaemia.

Tumour stage	Lymph node spread			
	N0 (None)	N1 (Ipsilateral hilar)	N2 (Ipsilateral mediastinal or subcarinal)	N3 (Contralateral or supraclavicular)
T1a (≤1 cm)	IA1 (92%)	IIB (53%)	IIIA (36%)	IIIB (26%)
T1b (>1 to ≤2 cm)	IA2 (83%)			
T1c (>2 to ≤3 cm)	IA3 (77%)			
T2a (>3 to ≤4 cm)	IB (68%)			
T2b (>4 cm to ≤5 cm)	IIA (60%)			
T3 (>5 cm)	IIB (53%)	IIIA (36%)	IIIB (26%)	IIIC (13%)
T4 (>7 cm or invading heart, vessels, oesophagus, carina etc.)				
M1a Lung metastasis/effusion	IVA (10%)			
M1b Single extrathoracic metastasis				
M1c Multiple extrathoracic metastases	IVB (0%)			

Fig. 9.9 Tumour stage and survival in non-small-cell lung cancer. For each clinical stage, percentage survival at 5 years is shown in brackets.

Tumours of the mediastinum

A variety of conditions can present radiologically as a mediastinal mass (Fig. 9.10). Benign tumours and cysts in the mediastinum are often an incidental finding. Malignant mediastinal tumours are distinguished by their power to invade, as well as compress, structures such as bronchi and lungs. CT (or MRI) is the investigation of choice for mediastinal tumours.

Interstitial and infiltrative pulmonary diseases

Diffuse parenchymal lung disease

DPLDs are a heterogeneous group of conditions affecting the pulmonary parenchyma (interstitium), which share a number of clinical, physiological and radiographic similarities. The current classification is shown in Fig. 9.11. They often present with a dry cough and breathlessness that is insidious in onset but relentlessly progressive. Examination reveals fine inspiratory crackles, and in many cases digital clubbing develops. Alternative conditions that may mimic DPLD include diffuse infections (e.g. viral, *Pneumocystis*, TB), malignancy (e.g. lymphoma or bronchoalveolar carcinoma), pulmonary oedema and aspiration.

Investigations

HRCT is central to the evaluation of interstitial lung disease. Appearances vary with diagnosis and stage, including diffuse ground glass infiltrates, nodules and reticular shadowing. Basal subpleural honeycomb shadowing is typical of usual interstitial pneumonia and is normally sufficient to diagnose idiopathic pulmonary fibrosis. Inconsistent clinical or CT findings

9

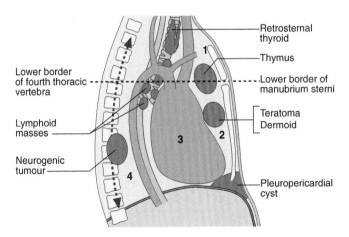

Fig. 9.10 The divisions of the mediastinum. (1) Superior mediastinum. (2) Anterior mediastinum. (3) Middle mediastinum. (4) Posterior mediastinum. Sites of the more common mediastinal tumours are also illustrated. *From Johnson N McL. Respiratory medicine. Oxford: Blackwell Science; 1986.*

should prompt consideration of bronchoalveolar lavage or transbronchial or surgical biopsy. CT may also reveal appearances diagnostic of alternative conditions, for example, subpleural nodules in sarcoid.

Pulmonary function tests in DPLD typically show a restrictive pattern with reduced lung volumes and reduced gas transfer (although gas transfer may be elevated in alveolar haemorrhage).

Idiopathic interstitial pneumonias

This is a subgroup of DPLD with unknown aetiology but distinguished by their radiological and histological appearances.

Idiopathic pulmonary fibrosis

IPF is the most common and important of the idiopathic interstitial pneumonias, characterised by pathological (or radiological) evidence of usual

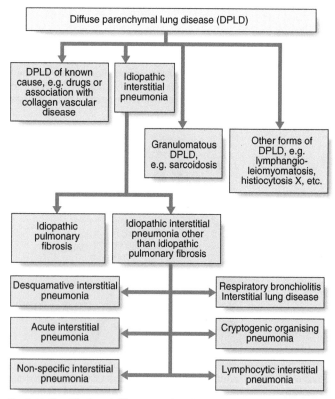

Fig. 9.11 Classification of diffuse parenchymal lung disease.

interstitial pneumonia (UIP). The aetiology remains unknown; speculation has included exposure to infectious agents (e.g. EBV) or to occupational dusts (metal or wood), drugs (antidepressants) or chronic gastro-oesophageal reflux. Some cases are familial. A strong association with smoking exists.

Clinical features

• Uncommon before the age of 50 years. • Usually presents with progressive breathlessness and a nonproductive cough, reduced expansion, tachypnoea and central cyanosis. • Finger clubbing may occur. • Fine inspiratory crackles likened to the parting of Velcro, classically heard at the lung bases. • May be discovered incidentally on CT done for other reasons.

Investigations

CXR demonstrates lower-zone peripheral reticular and reticulonodular shadowing. HRCT may be diagnostic, demonstrating a patchy, predominantly peripheral, subpleural and basal reticular pattern with subpleural cysts (honeycombing) and/or traction bronchiectasis. Pulmonary function tests show a restrictive defect with reduced lung volumes and gas transfer. Exercise tests are useful to demonstrate arterial hypoxaemia on exercise, but as IPF advances, hypoxia is present at rest. Blood tests may reveal a positive antinuclear antibody or evidence of underlying connective tissue disease. Patients with typical clinical features and HRCT appearances consistent with UIP do not require lung biopsy, particularly if other known causes of interstitial lung disease have been excluded.

Management

If the vital capacity is predicted to be between 50% and 80%, patients may be offered either pirfenidone (an antifibrotic agent) or nintedanib (a tyrosine kinase inhibitor). Both drugs reduce the rate of decline in lung function; however neither improves cough or breathlessness, and treatment should be discontinued if lung function declines by more than 10% in the first year. Medication to control gastro-oesophageal reflux may improve cough. Smokers should be advised to stop. Influenza and pneumococcal vaccination should be recommended. Pulmonary rehabilitation, using ambulatory oxygen if appropriate, is beneficial. Domiciliary oxygen may help to palliate breathlessness in hypoxic patients. Where appropriate, lung transplantation should be considered.

A median survival of 3 years is widely quoted; however, the rate of progression varies considerably, from death within a few months to survival for many years. Serial lung function may provide useful prognostic information, with relative preservation of lung function suggesting longer survival, and significantly impaired gas transfer and/or desaturation on exercise indicating a poorer prognosis.

Non-specific interstitial pneumonia

The clinical picture of NSIP is similar to that of IPF, although patients tend to be younger and female. It may present as an isolated idiopathic pulmonary condition, but is often associated with connective tissue disease, drugs, chronic hypersensitivity pneumonitis and HIV infection, and pulmonary symptoms may precede the appearance of connective tissue disease.

HRCT findings are less specific than with IPF, and lung biopsy may be required. The prognosis is better than in IPF (5-year mortality rate of <15%).

Sarcoidosis

Sarcoidosis is a multisystem disorder characterised by noncaseating epithelioid granulomas; it is more common in colder parts of Northern Europe. It tends to cause more severe disease in people of West Indian and Asian origin, sparing Inuit, Arab and Chinese populations. The aetiology is unknown, although atypical mycobacteria, viruses and genetic factors have been proposed. Sarcoidosis is less common in smokers.

Clinical features

Any organ may be affected, but 90% of cases affect the lungs. Otherwise, lymph glands, liver, spleen, skin, eyes, parotid glands and joints are the most frequently involved sites. Löfgren's syndrome—erythema nodosum, peripheral arthropathy, uveitis, bilateral hilar lymphadenopathy (BHL), lethargy and occasionally fever—presents in young adults. BHL may be detected in an otherwise asymptomatic individual undergoing CXR. Pulmonary disease may present insidiously with cough, exertional breathlessness and radiographic infiltrates. Fibrosis occurs in around 20%, and may cause a silent loss of lung function. Nephrocalcinosis attributed to hypercalcaemia is an important complication.

Investigations

• FBC: lymphopenia. • LFTs: may be mildly deranged. • Ca^{2+}: may be elevated. • Serum ACE: a nonspecific marker of disease activity. • CXR: used to stage sarcoid (Box 9.12). • HRCT: characteristic reticulonodular opacities that follow a perilymphatic distribution centred on bronchovascular bundles and the subpleural areas. • Pulmonary function: may show restriction and desaturation on exercise. • Bronchoscopy: may demonstrate a 'cobblestone' appearance of the mucosa, and bronchial and transbronchial biopsies usually show noncaseating granulomas.

i 9.12 CXR stage and outcomes in sarcoidosis	
Stage	Description
Stage I: BHL (usually symmetrical); paratracheal nodes often enlarged	Often asymptomatic, but may be associated with erythema nodosum and arthralgia; majority of cases resolve in <1 year
Stage II: BHL and parenchymal infiltrates	Patients may present with breathlessness or cough; majority of cases resolve spontaneously
Stage III: parenchymal infiltrates without BHL	Disease less likely to resolve spontaneously
Stage IV: pulmonary fibrosis	Can cause progression to ventilatory failure, pulmonary hypertension and cor pulmonale

The occurrence of erythema nodosum in patients in the second to third decades with BHL on CXR is often sufficient for a confident diagnosis.

Management

Most patients enjoy spontaneous remission, so in the absence of organ damage it is appropriate to withhold therapy for 6 months. Patients who present with acute illness with erythema nodosum should receive NSAIDs and, if systemically unwell, glucocorticoids. Systemic glucocorticoids are also indicated for hypercalcaemia, impaired pulmonary or renal function or uveitis. Mild uveitis responds to glucocorticoid eyedrops, and inhaled glucocorticoids can limit the need for systemic glucocorticoids in asymptomatic parenchymal sarcoid. Patients should be warned that sunlight may precipitate hypercalcaemia and renal impairment. Severe disease may respond to methotrexate or azathioprine, but generally the prognosis is good.

Lung diseases attributed to systemic inflammatory disease

Acute respiratory distress syndrome

See p. 82.

9

Respiratory involvement in connective tissue disorders

Pulmonary fibrosis is a recognised complication of many connective tissue diseases. The clinical features are usually indistinguishable from those of IPF (p. 348), and lung disease may precede the onset of other symptoms. Connective tissue disorders may also cause disease of the pleura, diaphragm and chest wall muscles. Pulmonary hypertension and cor pulmonale may complicate pulmonary fibrosis in connective tissue disorders and is particularly common in systemic sclerosis.

Patients with connective tissue disease may also develop respiratory complications because of pulmonary toxic effects of drugs used to treat the connective tissue disorder (e.g. gold and methotrexate), and secondary infection because of neutropenia or immunosuppressive drug regimens.

Rheumatoid disease: Pulmonary fibrosis is the most common pulmonary manifestation. All forms of interstitial disease have been described, but NSIP is probably the most common. Pleural effusion is common, especially in men with seropositive disease. Most resolve spontaneously. Biochemical testing shows an exudative effusion with markedly reduced glucose levels and raised LDH. Effusions that fail to resolve spontaneously may respond to prednisolone (30–40 mg daily), but some become chronic. Rheumatoid pulmonary nodules are usually asymptomatic and detected incidentally on CXR. They are usually multiple and subpleural in site and can mimic cancer. The combination of rheumatoid nodules and pneumoconiosis is known as Caplan's syndrome. Obliterative bronchiolitis and bronchiectasis are also recognised pulmonary complications of rheumatoid arthritis. Treatments given for rheumatoid arthritis may also be relevant; glucocorticoid therapy predisposes to infections, methotrexate may cause pulmonary fibrosis, and anti-TNF therapy has been associated with the reactivation of TB.

Systemic lupus erythematosus: Recurrent pleurisy is common in SLE, with or without effusions. Acute alveolitis, rarely associated with diffuse alveolar haemorrhage, is a life-threatening complication that requires immunosuppression. Pulmonary fibrosis is a relatively uncommon manifestation of SLE. Some patients with SLE present with exertional dyspnoea and orthopnoea, but without pulmonary fibrosis. Pulmonary function testing shows reduced lung volumes, and the CXR reveals elevated diaphragms. This condition ('shrinking lungs') probably represents a diaphragmatic myopathy. Antiphospholipid syndrome is associated with an increased risk of venous and pulmonary thromboembolism, and these patients require lifelong anticoagulation.

Systemic sclerosis: Most patients with systemic sclerosis eventually develop diffuse pulmonary fibrosis (up to 90% at autopsy). In some patients it is indolent, but when progressive, as in IPF, the median survival is around 4 years. Pulmonary fibrosis is rare in the CREST variant of progressive systemic sclerosis, but isolated pulmonary hypertension may develop. Other pulmonary complications include recurrent aspiration pneumonias secondary to oesophageal disease. Rarely, sclerosis of the skin of the chest wall may be so extensive as to restrict chest wall movement—the so-called *hidebound chest.*

Pulmonary eosinophilia and vasculitides

Pulmonary eosinophilia refers to a group of disorders of different aetiology (Box 9.13) in which CXR abnormalities are associated with eosinophilia on bronchoalveolar lavage with or without peripheral blood eosinophilia. Eosinophilic pneumonia may present as an acute febrile illness or with chronic peripheral CXR infiltrates but responds well to glucocorticoids.

Granulomatosis with polyangiitis (formerly Wegener's granulomatosis): This presents with cough, haemoptysis, chest pain and fever. Nasal discharge and crusting, as well as otitis media, also occur. Multiple cavitating nodules are seen on CXR. Nasal or lung biopsies show distinctive necrotising granulomas and vasculitis. Complications include subglottic stenosis and saddle nose deformity. Treatment is with immunosuppression. The differential includes eosinic granulomatosis with polyangiitis (Box 9.13).

 9.13 Pulmonary eosinophilia

Extrinsic

- Helminths, e.g. *Ascaris, Toxocara, Filaria*
- Drugs, e.g. nitrofurantoin, sulfasalazine, imipramine, chlorpropamide, phenylbutazone
- Fungi, e.g. *Aspergillus fumigatus* causing ABPA (p. 341)

Intrinsic

- Cryptogenic eosinophilic pneumonia
- Eosinic granulomatosis with polyangiitis (Churg–Strauss syndrome)–asthma, blood eosinophilia, neuropathy, pulmonary infiltrates, eosinophilic vasculitis
- Hypereosinophilic syndrome

Goodpasture's disease: The association of pulmonary haemorrhage and glomerulonephritis, in which IgG antibodies bind to the glomerular or alveolar basement membranes (p. 217). Pulmonary disease usually precedes renal involvement with radiographic infiltrates, hypoxia and haemoptysis. It occurs more commonly in men and almost exclusively in smokers.

Lung diseases attributed to irradiation and drugs

Acute radiation pneumonitis is typically seen within 6 to 12 weeks of lung irradiation, and causes cough and dyspnoea. This may resolve spontaneously but responds to glucocorticoid treatment. Chronic interstitial fibrosis may present several months later.

Drugs may cause a number of parenchymal reactions:

ARDS: Hydrochlorothiazide, streptokinase, aspirin and opiates (in overdose).

Pulmonary eosinophilia: See Box 9.13.

Noneosinophilic alveolitis: Amiodarone, gold, nitrofurantoin, bleomycin, methotrexate.

Pleural disease: Bromocriptine, amiodarone, methotrexate, methysergide or via induction of SLE (phenytoin, hydralazine, isoniazid).

Asthma: β-blockers, cholinergic agonists, aspirin, NSAIDs.

Occupational and environmental lung disease

Occupational airway disease

Occupational asthma: This should be considered in any individual of working age who develops new-onset asthma, particularly if the patient reports an improvement in asthma symptoms during absences from work, for example, at weekends or holidays. Sensitisation to the allergens may be demonstrated by skin testing or measurement of specific IgE. Serial recording of peak flow at work is crucial in confirming causation.

Reactive airways dysfunction syndrome: This is a persistent asthma-like syndrome with airway hyper-reactivity following the inhalation of an airway irritant: typically, a single exposure to a gas, smoke or vapour in very high concentrations. Management is similar to that of asthma.

COPD: Although smoking remains the dominant cause of COPD, occupational COPD is seen in workers exposed to coal dust, crystalline silica, cadmium and biomass fuel smoke.

Pneumoconiosis

This means a permanent alteration of lung structure because of the inhalation of mineral dust, excluding bronchitis and emphysema.

Coal worker's pneumoconiosis: Prolonged inhalation of coal dust overwhelms alveolar macrophages, leading to a fibrotic reaction.

Classification is based on the size and extent of radiographic nodularity. Simple CWP refers to the appearance of small radiographic nodules in an otherwise-well individual. Progressive massive fibrosis refers to the formation of conglomerate masses (mainly in the upper lobes), which may cavitate, associated with cough, sputum and breathlessness. PMF may progress after coal dust exposure ceases and, in extreme cases, causes respiratory failure.

Silicosis: This occurs in stonemasons who inhale crystalline silica, usually as quartz dust. Classic silicosis develops slowly after years of asymptomatic exposure. Accelerated silicosis is associated with shorter exposure (typically 5–10 years) and is more aggressive. Radiological features are similar to those of CWP, with multiple 3- to 5-mm nodular opacities, in the mid- and upper zones. As the disease progresses, PMF may develop. Enlargement of the hilar glands with an 'egg-shell' calcification is uncommon and nonspecific. The patient must be removed from further exposure, but fibrosis progresses even when exposure ceases. Individuals with silicosis are at increased risk of TB, lung cancer and COPD.

Lung diseases attributed to organic dusts

Hypersensitivity pneumonitis

HP (also called extrinsic allergic alveolitis) results from the inhalation of certain types of organic dust that give rise to a diffuse immune complex reaction in the walls of the alveoli and bronchioles. In the United Kingdom, 50% of reported cases of HP occur in farm workers; bird fanciers represent another important group.

Clinical features

The acute form of HP should be suspected when anyone exposed to organic dust complains of 'flu'-like symptoms (headache, malaise, myalgia, fever, dry cough, breathlessness) within a few hours of re-exposure to the same dust. Auscultation reveals widespread end-inspiratory crackles and squeaks. Disease onset is more insidious with chronic low-level exposure (e.g. from an indoor pet bird). If unchecked, the disease may progress to cause fibrosis, severe respiratory disability, hypoxaemia, pulmonary hypertension, cor pulmonale and eventually death.

Investigations

• CXR: demonstrates diffuse micronodular shadowing, which is usually more pronounced in the upper zones. • HRCT: in acute disease, shows bilateral areas of ground glass and consolidation with small centrilobar nodules and expiratory air-trapping. In chronic disease, fibrosis may predominate. • Pulmonary function tests: show a restrictive ventilatory defect with reduced lung volumes and gas transfer. • ABGs: hypoxia in advanced disease. • Serology: shows positive precipitating antibodies to the offending antigen, for example, *Micropolyspora faeni* (farmer's lung) or avian serum proteins (bird fancier's lung). However, precipitating antibodies are frequently present without evidence of HP. • Bronchoalveolar lavage: may show increased CD8+ T lymphocytes. • Lung biopsy: may be necessary for diagnosis.

Management

Whenever possible, the patient should avoid exposure to the inciting agent. This may be difficult, either because of implications for livelihood (e.g. farmers) or addiction to hobbies (e.g. pigeon breeders). Dust masks with appropriate filters may minimise exposure and may be combined with methods of reducing levels of antigen (e.g. drying hay before storage). In acute cases, prednisolone 40 mg/day should be given for 3 to 4 weeks. Most patients recover completely, but the development of interstitial fibrosis causes permanent disability when there has been prolonged exposure to antigen.

Asbestos-related lung and pleural diseases

Asbestos is a naturally occurring silicate, classified into chrysotile (white asbestos: 90% of world production) and serpentine types (crocidolite, blue asbestos and amosite–brown asbestos). It was used extensively as thermal insulation in industry in the mid-20th century. Asbestos exposure may lead to both pleural and pulmonary disease, after a lengthy latent period.

Pleural plaques: Discrete areas of fibrosis, frequently calcified, on the parietal pleura are the most common manifestation of past asbestos exposure. They are asymptomatic and are usually identified incidentally on CXR (Fig. 9.12) or CT scan. They do not impair lung function and are benign.

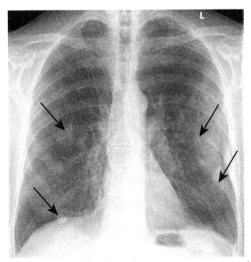

Fig. 9.12 Pleural plaques resulting from asbestos exposure appear as circumscribed calcified opacities (arrows) of similar density to ribs.

Acute benign asbestos pleurisy: Estimated to occur in 20% of asbestos workers, but many episodes are subclinical. When symptomatic, presents with pleurisy and mild fever. Diagnosis necessitates the exclusion of other known causes of pleurisy and effusion. Repeated episodes may lead to diffuse pleural thickening.

Diffuse pleural thickening: Affects the visceral pleura and, if extensive, may cause restrictive lung function impairment, exertional breathlessness and, occasionally, chest pain. The CXR shows extensive pleural thickening and obliteration of the costophrenic angles. CT may also show parenchymal bands and round atelectasis. The condition may progress in around one-third of individuals. In severe cases, surgical decortication may be considered. Pleural biopsy may be required to exclude mesothelioma.

Asbestosis: Lung fibrosis occurring after substantial asbestos exposure over several years; rare with low-level or bystander exposure. It presents with exertional breathlessness and fine, late inspiratory crackles over the lower zones. Finger clubbing may be present. Pulmonary function and HRCT appearances are similar to those of UIP. These features, accompanied by a history of substantial asbestos exposure, are generally sufficient to establish the diagnosis; lung biopsy is rarely necessary. Asbestosis is more slowly progressive and carries a better prognosis than idiopathic pulmonary fibrosis. About 40% of patients (usually smokers) develop lung cancer, and 10% develop mesothelioma.

Mesothelioma: A malignant tumour affecting the pleura or, rarely, the peritoneum. It almost invariably results from past asbestos exposure, which may be minor. There is a long interval between exposure and disease, so deaths from mesothelioma continue to increase, despite improved asbestos control. Pleural mesothelioma presents with increasing breathlessness resulting from pleural effusion, or unremitting chest pain because of chest wall involvement. As the tumour progresses, it encases the lung and may invade the parenchyma, the mediastinum and the pericardium. Metastatic disease is commonly found at postmortem. Prognosis is poor. Highly selected patients may benefit from radical surgery, but, in most, therapy aims to palliate symptoms. Chemotherapy may improve quality of life and yield a small survival benefit (~3 months). Radiotherapy is used to control pain and limit the risk of tumour seeding at biopsy sites. Pleural effusions are managed with drainage and pleurodesis. Survival from onset of symptoms is around 16 months for epithelioid tumours, 10 months for sarcomatoid tumours and 15 months for biphasic tumours.

Lung cancer: Substantial asbestos exposure causes an increased risk of lung cancer, particularly in smokers.

Pulmonary vascular disease

Venous thromboembolism

The majority (80%) of pulmonary emboli arise from the propagation of lower limb DVT. Rare causes include amniotic fluid, placenta, air, fat, tumour (especially choriocarcinoma) and septic emboli (from endocarditis affecting the tricuspid/pulmonary valves). PE is common, occurring in around 1% of all patients admitted to hospital and accounting for around 5% of in-hospital deaths.

Clinical features

Clinical presentation varies, depending on number, size and distribution of emboli and on underlying cardiorespiratory reserve. It is helpful to consider three questions:

• Is the clinical presentation consistent with PE? • Does the patient have risk factors for PE? • Is there any alternative diagnosis that can explain the patient's presentation?

A recognised risk factor for PE (Box 14.5) is present in 80% to 90% of patients. The clinical features (Box 9.14) depend largely upon the size of embolism and on comorbidity.

Investigations

CXR: PE may cause a variety of nonspecific appearances, but most cases have a normal CXR. A normal CXR in an acutely breathless and hypoxaemic patient should raise the suspicion of PE, as should bilateral atelectasis in a patient with unilateral pleuritic chest pain. CXR can also exclude alternatives such as heart failure, pneumonia or pneumothorax.

i	9.14 Features of pulmonary thromboemboli		
	Acute massive PE	**Acute small/ medium PE**	**Chronic PE**
Symptoms	Faintness or collapse, central chest pain, apprehension, severe dyspnoea	Pleuritic chest pain, restricted breathing, haemoptysis	Exertional dyspnoea; late symptoms of pulmonary hypertension or right heart failure
Signs	Major circulatory collapse: tachycardia, hypotension, ↑JVP, RV gallop rhythm, split P_2; severe cyanosis; ↓urinary output	Tachycardia, pleural rub, raised hemidiaphragm, crackles, effusion (often blood-stained), low-grade fever	Early: may be minimal Later: RV heave, loud, split P_2 Advanced: right heart failure
CXR	Usually normal; may be subtle oligaemia	Pleuropulmonary opacities, pleural effusion, linear shadows, raised hemidiaphragm	Enlarged pulmonary artery trunk, enlarged heart, prominent RV
ECG	$S_1Q_3T_3$, anterior T-wave inversion, right bundle branch block	Sinus tachycardia	RV hypertrophy and strain
ABGs	Markedly abnormal with ↓PaO_2 and ↓$PaCO_2$; metabolic acidosis	May be normal or ↓PaO_2	Exertional ↓PaO_2 or desaturation on exercise testing
Alternative diagnoses	Myocardial infarction, pericardial tamponade, aortic dissection	Pneumonia, pneumothorax, musculoskeletal chest pain	Other causes of pulmonary hypertension

ECG: ECG is often normal, but is helpful in excluding alternatives, for example, MI or pericarditis. The most common findings in PE are sinus tachycardia and anterior T-wave inversion; larger emboli may cause right heart strain with an $S_1Q_3T_3$ pattern, ST-segment and T-wave changes, or right bundle branch block.

ABGs: Typically show a reduced PaO_2 and a normal or low $PaCO_2$ but are occasionally normal. Metabolic acidosis may occur in acute massive PE with shock.

D-dimer: An elevated D-dimer is of limited value because it also occurs with myocardial infarction, pneumonia and sepsis. However, low levels, particularly when clinical risk is low, have a high negative predictive value, and further investigation is usually unnecessary (Fig. 9.13).

The D-dimer result should be disregarded in high-risk patients, as further investigation is mandatory even when normal. Serum troponin I may be elevated, reflecting right heart strain.

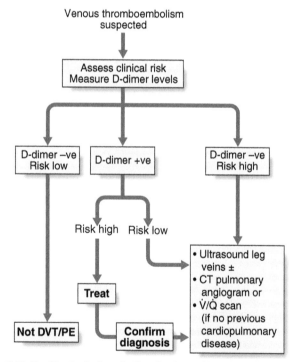

Fig. 9.13 Algorithm for the investigation of patients with suspected pulmonary thromboembolism. Clinical risk is based on the presence of risk factors for venous thromboembolism and the probability of another diagnosis. *DVT,* Deep vein thrombosis; *PE,* pulmonary embolism; *V/Q,* ventilation/perfusion.

CT pulmonary angiogram (CTPA): This is now the first-line diagnostic test (Fig. 9.14). It may not only exclude PE, but also reveal an alternative diagnosis. Contrast media, however, are nephrotoxic, and care should be taken in patients with renal impairment. In these patients, and in those with allergy to IV contrast, ventilation/perfusion scanning is an alternative.

Doppler USS of the leg veins: This may be used in patients with suspected PE, particularly if there are clinical signs in a limb, as many will have identifiable proximal leg vein thrombus.

Echocardiography: This is helpful in the differential diagnosis and assessment of acute circulatory collapse. Acute right heart dilatation is frequently present in massive PE, and thrombus may be visible. Alternative diagnoses, including left ventricular failure, aortic dissection and pericardial tamponade, can also be established.

Pulmonary angiography: This is still useful in selected settings or for the delivery of catheter-based therapies.

Management

General measures: Sufficient oxygen should be given to all hypoxaemic patients to restore SpO_2 to more than 90%. Hypotension should be treated using IV fluid or plasma expander; diuretics and vasodilators should be avoided. Opiates may be necessary to relieve pain and distress but should be used with caution. External cardiac massage may be successful in the moribund patient by dislodging and breaking up a large central embolus.

Anticoagulation: The principal treatment for PE is anticoagulation, which is discussed for PE and other forms of VTE on p. 588.

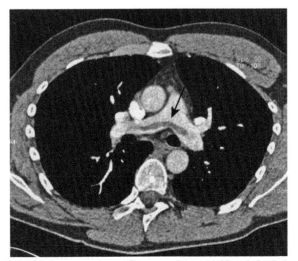

Fig. 9.14 CT pulmonary angiogram. The *arrow* points to a saddle embolism in the bifurcation of the pulmonary artery.

Thrombolytic therapy: Thrombolysis improves outcome when acute massive PE is accompanied by cardiogenic shock (systolic BP <90 mmHg), but has no clear benefits in normotensive patients. It carries a risk of intracranial haemorrhage, and patients must be screened carefully for haemorrhagic risk.

Caval filters: Selected patients with recurrent PE despite adequate anticoagulation or in whom anticoagulation is contraindicated may benefit from insertion of a filter in the inferior vena cava below the origin of the renal veins.

Prognosis

Immediate mortality is greatest in those with echocardiographic evidence of right ventricular dysfunction or cardiogenic shock. Once anticoagulation is commenced, however, the risk of mortality falls rapidly. The risk of recurrence is highest in the first 6 to 12 months after the initial event, and at 10 years around one-third of individuals will have suffered a further event.

Pulmonary hypertension

Pulmonary hypertension is defined as a mean pulmonary artery pressure of more than 25 mmHg at rest. The causes are listed in Box 9.15. Further classification is based on the degree of functional disturbance using the NYHA grades I to IV (Box 8.1, CH8 p1). Respiratory failure because of intrinsic pulmonary disease is the most common cause of pulmonary hypertension.

Primary pulmonary hypertension is a rare but important disease that predominantly affects women aged 20 to 30 years. It is usually sporadic but rarely is associated with an inherited mutation.

i	9.15 Classification of pulmonary hypertension	
Pulmonary arterial hypertension	Primary: sporadic and familial Secondary: connective tissue disease (limited cutaneous systemic sclerosis), congenital systemic to pulmonary shunts, portal hypertension, HIV infection, exposure to various drugs or toxins, persistent pulmonary hypertension of the newborn	
Pulmonary venous hypertension	Left-sided valvular or ventricular disease, pulmonary veno-occlusive disease	
Pulmonary hypertension associated with parenchymal lung disease and/or hypoxaemia	COPD; DPLD; sleep-disordered breathing; chronic high-altitude exposure, severe kyphoscoliosis	
Chronic thromboembolic disease	Recurrent thromboemboli, in situ thrombosis, sickle-cell disease	

(Modified from Dana Point 2008. Simmoneau G, et al. Updated clinical classification of pulmonary hypertension. J Am Coll Cardiol 2009; 54:S43–554.)

Presentation is with exertional breathlessness and syncope. Radiology shows enlarged pulmonary arteries, and echocardiography shows an enlarged right ventricle; pulmonary artery pressure can be estimated from the velocity of tricuspid regurgitation on Doppler echo.

The median survival from time of diagnosis (without heart–lung transplantation) is 2 to 3 years. Management should be guided by specialists and includes diuretics, oxygen, anticoagulation and vaccination against infection. Specific treatments include iloprost, epoprostenol, sildenafil and the oral endothelin receptor antagonist bosentan; these can dramatically improve exercise performance symptoms and prognosis in selected cases. Double lung transplantation may be considered in selected patients, and pulmonary thrombo-endarterectomy should be contemplated in patients with chronic proximal pulmonary thromboembolism.

Diseases of the upper airway

Diseases of the nasopharynx

Allergic rhinitis

In this disorder there are episodes of nasal congestion, watery nasal discharge and sneezing. It may be seasonal or perennial (continuous symptoms). It is because of an immediate hypersensitivity reaction to antigens including pollens from grasses (hay fever), flowers, weeds or trees. Perennial allergic rhinitis may be a reaction to antigens from house dust, fungal spores or animal dander, or to physical or chemical irritants. Skin hypersensitivity tests with the relevant antigen are usually positive in seasonal allergic rhinitis, but less useful in perennial rhinitis.

Management
Exposure to trigger antigens (e.g. pollen) should be minimised. The following medications may be used singly or in combination: an oral antihistamine, a topical glucocorticoid nasal spray and/or sodium cromoglicate nasal spray. When severe symptoms interfere with daily activities, immunotherapy (desensitisation) is also used, but carries the risk of serious reactions and must be managed in specialist centres.

Sleep-disordered breathing

A variety of respiratory disorders manifest themselves during sleep, for example, nocturnal cough and wheeze in asthma. Nocturnal hypoventilation may exacerbate respiratory failure in patients with restrictive lung disease such as that attributed to kyphoscoliosis, diaphragmatic palsy or muscle weakness (e.g. muscular dystrophy). In contrast, a small but important group of disorders cause problems only during sleep because of upper airway obstruction (obstructive sleep apnoea) or abnormalities of ventilatory drive (central sleep apnoea).

The sleep apnoea/hypopnoea syndrome

Recurrent upper airway obstruction during sleep, sufficient to cause sleep fragmentation and daytime sleepiness, is thought to affect 2% of women and 4% of men aged 30 to 60 years in Caucasian populations. Daytime sleepiness results in a threefold increased risk of road traffic accidents.

A reduction in upper airway muscle tone during sleep results in pharyngeal narrowing, which often manifests as snoring. Negative pharyngeal pressure during inspiration can then cause complete upper airway occlusion, usually at the level of the soft palate. This leads to transient wakefulness and recovery of upper airway muscle tone. The subject rapidly returns to sleep, snores and becomes apnoeic once more. This cycle repeats itself many times, causing severe sleep fragmentation (sleep apnoea/hypopnoea syndrome; SAHS). Predisposing factors include:

• Obesity. • Male gender. • Nasal obstruction. • Acromegaly. • Hypothyroidism. • Familial causes (back-set mandible and maxilla). • Alcohol and sedatives (relaxation of the upper airway dilating muscles).

Clinical features

Excessive daytime sleepiness is the principal symptom. Snoring is virtually universal; bed partners report loud snoring in all body positions, and often notice multiple breathing pauses (apnoeas). Sleep is unrefreshing. Patients have difficulty with concentration, impaired cognitive function and work performance, depression, irritability and nocturia.

Investigations

A quantitative assessment of daytime sleepiness can be obtained by questionnaire (e.g. Epworth Sleepiness Scale). Overnight studies of breathing, oxygenation and sleep quality are diagnostic (SAHS defined as ≥15 apnoeas/hypopnoeas per hour of sleep).

Differential diagnosis

Narcolepsy is a rare cause of sleepiness, occurring in 0.05% of the population, and is associated with cataplexy (when muscle tone is lost in fully conscious people in response to emotional triggers), hypnagogic hallucinations (hallucinations at sleep onset) and sleep paralysis.

Idiopathic hypersomnolence occurs in younger individuals and is characterised by long nocturnal sleeps.

Management

The major risk is traffic accidents, and all drivers must be advised not to drive until treatment has relieved their sleepiness. Weight reduction and avoidance of alcohol and sedatives are beneficial. Most patients need CPAP by nasal/face mask to prevent upper airway collapse during sleep. CPAP often leads to dramatic improvements in symptoms, daytime performance and quality of life. Unfortunately, 30% to 50% of patients are poorly compliant or intolerant of CPAP. Oral splints that hold the mandible forward (mandibular advancement devices) are an alternative approach. Palatal surgery is of no benefit.

Laryngeal disorders

The most common symptom of laryngeal disorders is hoarseness. The differential diagnosis of hoarseness that persists beyond a few days is:
• Laryngeal tumour. • Vocal cord paralysis. • Inhaled glucocorticoids.
• Chronic laryngitis because of overuse of the voice. • Heavy smoking.
• Chronic infection of nasal sinuses.

Laryngeal paralysis

Disease affecting the motor nerve supply of the larynx is nearly always unilateral and, because of the intrathoracic course of the left recurrent laryngeal nerve, usually left-sided. One or both recurrent laryngeal nerves may be damaged at thyroidectomy or by thyroid carcinoma. Symptoms are hoarseness, a 'bovine cough' and stridor, which may be severe if both vocal cords are affected. In some patients, a CXR may reveal an unsuspected lung cancer or pulmonary TB. If no such abnormality is found, laryngoscopy should be performed. In unilateral paralysis, the voice may be improved by injection of Teflon into the affected cord. In bilateral paralysis, tracheal intubation, tracheostomy or laryngeal surgery may be necessary.

Laryngeal obstruction

Laryngeal obstruction is more liable to occur in children than in adults because of the smaller size of the glottis. Sudden complete laryngeal obstruction by a foreign body causes acute asphyxia—violent but ineffective inspiratory efforts with indrawing of the intercostal spaces and the unsupported lower ribs, accompanied by cyanosis. Unrelieved, the condition is rapidly fatal. When, as in most cases, the obstruction is incomplete at first, the clinical features are progressive breathlessness accompanied by stridor and cyanosis.

Management

Urgent treatment to relieve obstruction is needed:
• When a foreign body causes laryngeal obstruction in children, it can often be dislodged by turning the patient head downwards and squeezing the chest vigorously.
• In adults this is often impossible, but a sudden forceful compression of the upper abdomen (Heimlich manœuvre) may be effective.
• In other circumstances, the cause should be investigated by direct laryngoscopy, which may also permit the removal of an unsuspected foreign body or the insertion of a tube past the obstruction into the trachea.
• Tracheostomy must be performed without delay if these procedures fail to relieve obstruction, but except in dire emergencies this operation should be performed in an operating theatre by a surgeon.
• In angioedema, complete laryngeal occlusion can usually be prevented by treatment with adrenaline (epinephrine) 0.5 to 1 mg (0.5–1 mL of 1:1000) IM, chlorphenamine maleate 10 to 20 mg by slow IV injection and IV hydrocortisone sodium succinate 200 mg.

Tracheal disorders

Tracheal obstruction

External compression by enlarged mediastinal lymph nodes containing metastatic deposits, usually from a lung cancer, is a more frequent cause of tracheal obstruction than the uncommon primary benign or malignant tumours. Rarely, the trachea may be compressed by an aneurysm of the aortic arch, by a retrosternal goitre or in children by tuberculous mediastinal lymph nodes. Tracheal stenosis is an occasional complication of tracheostomy, prolonged intubation, granulomatosis with polyangiitis or trauma.

Clinical features

Stridor can be detected in every patient with severe tracheal narrowing. Bronchoscopy should be undertaken without delay to determine the site, degree and nature of the obstruction.

Management

Localised tumours of the trachea can be resected but reconstruction after resection may be technically difficult. Endobronchial laser therapy, bronchoscopically placed tracheal stents, chemotherapy and radiotherapy are alternatives to surgery.

Tracheo-oesophageal fistula

This may be a congenital abnormality in newborn infants. In adults, it is usually because of malignant lesions in the mediastinum, such as carcinoma or lymphoma, eroding both the trachea and oesophagus to produce a communication between them. Swallowed liquids enter the trachea and bronchi through the fistula and provoke coughing.

Management

Surgical closure of a congenital fistula, if undertaken promptly, is usually successful. There is usually no curative treatment for malignant fistulae, and death from overwhelming pulmonary infection rapidly supervenes.

Pleural disease

Pleurisy, pleural effusion and empyema are described under presenting problems.

Pneumothorax

Pneumothorax is the presence of air in the pleural space, which can either occur spontaneously, or result from iatrogenic injury or trauma to the lung or chest wall. Primary spontaneous pneumothorax occurs in patients with no history of lung disease. Smoking, tall stature and the presence of apical subpleural blebs are known risk factors. Secondary pneumothorax affects patients with preexisting lung disease, especially COPD, bullous emphysema and asthma. It is most common in older patients and is associated with the highest mortality rates.

Clinical features

There is sudden-onset unilateral pleuritic chest pain or breathlessness (those with underlying chest disease may have severe breathlessness). With a small pneumothorax the physical examination may be normal; a larger pneumothorax (>15% of the hemithorax) results in decreased or absent breath sounds and a resonant percussion note. A tension pneumothorax occurs when a small communication acts as a one-way valve, allowing air to enter the pleural space from the lung during inspiration but not to escape on expiration; this causes raised intrapleural pressure, which leads to mediastinal displacement, compression of the opposite lung, impaired systemic venous return and cardiovascular compromise.

Investigations

CXR shows the sharply defined edge of the deflated lung with a complete lack of lung markings between this and the chest wall. CXR also shows any mediastinal displacement and gives information regarding the presence or absence of pleural fluid and underlying pulmonary disease. Care must be taken to differentiate between a large preexisting emphysematous bulla and a pneumothorax to avoid misdirected attempts at aspiration; where doubt exists, CT is useful in distinguishing bullae from pleural air.

Management (Fig. 9.15)

Primary pneumothorax, where the lung edge is less than 2 cm from the chest wall and the patient is not breathless, normally resolves without intervention. In young patients presenting with a moderate or large spontaneous primary pneumothorax, an attempt at percutaneous aspiration of air should be made in the first instance, with a 60% to 80% chance of avoiding the need for a chest drain. Patients with chronic lung disease usually require a chest drain and inpatient observation, as even a small pneumothorax may cause respiratory failure.

Intercostal drains should be inserted in the 4th, 5th or 6th intercostal space in the mid-axillary line, following blunt dissection through to the parietal pleura, or by using a guidewire and dilator ('Seldinger' technique). The tube should be advanced in an apical direction, connected to an underwater seal or one-way Heimlich valve, and secured firmly to the chest wall. Clamping of the drain is potentially dangerous and rarely indicated. The drain should be removed the morning after the lung has fully re-inflated and bubbling has stopped. Continued bubbling after 5 to 7 days is an indication for surgery.

Supplemental oxygen is given, as this accelerates the rate at which air is reabsorbed by the pleura. Patients with an unresolved pneumothorax should not fly until the pleural air is gone, as the trapped gas expands at altitude. Patients should be advised to stop smoking and informed about the risks of a recurrent pneumothorax (25% after primary spontaneous pneumothorax).

Recurrent spontaneous pneumothorax: Surgical pleurodesis, with thoracoscopic pleural abrasion or pleurectomy, is recommended in all patients following a second pneumothorax (even if ipsilateral) and should be considered following the first episode of secondary pneumothorax if low respiratory reserve makes recurrence hazardous. Patients who plan to continue activities where pneumothorax would be particularly dangerous (e.g. diving) should also undergo definitive treatment after the first episode of a primary spontaneous pneumothorax.

Diseases of the diaphragm

Congenital disorders: Congenital defects of the diaphragm (foramina of Bochdalek and Morgagni) can allow herniation of abdominal viscera. Abnormal elevation or bulging of one hemidiaphragm (eventration of the diaphragm), more often the left, may result from total or partial absence of muscular development of the septum transversum.

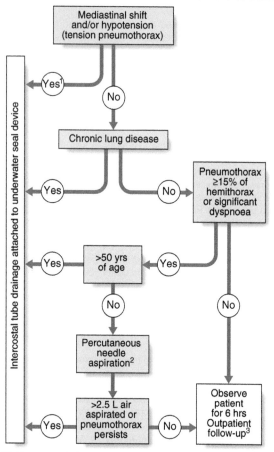

Fig. 9.15 Management of spontaneous pneumothorax. (1) Immediate decompression is required before insertion of an intercostal drain. (2) Aspirate in the second intercostal space anteriorly in the mid-clavicular line; discontinue if resistance is felt, the patient coughs excessively or more than 2.5 L is aspirated. (3) All patients should be told to attend again immediately in the event of noticeable deterioration.

Acquired disorders: Phrenic nerve damage leading to diaphragmatic paralysis may be idiopathic, but is most often because of lung cancer. Other causes include disease of cervical vertebrae, tumours of the cervical cord, shingles, trauma including road traffic and birth injuries, surgery and stretching of the nerve by mediastinal masses and aortic aneurysms. CXR demonstrates elevation of the hemidiaphragm. Screening USS can demonstrate paradoxical upward movement of the paralysed hemidiaphragm on sniffing. Bilateral diaphragmatic weakness occurs in neuromuscular disease of any type including Guillain–Barré syndrome, poliomyelitis, muscular dystrophies, motor neuron disease and connective tissue disorders, such as SLE and polymyositis.

Deformities of the chest wall

Thoracic kyphoscoliosis: Abnormalities of alignment of the dorsal spine and their consequent effects on thoracic shape may be congenital or caused by:

• Vertebral disease, including TB. • Osteoporosis. • Ankylosing spondylitis. • Trauma. • Previous lung surgery. • Neuromuscular disease such as poliomyelitis.

Kyphoscoliosis, if severe, restricts and distorts expansion of the chest wall. Patients with severe deformity may develop type II respiratory failure.

Pectus excavatum: In pectus excavatum (funnel chest), the body of the sternum, usually only the lower end, is curved backwards. This is rarely of any clinical consequence. Operative correction is usually only indicated for cosmetic reasons.

Pectus carinatum: Pectus carinatum (pigeon chest) is frequently caused by severe asthma during childhood.

9

10

Endocrinology

Endocrinology concerns the synthesis, secretion and action of hormones. These are chemical messengers released from endocrine glands that coordinate the activities of many different cells. Endocrine diseases can therefore affect multiple organs and systems.

Major endocrine functions and anatomy

Although some endocrine glands (e.g. the parathyroids and pancreas) respond directly to metabolic signals, most are controlled by hormones released from the pituitary gland. Anterior pituitary hormone secretion is controlled by substances produced in the hypothalamus and released into portal blood, flowing down the pituitary stalk. Posterior pituitary hormones are synthesised in the hypothalamus and transported down nerve axons to be released from the posterior pituitary. Hormone release in the hypothalamus and pituitary is regulated by numerous nervous, metabolic, physical or hormonal stimuli: in particular, feedback control by hormones produced by target glands (thyroid, adrenal cortex and gonads). These integrated endocrine systems are called 'axes' (Fig. 10.1).

Some hormones (e.g. insulin, adrenaline (epinephrine)) act on specific cell surface receptors. Others (e.g. steroids, triiodothyronine, vitamin D) bind to specific intracellular receptors forming a ligand-activated transcription factor, which regulates gene expression directly.

Classically, hormones that are synthesised in endocrine glands are released into the circulation, acting at distant sites. However, many other organs secrete hormones or contribute to the metabolism and activation of prohormones. Some hormones, such as neurotransmitters, act in a paracrine fashion to affect adjacent cells or act in an autocrine way to affect behaviour of the cell that produces the hormone.

Pathology arising within an endocrine gland is often called 'primary' disease (e.g. primary hypothyroidism in Hashimoto's thyroiditis), whereas abnormal stimulation of the gland is often called 'secondary' disease (e.g. secondary hypothyroidism in patients with TSH deficiency).

Clinical examination in endocrine disease

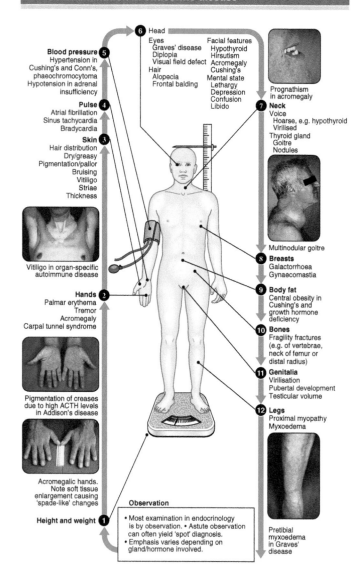

6 Head

Eyes
Graves' disease
Diplopia
Visual field defect

Hair
Alopecia
Frontal balding

Facial features
Hypothyroid
Hirsutism
Acromegaly
Cushing's

Mental state
Lethargy
Depression
Confusion
Libido

Prognathism in acromegaly

7 Neck

Voice
Hoarse, e.g. hypothyroid
Virilised
Thyroid gland
Goitre
Nodules

Multinodular goitre

8 Breasts
Galactorrhoea
Gynaecomastia

9 Body fat
Central obesity in Cushing's and growth hormone deficiency

10 Bones
Fragility fractures (e.g. of vertebrae, neck of femur or distal radius)

11 Genitalia
Virilisation
Pubertal development
Testicular volume

12 Legs
Proximal myopathy
Myxoedema

Pretibial myxoedema in Graves' disease

5 Blood pressure
Hypertension in Cushing's and Conn's, phaeochromocytoma
Hypotension in adrenal insufficiency

4 Pulse
Atrial fibrillation
Sinus tachycardia
Bradycardia

3 Skin
Hair distribution
Dry/greasy
Pigmentation/pallor
Bruising
Vitiligo
Striae
Thickness

Vitiligo in organ-specific autoimmune disease

2 Hands
Palmar erythema
Tremor
Acromegaly
Carpal tunnel syndrome

Pigmentation of creases due to high ACTH levels in Addison's disease

Acromegalic hands. Note soft tissue enlargement causing 'spade-like' changes

1 Height and weight

Observation
• Most examination in endocrinology is by observation. • Astute observation can often yield 'spot' diagnosis. • Emphasis varies depending on gland/hormone involved.

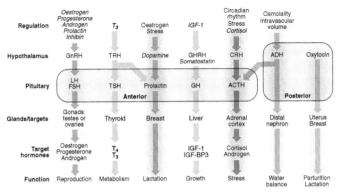

Fig. 10.1 The principal endocrine 'axes' and glands. Parathyroid glands, adrenal zona glomerulosa and endocrine pancreas are not controlled by the pituitary. Italics show negative regulation. *ACTH*, Adrenocorticotrophic hormone; *ADH*, antidiuretic hormone; *CRH*, corticotrophic releasing hormone; *FSH*, follicle-stimulating hormone; *GH*, growth hormone; *GHRH*, growth hormone releasing hormone; *GnRH*, gonadotrophin-releasing hormone; *IGF*, insulin-like growth factor; *LH*, lutenising hormone; *TRH*, thyroid-releasing hormone; *TSH*, thyroid-stimulating hormone.

i	10.1 Examples of nonspecific presentations of endocrine disease	
Symptom	**Most likely endocrine disorder(s)**	
Lethargy and depression	Hypothyroidism, diabetes mellitus, hyperparathyroidism, hypogonadism, adrenal insufficiency, Cushing's syndrome	
Weight gain	Hypothyroidism, Cushing's syndrome	
Weight loss	Thyrotoxicosis, adrenal insufficiency, diabetes mellitus	
Polyuria and polydipsia	Diabetes mellitus, diabetes insipidus, hyperparathyroidism, hypokalaemia (Conn's syndrome)	
Heat intolerance	Thyrotoxicosis, menopause	
Palpitation	Thyrotoxicosis, phaeochromocytoma	
Headache	Acromegaly, pituitary tumour, phaeochromocytoma	
Muscle weakness (usually proximal)	Thyrotoxicosis, Cushing's syndrome, hypokalaemia (e.g. Conn's syndrome), hyperparathyroidism, hypogonadism	
Coarsening of features	Acromegaly, hypothyroidism	

Presenting problems in endocrine disease

Patients with endocrine disease present in many ways, to many different specialists. Classical syndromes occur with dysfunction of individual glands; however, presentation is often with nonspecific symptoms or asymptomatic biochemical abnormalities. In addition, endocrine diseases are often part of the differential diagnosis of other disorders, including electrolyte abnormalities, hypertension, obesity and osteoporosis. Although diseases of the adrenal glands, hypothalamus and pituitary are relatively rare, their diagnosis often relies on astute clinical observation in a patient with nonspecific complaints, so it is important that clinicians are familiar with their key features.

The thyroid gland

Diseases of the thyroid affect 5% of the population, predominantly females. The thyroid axis is involved in the regulation of cellular differentiation and metabolism in virtually all nucleated cells, so that disorders of thyroid function have diverse manifestations. Follicular epithelial cells synthesise thyroid hormones by incorporating iodine into the amino acid tyrosine. The thyroid secretes predominantly thyroxine (T_4) and only a small amount of triiodothyronine (T_3), the more active hormone; around 85% of T_3 in blood is produced from peripheral conversion of T_4. They both circulate in plasma almost entirely (>99%) bound to transport proteins, mainly thyroxine-binding globulin (TBG). The unbound hormones diffuse into tissues and exert diverse metabolic actions. The advantage of measuring free over total hormone is that the former is not influenced by changes in TBG concentrations; with the contraceptive pill, for example, TBG rises and total T_3/T_4 may be raised, but free thyroid hormone levels are normal.

Production of T_3 and T_4 in the thyroid is stimulated by thyroid-stimulating hormone (TSH), a glycoprotein released from the thyrotroph cells of the anterior pituitary in response to the hypothalamic tripeptide thyrotrophin-releasing hormone (TRH). There is a negative feedback of thyroid hormones on the hypothalamus and pituitary such that in thyrotoxicosis, when plasma concentrations of T_3 and T_4 are raised, TSH secretion is suppressed. Conversely, in primary hypothyroidism, low T_3 and T_4 are associated with high circulating TSH levels. TSH is, therefore, regarded as the most useful investigation of thyroid function. However, TSH may take several weeks to 'catch up' with T_4/T_3 levels, for example, after prolonged suppression of TSH in thyrotoxicosis is relieved by antithyroid therapy. Common patterns of abnormal TFTs are shown in Box 10.2.

Presenting problems in thyroid disease

Thyrotoxicosis

Approximately 76% of cases are attributed to Graves' disease, 14% to multinodular goitre and 5% to toxic adenoma. Less common causes include transient thyroiditis (de Quervain's, postpartum), iodide-induced (drugs, supplementation), factitious and TSH-secreting pituitary tumour.

Clinical assessment

Manifestations of thyrotoxicosis are shown in Box 10.3. The most common symptoms are:
• Weight loss with a normal appetite. • Heat intolerance. • Palpitations.
• Tremor. • Irritability.

All causes of thyrotoxicosis can cause lid retraction and lid lag, but only Graves' disease causes exophthalmos, ophthalmoplegia and diplopia.

Investigations

Fig. 10.2 summarises the approach to establishing the diagnosis.

10.2 How to interpret thyroid function tests

TSH	T₄	T₃	Most likely interpretation(s)
UD	Raised	Raised	Primary thyrotoxicosis
UD or low	Raised	Normal	Over-treatment of hypothyroidism with T_4 Factitious thyrotoxicosis
UD	Normal[a]	Raised	Primary T_3-toxicosis
UD	Normal[a]	Normal[a]	Subclinical thyrotoxicosis
UD or low	Raised	Low or normal	Nonthyroidal illness, amiodarone therapy
UD or low	Low	Raised	Over-treatment of hypothyroidism with T_3
UD	Low	Low	Secondary hypothyroidism[d] Transient thyroiditis in evolution
Normal	Low	Low[b]	Secondary hypothyroidism[d]
Mildly elevated 5–20 mlU/L	Low	Low[b]	Primary hypothyroidism Secondary hypothyroidism[d]
Elevated >20 mlU/L	Low	Low[b]	Primary hypothyroidism
Mildly elevated 5–20 mlU/L	Normal[c]	Normal[b]	Subclinical hypothyroidism
Elevated 20–500 mlU/L	Normal	Normal	Artefact IgG interfering with TSH assay
Elevated	Raised	Raised	Nonadherence to T_4 replacement–recent 'loading' dose Secondary thyrotoxicosis[d] Thyroid hormone resistance

[a]Usually upper part of reference range.
[b]T_3 is not a sensitive indicator of hypothyroidism and should not be requested.
[c]Usually lower part of reference range.
[d]That is secondary to pituitary or hypothalamic disease.
UD = undetectable. Note TSH assays may report detectable TSH.

10

TFTs: T_3 and T_4 are elevated in most patients, but T_4 is normal and T_3 raised (T_3 toxicosis) in 5%. In primary thyrotoxicosis, serum TSH is undetectable (<0.05 mU/L).

Antibodies: TSH receptor antibodies (TRAb) are elevated in 80% to 95% of patients with Graves' disease. Other thyroid antibodies are nonspecific because they are present in many healthy people.

Imaging: [99m]Technetium scintigraphy scans indicate trapping of isotope in the gland (Fig. 10.2). In Graves' disease there is diffuse uptake. In multinodular goitre, there is low, patchy uptake within the nodules. A hot spot is seen in toxic adenoma, with no uptake in the dormant gland tissue. In low-uptake thyrotoxicosis, the cause is usually a transient thyroiditis,

i 10.3 Clinical features of thyrotoxicosis

Symptoms	Signs
Common	
Weight loss despite normal or increased appetite	Weight loss
Heat intolerance, sweating	Tremor
Palpitations, tremor	Palmar erythema
Dyspnoea, fatigue	Sinus tachycardia
Irritability, emotional lability	Lid retraction, lid lag
Less common	
Osteoporosis (fracture, loss of height)	Goitre with bruit[a]
Diarrhoea, steatorrhoea	Atrial fibrillation[b]
Angina	Systolic hypertension/in-
Ankle swelling	creased pulse pressure
Anxiety, psychosis	Cardiac failure[b]
Muscle weakness	Hyper-reflexia
Periodic paralysis (mainly in Chinese & Asian groups)	Ill-sustained clonus
Pruritus, alopecia	Proximal myopathy
Amenorrhoea/oligomenorrhoea	Bulbar myopathy[b]
Infertility, spontaneous abortion	
Loss of libido, impotence	
Excessive lacrimation	
Rare	
Vomiting	Gynaecomastia
Apathy	Spider naevi
Anorexia	Onycholysis
Exacerbation of asthma	Pigmentation

[a]In Graves' disease only.
[b]Features found particularly in elderly patients.

although rarely patients may induce 'factitious thyrotoxicosis' by consuming levothyroxine.

Management

Definitive treatment of thyrotoxicosis depends on the underlying cause (p. 382) and may include antithyroid drugs, radioactive iodine or surgery. A nonselective β-blocker (propranolol 160 mg daily) will alleviate symptoms within 24 to 48 hours.

Atrial fibrillation in thyrotoxicosis: AF is present in around 10% of all patients with thyrotoxicosis (more in the elderly). Subclinical thyrotoxicosis is also a risk factor for AF. Ventricular rate responds better to β-blockade than digoxin. Thromboembolic complications are particularly common, so anticoagulation is indicated. Once the patient is biochemically euthyroid, AF reverts to sinus rhythm spontaneously in around 50% of patients.

Thyrotoxic crisis ('thyroid storm'): This is a medical emergency with a mortality of 10%. The most prominent signs are fever, agitation, delirium,

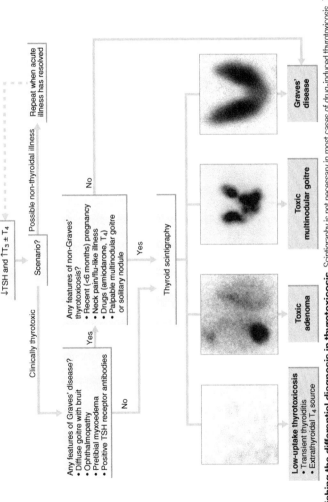

$\downarrow$ TSH and $\uparrow$ T$_3$ ± T$_4$

Clinically thyrotoxic

Scenario?

Possible non-thyroidal illness

Repeat when acute illness has resolved

Any features of Graves' disease?
• Diffuse goitre with bruit
• Ophthalmopathy
• Pretibial myxoedema
• Positive TSH receptor antibodies

Yes

No

Any features of non-Graves' thyrotoxicosis?
• Recent (<6 months) pregnancy
• Neck pain/flu-like illness
• Drugs (amiodarone, T$_4$)
• Palpable multinodular goitre or solitary nodule

Yes

No

Thyroid scintigraphy

Low-uptake thyrotoxicosis
• Transient thyroiditis
• Extrathyroidal T$_4$ source

Toxic adenoma

Toxic multinodular goitre

Graves' disease

Fig. 10.2 **Establishing the differential diagnosis in thyrotoxicosis.** Scintigraphy is not necessary in most cases of drug-induced thyrotoxicosis. *TSH*, Thyroid-stimulating hormone.

10

tachycardia or AF and cardiac failure. It is precipitated by infection in patients with unrecognised thyrotoxicosis and may develop after subtotal thyroidectomy or ^{131}I therapy. Patients should be rehydrated and given propranolol orally (80 mg four times daily) or intravenously (1–5 mg four times daily). Sodium ipodate (500 mg daily orally) restores serum T_3 levels to normal in 48 to 72 hours by inhibiting release of hormones and conversion of T_4 to T_3. Oral carbimazole 40 to 60 mg daily inhibits the synthesis of new thyroid hormone. In the unconscious patient, carbimazole can be administered rectally. After 10 to 14 days, maintenance with carbimazole alone is possible.

Hypothyroidism

Hypothyroidism is a common condition, with a female:male ratio of 6:1.

Autoimmune disease (Hashimoto's thyroiditis) and thyroid failure following ^{131}I or surgical treatment of thyrotoxicosis account for more than 90% of cases in regions where the population is not iodine-deficient.

Clinical assessment

Clinical features depend on the duration and severity of the hypothyroidism. The classical features (Box 10.4) occur when deficiency develops insidiously over months/years.

Investigations

In primary hypothyroidism, T_4 is low and TSH elevated (>20 mU/L) (Fig. 10.3). T_3 is not a sensitive indicator of hypothyroidism and should not be measured. Secondary hypothyroidism is rare and is caused by failure of TSH secretion because of hypothalamic or anterior pituitary disease, for example, pituitary macroadenoma. T_4 is low, and TSH is usually low but sometimes paradoxically detectable. Other biochemical abnormalities associated with hypothyroidism include ↑CK, ↑LDH, ↑AST, ↑cholesterol, ↓Na$^+$ and anaemia (macrocytic or normocytic). ECG may show sinus bradycardia with small complexes and ST–T abnormalities. Thyroid peroxidase antibodies are usually elevated in autoimmune causes but are also common in the healthy population.

Management

Most patients require lifelong levothyroxine therapy: levothyroxine 50 μg daily for 3 weeks, then 100 μg daily for 3 weeks then maintenance 100 to 150 μg daily.

Transient hypothyroidism occurs in the first 6 months after thyroidectomy or ^{131}I treatment of Graves' disease, in the postthyrotoxic phase of subacute thyroiditis and in postpartum thyroiditis. Levothyroxine treatment is not always necessary in these patients, as they may be asymptomatic during the short period of thyroid failure.

Levothyroxine has a half-life of 7 days, and so 6 weeks should pass before repeating TFTs following a dose change. Patients feel better within 2 to 3 weeks; resolution of skin and hair texture and effusions may take 3 to 6 months.

The dose of levothyroxine should be adjusted to maintain TSH within the reference range. This usually requires a T_4 level in the upper reference range because the necessary T_3 is derived exclusively from peripheral conversion of T_4 without the usual contribution from thyroid secretion. Some physicians advocate combined T_4/T_3 replacement, but this approach remains

i	10.4 Clinical features of hypothyroidism

Symptoms	Signs
Common	
Weight gain	Weight gain
Cold intolerance	
Fatigue, somnolence	
Dry skin	
Dry hair	
Menorrhagia	
Less common	
Constipation	Hoarse voice
Hoarseness	Facial features:
Carpal tunnel syndrome	Purplish lips
Alopecia	Malar flush
Aches and pains	Periorbital oedema
Muscle stiffness	Loss of lateral eyebrows
Deafness	Anaemia
Depression	Carotenaemia
Infertility	Erythema ab igne
	Bradycardia hypertension
	Delayed relaxation of reflexes
	Dermal myxoedema
Rare	
Psychosis (myxoedema madness)	Ileus, ascites
Galactorrhoea	Pericardial and pleural effusions
Impotence	Cerebellar ataxia
	Myotonia

10

controversial. TFTs should be checked every 1 to 2 years once the dose of thyroxine is stabilised.

Levothyroxine requirements may increase with co-administration of other drugs (e.g. phenytoin, ferrous sulphate, rifampicin) and during pregnancy. In nonadherence, if levothyroxine is taken just before clinic, the anomalous combination of a high T_4 and high TSH may result.

Levothyroxine replacement in ischaemic heart disease: Exacerbation of myocardial ischaemia, infarction and sudden death are well-recognised complications. In known ischaemic heart disease, levothyroxine should be introduced at low dose and increased under specialist supervision. Coronary intervention may be required to allow full replacement dosage.

Pregnancy: Most pregnant women with primary hypothyroidism require a 25 to 50 μg increase in levothyroxine dose. Inadequately treated hypothyroidism in pregnancy has been associated with impaired cognitive development in the fetus.

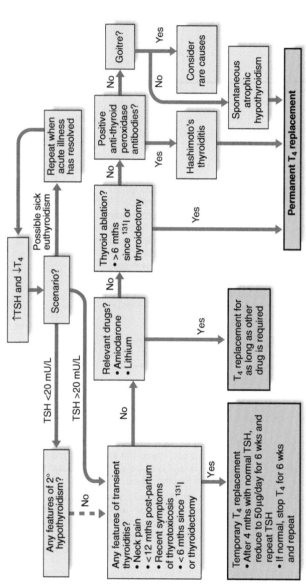

Fig. 10.3 Diagnostic approach to adults with suspected hypothyroidism. This scheme ignores congenital causes of hypothyroidism, such as thyroid aplasia and dyshormonogenesis. Rare causes of hypothyroidism with goitre include amyloidosis and sarcoidosis. *TSH*, Thyroid-stimulating hormone.

Myxoedema coma: This is a rare presentation of hypothyroidism in which there is depressed consciousness, usually in an elderly patient who appears myxoedematous. Body temperature may be low, convulsions are not uncommon, and CSF pressure and protein content are raised. The mortality rate is 50%, and survival depends on early recognition and treatment.

Myxoedema coma is an emergency, and treatment must begin before biochemical confirmation of diagnosis. Liothyronine is given as an IV bolus of 20 μg, followed by 20 μg three times daily until there is sustained clinical improvement. After 48 to 72 hours, oral levothyroxine (50 μg daily) may be substituted. Unless it is clear the patient has primary hypothyroidism, thyroid failure should be assumed to be secondary to hypothalamic or pituitary disease, and treatment given with hydrocortisone 100 mg IM three times daily, pending T_4, TSH and cortisol results. Other measures include slow rewarming, cautious IV fluids, broad-spectrum antibiotics and high-flow oxygen.

Symptoms of hypothyroidism with normal thyroid function tests

Individuals who believe they have hypothyroidism, despite normal thyroid function tests, require reassurance that organic disease has been carefully considered. If symptoms persist, referral to a team specialising in medically unexplained symptoms should be considered.

Asymptomatic abnormal thyroid function tests

Subclinical thyrotoxicosis: TSH is undetectable while T_3/T_4 is in the upper reference range. This condition is usually found in older patients with multinodular goitre. There is an increased risk of AF and osteoporosis; hence the consensus view is that such patients require therapy (usually ^{131}I). Otherwise, annual follow-up is required, as overt thyrotoxicosis occurs in 5% annually.

Subclinical hypothyroidism: TSH is raised while T_3/T_4 is in the lower reference range. Progression to overt thyroid failure is highest in those with antithyroid peroxidase antibodies or TSH greater than 10 mIU/L. This group should be treated with levothyroxine to normalise TSH.

Nonthyroidal illness ('sick euthyroidism'): TSH is low, T_4 raised and T_3 normal or low in a patient with systemic illness. Caused by decreased conversion of T_4 to T_3, alterations in levels and affinity to binding proteins and reduced TSH secretion. During convalescence, TSH may increase to levels found in primary hypothyroidism. TFTs should therefore not be checked during an acute illness in the absence of clear signs of thyroid disease. If an abnormal result is found, tests should be repeated after recovery.

Thyroid lump or swelling

A lump or swelling in the thyroid has many possible causes (Box 10.5). Most swellings are either a solitary nodule, a multinodular goitre or a diffuse goitre. Nodular thyroid disease is common in adult women. Most thyroid nodules are impalpable but are found incidentally on neck imaging, for example, Doppler USS of the carotid arteries or CT pulmonary angiography, or during staging of patients with cancer.

10.5 Causes of thyroid enlargement

Diffuse goitre

- Simple goitre
- Hashimoto's thyroiditis[a]
- Graves' disease
- Drugs: iodine, amiodarone, lithium
- Iodine deficiency (endemic goitre)[a]
- Suppurative thyroiditis[b]
- Transient thyroiditis[b]
- Dyshormonogenesis[a]
- Infiltrative: amyloidosis, sarcoidosis, etc.
- Riedel's thyroiditis[b]

Multinodular goitre

Solitary nodule

- Colloid cyst
- Hyperplastic nodule
- Follicular adenoma
- Papillary carcinoma
- Follicular carcinoma
- Medullary cell carcinoma
- Anaplastic carcinoma
- Lymphoma
- Metastasis

[a]Goitre likely to shrink with levothyroxine therapy.
[b]Usually tender.

Palpable thyroid nodules present as lumps in the neck in 4% to 8% of adult women and 1% to 2% of adult men. Multinodular goitre and solitary nodules sometimes present with acute painful swelling as a result of haemorrhage into a nodule.

Patients with thyroid nodules often worry about cancer, although in reality only 5% to 10% are malignant. Primary thyroid malignancy (p. 386) is more likely in:

• A nodule in childhood or adolescence, particularly with a past history of local irradiation. • A nodule presenting in an elderly patient. • Patients with cervical lymphadenopathy.

Rarely, a metastasis from renal, breast or lung carcinoma presents as a painful, enlarging thyroid nodule. Thyroid nodules identified on PET scanning have around a 33% chance of being malignant.

Clinical assessment and investigations

On examination, thyroid swellings move during swallowing, and palpation can often distinguish between the three main causes of thyroid swelling. The differential diagnosis includes lymphadenopathy, branchial cysts, dermoid cysts and thyroglossal duct cysts. USS should be performed urgently if there is any doubt about an anterior neck swelling.

T_3, T_4 and TSH should be measured, and hyper- or hypothyroidism treated as described earlier.

Thyroid scintigraphy: Scintigraphy with [99m]technetium should be performed in patients with low serum TSH and a nodular thyroid to confirm the presence of an autonomously functioning ('hot') nodule (see Fig. 10.2), for which fine needle aspiration is not necessary. 'Cold' nodules on scintigraphy are more likely to prove malignant; however, most are benign, and so scintigraphy is not routinely used to investigate thyroid nodules when TSH is normal.

Thyroid USS: If thyroid function is normal, ultrasound is used to distinguish generalised from localised thyroid swelling. Inflammatory disorders causing diffuse goitre (e.g. Graves' disease and Hashimoto's thyroiditis) cause diffuse hypoechogenicity and (in Graves' disease) increased thyroid blood flow on Doppler. Thyroid autoantibodies occur in both disorders, whereas their absence in younger patients with diffuse goitre and normal function suggests 'simple goitre' (p. 386). Ultrasound also reveals the size and number of thyroid nodules and can distinguish solid from cystic nodules. It cannot reliably differentiate between benign and malignant nodules, but features suggesting malignancy include hypoechoicity, intranodular vascularity, microcalcification and irregular, lobulated margins. A purely cystic nodule and a 'spongiform' appearance both predict a benign aetiology.

Fine needle aspiration cytology: This is recommended for most thyroid nodules that are suspicious of malignancy or radiologically indeterminate. Palpable nodules can be aspirated in clinic under ultrasound guidance. Aspiration may be therapeutic for cysts, although repeated recurrence is an indication for surgery. Fine needle aspiration cytology cannot differentiate between a follicular adenoma and a follicular carcinoma, and in 10% to 20% of cases an inadequate specimen is obtained.

Management

Nodules appearing benign on ultrasound may be observed by ultrasound surveillance; when the suspicion of malignancy is very low, the patient may be reassured and discharged. Where iodine-deficiency is common, levothyroxine sufficient to suppress TSH may shrink some nodules. This treatment is inappropriate in iodine-sufficient populations.

Nodules suspicious for malignancy are treated by surgical lobectomy or thyroidectomy. Nodules that are indeterminate often end up being surgically excised. Nodules in which malignancy is confirmed by formal histology are treated as described on p. 387.

A diffuse or multinodular goitre may also require surgery for cosmetic reasons or to relieve compression of adjacent structures (stridor or dysphagia). Levothyroxine may shrink the goitre of Hashimoto's disease, particularly if TSH is elevated.

Autoimmune thyroid disease

Graves' disease

Graves' disease most commonly affects women aged 30 to 50 years. The most common manifestation is thyrotoxicosis (see Box 10.3) with or without a diffuse goitre. Graves' disease also causes ophthalmopathy and, rarely, pretibial myxoedema. These features can occur in the absence of thyroid dysfunction.

Graves' thyrotoxicosis

IgG antibodies are directed against the TSH receptors on follicular cells, stimulating hormone production and goitre formation. These TRAbs can be detected in 80% to 95% of patients. The natural history of the disease follows one of three patterns:

• A prolonged period of hyperthyroidism of fluctuating severity. • Alternating relapse and remission. • A single, short-lived episode of hyperthyroidism, followed by prolonged remission and sometimes hypothyroidism.

There is a strong genetic component in Graves' disease, with 50% concordance between monozygotic twins. Smoking is weakly associated with Graves' thyrotoxicosis but strongly linked with the development of ophthalmopathy.

Management

Symptoms respond to β-blockade, but definitive treatment requires control of thyroid hormone secretion. The different options are compared in Box 10.6. Some clinicians prescribe a course of antithyroid drugs, resorting to ^{131}I or surgery if relapse occurs. In many centres, however, ^{131}I is used first line, given the high risk of relapse following antithyroid drugs. Some data suggest ^{131}I increases the incidence of malignancy; however, the association may be with Graves' disease rather than its therapy.

Antithyroid drugs: The most commonly used are carbimazole and propylthiouracil. These drugs reduce thyroid hormone synthesis by inhibiting tyrosine iodination. Antithyroid drugs are introduced at high doses (carbimazole 40–60 mg daily, propylthiouracil 400–600 mg daily). There is subjective improvement within 2 weeks, and the patient is biochemically euthyroid at 4 weeks, when the dose can be reduced. The maintenance

i 10.6 Comparison of treatments for the thyrotoxicosis of Graves' disease			
Management	Common indications	Contraindications	Disadvantages/ complications
Antithyroid drugs (carbimazole, propylthiouracil)	First episode in patients <40 years	Breastfeeding (propylthiouracil suitable)	Hypersensitivity rash 2% Agranulocytosis 0.2% Relapse (>50%)
Subtotal thyroid-ectomy	Large goitre Poor drug adherence Recurrence after drug treatment	Previous thyroid surgery Dependence on voice, for example, opera singer, lecturer	Hypothyroidism ~25% Transient hypocalcaemia 10% Hypoparathyroidism 1% Recurrent laryngeal nerve palsy 1%
Radioiodine	Patients >40 years Recurrence following surgery	Pregnancy Active Graves' opthalmopathy	Hypothyroidism: 40% in first year, 80% by 15 years Exacerbates ophthalmopathy

dose is determined by measurement of T_4 and TSH. Carbimazole is continued for 12 to 18 months in the hope that permanent remission will occur. In Graves' disease, 50% to 70% of patients will relapse, usually within 2 years of stopping treatment. Adverse effects of antithyroid drugs include rash and idiosyncratic but reversible agranulocytosis.

Thyroid surgery: Patients must be rendered euthyroid before operation. Potassium iodide, 60 mg three times daily orally, given for 10 days before surgery, inhibits thyroid hormone release and reduces the size and vascularity of the gland, making surgery easier. Complications are uncommon. One-year postsurgery, 80% of patients are euthyroid, 15% are hypothyroid and 5% remain thyrotoxic. 'Near-total' thyroidectomy, leaving a small portion adjacent to the recurrent laryngeal nerves, invariably results in permanent hypothyroidism, but maximises the chance of cure for thyrotoxicosis.

Radioactive iodine: [131]I is administered as a single oral dose (400–600 MBq, 10–15 mCi) and is trapped and organified in the thyroid. It is effective in 75% of patients within 4 to 12 weeks. Symptoms can initially be controlled by β-blockade or with carbimazole. However, carbimazole reduces the efficacy of ^{131}I therapy and should be avoided for 48 hours after radioiodine. If thyrotoxicosis persists after 6 months, a further dose of ^{131}I is indicated. Most patients eventually develop hypothyroidism, necessitating long-term follow-up.

Thyrotoxicosis in pregnancy

TFTs must be interpreted with caution in pregnancy. Thyroid-binding globulin, and hence total T_4/T_3 levels, are increased, and TSH reference ranges are lower; a fully suppressed TSH with elevated free hormone levels indicates thyrotoxicosis. The thyrotoxicosis is almost always caused by Graves' disease. Maternal thyroid hormones, TRAb and antithyroid drugs can all cross the placenta.

Propylthiouracil is the preferred treatment in the first trimester, as carbimazole is associated rarely with embryopathy, particularly the skin defect aplasia cutis. The smallest dose of propylthiouracil (<150 mg/day) is used that maintains maternal TFTs within the reference ranges, minimising fetal hypothyroidism and goitre. TRAb levels in the third trimester predict the likelihood of neonatal thyrotoxicosis; if they are not elevated, antithyroid drugs can be discontinued 4 weeks before delivery to avoid fetal hypothyroidism at the time of maximum brain development. During breastfeeding, propylthiouracil is used, as it is minimally excreted in the milk.

Graves' ophthalmopathy

Within the orbit, there is cytokine-mediated fibroblast proliferation, increased interstitial fluid and a chronic inflammatory cell infiltrate. This causes swelling and ultimately fibrosis of the extraocular muscles and a rise in retrobulbar pressure. The eye is displaced forwards (proptosis, exophthalmos) with optic nerve compression in severe cases.

Ophthalmopathy is typically episodic. It is detectable in around 50% of thyrotoxic patients at presentation, more commonly smokers, but may occur before or after thyrotoxic episodes (exophthalmic Graves' disease). Presenting symptoms are related to increased corneal exposure as a result of proptosis and lid retraction:

- Excessive lacrimation worsened by wind and sun. • 'Gritty' sensations.
- Pain as a result of corneal ulceration. • Reduced visual acuity/fields or colour vision as a result of optic nerve compression. • Diplopia resulting from extraocular muscle involvement.

Most patients require no treatment. Smoking cessation should be encouraged. Methylcellulose eye drops are used for dry eyes and sunglasses reduce the excessive lacrimation. Severe inflammatory episodes are treated with glucocorticoids (pulsed IV methylprednisolone) and sometimes orbital radiotherapy. Loss of visual acuity requires urgent surgical decompression of the orbit. Surgery to ocular muscles may improve diplopia.

Pretibial myxoedema

This infiltrative dermopathy occurs in less than 5% of patients with Graves' disease. Pink–purple plaques on the anterior leg and foot are seen. Lesions are itchy and the skin may have a 'peau d'orange' appearance with coarse hair. In severe cases, topical glucocorticoids may be helpful.

Hashimoto's thyroiditis

Hashimoto's thyroiditis increases in incidence with age. It is characterised by destructive lymphoid infiltration leading to a varying degree of fibrosis and thus a varying degree of thyroid enlargement. There is a slightly increased risk of thyroid lymphoma. The term 'Hashimoto's thyroiditis' has been reserved for patients with antithyroid peroxidase autoantibodies and a goitre (with or without hypothyroidism), whereas 'spontaneous atrophic hypothyroidism' has been used in hypothyroid patients without a goitre with TSH receptor–blocking antibodies. However, these syndromes are both variants of Hashimoto's.

At presentation, a small or moderately sized firm diffuse goitre may be palpable. Some 25% of patients are hypothyroid, and the remainder are at risk of developing hypothyroidism in future years. Antithyroid peroxidase antibodies are present in more than 90%. Levothyroxine therapy is given.

Transient thyroiditis

Subacute (de Quervain's) thyroiditis

Subacute thyroiditis is a virus-induced (e.g. Coxsackie, mumps) transient inflammation of the thyroid usually affecting 20- to 40-year-old females.

There is classically pain around the thyroid radiating to the jaw and ears, which is worsened by swallowing and coughing. The thyroid is enlarged and tender. Painless transient thyroiditis also occurs. Systemic upset is common. Inflammation in the thyroid causes release of colloid and stored hormones, and damages follicular cells. As a result, T_4/T_3 levels are raised for 4 to 6 weeks until depletion of colloid. A period of hypothyroidism follows, during which follicular cells recover, restoring thyroid function within 4 to 6 months. In the thyrotoxic phase, iodine uptake and technetium trapping are low because of follicular cell damage and TSH suppression. Pain and systemic upset respond to NSAIDs. Occasionally, prednisolone 40 mg daily for 3 to 4 weeks is required. Mild thyrotoxicosis is treated with propranolol. Monitoring of thyroid function is required so that levothyroxine can be prescribed temporarily in the hypothyroid phase.

Postpartum thyroiditis

The maternal immune response is enhanced after delivery and may unmask subclinical autoimmune thyroid disease. Transient asymptomatic disturbances of thyroid function occur in 5% to 10% of women postpartum. However, symptomatic thyrotoxicosis presenting within 6 months of childbirth is likely to be attributed to postpartum thyroiditis, and the diagnosis is confirmed by negligible radioisotope uptake. The clinical course is similar to that of painless subacute thyroiditis. Postpartum thyroiditis can recur after subsequent pregnancies and may progress to hypothyroidism.

Iodine-associated thyroid disease

Iodine deficiency

Iodine is an essential component of T_4 and T_3. Iodine deficiency is common in Central Africa, South-East Asia and the Western Pacific. Reduced iodine availability increases thyroid activity, stimulating goitre and nodule formation. Most affected patients are euthyroid with normal or raised TSH. In pregnancy, iodine deficiency is associated with impaired brain development. Iodine is commonly added to table salt as a preventive public health measure.

Iodine-induced dysfunction

Very high iodine levels inhibit thyroid hormone release; this is the rationale for iodine treatment in thyroid crisis and before surgery for thyrotoxicosis. Transient thyrotoxicosis may be precipitated in iodine deficiency following prophylactic iodinisation programmes. In individuals who have underlying thyroid disease predisposing to thyrotoxicosis (e.g. multinodular goitre or Graves' disease), thyrotoxicosis can be induced by iodine administration (e.g. radiocontrast media).

Amiodarone

The antiarrhythmic agent amiodarone contains large amounts of iodine. Amiodarone also has a cytotoxic effect on thyroid follicular cells and inhibits T_4 to T_3 conversion. Around 20% of patients develop hypothyroidism or thyrotoxicosis. TSH provides the best indicator of thyroid function.

Amiodarone-related thyrotoxicosis has been classified as:

- Type I: iodine-induced excess thyroid hormone synthesis.
- Type II: thyroiditis attributed to the cytotoxic effect of amiodarone.

Treatment of thyrotoxicosis is difficult. Excess iodine renders the gland resistant to radioiodine. Antithyroid drugs may be effective in patients with type I thyrotoxicosis, but not in those with type II, for which glucocorticoids are effective. Before amiodarone therapy, thyroid function should be measured and amiodarone avoided if TSH is suppressed. Thyroid function should be monitored regularly.

In hypothyroid patients, levothyroxine can be given while amiodarone is continued.

10

Simple and multinodular goitre

Simple diffuse goitre

This presents in 15- to 25-year-olds, often during pregnancy. The goitre is visible, soft and symmetrical, and the thyroid is two to three times its normal size. There is no tenderness, lymphadenopathy or bruit, and TFTs are normal. The goitre may regress without treatment or may progress to multinodular goitre.

Multinodular goitre

Patients with simple goitre as young adults may progress to develop nodules, which grow at varying rates and secrete thyroid hormone 'autonomously', suppressing the TSH-dependent growth and function in the remaining gland. Ultimately, complete TSH suppression occurs in around 25% of cases, with T_4 and T_3 levels often within the reference range (subclinical thyrotoxicosis) but sometimes elevated (toxic multinodular goitre).

Clinical features and investigations

Patients present with thyrotoxicosis, a large goitre or sudden painful swelling caused by haemorrhage into a nodule. The goitre is nodular or lobulated on palpation and may extend retrosternally. Very large goitres may cause stridor, dysphagia and superior vena cava obstruction. Hoarseness attributed to recurrent laryngeal nerve palsy is more suggestive of thyroid carcinoma. The diagnosis is confirmed by USS and/or thyroid scintigraphy. A flow-volume loop is a good screening test for tracheal compression. CT or MRI of the thoracic inlet can quantify the degree of tracheal compression and retrosternal extension. Nodules should be evaluated for neoplasia as described below.

Management

Small goitre: Annual thyroid function assessment is required, as progression to toxic multinodular goitre can occur.

Large goitre: Thyroid surgery is indicated for mediastinal compression or cosmetically unattractive goitres. [131]I is used in the elderly to reduce thyroid size, but recurrence is common after 10 to 20 years.

Toxic multinodular goitre: [131]I is used; hypothyroidism is less common than in Graves' disease. Partial thyroidectomy may be required for a large goitre. Antithyroid drugs are not usually used, as drug withdrawal invariably leads to relapse.

Subclinical thyrotoxicosis: This is increasingly being treated with ^{131}I, as a suppressed TSH is a risk factor for AF and osteoporosis.

Thyroid neoplasia

Patients with thyroid tumours usually present with a solitary nodule (p. 387). Most are benign, and a few (toxic adenomas) secrete excess thyroid hormones. Primary thyroid malignancy is rare (<1% of all carcinomas). As shown in Box 10.7, it can be classified according to the cell type of origin. With the exception of medullary carcinoma, thyroid cancer is more common in females.

i | 10.7 Malignant thyroid tumours

Origin of Tumour	Type of Tumour	Frequency (%)	Age at Presentation (years)	10-year Survival (%)
Follicular cells	Papillary	75–85	20–40	98
	Follicular	10–20	40–60	94
	Anaplastic	<5	>60	9
Parafollicular C cells	Medullary carcinoma	5–8	Childhood or >40	78
Lymphocytes	Lymphoma	<5	>60	45

Toxic adenoma

The presence of a toxic solitary nodule is the cause of less than 5% of cases of thyrotoxicosis. The nodule is a follicular adenoma, usually greater than 3 cm, which secretes excess thyroid hormones. The remaining gland atrophies following TSH suppression. Most patients are female and older than 40 years of age.

Diagnosis is by thyroid scintigraphy. Thyrotoxicosis is mild, and in 50% of patients T_3 alone is elevated (T_3 thyrotoxicosis). ^{131}I is highly effective and is an ideal treatment, because the atrophic cells surrounding the nodule do not take up iodine, making permanent hypothyroidism unusual. Hemi-thyroidectomy is an alternative.

Differentiated carcinoma

Papillary carcinoma: The most common thyroid malignancy. It may be multifocal, and spread is to regional lymph nodes.

Follicular carcinoma: A single encapsulated lesion. Cervical lymph nodes spread is rare. Metastases are blood-borne and are found in bone, lungs and brain.

Management

This should be individualised and planned by multidisciplinary teams. Total thyroidectomy is carried out, followed by a large dose of ^{131}I to ablate remaining thyroid tissue. Thereafter, long-term treatment is given with sufficient levothyroxine to suppress TSH (150–200 µg daily), as differentiated thyroid carcinomas are TSH-dependent. During follow-up, serum thyroglobulin should remain undetectable in patients whose thyroid has been ablated. Detectable thyroglobulin suggests tumour recurrence or metastases, which may respond to further surgery or ^{131}I. Carcinoma that is refractory to ^{131}I may respond to sorafenib or lenvatinib.

Most patients with papillary and follicular thyroid cancer will be cured with appropriate treatment. Adverse prognostic factors include older age, distant metastases, male sex and certain histological subtypes.

10

Anaplastic carcinoma and lymphoma

These two conditions are difficult to distinguish clinically. Patients are usually over 60 years of age and have rapid thyroid enlargement over 2 to 3 months. The goitre is hard and symmetrical, and may cause stridor (tracheal compression) and hoarseness (recurrent laryngeal nerve palsy). There is no effective treatment of anaplastic carcinoma, although surgery and radiotherapy are sometimes used.

The prognosis for lymphoma, which may arise from Hashimoto's thyroiditis, is better. External irradiation dramatically shrinks the goitre and, with chemotherapy, results in a median survival of 9 years.

Medullary carcinoma

This tumour arises from the parafollicular C cells of the thyroid and may secrete calcitonin, 5-HT (serotonin) and ACTH. As a consequence, carcinoid syndrome and Cushing's syndrome may occur.

Patients present with a firm thyroid mass and cervical lymphadenopathy. Distant metastases are rare. Serum calcitonin is raised and useful in monitoring treatment response. Hypocalcaemia is rare. Treatment is by total thyroidectomy with removal of cervical nodes. Vandetanib and cabozantinib are used for advanced cases. Medullary carcinoma occurs sporadically in 70% to 90% of cases; 10% to 30% have an inherited predisposition as part of the MEN type 2 syndrome (p. 418).

Riedel's thyroiditis

This rare, nonmalignant condition has a similar presentation to thyroid cancer, with a slow-growing goitre that is irregular, fibrous and hard. There may be mediastinal and retroperitoneal fibrosis. Tracheal and oesophageal compression often necessitate thyroidectomy.

The reproductive system

In the male, the testis has two principal functions:
• Synthesis of testosterone by the interstitial Leydig cells controlled by luteinising hormone (LH). • Spermatogenesis by Sertoli cells under the control of follicle-stimulating hormone (FSH).

Negative feedback suppression of LH is mediated principally by testosterone, while inhibin suppresses FSH.

In the female, FSH stimulates growth and development of ovarian follicles during the first 14 days of the menstrual cycle. This leads to a gradual increase in oestradiol production, which initially suppresses FSH secretion (negative feedback) but then, above a certain level, stimulates an increase in the frequency and amplitude of gonadotrophin-releasing hormone (GnRH) pulses, resulting in a surge in LH secretion (positive feedback), which induces ovulation. The follicle then differentiates into a corpus luteum, which secretes progesterone. Withdrawal of progesterone results in menstrual bleeding.

The cessation of menstruation (the menopause) occurs in developed countries at an average age of 50 years. In the 5 years before (the climacteric) there is an increase in the number of anovulatory cycles. Oestrogen and inhibin secretion falls, resulting in increased pituitary LH and FSH secretion.

Presenting problems in reproductive disease

Delayed puberty

Genetic factors influence the timing of puberty onset, although body weight acts as a trigger. Puberty is considered delayed if it has not begun by a chronological age greater than 2.5 SDs above the national average (>14 in boys, >13 in girls in the UK).

The differential diagnosis is considered in Box 10.8. The key distinction is between the 'clock running slow' (constitutional delay) and pathology in the hypothalamus/pituitary (hypogonadotrophic hypogonadism) or the gonads (hypergonadotrophic hypogonadism).

Constitutional delay of puberty: This should be considered a normal variant, and is the most common cause of delayed puberty, especially in boys. Affected children are typically shorter than their peers throughout childhood. There is often a family history, and bone age is lower than chronological age. Puberty will start spontaneously, but prolonged delay can have significant psychological consequences.

Hypogonadotrophic hypogonadism: This may be attributed to structural, inflammatory or infiltrative disorders of the pituitary/hypothalamus (p. 413). Other pituitary hormones are likely to be deficient. 'Functional' gonadotrophin deficiency is caused by a variety of factors (see Box 10.8). Isolated gonadotrophin deficiency is attributed to a genetic abnormality affecting GnRH or gonadotrophin synthesis. The most common form is Kallmann's syndrome, which also features olfactory bulb agenesis, resulting

10

---

i · 10.8 Causes of delayed puberty and hypogonadism

Constitutional delay

Hypogonadotrophic hypogonadism
- Structural hypothalamic/pituitary disease—see Box 10.16
- Functional gonadotrophin deficiency
  - Chronic systemic illness (e.g. asthma, coeliac disease, cystic fibrosis)
  - Psychological stress, anorexia nervosa, excessive exercise
  - Endocrine disease: hyperprolactinaemia, Cushing's syndrome hypothyroidism
- Isolated gonadotrophin deficiency (Kallman's syndrome)

Hypergonadotrophic hypogonadism

- Acquired damage to gonads
  - Chemotherapy/radiotherapy
  - Trauma/surgery
  - Autoimmune gonadal failure
  - Mumps, TB
  - Haemochromatosis
- Developmental/congenital disorders
  - Klinefelter's/Turner's syndrome
  - Anorchidism/cryptorchidism

in anosmia. If left untreated, the epiphyses fail to fuse, resulting in tall stature with disproportionately long arms and legs (eunuchoid habitus). Cryptorchidism (undescended testes) and gynaecomastia are seen in all forms of hypogonadotrophic hypogonadism.

Hypergonadotrophic hypogonadism: Hypergonadotrophic hypogonadism associated with delayed puberty is usually attributed to sex chromosome abnormalities (Klinefelter's/Turner's syndromes, p. 394). Other causes of gonadal failure are shown in Box 10.8.

Investigations

• LH/FSH, testosterone, oestradiol, FBC, renal, liver and thyroid function and coeliac disease autoantibodies: key measurements. • Elevated gonadotrophin concentrations: chromosome analysis. • Low gonadotrophin concentrations: differential diagnosis lies between constitutional delay and hypogonadotrophic hypogonadism. • X-ray of the wrist and hand: allows estimation of bone age. • Neuroimaging: required in hypogonadotrophic hypogonadism.

Management

Puberty can be induced using low dose oestrogen (in girls) or testosterone (in boys). Higher doses carry a risk of early fusion of epiphyses, so therapy should be monitored by a specialist. In constitutional delay, therapy is withdrawn once endogenous puberty is established. In other cases, hormone doses are gradually increased during puberty and full adult replacement doses given when development is complete.

Precocious puberty

PP means the development of secondary sexual characteristics under 9 years of age in boys and 6 to 8 years in girls. Central PP is caused by early maturation of the hypothalamic–pituitary–gonadal axis, and often no cause is identified. Structural causes occur more commonly in younger children and boys and include CNS tumours, injury and congenital abnormalities.

Peripheral PP is rarer and is as a result of excess sex steroids in the absence of gonadotrophins; causes include congenital adrenal hyperplasia and McCune–Albright syndrome.

Amenorrhoea

Primary amenorrhoea may be diagnosed in a female who has never menstruated. This is usually attributed to delayed puberty, but may be a consequence of anatomical defects, for example, endometrial hypoplasia, vaginal agenesis.

Secondary amenorrhoea describes the cessation of menstruation. The causes of this are:
• Physiological (pregnancy, menopause). • Hypogonadotrophic hypogonadism (see Box 10.8). • Ovarian dysfunction (hypergonadotrophic hypogonadism; see Box 10.8). • PCOS, androgen-secreting tumours. • Uterine dysfunction (Asherman's syndrome).

Premature ovarian failure (premature menopause) is defined as occurring before 40 years of age.

Clinical assessment

Hypothalamic/pituitary disease and premature ovarian failure result in oestrogen deficiency, which causes menopausal symptoms: hot flushes, sweating, anxiety, irritability, dyspareunia, vaginal infections. A history of galactorrhoea should be sought. Weight loss for any reason can cause amenorrhoea. Weight gain may suggest hypothyroidism or Cushing's syndrome. Hirsutism and irregular periods suggest PCOS.

Investigations

• Measurement of urinary hCG will exclude pregnancy. • LH, FSH, oestradiol, prolactin, testosterone, T_4 and TSH. • ↑LH, ↑FSH and ↓oestradiol: suggest primary ovarian failure. Ovarian autoantibodies suggest autoimmune ovarian failure. • ↑LH, ↑prolactin and ↑testosterone with normal oestradiol: common in polycystic ovararian syndrome (PCOS). • ↓LH, ↓FSH and ↓oestradiol: suggest hypothalamic/pituitary disease (pituitary MRI indicated). • Assessment of bone mineral density is appropriate in patients with low androgen and oestrogen levels.

Management

Where possible, the underlying cause should be treated. The management of structural pituitary/hypothalamic disease and PCOS is described later. In oestrogen deficiency, oestrogen replacement is necessary to treat symptoms and to prevent osteoporosis. Oestrogen should not be given without progesterone to a woman with a uterus because of the risk of endometrial cancer. It is administered most conveniently as an oral contraceptive pill. In postmenopausal females, HRT relieves menopausal symptoms and prevents osteoporotic fractures, but also causes adverse effects (e.g. stroke, breast cancer, pulmonary embolism). Many authorities recommend that women should take replacement therapy until the age of 50 years and continue only if there are unacceptable menopausal symptoms.

Male hypogonadism

The clinical features of both hypo- and hypergonadotrophic hypogonadism in men include:
• Loss of libido. • Lethargy. • Muscle weakness. • Decreased frequency of shaving. • Gynaecomastia. • Infertility. • Delayed puberty.

The causes of hypogonadism are listed in Box 10.8. Mild hypogonadism may also occur in older men in the context of central adiposity and metabolic syndrome.

Investigations

Male hypogonadism is confirmed by demonstrating a low serum testosterone level. Hypo- and hypergonadotrophic hypogonadism are distinguished by measurement of random LH and FSH. Patients with hypogonadotrophic hypogonadism should be investigated for pituitary disease (p. 412). Patients with hypergonadotrophic hypogonadism should have the testes examined for cryptorchidism or atrophy, and a karyotype should be performed (Klinefelter's syndrome).

Management

Testosterone replacement is indicated to prevent osteoporosis and to restore muscle power and libido. Testosterone administration should be avoided in prostatic carcinoma. In men over 50 years of age, PSA should be monitored.

Infertility

Infertility affects around 1 in 7 couples of reproductive age. Causes in women include anovulation or structural abnormalities preventing fertilisation or implantation. Male infertility may result from impaired quality or number of sperm. Azoospermia or oligospermia is usually idiopathic, but may result from hypogonadism (Box 10.8). In many couples no cause is found.

Clinical assessment

• History of previous illness/surgery. • Sensitive sexual history. • Menstrual history. • Scrotal examination for testicular size, vas deferens and varicocele.

Investigations

• Performed in both partners after failure to conceive for 12 months, unless there is an obvious abnormality (e.g. amenorrhoea). • Semen analysis for sperm count and quality. • Women with regular periods: ovulation is confirmed by elevated serum progesterone on day 21 of the cycle. • Transvaginal USS to assess uterine and ovarian anatomy. • Tubal patency: check using laparoscopy or hysterosalpingography.

Management

General advice: Couples are advised to have intercourse every 2 to 3 days throughout the menstrual cycle.

Ovulation induction:
• In PCOS with anovulatory cycles: clomifene.
• In gonadotrophin deficiency or if clomifene fails: daily FSH injections, then hCG to induce follicular rupture.
• In hypothalamic disease: pulsatile infusion of GnRH therapy to stimulate pituitary gonadotrophin secretion.

During ovulation induction, monitoring, including ultrasonography, it is essential to avoid multiple ovulation and ovarian hyperstimulation syndrome. Women who fail to respond to induction or who have primary ovarian failure may consider donated eggs or embryos, surrogacy and adoption.

In vitro fertilisation: IVF is widely used for many causes of idiopathic or prolonged (>3 years) infertility. The success rate falls in women older than 40 years.

Male infertility: Infertile men with hypogonadotrophic hypogonadism are usually given injections of hCG. Removal of a varicocele can improve semen quality. Sperm extraction from the epididymis and in vitro intracytoplasmic sperm injection into oöcytes (intracytoplasmic sperm injection (ICSI)) is used in men with oligospermia or poor sperm quality. Donated sperm is another option in azoospermia.

Gynaecomastia

Gynaecomastia is the presence of glandular breast tissue in males, resulting from an androgen/oestrogen imbalance (androgen deficiency or oestrogen excess). Causes are listed in Box 10.9. Physiological gynaecomastia is common, that is, in newborn babies (maternal oestrogens), pubertal boys (oestradiol reaches adult levels before testosterone) and elderly men (↓testosterone concentrations).

Take a drug history. On examination, gynaecomastia is often asymmetrical. Palpation should allow breast tissue to be distinguished from

> **10.9 Causes of gynaecomastia**
>
> - Idiopathic
> - Physiological
> - Drugs: cimetidine, digoxin, antiandrogens (cyproterone acetate, spironolactone), cannabis
> - Hypogonadism (see Box 10.8)
> - Androgen resistance syndromes
> - Oestrogen excess: liver failure (impaired steroid metabolism), oestrogen-secreting tumour (e.g. testis), hCG-secreting tumour (e.g. testis, lung)

adiposity in obesity, but if doubt remains then USS or mammography is required. The testes should be examined for cryptorchidism, atrophy or a tumour. Testosterone, LH, FSH, oestradiol, prolactin and hCG should be measured. Elevated oestrogen concentrations are found in testicular tumours and hCG-producing neoplasms. The underlying cause should be addressed, for example, change of drug treatment, excision of tumour. In physiological gynaecomastia, reassurance is usually sufficient, but if the condition is associated with significant psychological distress, surgical excision may be justified. Androgen replacement improves gynaecomastia in hypogonadal males.

Hirsutism

Hirsutism refers to the excessive growth of thick terminal hair in an androgen-dependent distribution in women (upper lip, chin, chest, back, lower abdomen, thigh, forearm). It should be distinguished from hypertrichosis, which is generalised excessive growth of thin vellus hair. Causes and treatment of hirsutism are shown in Box 10.10.

Important observations are a drug and menstrual history, BMI, BP, examination for virilisation (clitoromegaly, deep voice, male-pattern balding, breast atrophy) and associated features, for example, Cushing's syndrome. Recent hirsutism associated with virilisation is suggestive of an androgen-secreting tumour. Testosterone, prolactin, LH and FSH should be measured. If testosterone levels are over twice the upper limit of the normal female range, especially with ↓LH and ↓FSH, then causes other than idiopathic hirsutism and PCOS are more likely.

Polycystic ovarian syndrome

PCOS affects up to 10% of women of reproductive age. It is associated with obesity, and the primary cause remains uncertain. Genetic factors are important, as PCOS often affects several family members.

Clinical features

• Pituitary dysfunction: ↑LH, ↑prolactin. • Anovulatory menstrual cycles: oligomenorrhoea, secondary amenorrhoea, cystic ovaries, infertility. • Androgen excess: hirsutism, acne. • Obesity: hyperglycaemia, ↑oestrogens, dyslipidaemia, hypertension.

i 10.10	Causes of hirsutism	
Cause	**Investigation findings**	**Treatment**
Idiopathic	Normal	Cosmetic measures Antiandrogens
PCOS	LH:FSH ratio >2.5:1 Mild ↑androgens Mild hyperprolactinaemia	Weight loss Cosmetic measures Antiandrogens
Congenital adrenal hyperplasia (95% 21-hydroxylase deficiency)	↑Androgens that suppress with dexamethasone ACTH test causes ↑17OH-progesterone	Glucocorticoid replacement administered in reverse rhythm to suppress early morning ACTH
Exogenous androgen administration	↓LH/FSH Urinalysis detects drug of misuse	Stop steroid misuse
Androgen-secreting tumour of ovary or adrenal cortex	↑Androgens that do not suppress with dexamethasone/oestrogen↓ LH/FSH CT/MRI demonstrates tumour	Surgical excision
Cushing's syndrome	Normal or mild ↑adrenal androgens	Treat cause

Management

Weight loss can improve menstrual irregularity, hirsutism and diabetes risk.

Menses: Metformin reduces insulin resistance and can restore regular cycles. High oestrogen may cause endometrial hyperplasia. Inducing regular withdrawal bleeding using cyclical progestogens can reduce the risk of endometrial neoplasia.

Hirsutism: Many patients use shaving, bleaching and waxing. Electrolysis and laser treatment are effective but expensive. Eflornithine cream may reduce hair growth. Antiandrogen therapy may be employed if other measures have failed. Options include:

- Androgen receptor antagonists (e.g. cyproterone acetate).
- 5α-reductase inhibitors (e.g. finasteride): prevent activation of testosterone.
- Exogenous oestrogen: suppresses ovarian hormone production.

Infertility: See earlier.

Turner's syndrome

Turner's syndrome affects around 1 in 2500 females. The syndrome is classically associated with a 45XO karyotype. The genitals are female in character, although gonadal dysgenesis results in 'streak ovaries'. The lack of oestrogen causes loss of negative feedback and elevation of FSH and LH concentrations. There is a wide spectrum of associated somatic abnormalities, including:

• Short stature. • Webbing of the neck (25%–40%). • Widely spaced nipples. • Shield chest. • Horse-shoe kidney. • Lymphoedema of hands and feet (30%). • Autoimmune thyroid disease (20%). • Coarctation of the aorta. • Aortic root dilatation. • Psychological problems: low IQ. • Deafness.

Short stature may be helped by high doses of growth hormone. Pubertal development is induced with oestrogen therapy, and long-term oestrogen replacement is required.

Klinefelter's syndrome

Klinefelter's syndrome affects around 1 in 1000 males and is usually associated with a 47XXY karyotype. Leydig cell function is impaired, resulting in hypergonadotrophic hypogonadism. The diagnosis is often made in adolescents with gynaecomastia and delayed puberty. Affected individuals usually have small, firm testes and may have learning difficulties. Tall stature is apparent from early childhood, with a long leg length exacerbated by lack of epiphyseal closure in puberty. Individuals with androgen deficiency require androgen replacement.

10

The parathyroid glands

The four parathyroid glands lie behind the lobes of the thyroid. PTH interacts with vitamin D to control calcium metabolism. Calcium exists in serum as 50% ionised and 50% complexed with organic ions and proteins. The parathyroid chief cells respond directly to changes in calcium concentrations, secreting PTH in response to a fall in ionised calcium. PTH promotes reabsorption of calcium from renal tubules and bone, stimulating alkaline phosphatase and lowering plasma phosphate. PTH also promotes renal conversion of 25-hydroxycholecalciferol to the active metabolite 1,25-dihydroxycholecalciferol, which enhances calcium absorption from the gut.

To investigate disorders of calcium metabolism, measurement of calcium, phosphate, alkaline phosphatase and PTH should be undertaken. Most laboratories measure total calcium in serum. This needs to be corrected if serum albumin is low by adjusting the value for calcium upwards by 0.02 mmol/L (0.08 mg/dL) for each 1 g/L reduction in albumin below 40 g/L.

Presenting problems in parathyroid disease

Hypercalcaemia

Causes of hypercalcaemia are listed in Box 10.11. Primary hyperparathyroidism and malignant hypercalcaemia are the most common. Familial hypocalciuric hypercalcaemia (FHH) is a rare disorder that is important, as it may be misdiagnosed as primary hyperparathyroidism.

10.11 Causes of hypercalcaemia

With normal/elevated (inappropriate) PTH levels

- Primary or tertiary hyperparathyroidism
- Lithium-induced hyperparathyroidism
- Familial hypocalciuric hypercalcaemia

With low (Suppressed) PTH levels

- Malignancy—lung, breast, renal, thyroid, lymphoma, myeloma
- Elevated $1,25(OH)_2$ vitamin D—vitamin D intoxication, sarcoidosis, HIV
- Thyrotoxicosis
- Paget's disease with immobilisation
- Milk-alkali syndrome
- Thiazide diuretics
- Glucocorticoid deficiency

Clinical assessment

Symptoms and signs of hypercalcaemia include polyuria, polydipsia, renal colic, lethargy, anorexia, nausea, dyspepsia, peptic ulceration, constipation, depression and impaired cognition ('bones, stones and abdominal groans'). Patients with malignant hypercalcaemia can have a rapid onset of symptoms. Currently, more than 50% of patients are discovered incidentally on biochemical testing and are asymptomatic. Hypertension is common in hyperparathyroidism. Parathyroid tumours are almost never palpable. A family history of hypercalcaemia raises the possibility of FHH or multiple endocrine neoplasia (MEN).

Investigations

The most discriminatory investigation is serum PTH. If PTH levels are detectable or elevated in the presence of hypercalcaemia, then primary hyperparathyroidism is the likely diagnosis. High plasma phosphate and alkaline phosphatase with renal impairment suggest tertiary hyperparathyroidism. Hypercalcaemia may cause nephrocalcinosis and renal tubular impairment, resulting in hyperuricaemia and hyperchloraemia.

Low urine calcium excretion indicates likely FHH, confirmed by testing for mutations in the gene coding for the calcium-sensing receptor.

If PTH is low and no other cause is apparent, then malignancy with or without bony metastases is likely. The patient should be screened with a CXR, myeloma screen and CT as appropriate. PTH-related peptide, which causes hypercalcaemia associated with malignancy, can be measured by a specific assay.

Management

Treatment of severe hypercalcaemia is described on p. 796. For management of hyperparathyroidism, see p. 398. FHH does not require therapy.

i	**10.12 Differential diagnosis of hypocalcaemia**			
	Total serum calcium	Ionised serum calcium	Serum phosphate	Serum PTH concentration
Hypoalbuminaemia	↓	→	→	→
Alkalosis	→	↓	→	→ or ↑
Vitamin D deficiency	↓	↓	↓	↑
Chronic renal failure	↓	↓	↑	↑
Hypoparathyroidism	↓	↓	↑	↓
Pseudohypoparathyroidism	↓	↓	↑	↑
Acute pancreatitis	↓	↓	→ or ↓	↑
Hypomagnesaemia	↓	↓	Variable	↓ or →

Hypocalcaemia

The differential diagnosis of hypocalcaemia is shown in Box 10.12. The most common cause of hypocalcaemia is a low serum albumin with normal ionised calcium concentration. Ionised calcium may be low with a normal total serum calcium in alkalosis, for example, hyperventilation. Hypocalcaemia may also develop in magnesium deficiency, as this impairs PTH secretion.

Clinical assessment

Low ionised calcium increases excitability of peripheral nerves. Tetany can occur if total serum calcium is less than 2.0 mmol/L (8 mg/dL). In children, a characteristic triad of carpopedal spasm, stridor and convulsions occurs. Adults complain of tingling in the hands and feet and around the mouth. When overt signs are lacking, latent tetany may be revealed by Trousseau's sign (inflation of a sphygmomanometer cuff to more than the systolic BP causes carpal spasm) or Chvostek's sign (tapping over the facial nerve produces twitching of the facial muscles). Hypocalcaemia causes papilloedema and QT interval prolongation, predisposing to ventricular arrhythmias. Prolonged hypocalcaemia with hyperphosphataemia may cause calcification of the basal ganglia, epilepsy, psychosis and cataracts. Hypocalcaemia with hypophosphataemia (vitamin D deficiency) causes rickets in children and osteomalacia in adults.

Management

In hyperventilation with tetany, alkalosis is reversed by rebreathing expired air from a paperbag ($\uparrow PaCO_2$).

Injection of 20 mL of 10% calcium gluconate slowly into a vein will raise the serum calcium concentration immediately. IV magnesium is required to correct hypocalcaemia associated with hypomagnesaemia.

Primary hyperparathyroidism

Primary hyperparathyroidism is caused by autonomous secretion of PTH, usually by a single parathyroid adenoma, which can range from a few millimetres to several centimetres in diameter. It should be distinguished from secondary hyperparathyroidism, in which an increase in PTH secretion is caused by prolonged hypocalcaemia (e.g. in vitamin D deficiency, p. 397), and from tertiary hyperparathyroidism, in which prolonged parathyroid stimulation (usually in chronic kidney disease (Box 10.13) results in adenoma formation and autonomous PTH secretion (Box 10.13).

Primary hyperparathyroidism has a prevalence of 1 in 800 and is two to three times more common in women; 90% of patients are aged over 50 years. It also occurs in MEN syndromes. Clinical presentation is described earlier (p. 396).

Skeletal and radiological changes include:

• Osteoporosis-reduced bone mineral density on DEXA scanning. • Osteitis fibrosa resulting from increased bone resorption by osteoclasts with fibrous replacement. It presents as bone pain, fracture and deformity. • Chondrocalcinosis because of deposition of calcium pyrophosphate crystals within articular cartilage, typically the knee, leading to osteoarthritis or acute pseudogout. • X-ray changes: subperiosteal erosions, terminal resorption in the phalanges, 'pepper-pot' skull and renal calcification.

^{99m}Tc-sestamibi scintigraphy or ultrasound can be performed before surgery to localise the adenoma but may be negative.

Management

The treatment of choice for primary hyperparathyroidism is surgical excision of a solitary parathyroid adenoma or hyperplastic glands. Experienced surgeons will identify solitary tumours in more than 90% of cases. Patients with parathyroid bone disease run a significant risk of developing hypocalcaemia postoperatively, but this risk can be reduced by correcting vitamin D deficiency preoperatively.

Surgery is indicated for patients under 50 and for those with symptoms or complications, for example, renal stones, renal impairment or osteopenia. The remainder can be reviewed annually, with assessment of symptoms, renal function, serum calcium and bone mineral density.

i 10.13 **Hyperparathyroidism**		
Type	Serum calcium	PTH
Primary Single adenoma (90%), multiple adenomas (4%), nodular hyperplasia (5%), carcinoma (1%)	Raised	Not suppressed
Secondary Chronic renal failure, malabsorption, osteomalacia and rickets	Low	Raised
Tertiary	Raised	Not suppressed

Treatment of severe hypercalcaemia is described on p. 796.

Cinacalcet is a calcimimetic that enhances the sensitivity of the calcium-sensing receptor, so reducing PTH levels, and is licensed for tertiary hyperparathyroidism and for patients with primary hyperparathyroidism who are unwilling or unfit to have surgery.

Hypoparathyroidism

Causes of hypoparathyroidism include:
• Parathyroid gland damage during thyroid surgery. • Rarely, infiltration of the glands, for example, haemochromatosis, Wilson's disease. • Congenital/inherited (rare), for example autoimmune polyendocrine syndrome type I, autosomal dominant hypoparathyroidism.

Pseudohypoparathyroidism

PTH levels are high, but there is tissue resistance to PTH. Clinical features include:
• Short stature. • Short fourth metacarpals and metatarsals. • Rounded face. • Obesity. • Subcutaneous calcification.

The term *pseudo-pseudohypoparathyroidism* describes the condition of individuals with these clinical features in whom serum calcium and PTH concentrations are normal. Because of genomic imprinting, pseudohypoparathyroidism results from inheritance of the gene defect from the mother, but inheritance from the father results in pseudo-pseudohypoparathyroidism.

Persistent hypoparathyroidism and pseudohypoparathyroidism are treated with oral calcium salts and vitamin D analogues (alfacalcidol or calcitriol). Monitoring of therapy is required because of the risks of iatrogenic hypercalcaemia, hypercalciuria and nephrocalcinosis.

The adrenal glands

The adrenals comprise separate endocrine glands within one anatomical structure.

The adrenal medulla is an extension of the sympathetic nervous system that secretes catecholamines. Most of the adrenal cortex is made up of cells that secrete cortisol and adrenal androgens, and form part of the HPA axis. The small outer glomerulosa of the cortex secretes aldosterone under the control of the renin–angiotensin system.

Adrenal anatomy and function are shown in Fig. 10.4.

Glucocorticoids: Cortisol is the major glucocorticoid in humans. Levels are highest in the morning and lowest in the middle of the night. Over 95% of circulating cortisol is bound to cortisol-binding globulin; it is the free fraction that is active. Cortisol rises during stress, including illness. This elevation protects key metabolic functions and cortisol deficiency is, therefore, most obvious during stress.

Mineralocorticoids: Aldosterone is the most important mineralocorticoid. It binds to renal mineralocorticoid receptors, causing sodium retention and increased excretion of potassium and protons. The principal stimulus to aldosterone secretion is angiotensin II, a peptide produced by activation of the renin–angiotensin system (see Fig. 10.4). Renin activity in the

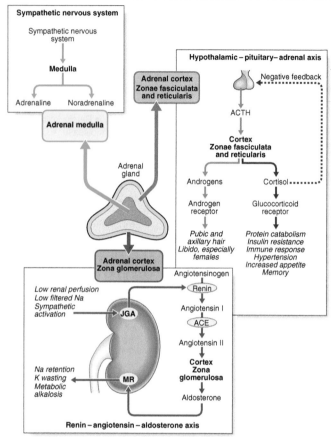

Fig. 10.4 Structure and function of the adrenal glands. *ACE,* Angiotensin-converting enzyme: *ACTH,* adrenocorticotrophic hormone; *JGA,* juxtaglomerular apparatus: *MR,* mineralocorticoid receptor.

juxtaglomerular apparatus of the kidney is stimulated by low perfusion pressure in the afferent arteriole, low sodium filtration or increased sympathetic nerve activity.

Catecholamines: In humans, most circulating noradrenaline (norepinephrine) is derived from sympathetic nerve endings. However, noradrenaline is converted to adrenaline (epinephrine) in the adrenal medulla by an enzyme induced by glucocorticoids. The medulla is thus the major source of circulating adrenaline.

Adrenal androgens: Adrenal androgens are secreted in response to ACTH. They are probably important in the initiation of puberty (adrenarche), are the major source of androgens in females and may be important in female libido.

> ## 10.14 Classification of endogenous cushing's syndrome
>
> **ACTH-dependent—80%**
>
> - Pituitary adenoma secreting ACTH (Cushing's disease) —70%
> - Ectopic ACTH syndrome (e.g. bronchial carcinoid, small-cell lung carcinoma) —10%
>
> **Non-ACTH-dependent—20%**
>
> - Adrenal adenoma—15%
> - Adrenal carcinoma—5%
>
> **Hypercortisolism attributed to other causes (Pseudo-Cushing's syndrome)**
>
> - Alcohol excess (clinical and biochemical features)
> - Major depressive illness (biochemical features)
> - Primary obesity (mild biochemical features)

Presenting problems in adrenal disease

Cushing's syndrome

Cushing's syndrome is caused by excessive activation of glucocorticoid receptors. Endogenous causes are shown in Box 10.14; by far the most common cause is iatrogenic, however, caused by prolonged administration of synthetic glucocorticoids such as prednisolone.

Clinical assessment

The diverse manifestations of glucocorticoid excess are indicated in Fig. 10.5. Some common disorders can be confused with Cushing's syndrome because they are associated with alterations in cortisol secretion, for example, obesity and depression.

A careful drug history is vital to exclude iatrogenic causes; even inhaled or topical glucocorticoids can induce Cushing's syndrome. Some clinical features are more common in ectopic ACTH syndrome. Ectopic tumours lack negative feedback sensitivity to cortisol, resulting in very high ACTH levels associated with marked pigmentation and hypokalaemic alkalosis, aggravating myopathy and hyperglycaemia. When the tumour secreting ACTH is malignant, the onset is usually rapid and may be associated with cachexia.

In Cushing's disease, the pituitary tumour is usually a microadenoma (<10 mm diameter); hence other features of a pituitary macroadenoma (hypopituitarism, visual failure or disconnection hyperprolactinaemia) are rare.

Investigations

This is a two-step process; firstly establishing whether the patient has Cushing's syndrome and secondly defining its cause. Additional tests include plasma electrolytes, glucose, glycosylated haemoglobin and bone mineral density.

Does the patient have Cushing's syndrome? Cushing's syndrome is confirmed by the demonstration of increased secretion of cortisol (24-hour urinary cortisol) and serum cortisol that fails to suppress either with a 1-mg overnight dexamethasone suppression test or with the 48-hour low-dose dexamethasone suppression test (0.5 mg four times daily for 48 hours).

10

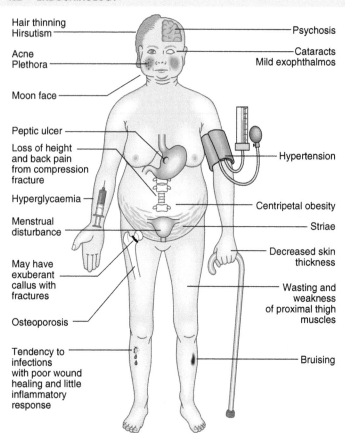

Hair thinning
Hirsutism

Acne
Plethora

Moon face

Peptic ulcer

Loss of height
and back pain
from compression
fracture

Hyperglycaemia

Menstrual
disturbance

May have
exuberant
callus with
fractures

Osteoporosis

Tendency to
infections
with poor wound
healing and little
inflammatory
response

Psychosis

Cataracts
Mild exophthalmos

Hypertension

Centripetal obesity

Striae

Decreased skin
thickness

Wasting and
weakness
of proximal thigh
muscles

Bruising

Fig. 10.5 Clinical features of Cushing's syndrome.

Loss of diurnal variation, with elevated late night salivary or serum corti-sol, is also characteristic of Cushing's syndrome. In iatrogenic Cushing's syndrome, cortisol levels are low unless the glucocorticoid cross-reacts in immunoassays with cortisol (e.g. prednisolone).

What is the cause of the Cushing's syndrome? Plasma ACTH lower than 1.1 pmol/L indicates an adrenal tumour, whereas ACTH greater than 3.3 pmol/L indicates a pituitary or ectopic source. Tests to discrimi-nate pituitary from ectopic ACTH rely on the fact that pituitary tumours, but not ectopic tumours, retain some features of normal regulation. Thus, in pituitary disease, ACTH and cortisol are stimulated by CRH injection and suppressed during a 48-hour high-dose dexamethasone suppression test (2 mg four times daily for 48 hours). CT/MRI detects most adrenal adeno-mas. Adrenal carcinomas are usually large (>5 cm). Tumours not imaged are localised with selective adrenal vein catheterisation with cortisol sampling. Pituitary MRI detects around 60% of pituitary microadenomas. Venous catheterisation with inferior petrosal sinus ACTH measurement is used if the MRI is nondiagnostic.

Management

Untreated Cushing's syndrome has a 50% 5-year mortality. Most patients are treated surgically, and glucocorticoid biosynthesis can be inhibited by metyrapone or ketoconazole pending operation.

Cushing's disease: Trans-sphenoidal selective excision of the adenoma is the treatment of choice. Bilateral adrenalectomy is an alternative, but there is a risk that the pituitary tumour will grow in the absence of negative feedback. This can result in Nelson's syndrome, with an aggressive pituitary macroadenoma and very high ACTH levels causing pigmentation. Nelson's syndrome may be prevented by pituitary irradiation. The somatostatin analogue pasireotide suppresses ACTH secretion, causing tumour shrinkage. It may be useful in inoperable patients.

Adrenal tumours: Laparoscopic surgery is the treatment of choice for adrenal adenomas. Adrenal carcinomas are resected if possible, then the tumour bed is irradiated and the adrenolytic drug mitotane is given, but recurrence remains common.

Ectopic ACTH syndrome: Localised tumours causing this syndrome should be removed. In unresectable malignancies, the severity of the Cushing's syndrome can be reduced with medical therapy (see earlier).

Therapeutic use of glucocorticoids

Glucocorticoids are used for many conditions, but even topical preparations (dermal, rectal and inhaled) can cause significant suppression of endogenous ACTH and cortisol secretion. Doses equivalent to 5 mg prednisolone are:
• Hydrocortisone 20 mg. • Cortisone acetate 25 mg. • Dexamethasone 0.5 mg.

Adverse effects of glucocorticoids

The clinical features of glucocorticoid excess are illustrated in Fig. 10.5 and are related to dose and duration of therapy.

Diabetes mellitus or glucose intolerance can be worsened. Rapid changes in cortisol can cause marked mood disturbance, depression or mania and insomnia. Fracture risk is greater in glucocorticoid-induced osteoporosis than in postmenopausal osteoporosis, so when systemic glucocorticoids are prescribed for more than 3 months, bone-protective therapy (p. 631) should be considered. Signs of perforation of a viscus may be masked, and the patient may show no febrile response to an infection. Glucocorticoids act synergistically with NSAIDs, including aspirin, to increase the risk of gastric erosions and ulceration. Latent TB may be reactivated, and patients on glucocorticoids are at risk of severe varicella zoster virus if they are not immune.

Management of glucocorticoid withdrawal

All glucocorticoid therapy can suppress the HPA axis; however, a crisis because of adrenal insufficiency on withdrawal of glucocorticoids occurs only after prolonged (>3 weeks) or repeated courses, or doses of predniso-lone greater than 7.5 mg/day. In these circumstances, glucocorticoid with-drawal must be slow because the HPA axis may take months to recover. Patients must avoid sudden withdrawal, carry a steroid card and/or wear an engraved bracelet.

To confirm that the HPA axis is recovering, reduce the dose to 5 mg prednisolone then measure cortisol at 9:00 AM before the next dose. If cor-tisol is less than 100 nmol/L, continue slow reduction and repeat a morning cortisol on 3 mg/day. Once morning cortisol is greater than 100 nmol/L, perform an ACTH stimulation test to confirm that glucocorticoids can be withdrawn completely.

Adrenal insufficiency

Adrenal insufficiency results from inadequate secretion of cortisol and/or aldosterone. Causes are shown in Box 10.15. The most common is ACTH deficiency (secondary adrenocortical failure), usually because of withdrawal of chronic glucocorticoid therapy or a pituitary tumour. Congenital adrenal hyperplasia and Addison's disease are rare.

Clinical assessment

Patients may present with chronic features or in acute circulatory shock.

With a chronic presentation, initial symptoms of weight loss, fatigue and anorexia are often misdiagnosed as depression or chronic fatigue. The diagnosis should be considered in all patients with hyponatraemia. Fea-tures of an acute adrenal crisis include circulatory shock with severe hypo-tension, hyponatraemia, hyperkalaemia and, occasionally, hypoglycaemia and hypercalcaemia. Muscle cramps, vomiting, diarrhoea and fever may be present. The crisis is often precipitated by intercurrent disease, surgery or infection. Pigmentation because of excess ACTH may be prominent, par-ticularly in recent scars and pressure areas. Vitiligo occurs in 10% to 20% of patients with autoimmune Addison's disease.

10.15 Causes of adrenocortical insufficiency

Secondary (↓ACTH)

- Withdrawal of glucocorticoid therapy
- Hypothalamic/pituitary disease

Primary (↑ACTH)

- Addison's disease
  - Common: autoimmune, TB, HIV/AIDS, metastatic carcinoma, bilateral adrenalectomy
  - Rare: lymphoma, intra-adrenal haemorrhage (Waterhouse–Friderichsen syn-drome in meningococcal septicaemia), amyloidosis, haemochromatosis
- Corticosteroid biosynthetic enzyme defects
  - Congenital adrenal hyperplasias
  - Drugs: metyrapone, ketoconazole

Investigations

In an acute crisis, a random blood sample should be stored for measurement of cortisol and ACTH, but other tests are deferred until after treatment. In chronic illness, investigations may be performed before any treatment.

Assessment of glucocorticoids: Random plasma cortisol is usually low in adrenal insufficiency but may be inappropriately within the reference range for a seriously ill patient. The short ACTH stimulation test (tetracosactide, short Synacthen test) requires administration of 250 µg ACTH (Synacthen) IM with serum cortisol measured at 0 and 30 minutes. A cortisol level greater than 500 nmol/L (>18 µg/dL) at either time excludes adrenal insufficiency. A cortisol level that fails to increase occurs with primary or secondary adrenal insufficiency. These can be distinguished by measurement of ACTH, which is low in ACTH deficiency and high in Addison's disease.

Assessment of mineralocorticoids: Hyponatraemia occurs in both aldosterone and cortisol deficiency. Hyperkalaemia is common in aldosterone deficiency. Plasma renin and aldosterone should be measured in the supine position. In mineralocorticoid deficiency, plasma renin activity is high, with a low or low normal plasma aldosterone.

Other tests to establish the cause: Patients with unexplained secondary adrenocortical insufficiency should be investigated as described on p. 404. In patients with elevated ACTH, further investigation of the adrenals is required. Adrenal autoantibodies are frequently positive in autoimmune adrenal failure, and other autoimmune diseases may be present. If negative, adrenal imaging with CT or MRI may reveal malignancy, and an AXR may show adrenal calcification in TB. An HIV test should be performed.

Management

Glucocorticoid replacement: Oral hydrocortisone (cortisol) is the drug of choice. In the noncritically ill, cortisol is given 10 mg on waking and 5 mg at around 1500 hours. Replacement doses should not cause Cushingoid side effects. Excess weight gain usually indicates over-replacement, whereas persistent lethargy or hyperpigmentation may indicate an inadequate dose. Patients on glucocorticoid replacement should be advised to: • Double the dose of hydrocortisone during intercurrent infection. • Increase the dose perioperatively (major operation, 100 mg four times daily). • Keep parenteral hydrocortisone at home in case of vomiting. • Carry a steroid card and wear a medical bracelet.

Adrenal crisis is a medical emergency and requires IV hydrocortisone succinate 100mg, normal saline to correct volume depletion and 10% glucose if there is hypoglycaemia. Parenteral hydrocortisone should be continued (100 mg IM four times daily) until the patient is able to take oral therapy. The precipitating cause should be treated.

Mineralocorticoid replacement: Needed for primary, not secondary adrenal insufficiency. Fludrocortisone is administered (0.05–0.15 mg daily). Adequacy of replacement can be assessed with measurement of BP, plasma electrolytes and plasma renin activity.

Androgen replacement: Dehydroepiandrosterone sulphate (DHEAS, 50 mg/day) may be given to women with primary adrenal insufficiency for reduced libido and fatigue, but evidence is not robust.

Incidental adrenal mass

Adrenal 'incidentalomas' are present in up to 10% of adults. They are identified on an abdominal CT or MRI scan that has been performed for another indication. Some 85% are nonfunctioning adrenal adenomas. The remainder includes functional tumours of the adrenal cortex, phaeochromocytomas, primary/secondary carcinomas or hamartomas.

Investigations should include a dexamethasone suppression test, urine or plasma metanephrines and, in virilised women, serum testosterone, DHEAS and androstenedione. CT and MRI can be used to assess malignant potential (from size, homogeneity, lipid content and enhancement). Biopsy cannot distinguish adenoma from carcinoma, but can help to diagnose metastases. Functional lesions and tumours greater than 4 cm in diameter are usually removed by laparoscopic adrenalectomy. In nonfunctioning lesions, less than 4 cm excision is only required if serial imaging suggests growth.

Primary hyperaldosteronism

This may occur in up to 10% of people with hypertension. Indications to test for mineralocorticoid excess in hypertensive patients include:
• Hypokalaemia. • Poor control of BP with conventional therapy. • Presentation at a young age.

Causes of mineralocorticoid excess include:

High renin and aldosterone (secondary hyperaldosteronism): Renin secretion is increased in response to inadequate renal perfusion and hypotension, for example, diuretic therapy, cardiac failure, liver failure, renal artery stenosis or very rarely, renin-secreting renal tumours.

Low renin and high aldosterone (primary hyperaldosteronism): Presents with hypertension; most patients have idiopathic bilateral adrenal hyperplasia and only a minority have an aldosterone-producing adenoma (Conn's syndrome).

Low renin and aldosterone: The mineralocorticoid receptor pathway in the distal nephron is activated, even though aldosterone levels are low. This can occur with ectopic ACTH syndrome, liquorice misuse, an 11-deoxycorticosterone-secreting adrenal tumour or Liddle's syndrome.

Clinical assessment

Patients with primary hyperaldosteronism are usually asymptomatic, but they may have features of sodium retention or potassium loss. Sodium retention may cause oedema. Hypokalaemia causes muscle weakness (or even paralysis), polyuria (renal tubular damage producing nephrogenic diabetes insipidus) and occasionally tetany (associated metabolic alkalosis and low ionised calcium). BP is elevated.

Investigations

Biochemical: Plasma electrolytes: hypokalaemia, ↑bicarbonate, sodium upper normal (primary hyperaldosteronism), hyponatraemia (secondary hyperaldosteronism: hypovolaemia stimulates ADH release, and high angiotensin II levels stimulate thirst). Renin and aldosterone levels distinguish the patterns above.

Localisation: Abdominal CT/MRI can localise an aldosterone-producing adenoma, but nonfunctioning adrenal adenomas are common and small adenomas may be missed. If the scan is inconclusive, adrenal vein catheterisation with measurement of aldosterone may be helpful.

Management

Mineralocorticoid receptor antagonists (spironolactone and eplerenone) treat both hypokalaemia and hypertension because of mineralocorticoid excess. Spironolactone can be changed to the sodium channel blocker amiloride (10–40 mg/day) if gynaecomastia develops (~20%). In patients with aldosterone-producing adenoma, preoperative therapy to normalise whole-body electrolyte balance should be undertaken before unilateral adrenalectomy. Postoperatively, hypertension remains in as many as 70% of cases.

Phaeochromocytoma and paraganglioma

These rare neuro-endocrine tumours may secrete catecholamines (adrenaline/epinephrine, noradrenaline/norepinephrine). Approximately 80% occur in the adrenal medulla (phaeochromocytomas), whereas 20% arise in sympathetic ganglia (paragangliomas). Most are benign, but around 15% show malignant features. Around 30% are associated with inherited disorders, including neurofibromatosis (p. 697), von Hippel–Lindau syndrome (p. 697) and MEN 2 (p. 417).

Clinical features

These can be paroxysmal and include:
• Hypertension (with postural hypotension). • Palpitations. • Pallor.
• Sweating. • Headache. • Anxiety (with fear of death). • Abdominal pain.
• Glucose intolerance.

Some patients present with a complication of hypertension, for example, stroke. There may be features of associated familial syndromes (see earlier).

Investigations

Excessive secretion of catecholamines can be confirmed by measuring metabolites (metanephrine and normetanephrine) in serum and/or urine. False positives occur in stressed patients and with some drugs (e.g. tricyclic antidepressants). False-negative results also occur because of intermittent catecholamine secretion. Phaeochromocytomas are identified by abdominal CT/MRI often combined with scintigraphy using meta-iodobenzyl guanidine (MIBG). [68]Gallium dotatate PET/CT imaging has high sensitivity for paraganglioma.

Management

Medical therapy is required preoperatively, preferably for a minimum of 6 weeks. The noncompetitive α-blocker phenoxybenzamine (10–20 mg orally three to four times daily) is used with a β-blocker (e.g. propranolol). β-Blockers must not be given before the α-blocker, as this may cause a paradoxical rise in BP. Careful pharmacological control of BP is essential during surgery for phaeochromocytoma.

10

Congenital adrenal hyperplasia

This rare autosomal recessive defect of cortisol biosynthesis causes insufficiency of hormones downstream of the block, with reduced feedback and increased ACTH causing over-production of steroids upstream of the block.

The most common example is 21-hydroxylase deficiency. This causes impaired synthesis of cortisol and aldosterone with accumulation of 17-OH-progesterone, which is converted into adrenal androgens. About 30% of cases present in infancy with features of glucocorticoid and mineralocorticoid deficiency and androgen excess, including ambiguous genitalia in girls. The remainder have milder cortisol deficiency and/or ACTH and androgen excess, causing precocious pseudo-puberty. The mildest defects may present in adult females as amenorrhoea and/or hirsutism (p. 393).

Investigations

Circulating 17-OH-progesterone levels are raised in 21-hydroxylase deficiency. Assessment is otherwise as described for adrenal insufficiency on p. 404. Antenatal diagnosis should be offered to families of affected children.

Management

Replacement of deficient corticosteroids suppresses ACTH-driven adrenal androgen production.

In hirsute women with late-onset 21-hydroxylase deficiency, antiandrogen therapy is equally effective.

The endocrine pancreas and GI tract

Presenting problems in endocrine pancreas disease

Spontaneous hypoglycaemia

Hypoglycaemia most commonly complicates treatment of diabetes mellitus with insulin or sulphonylureas. Spontaneous hypoglycaemia should only be diagnosed if all three conditions of Whipple's triad are met:

• Symptoms of hypoglycaemia. • Low blood glucose measured at the time of symptoms. • Symptoms resolving on correction of hypoglycaemia.

There is no specific blood glucose at which spontaneous hypoglycaemia occurs, but investigations are not needed unless values less than 3.0 mmol/L are observed.

Clinical assessment

Clinical features of hypoglycaemia are described on p. 430. Symptoms are episodic, and key questions include symptom frequency on fasting/exercise and symptom relief by consumption of sugar. Hypoglycaemia should be considered in all comatose patients, even if there is an apparently obvious cause such as alcohol intoxication.

Investigations

Does the patient have a hypoglycaemic disorder? In an acute presentation, hypoglycaemia is usually tested with capillary blood glucose strips. However, because of their relative inaccuracy, hypoglycaemia should be confirmed

by laboratory measurement. Establishing the existence of a hypoglycaemic disorder in outpatient clinics requires a prolonged (72-hour) fast:
If symptoms develop, blood is taken to confirm hypoglycaemia and to measure insulin and C-peptide. If symptoms resolve with glucose, Whipple's triad is completed. Absence of clinical and biochemical hypoglycaemia during the test excludes the diagnosis of hypoglycaemia.

What is causing the hypoglycaemia? Causes can be classified by the level of insulin and C-peptide measured in serum sampled during hypoglycaemia:

- ↓Insulin and ↓C-peptide: impaired liver glucose release because of alcohol (the most common cause in nondiabetics), drugs, critical illnesses, hypopituitarism, adrenocortical failure, nonislet cell tumours.
- ↑Insulin and ↓C-peptide: exogenous insulin.
- ↑Insulin and ↑C-peptide: insulinoma, drugs (sulphonylureas, pentamidine).

Insulinomas in the pancreas are usually small (<5 mm) and can be identified by CT, MRI or endoscopic/laparoscopic ultrasound. About 10% of insulinomas are malignant. Rarely, sarcomas may cause recurrent hypoglycaemia because of production of IGF-2.

Management

Acute hypoglycaemia should be treated as soon as blood samples have been taken. IV dextrose (5% or 10%) should be followed with oral carbohydrate. Continuous dextrose infusion may be necessary, especially in sulphonylurea poisoning. IM glucagon (1 mg) stimulates hepatic glucose release but is ineffective when glycogen reserves are depleted (alcohol excess, liver disease). Chronic recurrent hypoglycaemia in insulin-secreting tumours can be treated by regular carbohydrate consumption combined with inhibitors of insulin secretion (diazoxide or somatostatin analogues). Benign insulinomas are usually resected.

Gastroenteropancreatic neuro-endocrine tumours

Neuro-endocrine tumours (NETs) are a heterogeneous group derived from neuro-endocrine cells in many organs, including the GI tract, lung, adrenals (phaeochromocytoma) and thyroid (medullary carcinoma). They range from benign (e.g. most insulinomas) to aggressively malignant. Most GI and pancreatic NETs are nonsecretory and grow slowly but can metastasise, for example, to the liver. NETs may be single or multifocal (typically as part of MEN 1).

GI carcinoid tumours can secrete 5-hydroxyindoleacetic acid (5-HIAA), but this only produces carcinoid syndrome (flushing, wheezing and diarrhoea) when hepatic or peritoneal metastases allow vasoactive hormones to reach the systemic circulation. Secretory pancreatic NETs include:
• Gastrinoma: Zollinger–Ellison syndrome. • Insulinoma: recurrent hypoglycaemia. • Vipoma: watery diarrhoea, hypokalaemia. • Glucagonoma: diabetes mellitus, necrolytic migratory erythema. • Somatostatinoma: diabetes mellitus, steatorrhoea.

Investigations

A combination of imaging with ultrasound, CT, MRI and/or radio-labelled somatostatin analogue is used to identify the primary and allow staging.

Biopsy of the tumour or a metastasis is required to confirm the histological type. Carcinoid syndrome is confirmed by elevated concentrations of 5-HIAA in a 24-hour urine collection. False positives can occur after certain foods, for example, avocado and pineapple. Plasma chromogranin A can be measured in a fasting blood sample, and the pathologically secreted hormones can be useful as tumour markers.

Management

Treatment of solitary tumours is by surgical resection. Diazoxide may reduce insulin secretion in insulinomas, and high-dose proton pump inhibitors suppress acid in gastrinomas. Somatostatin analogues reduce the symptoms of carcinoid syndrome and of excess glucagon and vasoactive intestinal peptide. Cytotoxic chemotherapy, targeted radionuclide therapy with ^{131}I-MIBG, sunitinib, everolimus and resection/embolisation of hepatic metastases are used in advanced disease.

The hypothalamus and the pituitary gland

Diseases of the hypothalamus and pituitary are rare (annual incidence ~3:100000). The gland is composed of two lobes, anterior and posterior, and is connected to the hypothalamus by the infundibular stalk, which has portal vessels carrying blood from the median eminence of the hypothalamus to the anterior lobe and nerve fibres to the posterior lobe. The functions of the pituitary are summarised in Fig. 10.1.

Presenting problems in hypothalamic and pituitary disease

The clinical features of pituitary disease are shown in Fig. 10.6. The most common problem is an adenoma of the anterior pituitary.

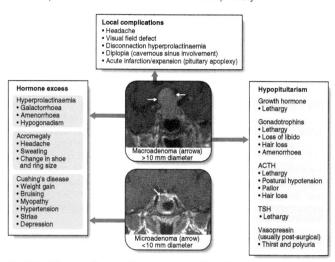

Fig. 10.6 Clinical effects of large and small pituitary tumours. *ACTH*, Adrenocorticotrophic hormone; *TSH*, thyroid-stimulating hormone.

Young women with pituitary disease most commonly present with secondary amenorrhoea or galactorrhoea (in hyperprolactinaemia). Men and postmenopausal women are less likely to report symptoms of hypogonadism, and so are more likely to present late with larger tumours causing visual field defects. Pituitary tumours are increasingly discovered incidentally on CT/MRI scans. Size and effect on secretory function determine symptoms:

- Microadenomas (<10 mm diameter) are common incidental findings and should only be treated if they are secreting excess hormones (examples include Cushing's, acromegaly and hyperprolactinaemia).
- Macroadenomas may also compress adjacent neural tissue and normal pituitary tissue, causing neurological symptoms and hypopituitarism (see Fig. 10.6).

Hypopituitarism

Hypopituitarism describes the combined deficiency of any of the anterior pituitary hormones. The most commonly cause is a pituitary macroadenoma, but other causes are shown in Box 10.16.

Clinical assessment

With progressive pituitary lesions, onset of symptoms is insidious. Pituitary functions are lost in a characteristic sequence:

1. Growth hormone: lethargy, muscle weakness and increased fat mass.
2. Gonadotrophins (LH and FSH): loss of libido, gynaecomastia, decreased shaving in men and oligomenorrhoea or amenorrhoea in women.
3. ACTH: symptoms of cortisol deficiency but maintenance of aldosterone secretion. Serum potassium is normal, but postural hypotension and

10

---

i **10.16 Causes of anterior pituitary hormone deficiency**

Structural

- Primary pituitary tumour (adenoma[a]), craniopharyngioma[a], meningioma[a], haemorrhage (apoplexy), arachnoid cyst

Inflammatory/infiltrative

- Sarcoidosis, infections (e.g. pituitary abscess, TB, syphilis, encephalitis), haemochromatosis, Langerhans cell histiocytosis

Congenital deficiencies

- GnRH (Kallmann's syndrome)[a], TRH, GHRH[a], CRH

Functional[a]

- Chronic systemic illness, excessive exercise, anorexia nervosa

Other

- Head injury[a], (para-)sellar radiotherapy[a], (para-)sellar surgery[a], postpartum necrosis (Sheehan's syndrome)

[a]Most common causes of pituitary hormone deficiency.

dilutional hyponatraemia may occur. Pallor caused by lack of stimulation of melanocytes by β-lipotrophic hormone (a fragment of the ACTH precursor).

4. TSH: secondary hypothyroidism contributes further to apathy and cold intolerance.

Investigations

The investigation of pituitary disease is described in Box 10.17. In acutely unwell patients, the priority is to diagnose and treat cortisol deficiency (see earlier), followed later by other tests. All patients with pituitary hormone deficiency should have an MRI or CT scan to identify pituitary or hypothalamic tumours. If no tumour is identified, further investigations are indicated to exclude infectious or infiltrative causes.

Management

Treatment of acutely ill patients is similar to that described for adrenocortical insufficiency (see earlier). Once the cause of hypopituitarism is established, specific treatment, for example, of a pituitary macroadenoma, may be required.

Cortisol replacement: Hydrocortisone is used. Mineralocorticoid replacement is not required.

Thyroid hormone replacement: Levothyroxine 50 to 150 μg once daily should be given. The aim is to maintain serum T_4 in the upper part of the reference range. It is dangerous to give thyroid replacement in adrenal insufficiency without first giving glucocorticoid therapy because this may precipitate adrenal crisis.

 10.17 Investigation of pituitary and hypothalamic disease

Identify pituitary hormone deficiency

- ACTH deficiency: short ACTH stimulation test; insulin tolerance test (if uncertainty in interpretation of short ACTH stimulation test)
- LH/FSH deficiency: male—random serum testosterone, LH, FSH; premenopausal female—ask if menses are regular; postmenopausal female—random serum LH (usually >20 IU/L), FSH (usually >30 mU/L)
- TSH deficiency: serum T_4; Note—TSH often detectable in secondary hypothyroidism (inactive isoforms)
- GH deficiency (only investigate if GH replacement contemplated): measure immediately after exercise; consider other stimulatory tests
- Cranial diabetes insipidus (may be masked by ACTH/TSH deficiency): exclude other causes of polyuria (blood glucose, potassium and calcium measurements); water deprivation test or 5% saline infusion test

Identify hormone excess

- Measure serum prolactin; investigate for acromegaly (glucose tolerance test) or Cushing's syndrome if indicated

Establish the anatomy and diagnosis

- Visual field testing; image pituitary/hypothalamus by MRI/CT

Sex hormone replacement: This is indicated for gonadotrophin deficiency in women under 50 years old and in men.

GH replacement: GH is administered by daily subcutaneous self-injection to children and adolescents with GH deficiency, and until recently was discontinued once the epiphyses had fused. There is now evidence that GH improves quality of life and exercise capacity in adults. It also helps young adults to achieve a higher peak bone mineral density. GH replacement is monitored by measurement of serum IGF-1 levels.

Pituitary tumour

Pituitary tumours may produce various local mass effects and may be discovered incidentally on CT/MRI or present with hypopituitarism. A wide variety of disorders can present as a mass in the pituitary/hypothalamus region:
• The majority of intrasellar tumours are pituitary macroadenomas (most commonly nonfunctioning adenomas). • Most suprasellar masses are craniopharyngiomas. • Parasellar masses are most commonly meningiomas.

Clinical assessment

A common presentation is headache as a result of stretching of the dura. Although, classically, compression of the optic chiasm causes bitemporal hemianopia or upper quadrantanopia, any visual field defect can result from suprasellar extension because tumour may compress the optic nerve (scotoma) or tract (homonymous hemianopia). Optic atrophy may be apparent on ophthalmoscopy. Lateral extension may compress the 3rd, 4th or 6th cranial nerve, causing diplopia and strabismus, although this is unusual in anterior pituitary tumours.

Occasionally, pituitary tumours infarct or there is bleeding into cystic lesions. This is termed *pituitary apoplexy* and may result in sudden localised compression and acute-onset hypopituitarism. Nonhaemorrhagic pituitary infarction may occur in obstetric haemorrhage (Sheehan's syndrome), diabetes mellitus and raised intracranial pressure.

Investigations

A precise diagnosis requires surgical biopsy, but this is usually performed as part of a therapeutic procedure. All patients should have pituitary function assessed (see Box 10.17).

Management

Specific treatments are described in the sections on hyperprolactinaemia, acromegaly and Cushing's disease. If serum prolactin is raised, dopamine agonists may shrink the lesion, avoiding the need for surgery. Nonfunctioning pituitary macroadenomas and craniopharyngiomas should be managed surgically, if needed, with radiotherapy reserved for second-line treatment. If there is evidence of pressure on visual pathways, urgent treatment is required. Most operations on the pituitary are performed using the transsphenoidal approach, from an incision under the upper lip or through the nose. Transfrontal surgery (craniotomy) is occasionally required for suprasellar tumours. All operations on the pituitary carry a risk of damaging endocrine function. Associated hypopituitarism should be treated as described.

Pituitary function (see Box 10.17) should be retested 4 to 6 weeks following surgery to detect the development of new hormone deficits. Imaging is repeated after a few months and, if there is any residual tumour, external radiotherapy may reduce recurrence, but the risk:benefit ratio needs individualised discussion. Radiotherapy is not useful in patients requiring urgent therapy, because it takes many months to be effective. It carries a lifelong risk of hypopituitarism (50%–70% in first 10 years), and annual pituitary function tests are obligatory. Nonfunctioning tumours are followed up by repeated imaging. For smaller lesions, therapeutic surgery may not be indicated, and the lesion may be monitored by serial neuroimaging.

Hyperprolactinaemia/galactorrhoea

Hyperprolactinaemia presents with hypogonadism and/or galactorrhoea. Galactorrhoea means lactation without breastfeeding. Prolactin stimulates milk secretion but not breast development; galactorrhoea therefore rarely occurs in men.

The causes of hyperprolactinaemia may be:

Physiological: Pregnancy, lactation, sleep, coitus, stress (e.g. postseizure).

Drugs: Dopamine antagonists (phenothiazines, antidepressants, metoclopramide); dopamine-depleting drugs (reserpine, methyldopa); oestrogens (contraceptive pill).

Pathological: Pituitary tumours secreting prolactin (prolactinoma) or compressing the infundibular stalk, interrupting the hypothalamic dopaminergic inhibition of prolactin secretion ('disconnection' hyperprolactinaemia).

Other causes of hyperprolactinaemia include primary hypothyroidism, PCOS, hypothalamic disease and macroprolactinaemia. Macroprolactin is prolactin bound to IgG antibodies, which cross-reacts with some prolactin assays. Because macroprolactin cannot cross blood vessel walls to reach prolactin receptors, it is of no pathological significance.

Clinical assessment

In women, in addition to galactorrhoea, the associated hypogonadism causes secondary amenorrhoea and anovulation with infertility. History should include drug use, recent pregnancy and menstrual history. Breast examination is important to exclude malignancy with discharge. In men, there is decreased libido, reduced shaving frequency and lethargy. Further assessment should address the features of any pituitary disease (p. 410).

Investigations

Pregnancy should be excluded. Macroprolactin should be measured and, if present with a normal unbound prolactin concentration, then further investigation is not necessary in the absence of clinical features. Prolactin levels may indicate underlying pathology:
• Normal: less than 500 mIU/L. • 500 to 1000 mIU/L: stress or drugs most likely in nonpregnant/nonlactating patients. Repeat the measurement. • 1000 to 5000 mU/L: drugs, microprolactinoma or 'disconnection' hyperprolactinaemia. • More than 5000 mU/L: suggests a macroprolactinoma.

Other investigations include:
• Test of gonadal function (see earlier) • TFTs to exclude primary hypothyroidism (TRH-induced prolactin excess). • MRI/CT of hypothalamus/pituitary if prolactin remains raised after drugs excluded. • Patients with a macroadenoma need tests for hypopituitarism (Box 10.17).

Management

Any underlying cause should be corrected (stop offending drugs; give levothyroxine in primary hypothyroidism). Physiological galactorrhoea can be treated with dopamine agonists. These include bromocriptine 2.5 to 15 mg/day, cabergoline 250 to 1000 µg/week and quinagolide 50 to 150 µg/day.

Prolactinoma

Most prolactinomas in premenopausal women are microadenomas, because symptoms trigger early presentation. Occasionally, prolactinomas also secrete GH and cause acromegaly. Prolactin concentration correlates with tumour size: the higher the level, the bigger the tumour.

Management

Dopamine agonists are first-line treatment and shrink most prolactin-secreting macroadenomas, rendering surgery unnecessary. In microprolactinomas, it may be possible to withdraw therapy without recurrence of hyperprolactinaemia after a few years. In macroadenomas, drugs can be withdrawn only after curative surgery or radiotherapy.

If dopamine agonists fail to shrink a prolactinoma, trans-sphenoidal surgery is effective. It cures 80% of microadenomas, although cure rates in macroadenomas are lower. Radiotherapy may be required for some macroadenomas to prevent regrowth if dopamine agonists are stopped.

Pregnancy

Patients with microadenomas should have dopamine agonist therapy withdrawn as soon as pregnancy is confirmed. In contrast, macroprolactinomas may enlarge rapidly under oestrogen stimulation. Dopamine agonist therapy should be continued with monitoring of prolactin levels and visual fields during pregnancy.

Acromegaly

Acromegaly is caused by GH secretion, usually from a macroadenoma.

Clinical features

If GH hypersecretion occurs before epiphyseal fusion, then gigantism will result. More commonly, GH excess occurs after epiphyseal closure and acromegaly ensues. The most common complaints are headache and sweating. Other clinical features include:
• Skull growth with prominent supraorbital ridges. • Prognathism. • Enlargement of lips, nose and tongue. • Enlargement of hands and feet. • Carpal tunnel syndrome. • Cardiomyopathy. • Increased incidence of diabetes mellitus, hypertension, cardiovascular disease and colonic cancer. Additional features include those of any pituitary tumour (Fig. 10.6).

10

Investigations

An oral glucose tolerance test with GH measurement confirms the diagnosis. In normal subjects, plasma GH suppresses to less than 0.5 µg/L (<2 mIU/L). In acromegaly, it does not suppress, and in around 30% of patients there is a paradoxical rise; IGF-1 is also elevated. Remaining pituitary function should be investigated (see Box 10.17). Prolactin is elevated in around 30% because of tumour co-secretion of prolactin. Screening for colonic neoplasms with colonoscopy may also be undertaken.

Management

Surgical: Trans-sphenoidal surgery is first-line treatment and may result in cure of GH excess, especially in microadenomas. However, surgery usually debulks the tumour, and further second-line therapy is required, according to postoperative imaging and glucose tolerance test results.

Radiotherapy: External radiotherapy is usually employed as second-line treatment if acromegaly persists after surgery, to stop tumour growth and lower GH. However, GH falls slowly (over many years), and there is a risk of hypopituitarism.

Medical: Somatostatin analogues (octreotide, lanreotide), administered as slow-release injections, are used to lower GH levels to less than 1.0 µg/L (<3 mIU/L) following surgery. These may be discontinued after several years in patients who have received radiotherapy. Dopamine agonists are less potent in lowering GH but may be helpful in patients with associated hyperprolactinaemia. A GH receptor antagonist (pegvisomant) is available for daily self-injection for patients unresponsive to somatostatin analogue therapy.

Craniopharyngioma

Craniopharyngiomas are benign tumours within the sella or suprasellar space. They usually present because of pressure on the pituitary or adjacent structures and are managed by surgery followed by radiotherapy to reduce relapse rate.

Diabetes insipidus

This uncommon disorder is characterised by the excretion of excessive dilute urine and by thirst. It can be classified as cranial diabetes insipidus (deficient vasopressin production by hypothalamus) or nephrogenic diabetes insipidus (renal tubules unresponsive to vasopressin). Causes are listed in Box 10.18. Clinical features include polyuria (5–20 L/24 hours) and polydipsia. Urine is of low specific gravity and osmolality. Adequate fluid intake can be maintained with an intact thirst mechanism in a conscious individual. However, in unconsciousness or hypothalamic thirst centre damage, DI is potentially lethal. The differential diagnosis includes diabetes mellitus and primary polydipsia (usually in patients with established psychiatric disease).

Investigations

DI is confirmed if, with an elevated plasma osmolality (>300 mOsm/kg), either serum vasopressin is undetectable or urine is not maximally concentrated

10.18 Causes of diabetes insipidus

Cranial

- Structural hypothalamic or high stalk lesion: see Box 10.16
- Idiopathic
- Genetic defect:
  Dominant
  Recessive (DIDMOAD syndrome)

Nephrogenic

- Genetic defect: V2 receptor mutation; aquaporin-2 mutation
- Metabolic abnormality: hypercalcaemia; hypokalaemia
- Drug therapy: lithium; demeclocycline
- Poisoning: heavy metals
- Chronic kidney disease: polycystic kidney disease, infiltrative disease, sickle-cell anaemia

(i.e., <600 mOsm/kg). Random simultaneous samples of blood and urine may exclude the diagnosis but, more often, the water deprivation test is required: no fluids are allowed for 8 hours, and body weight, plasma and urine osmolality are measured every 2 hours; the test is stopped if more than 3% of body weight is lost. DI is confirmed by plasma osmolality greater than 300 mOsm/kg with urine osmolality less than 600 mOsm/kg.

Desmopressin (DDAVP), an analogue of vasopressin with a longer half-life move earlier for clarity is then given to distinguish cranial and nephrogenic DI:
• Cranial DI: confirmed if urine osmolality rises by more than 50% after DDAVP. • Nephrogenic DI: DDAVP does not concentrate urine. • Primary polydipsia: suggested by low plasma osmolality at the start of the test.

Anterior pituitary function and suprasellar anatomy should be assessed in patients with cranial diabetes insipidus, as indicated in Box 10.17.

Management

Treatment of cranial DI is with DDAVP, usually administered via the nasal mucous membrane as a spray, although it can be given orally or intramuscularly. The ideal dose prevents nocturia but avoids hyponatraemia, for example, DDAVP nasal dose 5 μg in the morning and 10 μg at night. Polyuria in nephrogenic DI is improved by thiazide diuretics (bendroflumethiazide 5 mg/day) or amiloride (5–10 mg/day).

Diseases affecting multiple endocrine glands

Multiple endocrine neoplasia

MEN syndromes are rare autosomal dominant syndromes characterised by hyperplasia and tumours in multiple glands.
• MEN 1 (Wermer's syndrome): the association of primary hyperparathyroidism, pituitary tumours and pancreatic neuro-endocrine tumours.

• MEN 2 (Sipple's syndrome): primary hyperparathyroidism, thyroid medullary carcinoma and phaeochromocytoma.

• MEN 3: As for MEN 2 plus marfanoid habitus, skeletal and dental abnormalities and mucosal neuromas.

MEN 1 results from inactivating mutations in *MENIN*, a tumour suppressor gene on chromosome 11. In MEN 2 and 3, mutations are found in the *RET* proto-oncogene on chromosome 10. Genetic testing can be performed on relatives of affected individuals.

Individuals with MEN should have regular surveillance:

• MEN 1: annual measurements of calcium, GI hormones and prolactin; pituitary and pancreatic MRI is performed every 2 years. • MEN 2 and 3: measurement of calcium, calcitonin and urinary catecholamines. The penetrance of thyroid medullary carcinoma is 100% in individuals with a *RET* mutation. Prophylactic thyroidectomy is therefore performed in childhood.

Autimmune polyendocrine syndromes

Two distinct autoimmune polyendocrine syndromes are known: APS types 1 and 2.

• APS type 2 (Schmidt's syndrome): more common and observed in women aged 20 to 60 years. It is defined as the occurrence of two or more autoimmune endocrine disorders, for example, Addison's disease, hypoparathyroidism, type 1 diabetes, Graves's disease and coeliac disease. Inheritance is autosomal dominant with incomplete penetrance, and there is a strong association with HLA-DR3.

• APS type 1 Autoimmune polyendocrinopathy-candidiasis-ectodermal dystrophy (APECED): much rarer and displays autosomal recessive inheritance. In addition to autoimmune diseases, nail dystrophy, dental enamel hypoplasia and mucocutaneous candidiasis are seen.

Diabetes mellitus

Diabetes mellitus is a clinical syndrome characterised by hypergly-caemia caused by absolute or relative deficiency of insulin. Long-standing metabolic derangement can lead to the development of complications of diabetes, which characteristically affect the eyes, kidneys and nervous system. Diabetes occurs worldwide, and its prevalence is rising: 415 million people had diabetes in 2015, and this is expected to reach 642 million by 2040. Diabetes is a major burden upon health-care facilities in all countries.

Functional anatomy and physiology

Regulation of insulin secretion

Insulin is secreted from pancreatic β cells into the portal circulation in response to glucose and other nutrient stimuli. In addition, insulin release can be modulated by the autonomic nervous system and augmented by gut peptides following ingestion of food (the 'incretin' effect).

Insulin is synthesised as a prohormone (proinsulin) that is cleaved by β-cell peptidases to create insulin and C-peptide. Insulin secretion in response to a glucose stimulus is biphasic: an initial rapid phase repre-senting secretion of preformed insulin and a prolonged second phase representing newly synthesised insulin.

Regulation of glucagon secretion

Pancreatic islets also contain α cells that secrete glucagon. Glucagon has opposite effects to insulin and acts on the liver (and kidney) to stimulate gly-cogenolysis, increasing hepatic glucose production. Insulin and glucagon secretion are tightly and reciprocally regulated.

Blood glucose homeostasis

Blood glucose concentration is maintained within a narrow range. The brain cannot store energy as glycogen or triglyceride, nor can it utilise fatty acids, so it depends on a supply of glucose from the liver for generation of ATP. Glucose homeostasis reflects a balance between the entry of glucose into the circulation from the liver and intestine and the uptake of glucose by peripheral tissues, particularly muscle and brain.

Clinical examination of the patient with diabetes

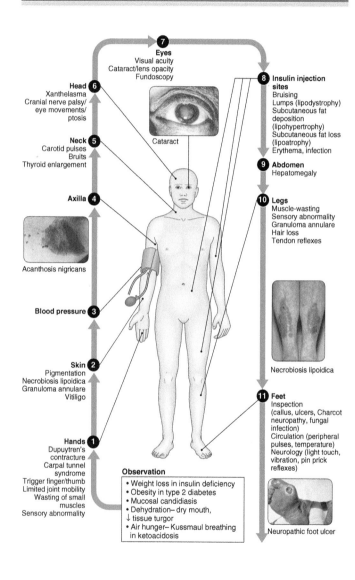

7 Eyes
Visual acuity
Cataract/lens opacity
Fundoscopy

Cataract

6 Head
Xanthelasma
Cranial nerve palsy/
eye movements/
ptosis

5 Neck
Carotid pulses
Bruits
Thyroid enlargement

4 Axilla

Acanthosis nigricans

3 Blood pressure

2 Skin
Pigmentation
Necrobiosis lipoidica
Granuloma annulare
Vitiligo

1 Hands
Dupuytren's
contracture
Carpal tunnel
syndrome
Trigger finger/thumb
Limited joint mobility
Wasting of small
muscles
Sensory abnormality

**8 Insulin injection
sites**
Bruising
Lumps (lipodystrophy)
Subcutaneous fat
deposition
(lipohypertrophy)
Subcutaneous fat loss
(lipoatrophy)
Erythema, infection

9 Abdomen
Hepatomegaly

10 Legs
Muscle-wasting
Sensory abnormality
Granuloma annulare
Hair loss
Tendon reflexes

Necrobiosis lipoidica

11 Feet
Inspection
(callus, ulcers, Charcot
neuropathy, fungal
infection)
Circulation (peripheral
pulses, temperature)
Neurology (light touch,
vibration, pin prick
reflexes)

Neuropathic foot ulcer

Observation
- Weight loss in insulin deficiency
- Obesity in type 2 diabetes
- Mucosal candidiasis
- Dehydration– dry mouth,
  ↓ tissue turgor
- Air hunger– Kussmaul breathing
  in ketoacidosis

Fat metabolism

Insulin also regulates fatty acid metabolism. Adipocytes (and hepatocytes) synthesise triglycerides from FFAs and glycerol. High insulin levels after meals promote triglyceride accumulation. During fasting, low insulin levels permit lipolysis, releasing FFAs and glycerol, which can be oxidised by many tissues. Partial oxidation in the liver drives gluconeogenesis and also produces ketone bodies, which may accumulate in starvation.

Investigations

Urine glucose

Urine dipsticks are used to screen for diabetes. Testing should ideally use urine passed 1 to 2 hours after a meal, as this will maximise sensitivity. Glycosuria always warrants further assessment by blood testing; however, glycosuria can be caused by a low renal threshold. This is a benign condition unrelated to diabetes that is common during pregnancy and in young people. Another disadvantage is that some drugs (such as β-lactam antibiotics, levodopa and salicylates) may interfere with urine glucose tests.

Blood glucose

Laboratory blood glucose testing is cheap and highly reliable. Capillary blood glucose can also be measured with a portable electronic meter used to monitor diabetes treatment. Glucose concentrations are lower in venous blood than in arterial or capillary (fingerprick) blood. Whole-blood glucose concentrations are lower than plasma concentrations because red blood cells contain relatively little glucose. Venous plasma values are the most reliable for diagnostic purposes.

Interstitial glucose

Subcutaneously implanted sensors can now be used for interstitial CGM, providing real-time glucose measurements every 1 or 5 minutes. CGM is not as accurate as blood glucose testing, particularly when levels are low or changing rapidly, but convenience and ease of measurement are leading to increased use.

Urine and blood ketones

Ketonuria may be found in normal people who have been fasting, exercising or vomiting repeatedly, or consuming a high-fat, low-carbohydrate diet. Ketonuria is therefore not pathognomonic of diabetes; but if there is also glycosuria, diabetes is highly likely. Beta-hydroxybutyrate (β-OHB) can be measured in blood in the laboratory, and also in a fingerprick specimen of capillary blood with a test stick and electronic meter. Blood β-OHB monitoring is useful in guiding insulin adjustment during intercurrent illness or sustained hyperglycaemia to prevent or detect diabetic ketoacidosis (p. 427).

Glycated Hb

Glycated Hb provides a measure of glycaemic control over a period of weeks to months. The nonenzymatic covalent attachment of glucose to Hb (glycation) increases the amount in the HbA_{1c} fraction relative to nonglycated adult Hb (HbA_0). The rate of formation of HbA_{1c} is proportional to the blood glucose concentration; for example, a rise of 11 mmol/mol in HbA_{1c} corresponds to an increase of 2 mmol/L (36 mg/dL) in blood glucose. HbA_{1c} concentration reflects blood glucose over the erythrocyte lifespan (120 days); it is most sensitive to glycaemic control in the past month.

HbA_{1c} estimates may be erroneously diminished in anaemia and pregnancy and may be difficult to interpret in uraemia and haemoglobinopathy.

Islet autoantibodies

Because type 1 diabetes is characterised by autoimmune destruction of the pancreatic β cells, it can be useful in the differential diagnosis of diabetes (see later) to establish evidence of such an autoimmune process.

C-Peptide

Serum C-peptide is a marker of endogenous insulin secretion that is not influenced by injected insulin treatment. It is very low in long-standing type 1 diabetes and very high in severe insulin resistance.

Urine protein

Standard dipstick testing will detect urinary albumin less than 300 mg/L, but lower levels require specific sticks or laboratory urinalysis. Microalbuminuria or proteinuria, in the absence of UTI, is an indicator of diabetic nephropathy and increased risk of macrovascular disease (p. 444).

Establishing the diagnosis of diabetes

Glycaemia can be classified as either normal, impaired (prediabetes) or diabetes. The glycaemia cut-off that defines diabetes is the level above which there is a significant risk of microvascular complications (retinopathy, nephropathy, neuropathy). Those with prediabetes have a negligible risk of microvascular complications but are at increased risk of developing diabetes. Also, because there is a continuous risk of macrovascular disease (atheroma of large blood vessels) with increasing glycaemia in the population, people with prediabetes have an increased risk of cardiovascular disease (myocardial infarction, stroke and peripheral vascular disease).

In symptomatic patients, diabetes can be diagnosed from a fasting glucose test, a random glucose test, a glucose tolerance test or an HbA_{1c} measurement (Box 11.1). Asymptomatic individuals should have a second confirmatory test. Diabetes should not be diagnosed by capillary blood glucose results.

Prediabetes can be subclassified as 'impaired fasting glucose' or 'impaired glucose tolerance' based on fasting and 2-hour glucose tolerance test results. Patients with prediabetes should be advised of their risk of developing diabetes and be given lifestyle advice and aggressive management for hypertension and dyslipidaemia to reduce this risk.

Stress hyperglycaemia occurs during acute severe illness, when cortisol and catecholamines antagonise the action of insulin. Glucocorticoid treatment can also cause hyperglycaemia. It usually disappears after the acute illness has resolved, but blood glucose should be remeasured.

> # i 11.1 Diagnosis of diabetes and prediabetes
>
> **Diabetes is confirmed by either:**
>
> - Plasma glucose in random sample or 2 hours after a 75 g glucose load ≥11.1 (200 mg/dL) *or*
> - Fasting plasma glucose ≥7.0 mmol/L (126mg/dL) *or*
> - HbA$_{1c}$ ≥48 mmol/mol
>
> In asymptomatic patients, two diagnostic tests are required to confirm diabetes.
>
> **'Prediabetes' is classified as:**
>
> - Impaired fasting glucose = fasting plasma glucose ≥6.1 mmol/L (110 mg/dL) and <7.0 mmol/L (126 mg/dL)
> - Impaired glucose tolerance = fasting plasma glucose <7.0 mmol/L (126 mg/dL) **and** 2-hour glucose after 75 g oral glucose drink 7.8–11.1 mmol/L (140–200 mg/dL)

When diabetes is confirmed, other investigations should include:

- U&Es. • Creatinine. • LFTs. • TFTs. • Lipids. • Urine: ketones, protein.

Aetiology and pathogenesis of diabetes

In both of the common types of diabetes, environmental factors interact with genetic susceptibility to determine who develops the clinical syndrome and the timing of its onset. However, the underlying genes, precipitating environmental factors and pathophysiology differ substantially between type 1 and type 2 diabetes.

Type 1 diabetes

Type 1 diabetes is invariably associated with profound insulin deficiency requiring replacement therapy. It is a T cell–mediated autoimmune disease leading to progressive destruction of the insulin-secreting pancreatic β cells. Classical symptoms of diabetes occur only when 80% to 90% of β cells have been destroyed. Pathology shows insulitis (infiltration of the islets with mononuclear cells), in which β cells are destroyed, but cells secreting glucagon and other hormones remain intact. Islet cell antibodies can be detected before clinical diabetes develops, and disappear with increasing duration of diabetes; however, they are not suitable for screening or diagnostic purposes. Glutamic acid decarboxylase (GAD) antibodies may have a role in identifying late-onset type 1 autoimmune diabetes in adults (LADA). Type 1 diabetes is associated with other autoimmune disorders, including thyroid disease (p. 381), coeliac disease (p. 479), Addison's disease (p. 418), pernicious anaemia (p. 567) and vitiligo (p. 763).

Genetic predisposition

Genetic factors account for about one-third of the susceptibility to type 1 diabetes, with 30% to 50% concordance between monozygotic twins. The HLA haplotypes *DR3* and/or *DR4* on chromosome 6 are associated with increased susceptibility to type 1 diabetes.

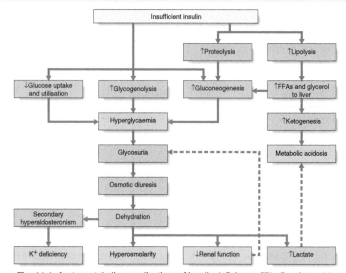

Fig. 11.1 Acute metabolic complications of insulin deficiency. *FFAs,* Free fatty acids.

Environmental predisposition

Wide geographic and seasonal variations in incidence suggest that environmental factors have an important role in type 1 diabetes. Viral infections implicated in the aetiology include mumps, coxsackie B4, retroviruses, congenital rubella, cytomegalovirus and Epstein-Barr virus. Various dietary nitrosamines (found in smoked and cured meats) and coffee have been proposed as potentially diabetogenic toxins. Bovine serum albumin (a constituent of cow's milk) has been implicated, as infants who are given cow's milk are more likely to develop type 1 diabetes than those who are breastfed. Reduced exposure to microorganisms in early childhood may limit maturation of the immune system and increase susceptibility to autoimmune disease (the 'hygiene hypothesis').

Metabolic disturbances in type 1 diabetes

Patients with type 1 diabetes present when adequate insulin secretion can no longer be sustained. High glucose levels may be toxic to the remaining β cells, so that profound insulin deficiency rapidly ensues. Insulin deficiency is associated with the metabolic sequelae shown in Fig. 11.1. Hyperglycaemia leads to glycosuria and dehydration, which induces secondary hyperaldosteronism. Unrestrained lipolysis and proteolysis result in weight loss, increased gluconeogenesis and ketogenesis. When generation of ketone bodies exceeds their metabolism, ketoacidosis results. Secondary hyperaldosteronism encourages urinary loss of potassium. Patients usually present with a short history of hyperglycaemic symptoms (thirst, polyuria, nocturia and fatigue), infections and weight loss, and may have developed ketoacidosis. Although classically regarded as a disease presenting in childhood and adolescence, about 50% of cases arise in adults.

> ### 11.2 Features of the insulin resistance (metabolic) syndrome
>
> - Hyperinsulinaemia
> - Type 2 diabetes or impaired glucose tolerance
> - Hypertension
> - Dyslipidaemia (↑LDL cholesterol, ↑triglycerides, ↓HDL cholesterol)
> - Nonalcoholic fatty liver
> - Central (visceral) obesity
> - Increased fibrinogen, uric acid
> - Polycystic ovarian syndrome (in women)

Type 2 diabetes

Type 2 diabetes is only diagnosed after excluding other causes of hyperglycae-mia, including type 1 diabetes. Patients retain some capacity to secrete insulin, but there is a combination of resistance to the actions of insulin followed by impaired pancreatic β cell function, leading to 'relative' insulin deficiency.

Insulin resistance and the metabolic syndrome

Type 2 diabetes is often associated with other medical disorders; when these coexist, they are termed 'metabolic syndrome' (Box 11.2), with a predisposition to insulin resistance being the primary defect. It is strongly associated with macrovascular disease (coronary, cerebral, peripheral) and excess mortality.

The primary cause of insulin resistance remains unclear, and multiple defects in insulin signalling are found. 'Central' adipose tissue may amplify insulin resistance by releasing FFAs and hormones (adipokines). Sedentary people are more insulin-resistant than active people with similar obesity. Inactivity down-regulates insulin-sensitive kinases and may also increase FFA accumulation within skeletal muscle. Exercise also allows non-insulin-dependent glucose uptake into muscle, reducing the 'demand' on pancreatic β cells to produce insulin. Many patients also develop non-alcoholic fatty liver disease.

Pancreatic β cell failure

In early type 2 diabetes, only around 50% of β cell function is lost. Amyloid deposits are found around pancreatic islet cells. Although β cell numbers are typically reduced, β cell mass is unchanged, and glucagon secretion is increased, which may contribute to the hyperglycaemia.

Genetic predisposition

Genetic factors are important in type 2 diabetes; different ethnic groups have different susceptibility, but monozygotic twins have concordance rates approaching 100%. However, many genes are involved, and individual risk of diabetes is also influenced by environmental factors.

Environmental and other risk factors

Diet and obesity: Epidemiology indicates that type 2 diabetes is associated with overeating, especially combined with obesity and under-activity. The risk of type 2 diabetes increases tenfold when BMI exceeds 30 kg/m². However, only a minority of obese people develop diabetes. Obesity probably acts as a diabetogenic factor in those who are genetically predisposed both to insulin resistance and β-cell failure.

Age: Type 2 diabetes is principally a disease of the middle-aged and elderly. In the UK, it affects 10% of the population older than 65 years, and less than 70% of all cases of diabetes occur after the age of 50 years.

Metabolic disturbances in type 2 diabetes

Relatively small amounts of insulin are required to suppress lipolysis, and some glucose uptake is maintained in muscle, so that weight loss and ketoacidosis are rare. Hyperglycaemia develops slowly, so the diagnosis may be overlooked or discovered incidentally. Initially, patients are often asymptomatic or give a long history (typically many months) of fatigue, with or without osmotic symptoms (thirst and polyuria). Some patients present late when pancreatic β cell function has declined to the point of profound insulin deficiency. These patients may present with weight loss, although ketoacidosis remains uncommon. In some ethnic groups, such as African Americans, however, half of those first presenting with DKA have type 2 diabetes.

Intercurrent illness, for example, infection, increases the production of stress hormones that oppose insulin (cortisol, growth hormone, catecholamines). This can precipitate more severe hyperglycaemia and dehydration.

Other forms of diabetes

These include:

• Pancreatic disease (e.g. pancreatitis, haemochromatosis, cystic fibrosis).
• Excess endogenous production of insulin antagonists (acromegaly, Cushing's disease, thyrotoxicosis). • Genetic defects of β cell function (e.g. maturity-onset diabetes of the young, a rare autosomal dominant disease representing <5% of diabetes cases). • Genetic defects of insulin action.
• Drug-induced diabetes (glucocorticoids, thiazides, phenytoin). • Diabetes associated with genetic syndromes (e.g. Down's syndrome, diabetes insipidus, diabetes mellitus, optic atrophy, deafness (DIDMOAD)).

Presenting problems in diabetes mellitus

Hyperglycaemia

Following the identification of hyperglycaemia and subsequent diagnosis of diabetes (Box 11.1), it is important to distinguish type 1 from type 2 diabetes, as the former is fatal without insulin treatment. The clinical features of type 1 and type 2 diabetes are compared in Box 11.3. Hyperglycaemia causes a wide variety of symptoms:

• Thirst. • Polyuria/nocturia. • Fatigue. • Blurred vision. • Pruritus vulvae/balanitis. • Nausea. • Hyperphagia. • Irritability, poor concentration, headache.

i	**11.3 Comparative clinical features of type 1 and type 2 diabetes**	
	Type 1	**Type 2**
Typical age at onset	<40 years	>50 years
Duration of symptoms	Weeks	Months to years
Body weight	Normal or low	Obese
Ketonuria	Yes	No
Rapid death without treatment with insulin	Yes	No
Autoantibodies	Positive in 80%–90%	No
Diabetic complications at diagnosis	No	25%
Family history of diabetes	Uncommon	Common
Other autoimmune disease	Common	Uncommon

Patients with type 2 diabetes may be asymptomatic or present with chronic fatigue or malaise. Uncontrolled diabetes is associated with susceptibility to infection, and patients may present with skin infections. A history of pancreatic disease (particularly with alcohol excess) makes insulin deficiency more likely.

Overlap occurs, particularly in age at onset, duration of symptoms and family history. Typical type 2 diabetes occurs increasingly in obese young people. Older adults may have evidence of autoimmune activity against β cells, a slowly-evolving variant of type 1 diabetes (LADA). More than 80% of patients with type 2 diabetes are overweight, 50% have hypertension, and hyperlipidaemia is common.

Diabetes presenting through complications

Diabetic complications (Box 11.9, p. 438) may be the presenting finding in a patient not known to have diabetes. Around 25% of people with type 2 diabetes have established complications at the time of diagnosis. Patients presenting with hypertension or a vascular event should have coexistent diabetes excluded.

Diabetes emergencies

Diabetic ketoacidosis

DKA is a medical emergency that principally occurs in people with type 1 diabetes. Mortality is low in the UK (~2%), but higher in developing countries and among nonhospitalised patients. It may be the presenting feature of diabetes, or may be precipitated by stress, particularly infection, in those

11.4 Average fluid and electrolyte loss in adult diabetic ketoacidosis of moderate severity

• Water: 6 L	3 L extracellular
• Sodium: 500 mmol	- replace with saline
• Chloride: 400 mmol	3 L intracellular
• Potassium: 350 mmol	- replace with dextrose

with established diabetes. Although DKA is typical of type 1 diabetes, an increasing number of patients presenting with DKA have underlying type 2 diabetes. This appears to be particularly prevalent in black populations. Sometimes, DKA develops because of errors in self-management. In young patients with recurrent episodes of DKA, up to 20% may have psychological problems complicated by eating disorders.

The cardinal biochemical features of DKA are:

• Hyperglycaemia. • Hyperketonaemia. • Metabolic acidosis.

Hyperglycaemia causes an osmotic diuresis leading to dehydration and electrolyte loss. Ketosis is caused by insulin deficiency exacerbated by stress hormones (e.g. catecholamines), leading to unrestrained lipolysis and supply of FFAs for hepatic ketogenesis. When this exceeds the capacity to metabolise acidic ketones, these accumulate in the blood. The resulting acidosis forces hydrogen ions into cells, displacing potassium ions, which are lost in urine or through vomiting. The average loss of fluid and electrolytes in moderately severe DKA in an adult is shown in Box 11.4. Patients with DKA have a total body potassium deficit, but this is not reflected by plasma potassium levels, which may initially be raised as a result of disproportionate water loss. Once insulin is started, however, plasma potassium can fall precipitously as a result of dilution by IV fluids, potassium movement into cells and continuing renal loss of potassium.

Clinical assessment

Clinical features of DKA are listed in Box 11.5.

Investigations

The following are important, but should not delay IV fluid and insulin replacement:

• U&Es, blood glucose, plasma bicarbonate and acid–base status (venous blood can be used, as differences from arterial pH and bicarbonate are minor). • Urine and plasma for ketones. • ECG. • Infection screen: FBC, blood/urine culture, CRP, CXR. Leucocytosis invariably occurs, representing a stress response rather than infection.

Management

Guidelines for the management of DKA are shown in Box 11.6. Patients should be treated in hospital, preferably in a high-dependency area, and

11.5 Clinical features of diabetic ketoacidosis

Symptoms

- Polyuria, thirst
- Weight loss
- Weakness
- Nausea, vomiting
- Blurred vision
- Abdominal pain, leg cramps

Signs

- Dehydration
- Hypotension (postural or supine), tachycardia
- Cold extremities/peripheral cyanosis
- Air hunger (Kussmaul breathing)
- Smell of acetone
- Hypothermia
- Delirium, drowsiness, coma (10%)

11.6 Management of diabetic ketoacidosis

First hour

- Give 0.9% saline IV: 1 L in 60 minutes, faster if systolic BP <90 mmHg
- Give insulin: 50 U human soluble insulin in 50 mL saline IV at 0.1 U/kg/hour
- Perform initial investigations and treat any precipitating cause–see text
- Monitor: *hourly*–capillary glucose and ketones, venous bicarbonate and potassium, pulse, BP, O_2 saturation, urine output; *4-hourly*–plasma electrolytes

1–12 hours

- Give 0.9% saline IV: 2 L over 4 hours, then 2 L over 8 hours; less in elderly, young and patients with renal or cardiac failure; 0.45% saline if sodium >155 mmol/L
- Add potassium chloride according to plasma potassium: >5.5 mmol/L–nil; 3.5–5.5 mmol/L–40 mmol potassium chloride/L infusion; <3.5 mmol/L–additional potassium chloride required–senior review
- Add 10% glucose 125 mL/hour IV when glucose <14 mmol/L (252 mg/dL)

12–24 hours

- Check that ketonaemia and acidosis have resolved–senior review if not
- Continue IV fluids and insulin (2–3 U/hour) until patient is eating and drinking
- If ketonaemia and acidosis have resolved and patient is eating, commence SC insulin with advice from diabetes team

Additional procedures

Catheterisation if anuric at 3 hours, CVP line if cardiovascular compromise, NG tube if obtunded or vomiting, ABGs and repeat CXR if oxygen saturation <92%, ECG monitoring if severe, thromboprophylaxis with low molecular weight heparin

Modified from Joint British Diabetes Society Inpatient Care Group, (2013).

the diabetes specialty team should be involved. Regular clinical and biochemical monitoring is essential. The principal components of treatment are insulin, fluid and potassium.

Insulin: The preferred route is IV infusion at 0.1 U/kg/hour, but (exceptionally) if this is not possible, 10 to 20 U can be given IM, followed by 5 U IM hourly thereafter. Blood glucose should ideally fall at a rate of 3 to 6 mmol/L/hour (~55–110 mg/dL/hour); a more rapid fall in blood glucose should be avoided, as this can cause cerebral oedema, particularly in children. Failure of blood glucose to fall within 1 hour of commencing insulin infusion should lead to a re-assessment of the insulin dose. When the blood glucose has fallen, 10% dextrose is introduced, and insulin infusion is continued to encourage glucose uptake into cells and restoration of normal metabolism. Short-acting SC insulin should be delayed until the patient is eating and drinking normally.

Fluid replacement: Large volumes are required; details are given in Box 11.6.

Potassium: Hyperkalaemia is often present initially, so replacement is not usually recommended with the initial litre of fluid treatment. Later, large amounts are usually required (100–300 mmol in the first 24 hours). Cardiac rhythm should be monitored in severe DKA because of the risk of arrhythmia.

Bicarbonate: Adequate fluid and insulin replacement should resolve the acidosis, so IV bicarbonate is not recommended. Acidosis may reflect an adaptive response, improving oxygen delivery to the tissues, and excessive bicarbonate has been implicated in the pathogenesis of cerebral oedema in children and young adults.

Hyperglycaemic hyperosmolar state

Hyperglycaemic hyperosmolar state is characterised by hypovolaemia, severe hyperglycaemia (>30 mmol/L (600 mg/dL)) and hyperosmolality (serum >320 mOsm/L) without significant ketoacidosis. It typically affects elderly patients, but is seen increasingly in younger adults. The onset is slow (days to weeks), and dehydration and hyperglycaemia are profound. Mortality is higher than in DKA—up to 20% in the United States.

Plasma osmolality should be measured, or osmolarity calculated, using the formula:

$$\text{Plasma osmolarity} = 2[\text{Na}^+] + [\text{glucose}] + [\text{urea}] \text{ (all mmol/L)}$$

The normal value is 280 to 296 mOsmol/L, and the conscious level is depressed when it is greater than 340 mOsmol/L. Treatment is different from DKA; in particular, rapid shifts in osmolality should be avoided by slower fluid replacement using only 0.9% saline, and guided by serial calculations of serum osmolality. Insulin is introduced only when the rate of fall in blood glucose has plateaued. Give prophylactic heparin (thromboembolic complications).

Hypoglycaemia

Hypoglycaemia in a nondiabetic person is covered on p. 408. Hypoglycaemia in diabetes (blood glucose less than 3.9mmol/L (70mg/dL) occurs as a result of treatment with insulin, and occasionally sulphonylureas. The risk of hypoglycaemia limits the attainment of near-normal glycaemia; fear of hypoglycaemia is common among patients and their relatives.

Clinical assessment

• Symptoms of autonomic nervous system activation: sweating, trembling, palpitation, hunger and anxiety. • Symptoms of glucose deprivation of the brain (neuroglycopenia), including delirium, drowsiness, poor coordination and speech difficulty.

Hypoglycaemia also affects mood, inducing a state of increased tension and low energy. Educating patients to recognise the onset of hypoglycaemia is important in insulin-treated patients. The severity of hypoglycaemia is defined by the ability to self-treat; 'mild' episodes are self-treated, while 'severe' episodes require assistance for recovery.

Circumstances of hypoglycaemia: Risk factors and causes of hypoglycaemia in patients taking insulin or sulphonylurea drugs are listed in Box 11.7. Severe hypoglycaemia can have serious morbidity (e.g. convulsions, coma, focal neurological lesions) and has a mortality of up to 4% in insulin-treated patients. Rarely, sudden death during sleep occurs in otherwise healthy young patients with type 1 diabetes. Severe hypoglycaemia is very disruptive, and impinges on employment, driving, travel, sport and personal relationships. Nocturnal hypoglycaemia in type 1 diabetes is common, but often undetected, as hypoglycaemia does not usually waken a person. Patients may describe poor sleep quality, morning headaches and vivid dreams or nightmares, or a partner may observe profuse sweating, restlessness, twitching or even seizures. The only reliable way to identify this problem is to measure blood glucose during the night. Exercise-induced hypoglycaemia occurs in people with well-controlled, insulin-treated diabetes because of hyperinsulinaemia. In healthy people, exercise suppresses endogenous insulin secretion to allow increased hepatic glucose production to meet the increased metabolic demand. In patients with insulin-treated diabetes, insulin levels may increase with exercise because of improved blood flow at injection sites, leading to hypoglycaemia.

Awareness of hypoglycaemia: For most individuals, the glucose threshold at which they become aware of hypoglycaemia varies according to the circumstances (e.g. during the night or during exercise). In addition, with longer duration of disease and in response to frequent hypoglycaemia, the threshold for symptoms shifts to a lower glucose concentration. This cerebral adaptation has a similar effect on the counter-regulatory hormonal response to hypoglycaemia. Taken together, this means that individuals with type 1 diabetes may have reduced (impaired) awareness of hypoglycaemia. Symptoms can be experienced less intensely, or even be absent, despite blood glucose concentrations <3.0 mmol/L (55 mg/dL). Impaired awareness of hypoglycaemia affects around 20% to 25% of people with type 1 diabetes and less than 10% with insulin-treated type 2 diabetes.

Management

Treatment of acute hypoglycaemia depends on its severity and on whether the patient is conscious. If hypoglycaemia is recognised early, oral

11.7 Hypoglycaemia: common causes and risk factors

Causes of hypoglycaemia

- Missed/delayed meal
- Unexpected or unusual exercise
- Alcohol
- Error in oral hypoglycaemic or insulin dose/timing
- Lipohypertrophy causing variable insulin absorption
- Gastroparesis as a result of autonomic neuropathy
- Malabsorption, e.g. coeliac disease
- Unrecognised other endocrine disorder, e.g. Addison's disease
- Factitious (deliberately induced)
- Breastfeeding

Risk factors for severe hypoglycaemia

- Strict glycaemic control
- Impaired awareness of hypoglycaemia
- Extremes of age
- Long duration of diabetes
- History of previous hypoglycaemia
- Renal or hepatic impairment

fast-acting carbohydrate, followed by a complex carbohydrate snack, is sufficient. In those unable to swallow, IV glucose (75 mL of 20% dextrose over 15 minutes, 0.2 g/kg in children) or IM glucagon (1 mg, 0.5 mg in children) should be administered. Viscous glucose gel solution or jam can be applied into the buccal cavity but should not be used if the person is unconscious. Full recovery may not occur immediately; reversal of cognitive impairment may take 60 minutes. The possibility of recurrence should be anticipated in those on long-acting insulins or sulphonylureas; a 10% dextrose infusion, titrated to the patient's blood glucose, may be necessary. In patients who fail to regain consciousness after blood glucose is restored to normal, cerebral oedema (which has a high mortality and morbidity) may have developed.

Following recovery, it is important to try to identify a cause, make appropriate adjustments to therapy and educate the patient. The management of self-poisoning with oral antidiabetic agents is given on p. 48.

Prevention of hypoglycaemia

Patient education must cover risk factors for and treatment of hypoglycaemia. The importance of regular blood glucose monitoring and the need to have glucose (and glucagon) readily available should be stressed. A review of insulin and carbohydrate management during exercise is particularly useful.

Relatives and friends also need to know the symptoms and signs of hypoglycaemia and should be instructed in how to help (including how to inject glucagon).

Management of diabetes

Aims are to improve symptoms and minimise complications:

- Type 1 diabetes: urgent therapy with insulin and prompt referral to a specialist.
- Type 2 diabetes: advice about dietary and lifestyle modification, followed by initiation of oral antidiabetic drugs/insulin if needed.
- Hypertension, dyslipidaemia and smoking cessation.

Diabetes is a complex disorder that progresses in severity with time. Patients with diabetes should therefore be seen by staff trained in diabetes care at regular intervals for life. A checklist for follow-up visits is given in Box 11.8. The frequency of visits varies from weekly during pregnancy to annually in well-controlled type 2 diabetes.

Self-assessment of glycaemic control: Patients with type 2 diabetes do not usually need regular self-assessment of blood glucose, unless they use insulin or are at risk of hypoglycaemia resulting from taking sulphonylureas. Insulin-treated patients should be taught to monitor blood glucose using capillary blood glucose meters, and to use the results to guide insulin dosing and to manage exercise and illness. A fasting glucose of 5-7 mmol/L (90–126 mg/dL), premeal glucose of 4-7 mmol/L (72–126 mg/dL) and 2-hour postmeal glucose of 4-8 mmol/L (72-144 mg/dL) represent optimal control. Continuous glucose monitoring is being used increasingly in place of fingerprick testing. Urine testing for glucose is not recommended.

Therapeutic goals

The target HbA_{1c} depends on the patient. Early in diabetes (i.e., patients managed by diet or one or two oral agents), a target of 48 mmol/mol or less may be appropriate. However, a higher target of 58 mmol/mol may be more appropriate in older patients with preexisting cardiovascular disease, or in those treated with insulin and therefore at risk of hypoglycaemia. The benefits of a lower target HbA_{1c} (primarily a lower risk of microvascular disease) need to be weighed against increased risks (primarily hypoglycaemia in insulin-treated patients). Type 2 diabetes is usually a progressive condition, so there is normally a need to increase medication over time to achieve the individualised target HbA_{1c}.

Treatment of hypertension (target <140/80) and dyslipidaemia is important to reduce cardiovascular risk. Statins are indicated when the 10-year cardiovascular event risk is at least 20%, and in all patients with type 2 diabetes aged over 40. In all diabetic patients, total cholesterol should be less than 4 mmol/L (150 mg/dL), and LDL cholesterol should be less than 2 mmol/L (75 mg/dL).

Patient education, diet and lifestyle

This can be achieved by a multidisciplinary team (doctor, dietitian, specialist nurse and podiatrist) in the outpatient setting. Lifestyle changes, such as taking regular exercise, observing a healthy diet, reducing alcohol consumption and stopping smoking, are important but difficult for many to sustain.

11.8 How to follow up patients with diabetes mellitus

Lifestyle issues	Smoking, alcohol, stress, sexual health, exercise
Body weight	
BP	Individualised target 130–140/70–80 mmHg based on risk
Urinalysis (fasting)	Glucose, ketones, macro- and microalbuminuria
Biochemistry	Renal, liver and thyroid function; lipid profile
Glycaemic control	HbA_{1c}, inspection of home blood glucose monitoring record
Hypoglycaemic episodes	Number and cause of severe and mild episodes, nature of symptoms, awareness, driving
Injection sites if on insulin	
Eye examination	Visual acuity, ophthalmoscopy, digital photography
Lower limbs and feet	Signs of peripheral neuropathy, ulceration, deformity, nails

Healthy eating

People with diabetes should have access to dietitians at diagnosis, at review and at times of treatment change. Nutritional advice should be tailored to individuals and take account of their age and lifestyle. The aims are to improve glycaemic control, manage weight and avoid both acute and long-term complications.

Carbohydrate

Both the amount and type of carbohydrate determine postprandial glucose. The effect of a particular ingested carbohydrate on blood glucose relative to the effect of a glucose drink is termed the glycaemic index. Starchy foods such as rice, porridge and noodles have a low glycaemic index and may reduce postprandial glucose excursions. However, food processing and preparation can influence the glycaemic index of foods, and this may limit their benefit.

Low-carbohydrate diets can cause weight loss and improved glycaemic control in the short term, but high dropout rates and poor adherence have limited widespread application of this approach. Increased consumption of whole grains has not been shown to improve glycaemic control.

For people with type 2 diabetes, avoidance of refined carbohydrates and restriction of carbohydrates to no more than 50% of total energy intake is recommended.

Fat

Total fat intake should be restricted to less than 35% of energy intake, of which not more than 11% should be polyunsaturated fats. Mediterranean diets rich in monounsaturated fats appear beneficial.

Salt

People with diabetes should follow general population advice: namely, adults should not consume more than 6 g of sodium daily.

Weight management

A high percentage of people with type 2 diabetes are overweight or obese, and administration of many antidiabetic medications and insulin encourages weight gain. Abdominal obesity also predicts insulin resistance and cardiovascular risk. Weight loss is achieved through a reduction in energy intake and an increase in energy expenditure through physical activity. In extreme cases, bariatric surgery can induce marked weight loss and improvement in HbA_{1c} in patients with type 2 diabetes, sometimes enabling treatment withdrawal.

Exercise

All patients with diabetes should be advised to maintain a significant level of physical activity (e.g. walking, gardening, swimming or cycling) in the long term. Supervised exercise programmes may be of particular benefit in type 2 diabetes. US guidelines suggest that adults aged over 18 years should do either 150 minutes per week of moderate-intensity exercise or 75 minutes per week of vigorous-intensity exercise, or a combination thereof. Muscle-strengthening (resistance) exercise is recommended on two or more days of the week. Recent evidence also indicates that extended sedentary time (>90 minutes) should be avoided.

Alcohol

Alcohol can be consumed in moderation. As alcohol suppresses gluconeo-genesis, it can precipitate or prolong hypoglycaemia, particularly in patients taking insulin or sulphonylureas. Drinks containing alcohol can be a substantial source of calories, and their intake may have to be reduced to assist weight reduction.

Driving

Legislation on driving with diabetes varies between countries. In the UK, people using insulin therapy must notify the DVLA. They must have adequate awareness of hypoglycaemia, have acceptable visual acuity and fields and not be regarded as a likely risk to the public while driving. Blood glucose testing before and during journeys is also required.

Ramadan

The Qur'an requires Muslims to fast during the month of Ramadan from sunrise to sunset. Although people with diabetes are a recognised exception to this, many still choose to fast. Diabetes therapies that do not cause hypoglycaemia are safest during Ramadan if glycaemic control permits.

Drugs to reduce hyperglycaemia

Most drugs used in type 2 diabetes depend upon a supply of endogenous insulin, and therefore have no effect in type 1 diabetes. The sulphonylureas and biguanides have been the mainstay of treatment in the past, but a variety of newer agents are now available, and the optimal place for these in treatment is yet to be determined.

Current US and European guidelines position metformin as the first-line treatment, then encourage choice of second-line treatment to be per-sonalised for each patient, taking into account the adverse risks of each drug—in particular, the risk of hypoglycaemia and weight gain. There is little evidence to guide the clinician and patient in choosing the second- or third-line treatment.

Biguanides

Metformin is now used widely as first-line therapy in type 2 diabetes. Approximately 25% of patients develop mild gastrointestinal side effects (diarrhoea, abdominal cramps, bloating and nausea) with metformin, but only 5% are unable to tolerate it even at a low dose. It improves insulin sen-sitivity and peripheral glucose uptake, and impairs both glucose absorption by the gut and hepatic gluconeogenesis. Endogenous insulin is required for its glucose-lowering action, but it does not increase insulin secretion or cause hypoglycaemia. Metformin does not increase body weight, and it is therefore preferred for obese patients. It acts synergistically with sulphonyl-ureas, allowing the two to be combined. Metformin is given with food two to three times daily. The usual starting dose is 500 mg twice daily (usual maintenance 1 g twice daily). Its use is contraindicated in alcohol excess and in impaired renal or hepatic function as a result of the increased risk of lactic acidosis. It should be discontinued temporarily if another serious medical condition develops (especially shock or hypoxaemia).

Sulphonylureas

Sulphonylureas are 'insulin secretagogues', that is they promote pancreatic β cell insulin secretion. They effectively lower blood glucose and are often used as an add-on to metformin, if glycaemia is inadequately controlled on metformin alone. They are known to reduce microvascular complications with long-term use.

Gliclazide and glipizide cause few side effects, but glibenclamide is long-acting and prone to inducing hypoglycaemia, so should be avoided in the elderly.

α-Glucosidase inhibitors

These delay carbohydrate absorption in the gut by selectively inhibiting disaccharidases. Acarbose or miglitol are taken with each meal, and lower postprandial blood glucose. Side effects are flatulence, abdominal bloating and diarrhoea.

Thiazolidinediones

These drugs ('glitazones' or PPARγ agonists) bind and activate a recep-tor found in adipose tissue, enhancing the actions of endogenous insulin.

Plasma insulin concentrations are not increased, and hypoglycaemia does not occur.

TZDs have been prescribed widely since the late 1990s, but a number of adverse effects have become apparent, and their use has declined. Rosiglitazone was reported to increase the risk of myocardial infarction, and was withdrawn in 2010. The other TZD in common use, pioglitazone, does not appear to increase the risk of myocardial infarction, but may exacerbate cardiac failure by causing fluid retention, and recent data show that it increases the risk of bone fracture and possibly bladder cancer. These observations have reduced the use of pioglitazone dramatically.

Pioglitazone can be effective in patients with insulin resistance, and also has a beneficial effect in reducing fatty liver and nonalcoholic steatohepatitis (p. 425). Pioglitazone is usually added to metformin with or without sulphonylurea therapy. It may be given with insulin, when it can be very effective, but the combination of insulin and TZDs markedly increases fluid retention and risk of cardiac failure, so should be used with caution.

Incretin-based therapies: DPP-4 inhibitors and GLP-1 receptor agonists

The incretin effect is the augmentation of insulin secretion seen when glucose is given orally rather than IV, as a result of the release of gut peptides (GLP-1 and GIP). These are broken down by DPP-4.

DPP-4 inhibitors: Prevent breakdown and therefore increase endogenous GLP-1 and GIP levels. Examples include sitagliptin, vildagliptin, saxagliptin and linagliptin. They are well tolerated and weight neutral.

GLP-1 receptor agonists: Mimic GLP-1 but are modified to resist DPP-4. They have to be given by SC injection, but have a key advantage over DPP-4 inhibitors in that they decrease appetite at the level of the hypothalamus. Thus GLP-1 analogues lower blood glucose and result in weight loss—a major advantage in obese patients with type 2 diabetes. Examples include exenatide (twice daily), exenatide modified-release (once weekly) and liraglutide (once daily).

Incretin-based therapies do not cause hypoglycaemia.

Sodium and glucose transporter 2 inhibitors

The SGLT2 reabsorbs glucose in the proximal tubules, and its inhibition results in glycosuria. The SGLT2 inhibitors dapagliflozin, canagliflozin and empagliflozin help to lower blood glucose, resulting in calorie loss and weight loss; however, the resulting glycosuria can cause genital fungal infections. SGLT2 inhibitors also reduce cardiovascular mortality and may be particularly useful in patients with vascular disease.

Insulin

The duration of action of the main groups of insulin preparations is given in Box 11.9.

i | **11.9 Duration of action (hours) of insulin preparations**

Insulin	Onset	Peak	Duration
Rapid-acting (insulin analogues: lispro, aspart, glulisine)	<0.5	0.5–2.5	3–4.5
Short-acting (soluble (regular))	0.5–1	1–4	4–8
Intermediate-acting (isophane, lente)	1–3	3–8	7–14
Long-acting (bovine ultralente)	2–4	6–12	12–30
Long-acting (insulin analogues: glargine, detemir)	1–2	None	18–26

Subcutaneous multiple dose insulin therapy

Insulin is injected SC into the anterior abdominal wall, upper arms, outer thighs and buttocks. The rate of absorption of insulin may be influenced by the insulin formulation; the site, depth and volume of injection; skin temperature (warming); local massage; and exercise. Absorption is delayed from areas of lipohypertrophy at injection sites.

Once absorbed into the blood, insulin has a half-life of just a few minutes. Excretion is hepatic and renal, so insulin levels are elevated in hepatic or renal failure.

Insulin delivered by re-usable syringe has largely been replaced by that delivered by pen injectors containing sufficient insulin for multiple dosing.

Insulin analogues have largely replaced soluble and isophane insulins, especially for type 1 diabetes, because they allow greater flexibility and convenience. Unlike soluble insulin, which should be injected 30 to 60 minutes before eating, rapid-acting insulin analogues can be administered immediately before, during or even after meals. Long-acting insulin analogues are better able than isophane insulin to maintain 'basal' insulin levels for up to 24 hours.

The complications of insulin therapy include:

• Hypoglycaemia. • Weight gain. • Peripheral oedema (insulin treatment causes salt and water retention in the short term). • Insulin antibodies. Local allergy (rare). • Lipodystrophy at injection sites.

A common problem is fasting hyperglycaemia (the 'dawn phenomenon') caused by the release of growth hormone and cortisol during the night and the waning of overnight isophane insulin.

Insulin dosing regimens

The choice of regimen depends on the desired degree of glycaemic control, the severity of insulin deficiency, the patient's lifestyle and the patient's ability to adjust the insulin dose. Most people with type 1 diabetes usually need multiple insulin injections daily. In type 2 diabetes, insulin is usually initiated as a once-daily long-acting insulin, with or without oral antidiabetic agents.

The plasma insulin profiles associated with various insulin regimens are illustrated in Fig. 11.2.

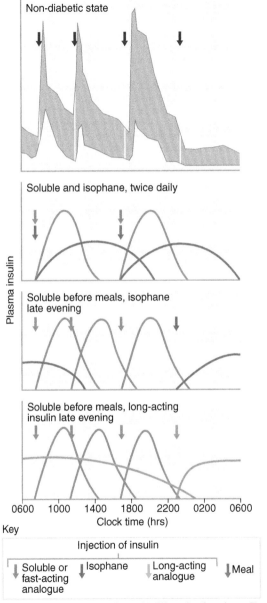

Fig. 11.2 Plasma insulin profiles associated with different insulin regimens. The schematic profiles are compared with the insulin responses (mean ± 1 standard deviation) observed in nondiabetic adults shown in the top panel (*shaded area*). These are theoretical patterns of plasma insulin and may differ considerably in magnitude and duration of action between individuals.

Twice-daily administration: A short-acting and an intermediate-acting insulin (usually soluble and isophane), given before breakfast and the evening meal, is the simplest regimen. Initially, two-thirds of the daily insulin is given in the morning in a ratio of short- to intermediate-acting of 1:2; the remainder is given in the evening. Premixed formulations containing fixed proportions of soluble and isophane insulins are useful if patients have difficulty mixing insulins, but the individual components cannot be adjusted independently. Fixed-mixture insulins also have altered pharmacokinetics, that is the peak insulin and time to peak effect are significantly reduced compared with the same insulins injected separately.

Multiple injection regimens: These are popular, with short-acting insulin injected before each meal, plus intermediate- or long-acting insulin injected once or twice daily (basal-bolus regimen). This regimen is more physiological and allows for variable meal timing and day-to-day physical activity.

Subcutaneous continuous insulin (insulin pump): Battery pumps infusing continuous SC insulin allow flexibility of bolus timing and shape and basal rate, allowing excellent glycaemic control. If integrated with continuous glucose monitoring systems, they form a 'closed loop' or artificial pancreas system. Widespread use of these systems is currently limited by cost.

Transplantation

Whole-pancreas transplantation presents problems relating to exocrine pancreatic secretions, and long-term immunosuppression is necessary. The procedure is often undertaken in patients with end-stage renal failure as a combined pancreas/kidney transplant, and posttransplant prognosis is good.

Transplantation of allogenic pancreatic islets (usually into the liver via the portal vein) has been adopted successfully in a number of centres around the world. Progress is being made regarding supply, purification and storage of islets, but the problems of transplant rejection and islet destruction by the patient's autoantibodies against β cells remain.

Management of diabetes in special situations

Diabetes in pregnancy

It is important to institute meticulous glucose control in pregnancy, as maternal diabetes is associated with increased risks of congenital malformations, stillbirth, preeclampsia, preterm delivery, operative delivery, neonatal hypoglycaemia and admission to neonatal intensive care.

Gestational diabetes

This is defined as diabetes with first onset or recognition during pregnancy. Occasionally, type 1 or type 2 diabetes develops during pregnancy, but the majority of these patients can expect to return to normal glucose tolerance immediately after pregnancy. Patients at high risk include those with a BMI greater than 30, those with previous macrosomia or gestational diabetes, those with a family history of diabetes or those belonging to a high-risk ethnic group (South Asian, black Caribbean, Middle Eastern).

The definitions of diabetes in pregnancy are based on maternal glucose levels associated with increased fetal growth, and are lower than the definitions for nongestational diabetes. The definition is either:

• Fasting venous plasma glucose greater than 5.1 mmol/L (92 mg/dL); or • Greater than 10 mmol/L (>180 mg/dL) at 1 hour or greater than 8.0 mmol/L (144 mg/dL) at 2 hours after a 75-gram glucose load.

Management of gestational diabetes

The aim is to normalise maternal blood glucose to prevent excessive fetal growth. Dietary restriction of refined carbohydrates is important. Women with gestational diabetes should regularly check pre- and postprandial blood glucose, aiming for premeal levels of less than 5.3 mmol/L (95 mg/dL) and 2-hour postmeal levels of less than 6.4 mmol/L (114 mg/dL). If treatment is necessary, metformin, glibenclamide or insulin can all be used, but other therapies should be avoided.

After delivery, maternal glucose usually returns rapidly to prepregnancy levels. These women should have fasting glucose measured 6 weeks postpartum and undergo annual HbA$_{1c}$ checks, because they remain at considerable risk for developing type 2 diabetes (5-year risk 15%–50% depending on the population) They should also be given diet and lifestyle advice (p. 433) to reduce this risk.

Pregnancy in women with established diabetes

Maternal hyperglycaemia early in pregnancy can lead to fetal abnormalities, including cardiac, renal and skeletal malformations, of which caudal regression syndrome is the most characteristic. Diabetic women should receive prepregnancy counselling and be encouraged to achieve excellent glycaemic control before conceiving. High-dose folic acid (5 mg, rather than the usual 400 μg daily) should be initiated before conception to reduce the risk of neural tube defects.

Glucose targets are as for gestational diabetes, but are often difficult to achieve. Pregnancy carries an increased risk of ketosis, which is dangerous for the mother and is associated with a high rate (10%–35%) of fetal mortality.

Pregnancy is associated with worsening of diabetic retinopathy and nephropathy. Heavy proteinuria and/or renal dysfunction before pregnancy indicates an increased risk of preeclampsia and irreversible loss of renal function. These risks need to be carefully discussed before considering a pregnancy. Diabetes increases perinatal mortality three- to fourfold and congenital malformation five- to sixfold.

Surgery and diabetes

Surgery causes catabolic stress and secretion of counter-regulatory hormones, resulting in increased glycogenolysis, gluconeogenesis, lipolysis, proteolysis and insulin resistance. This normally leads to increased secretion of insulin, which exerts a restraining and controlling influence. In diabetic patients, insulin deficiency leads to increased catabolism and ultimately metabolic decompensation. In addition, hyperglycaemia increases infection risk and impairs wound healing. Hypoglycaemia risk, which is particularly dangerous in the semiconscious patient, should be minimised.

Preoperative assessment

This includes assessment of:

• Glycaemic control (HbA$_{1c}$ and preprandial glucose). • Cardiovascular and renal function. • Foot risk (perioperative pressure relief).

Ideally, HbA$_{1c}$ should be less than 75 mmol/mol, and higher values should be optimised before surgery. For emergency patients with significant hyperglycaemia or ketoacidosis, this should be corrected first with an IV infusion of saline and/or dextrose plus insulin, 6 U/hour, and potassium as required.

Perioperative management

The management of patients with diabetes undergoing surgery who require general anaesthesia is summarised in Fig. 11.3. Low-risk patients can attend as day cases or be admitted on the day of surgery.

Patients who need to continue fasting after surgery should be maintained on an insulin and dextrose infusion with sodium and potassium supplementation. UK guidelines recommend the use of dextrose/saline (0.45% saline with 5% dextrose and 0.15% potassium chloride).

Complications of diabetes

People with diabetes have a mortality rate over twice that of age- and sex-matched controls. The range of complications of diabetes is summarised in Box 11.10. Cardiovascular disease accounts for 70% of all deaths. Atherosclerosis in diabetic patients occurs earlier and is more extensive and severe. Diabetes amplifies the effects of the other major cardiovascular risk factors: smoking, hypertension and dyslipidaemia.

Disease of small blood vessels (diabetic microangiopathy) is a specific complication of diabetes. It damages the kidneys, the retina and the peripheral and autonomic nerves, causing substantial morbidity and disability: blindness, difficulty in walking, chronic foot ulceration and bowel and bladder dysfunction. The risk of microangiopathy is related to the duration and degree of hyperglycaemia.

Preventing diabetes complications

The evidence that improved glycaemic control decreases the risk of microvascular complications of diabetes comes from the DCCT in type 1 diabetes, and the UKPDS in type 2 diabetes. The DCCT lasted 9 years and showed a 60% overall reduction in the risk of diabetic complications in patients with type 1 diabetes on intensive therapy with strict glycaemic control, compared with conventional therapy. However, the intensively treated group had three times the rate of severe hypoglycaemia. The UKPDS showed that, in type 2 diabetes, the frequency of diabetic complications is lower and progression is slower with good glycaemic control and effective treatment of hypertension, irrespective of the type of therapy used. Extrapolation from the UKPDS suggests that, for every 11 mmol/mol reduction in HbA$_{1c}$, there is a 21% reduction in deaths related to diabetes, a 14% reduction in myocardial

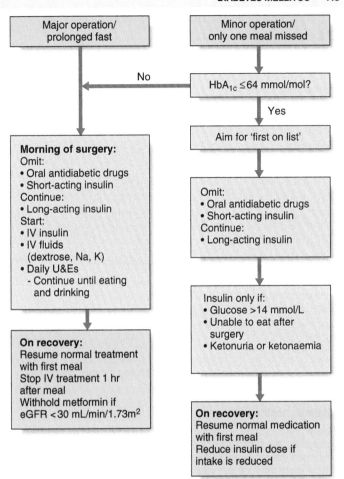

Fig. 11.3 Management of diabetic patients undergoing surgery and general anaesthesia. (Glucose >14 mmol/L = 250 mg/dL)

infarction and a 30% to 40% reduction in the risk of microvascular complications.

These trials demonstrate that diabetic complications are preventable, and that the aim of treatment should be 'near-normal' glycaemia. However, the recent Action to Control Cardiovascular Risk in Diabetes study showed increased mortality in a high-risk subgroup of patients who were treated aggressively to lower HbA_{1c} to less than 48 mmol/mol. Therefore, although a low target HbA_{1c} is appropriate in younger patients with earlier diabetes without underlying cardiovascular disease, aggressive glucose-lowering is

---

11.10 Complications of diabetes

Microvascular/neuropathic

Retinopathy, cataract	Impaired vision
Nephropathy	Renal failure
Peripheral neuropathy	Sensory loss, motor weakness
Autonomic neuropathy	Postural hypotension, gastrointestinal problems (gastroparesis; altered bowel habit)
Foot disease	Ulceration, arthropathy

Macrovascular

Coronary circulation	Myocardial ischaemia/infarction
Cerebral circulation	Transient ischaemic attack, stroke
Peripheral circulation	Claudication, ischaemia

---

not beneficial in older patients with a long duration of diabetes and with multiple comorbidities.

RCTs have also shown that aggressive management of lipids and BP limits complications. ACE inhibitors are valuable in improving outcomes in heart disease and in preventing diabetic nephropathy.

Diabetic eye disease

Diabetic retinopathy is a common cause of blindness in adults in developed countries. The complications of diabetes affecting the eyes are covered in detail in Chapter 17.

Diabetic nephropathy

Diabetic nephropathy is among the most common causes of ESRF in developed countries. About 30% of patients with type 1 diabetes have developed diabetic nephropathy after 20 years, but the risk after this time falls to lower than 1% per year. Risk factors for developing nephropathy include:

• Poor glycaemic control. • Duration of diabetes. • Other microvascular complications. • Ethnicity: Asian, Pima Indians. • Hypertension. • Family history of nephropathy or hypertension.

Pathologically, thickening of the glomerular basement membrane is followed by nodular deposits. As glomerulosclerosis worsens, heavy proteinuria develops, and renal function progressively deteriorates.

Diagnosis and screening

Microalbuminuria (defined as a urine albumin:creatinine ratio of 2.5–30 mg/mmol creatinine in men and 3.5–30 mg/creatinine mmol in women; undetectable by dipstick) is a risk factor for developing overt diabetic nephropathy in type 1 diabetes, although it also has other causes in type

2 diabetes. Overt nephropathy is defined as the presence of macroalbuminuria (urinary albumin >300 mg/day; detectable by urine dipstick). Patients with type 1 diabetes should be screened annually from 5 years after diagnosis; those with type 2 diabetes should be screened annually from the time of diagnosis.

Management

Progression of nephropathy can be reduced by improved glycaemic control and aggressive reduction of BP and other cardiovascular risk factors.

Blockade of the renin–angiotensin system using either ACE inhibitors or ARBs provides additional benefit over equal BP reduction achieved with other drugs, and is recommended as the first-line therapy. Treatment with ACE inhibitors or ARBs, however, may provoke renal impairment in renal artery stenosis. Calcium antagonists (diltiazem, verapamil) are second-line alternatives.

Halving the amount of albuminuria with an ACE inhibitor or an ARB reduces the risk of progression to ESRD by nearly 50%. However, in those who do progress, renal replacement therapy is of value at an early stage in diabetes.

Renal transplantation dramatically improves the life of many, and recurrence of diabetic nephropathy in the allograft is rare.

Diabetic neuropathy

This complication affects 50% to 90% of patients. It is symptomless in the majority, and can involve motor, sensory and autonomic nerves. Prevalence is related to the duration of diabetes and the degree of metabolic control.

Clinical features

Symmetrical sensory polyneuropathy: This is commonly asymptomatic. The most common signs are diminished perception of vibration distally, 'glove-and-stocking' impairment of all sensory modalities and loss of tendon reflexes in the legs. Symptoms may include paraesthesia in the feet or hands, pain on the anterior aspect of the legs (worse at night), burning sensations in the soles of the feet, hyperaesthesia and (when severe) a wide-based gait. Toes may be clawed, with wasting of the interosseous muscles. A diffuse small-fibre neuropathy causes altered pain and temperature sensation, and is associated with symptomatic autonomic neuropathy; characteristic features include foot ulcers and Charcot neuroarthropathy.

Asymmetrical motor diabetic neuropathy (diabetic amyotrophy): This presents as severe, progressive weakness and wasting of the proximal muscles of the legs (occasionally arms), accompanied by severe pain, hyperaesthesia and paraesthesia. There may also be marked loss of weight ('neuropathic cachexia') and absent tendon reflexes; the CSF protein level is often raised. This condition is thought to involve acute infarction of the lumbosacral plexus. Although recovery usually occurs within 12 months, some deficits become permanent. Management is mainly supportive.

Mononeuropathy: Either motor or sensory function can be affected within a single peripheral or cranial nerve. Unlike other neuropathies, mononeuropathies are severe and of rapid onset. The patient usually recovers.

11

Most commonly affected are the third and sixth cranial nerves (causing diplopia), and the femoral and sciatic nerves. Multiple nerves are affected in mononeuritis multiplex. Nerve compression palsies commonly affect the median nerve and lateral popliteal nerve (foot drop).

Autonomic neuropathy: This is less clearly related to poor metabolic control, and improved control rarely improves symptoms. Within 10 years of developing autonomic neuropathy, 30% to 50% of patients are dead. Postural hypotension indicates a poor prognosis.

Gastroparesis: This means an objectively measured delay in gastric emptying in the absence of mechanical obstruction. It usually represents autonomic neuropathy in diabetes, but can complicate anorexia nervosa or bulimia, which are also associated with diabetes. It causes chronic nausea, vomiting (especially of undigested food), abdominal pain and a feeling of early satiety. Diagnosis is by [99m]-technetium scintigraphy following a solid-phase meal.

Erectile dysfunction: This affects 30% of diabetic males and is often multifactorial. Psychological problems, depression, alcohol and drug therapy may contribute (p. 248).

Management
See Box 11.11.

11.11 Management of peripheral sensorimotor and autonomic neuropathies		
Type of neuropathy	**Symptom/sign**	**Management**
Peripheral somatic neuropathies	Pain and paraesthesiae	Strict glycaemic control Anticonvulsants (e.g. gabapentin) Antidepressants (e.g. amitriptyline, duloxetine) Substance P depleter (capsaicin–topical) Opiates (tramadol, oxycodone) Membrane stabilisers (mexiletine, IV lidocaine) Antioxidant (α-lipoic acid)
Autonomic neuropathy	Postural hypotension	Fludrocortisone, NSAIDs, midodrine Support stockings
	Gastroparesis	Metoclopramide, erythromycin Gastric pacemaker, enterostomy feeding
	Motility disorders	Diarrhoea: loperamide, octreotide Constipation: stimulant laxatives
	Atonic bladder	Intermittent self-catheterisation
	Excessive sweating	Propantheline, clonidine Topical antimuscarinics (e.g. glycopyrrolate)
	Erectile dysfunction	Sildenafil Prostaglandin injections

The diabetic foot

Tissue necrosis in the feet is a common reason for hospital admission in diabetic patients. Foot ulceration occurs as a result of often trivial trauma in the presence of neuropathy (peripheral and autonomic) and/or peripheral vascular disease; infection occurs as a secondary phenomenon. Most ulcers are neuropathic or neuro-ischaemic in type. They usually develop at the site of a plaque of callus skin, beneath which tissue necrosis occurs, eventually breaking through to the surface. Charcot neuro-arthropathy, with destructive inflammation of neuropathic joints, is usually caused by diabetes.

Management

Preventative treatment is the most effective method of managing the diabetic foot. Patient education is crucial. Annual screening should include formal testing of sensation and removal of callus (by podiatrist). Further management includes:

- Debridement of dead tissue.
- Prompt and prolonged antibiotics in the presence of infection.
- Bespoke orthotic footwear (preventing pressure and deformity).
- Vascular assessment: angiography/vascular reconstruction if the foot is ischaemic.
- Charcot foot: cast immobilisation and avoidance of weight-bearing.
- Amputation: if there is extensive tissue/bony destruction, or intractable ischaemic pain when vascular reconstruction is not possible or has failed.

11

Gastroenterology

Diseases of the GI tract are a major cause of morbidity and mortality. Approximately 10% of all GP consultations in the UK are for indigestion, and 1 in 14 is for diarrhoea. Infective diarrhoea and malabsorption are responsible for much ill health and many deaths in the developing world.

Presenting problems in gastrointestinal disease

Dysphagia

Dysphagia means difficulty in swallowing, as distinct from globus sensation (a 'lump' in the throat without organic cause) and odynophagia (pain during swallowing). Oropharyngeal dysphagia results from neuromuscular dysfunction that affects swallowing, causing choking, nasal regurgitation or tracheal aspiration. Drooling, dysarthria, hoarseness and other neurological signs may be present. Oesophageal causes include benign or malignant strictures and oesophageal dysmotility. Patients complain of food 'sticking' after swallowing, although swallowing of liquids is normal until strictures become extreme.

Endoscopy is preferred to facilitate biopsy and dilatation of strictures. Videofluoroscopic barium swallow will detect most motility disorders. Oesophageal manometry is occasionally required.

Dyspepsia

Dyspepsia describes symptoms of discomfort, bloating and nausea in the upper abdomen. There are many causes (Box 12.1). Although symptoms correlate poorly with diagnosis, careful history may reveal classical symptoms of peptic ulcer, 'alarm' features requiring urgent investigation (Box 12.2) or symptoms of other disorders. Dyspepsia affects up to 80% of the population at some time, often with no abnormality on investigation, especially in younger patients.

Examination may reveal anaemia, weight loss, lymphadenopathy, abdominal masses or liver disease. Patients with 'alarm' symptoms, and those older than 55 years with new dyspepsia require prompt endoscopy.

Clinical examination of the gastrointestinal tract

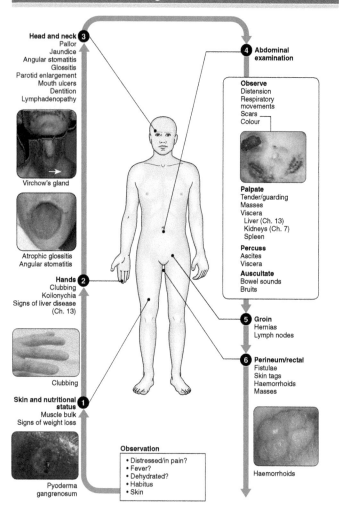

Head and neck ❸
Pallor
Jaundice
Angular stomatitis
Glossitis
Parotid enlargement
Mouth ulcers
Dentition
Lymphadenopathy

Virchow's gland

Atrophic glossitis
Angular stomatitis

Hands ❷
Clubbing
Koilonychia
Signs of liver disease
(Ch. 13)

Clubbing

**Skin and nutritional
status** ❶
Muscle bulk
Signs of weight loss

Pyoderma
gangrenosum

Observation
• Distressed/in pain?
• Fever?
• Dehydrated?
• Habitus
• Skin

❹ **Abdominal
examination**

Observe
Distension
Respiratory
movements
Scars
Colour

Palpate
Tender/guarding
Masses
Viscera
  Liver (Ch. 13)
  Kidneys (Ch. 7)
  Spleen
Percuss
Ascites
Viscera
Auscultate
Bowel sounds
Bruits

❺ **Groin**
Hernias
Lymph nodes

❻ **Perineum/rectal**
Fistulae
Skin tags
Haemorrhoids
Masses

Haemorrhoids

Younger patients should be tested for *Helicobacter pylori*; if symptoms persist after treatment, they should have endoscopy.

Heartburn and regurgitation

Heartburn describes retrosternal, burning discomfort, sometimes with regurgitation of bitter fluid into the throat. Symptoms occur after meals, on lying down or with bending, straining or heavy lifting, and are typical

12.1 Causes of dyspepsia

GI disorders

- Peptic ulcer disease
- Acute gastritis
- Gallstones
- Motility disorders, e.g. oesophageal spasm
- Colonic carcinoma
- 'Functional' (nonulcer dyspepsia and irritable bowel syndrome)
- Pancreatic disease (cancer, chronic pancreatitis)
- Hepatic disease (hepatitis, metastases)

Systemic disease

- Renal failure
- Hypercalcaemia

Drugs

- NSAIDs
- Iron and potassium supplements
- Glucocorticoids
- Digoxin

Others

- Psychological, e.g. anxiety, depression
- Alcohol

12

12.2 'Alarm' features in dyspepsia

- Weight loss
- Anaemia
- Vomiting
- Haematemesis and/or melaena
- Dysphagia
- Palpable abdominal mass

of gastro-oesophageal reflux. However, nearly half of patients with reflux present atypically, with chest pain, belching, halitosis, chronic cough or sore throats. Young patients responding to dietary changes, antacids or acid suppression do not need investigation. Patients aged over 55 years and those with alarm symptoms or atypical features need urgent endoscopy.

Vomiting

Vomiting is a complex reflex involving contraction of the diaphragm and intercostal and abdominal muscles and simultaneous relaxation of the lower oesophageal sphincter, causing forcible ejection of gastric contents.

> ### 12.3 Common causes of acute upper GI haemorrhage
>
> - Oesophagitis (10%)
> - Mallory–Weiss tear (5%)
> - Varices (2%–9%)
> - Peptic ulcer (*H. pylori* or NSAID) (35%–50%)
> - Gastric erosions (NSAID or alcohol) (10%–20%)
> - Vascular malformation (5%)
> - Carcinoma of stomach or oesophagus (2%)

The history helps to distinguish the main causes:

- Alcoholism
- Gastroduodenal—peptic ulcer, cancer, gastroparesis
- CNS—vestibular neuronitis, migraine, raised ICP, meningitis
- Metabolic—diabetic ketoacidosis, Addison's disease
- Acute abdomen—appendicitis, cholecystitis, pancreatitis, intestinal obstruction
- Infections—gastroenteritis, hepatitis, urinary tract infection
- Drugs—digoxin, opiates, NSAIDs, antibiotics, cytotoxics
- Psychogenic

GI bleeding

Acute upper GI haemorrhage

This is the most common GI emergency, accounting for 50 to 170 hospital admissions per 100 000 each year in the UK.

Haematemesis may be red with clots when bleeding is profuse, or black ('coffee grounds') when less severe. Syncope may occur with rapid bleeding. Anaemia suggests chronic bleeding. Melaena is the passage of black, tarry stools containing altered blood. This is usually because of upper GI bleeding, although the ascending colon is occasionally responsible. Severe acute upper GI bleeding occasionally causes maroon or bright red stool. Causes of acute upper GI haemorrhage are shown in Box 12.3.

Management

IV access: should be secured with a large-bore cannula.

Clinical assessment: • Circulatory–tachycardia, hypotension and oliguria indicate severe bleeding. • Liver disease–jaundice, cutaneous stigmata, hepatosplenomegaly and ascites. • Comorbidity—cardiorespiratory, cerebrovascular or renal disease may be worsened by bleeding and also increase the hazards of endoscopy and surgery.

Blood tests: Full blood count: bleeding causes anaemia, although haemoglobin may be normal after sudden, major bleeding. Cross-match at least 2 U of blood in significant bleeding. U&Es—shock may cause kidney injury; urea also rises as luminal blood is digested. LFTs and prothrombin time, to detect liver disease or in anticoagulated patients.

Resuscitation: IV crystalloid infusion restores BP, and blood transfusion is indicated if there is shock and active bleeding. Antibiotics are given in chronic liver disease. Oxygen should be given to all shocked patients.

Endoscopy: After resuscitation, this will reveal a diagnosis in 80% of cases. Patients with a visible bleeding vessel can be treated by thermal probe or metal clips, combined with adrenaline (epinephrine) injection. This may stop bleeding and, combined with IV PPI therapy, prevent rebleeding, thus avoiding surgery. Variceal bleeding is covered on p. 525.

Monitoring: Hourly pulse, BP and urine output should be monitored.

Surgery: This is indicated when endoscopic haemostasis fails to stop the bleeding, or rebleeding occurs once in an elderly or frail patient/twice in younger, fitter patients.

Following successful treatment for ulcer bleeding, all patients should avoid NSAIDs, and those who test positive for *H. pylori* should receive eradication therapy.

Lower GI bleeding

This may be the result of haemorrhage from the small bowel, colon or anal canal.

Severe acute lower GI bleeding

Patients present with profuse red or maroon diarrhoea and shock.

Diverticular disease: This is the most common cause. Bleeding almost always stops spontaneously, but if not, the diseased segment is located by angiography or colonoscopy and resected.

Angiodysplasia: Vascular malformations in the proximal colon of elderly patients cause bleeding, which usually stops spontaneously but commonly recurs. Treatment is by colonoscopic thermal ablation, or by resection if bleeding continues.

Ischaemia because of inferior mesenteric artery occlusion: Presents with abdominal colic and rectal bleeding. It occurs in elderly patients with atherosclerosis and is diagnosed by colonoscopy. Resection is required only if peritonitis develops.

Meckel's diverticulum: May erode into a major artery and cause profuse lower GI bleeding in children or adolescents. The diagnosis is commonly made only by resection at laparotomy.

Subacute or chronic lower GI bleeding

This is extremely common and is usually as a result of haemorrhoids or anal fissure. Proctoscopy reveals the diagnosis, but if there is altered bowel habit, and in all patients presenting at age 40 years and over, colonoscopy is necessary to exclude colorectal cancer.

Major GI bleeding of unknown cause

If upper endoscopy and colonoscopy are inconclusive, CT mesenteric angiography usually identifies the site, and angiographic embolisation can often stop the bleeding. If angiography is negative, double balloon enteroscopy or wireless capsule endoscopy can be employed to identify a bleeding source in the small intestine. When all else fails, laparotomy with on-table endoscopy is indicated.

Occult GI bleeding

Occult bleeding (no visible blood) may reach 200 mL/day, cause iron deficiency anaemia and signify serious disease. The most important cause is colorectal cancer, which may have no GI symptoms. GI investigations should be considered in any patient with unexplained iron deficiency anaemia. A negative faecal occult blood (FOB) test does not exclude important GI disease. FOB is now only used in population screening for colonic neoplasia.

Diarrhoea

Diarrhoea is defined as the passage of more than 200 g of stool daily, commonly with increased frequency and loose or watery stools. In severe cases, urgency of defecation and faecal incontinence occur.

Acute diarrhoea

Infective diarrhoea is usually caused by faecal–oral transmission of bacteria, viruses or parasites, and is normally short-lived. Diarrhoea lasting more than 10 days is rarely caused by infection. Drugs, including antibiotics, cytotoxics, PPIs and NSAIDs, may cause acute diarrhoea.

Chronic or relapsing diarrhoea

The most common cause is irritable bowel syndrome, in which frequent watery or pellety stools are passed mainly before and after breakfast, rarely at night. At other times the patient is constipated. The stool often contains mucus but never blood, and 24-hour stool volume is less than 200 g. Chronic diarrhoea can also be caused by inflammatory or neoplastic disease of the colon or small bowel, or by malabsorption. Negative investigations suggest irritable bowel syndrome.

Malabsorption

Diarrhoea and weight loss in patients with a normal diet suggest malabsorption. Bulky, pale and offensive stools that float (steatorrhoea) signify fat malabsorption. Abdominal distension, borborygmi, cramps and undigested food in the stool may be present. Malaise, lethargy, peripheral neuropathy and symptoms related to vitamin or mineral deficiencies may occur.

Malabsorption results from abnormalities of the three components of normal digestion:

• Intraluminal maldigestion caused by deficiency of bile or pancreatic enzymes. • Mucosal malabsorption from small bowel resection or damage to the small intestinal epithelium. • 'Postmucosal' lymphatic obstruction preventing the uptake of absorbed lipids into lymphatic vessels.

Investigation of malabsorption is outlined in Fig 12.1.

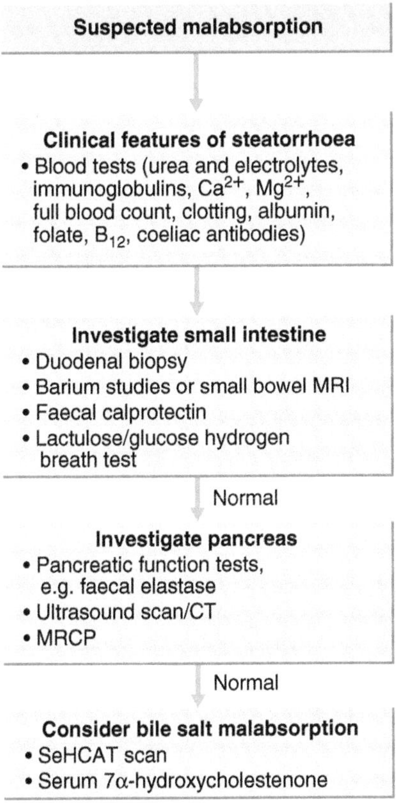

Suspected malabsorption

↓

Clinical features of steatorrhoea
- Blood tests (urea and electrolytes, immunoglobulins, Ca^{2+}, Mg^{2+}, full blood count, clotting, albumin, folate, B_{12}, coeliac antibodies)

↓

Investigate small intestine
- Duodenal biopsy
- Barium studies or small bowel MRI
- Faecal calprotectin
- Lactulose/glucose hydrogen breath test

↓ Normal

Investigate pancreas
- Pancreatic function tests, e.g. faecal elastase
- Ultrasound scan/CT
- MRCP

↓ Normal

Consider bile salt malabsorption
- SeHCAT scan
- Serum 7α-hydroxycholestenone

Fig. 12.1 Investigation for suspected malabsorption. *CT,* Computed tomography; *MRCP,* magnetic resonance cholangiopancreatography; *MRI,* magnetic resonance imaging; [75]*SeHCAT,* ^{75}Se-homocholic acid taurine.

Weight loss

Unplanned weight loss of more than 3 kg over 6 months is significant. Previous weight records are useful confirmation. Pathological weight loss can be caused by psychiatric illness, systemic disease, GI causes or advanced disease of any specific organ system.

History and examination

Physiological causes: Change in diet, activity or social circumstances are revealed by the history, although in older patients the dietary history may be unreliable; a dietitian's opinion is often valuable.

Psychiatric illness: Features of anorexia nervosa, bulimia and depression may be apparent only after formal psychiatric input. Alcoholic patients lose weight through self-neglect and poor diet.

12.4 Causes of constipation

GI–

- Lack of dietary fibre +/– fluid intake
- Altered motility, e.g. irritable bowel syndrome
- Structural, e.g. colonic carcinoma, diverticular disease, Hirschsprung's disease
- Obstructed defecation, e.g. anal fissure, Crohn's disease

Non-GI

- Drugs, e.g. opiates, anticholinergics
- Neurological, e.g. multiple sclerosis, paraplegia
- Metabolic/endocrine, e.g. hypercalcaemia, hypothyroidism
- Others: any serious illness, especially in the elderly, depression

Systemic diseases: Chronic infections lead to weight loss, and a history of foreign travel, fever, night sweats, rigours, productive cough and dysuria must be sought. Promiscuous sexual activity and drug misuse suggest HIV-related illness. Weight loss is a late feature of disseminated malignancy (carcinoma, lymphoma or other haematological disorders), which may be revealed on examination.

GI disease: Dysphagia and gastric outflow obstruction cause defective intake. Malignancy may cause weight loss by mechanical obstruction, anorexia or systemic effects. Pancreatic or small bowel malabsorption causes profound weight loss and nutritional deficiencies. Crohn's disease and ulcerative colitis cause anorexia, fear of eating and loss of protein, blood and nutrients from the gut.

Metabolic and miscellaneous causes: Weight loss may occur in many endocrine or metabolic disorders, as well as end-stage respiratory and cardiac disease.

Investigations

• Urinalysis for glucose, protein and blood. • Blood tests: LFTs, random blood glucose and TFTs; CRP and ESR (often raised in infections, connective tissue disorders and malignancy). • Bone marrow aspiration or liver biopsy: to identify cryptic miliary TB when there is strong clinical suspicion. • Abdominal and pelvic CT: occasionally help, but only after careful history and reweighing.

Constipation

Constipation is the infrequent passage of hard stools, often with straining, a sensation of incomplete evacuation and perianal or abdominal discomfort. It occurs in many disorders.

In the absence of a history suggesting a specific cause (Box 12.4), it is not necessary to investigate every person with constipation. Most respond to dietary fibre supplementation and the judicious use of laxatives. Middle-aged or elderly patients with a short history or worrying symptoms (rectal bleeding, pain or weight loss) must be investigated

promptly, by either barium enema or colonoscopy. Others should be investigated as follows:
• Initially, digital rectal examination, proctoscopy and sigmoidoscopy, routine biochemistry, including serum calcium and thyroid function, and an FBC. • If normal: a 1-month trial of dietary fibre and/or laxatives. • If symptoms persist: examination of the colon by barium enema or CT colonography to look for structural disease.

Abdominal pain

Abdominal pain may be:
• Visceral: usually midline, because of stretching or torsion of a viscus.
• Parietal: usually sharp, lateralised and localised, because of peritoneal irritation. • Referred: for example, gallbladder pain referred to the back or shoulder tip. • Psychogenic: cultural, emotional and psychosocial factors influence the experience of pain. In some patients, no organic cause is found despite investigation.

The acute abdomen

This accounts for around 50% of all urgent surgical admissions, and is a consequence of one or more pathological processes:

Inflammation (e.g. appendicitis, pancreatitis, diverticulitis): Diffuse pain develops gradually, over hours. If the parietal peritoneum is involved, pain becomes localised. Movement exacerbates it; rigidity and guarding occur.

Perforation (e.g. peptic ulcer, ovarian cyst, diverticular disease): Pain starts abruptly, is severe and leads to generalised peritonitis.

Obstruction (intestinal, biliary or ureteric): Pain is colicky, with spasms causing the patient to writhe around. If it does not disappear between spasms, this suggests complicating inflammation.

If there are signs of peritonitis (i.e. guarding and rebound tenderness with rigidity), resuscitation with IV fluids, oxygen and antibiotics is needed. Further investigations should include:
• FBC: may demonstrate leucocytosis. • U&Es: reveal dehydration.
• Serum amylase: raised in acute pancreatitis. • Erect CXR: shows air under the diaphragm in perforation; an AXR reveals obstruction. • USS: may reveal free fluid or intra-abdominal abscess. • Contrast studies, by either mouth or anus: useful to evaluate obstruction, and essential to distinguish pseudo-obstruction from mechanical large bowel obstruction.
• CT: useful for pancreatitis, retroperitoneal collections or masses, renal calculi and aortic aneurysm. • Angiography: used in mesenteric ischaemia.
• Diagnostic laparoscopy: may be useful if the cause remains obscure.

Management

Perforations are closed, inflammatory conditions are treated with antibiotics or resection, and obstructions are relieved. Most but not all patients require surgery. The need for, and urgency of, surgical intervention depends on clinical severity and stability, and the presence or absence of peritonitis.

12

i	**12.5 Investigation of chronic or recurrent abdominal pain**

Symptom	Probable diagnosis	Investigation
Epigastric pain; dyspepsia; relationship to food	Gastroduodenal or biliary disease	Endoscopy and USS
Altered bowel habit; rectal bleeding; features of obstruction	Colonic disease	Barium enema and sig-moidoscopy/colonoscopy
Pain provoked by food in widespread atherosclerosis	Mesenteric ischaemia	Mesenteric angiography
Upper abdominal pain radiating to the back; history of alcohol misuse; weight loss; diarrhoea	Chronic pancreatitis or pancreatic cancer	USS, CT and pancreatic function tests
Recurrent loin or flank pain with urinary symptoms	Renal or ureteric stones	USS and IV urography

Acute appendicitis: The risk of perforation or recurrence is high with conservative treatment, so surgery is usually advisable.

Small bowel obstruction: If the cause is obvious and surgery inevitable (e.g. a strangulated hernia), early operation is appropriate. If the suspected cause is adhesions from previous surgery, only patients who do not resolve within 48 hours or who develop signs of strangulation (colicky pain becoming constant, peritonitis, tachycardia, fever, leucocytosis) should have surgery.

Large bowel obstruction: Pseudo-obstruction is treated nonoperatively. Some patients benefit from colonoscopic decompression, but mechanical obstruction merits surgery. Differentiation between the two is by a water-soluble contrast enema.

Acute cholecystitis: See p. 549.

Acute diverticulitis: See p. 499.

Perforated peptic ulcer: See p. 474.

Chronic or recurrent abdominal pain

A detailed history, including fever, weight loss and mood, is essential. If abdominal and rectal examination is normal, a careful search should be made for disease affecting the vertebral column, spinal cord, lungs and cardiovascular system.

The choice of investigations depends on the history and examination (Box 12.5). Persistent symptoms require exclusion of colonic or small bowel disease. A history of psychiatric disturbance, repeated negative investigations or vague symptoms not fitting any particular disease or organ pattern may point to a psychological origin.

Constant abdominal pain

Patients with constant abdominal pain usually have features to suggest the underlying diagnosis, for example, malignancy, chronic pancreatitis or intra-abdominal abscess. Occasionally no cause will be found, leading to the diagnosis of 'chronic functional abdominal pain'. In these patients a psychological cause is highly likely, and treatment is aimed at symptom control, psychological support and minimising disease impact.

Disorders of nutrition

Obesity

Obesity is a pandemic with potentially disastrous consequences for health. Over 25% of adults in the UK are obese (BMI >30), compared with 7% in 1980. Some 66% of UK adults are overweight (BMI >25).

Aetiology

The pandemic reflects changes in both energy intake and expenditure. The estimated average global daily supply of food energy per person increased from around 2350 kcal in the 1960s to around 2800 kcal in the 1990s. Portion sizes, particularly of sugary drinks and high-fat snacks, have increased. Corresponding changes in energy expenditure are important; obesity is correlated positively with hours spent watching television, and inversely with physical activity.

Susceptibility to obesity varies between individuals. Twin studies confirm a genetic pattern of inheritance, suggesting a polygenic disorder. In a few cases, specific causal factors can be identified, such as hypothyroidism, Cushing's syndrome or insulinoma. Drugs implicated include: tricyclic antidepressants, sulphonylureas, sodium valproate and β-blockers.

Complications

Health consequences of obesity include:
• Metabolic syndrome (p. 425). • Nonalcoholic steatohepatitis. • Cirrhosis.
• Sleep apnoea. • Osteoarthritis. • Psychosocial disadvantage.

Obesity has adverse effects on both mortality and morbidity; life expectancy is reduced by 13 years amongst obese smokers. CAD is the major cause of death, but some cancer rates are also increased.

Clinical features and investigations

Obesity can be quantified using the body mass index (BMI = weight in kilograms divided by the height in metres squared (kg/m^2)):
• Normal 18.5 to 25. • Overweight 25 to 30. • Obese over 30.

Risk of complications rises steeply for BMI greater than 40. High waist circumference also correlates with metabolic and cardiovascular complications of obesity.

A dietary history may be helpful in guiding dietary advice but is susceptible to under-reporting of consumption. Alcohol is an important source of energy intake. All obese patients should have TFTs performed, and an overnight dexamethasone suppression test or 24-hour urine free cortisol test if Cushing's syndrome is suspected. Assessment of other cardiovascular risk factors is important. BP should be measured, and type 2 diabetes and dyslipidaemia detected by measuring blood glucose and serum lipids. Elevated transaminases suggest nonalcoholic fatty liver disease.

Management

The health risks of obesity are largely reversible if identified and treated early. Interventions that reduce weight in studies in obese patients have also been shown to ameliorate cardiovascular risk factors. Lifestyle advice that lowers body weight and increases physical exercise reduces the incidence of type 2 diabetes.

Most patients seeking assistance will have attempted weight loss previously, sometimes repeatedly. An empathetic explanation of energy balance, recognising that some individuals are more susceptible to obesity, is important. Appropriate weight loss goals (e.g. 10% of body weight) should be agreed.

Lifestyle advice: All patients should be advised to maximise their physical activity by incorporating it into the daily routine (e.g. walking rather than driving to work). Changes in eating behaviour (including controlling portion size, avoiding snacking, eating regular meals to encourage satiety and using artificial sweeteners) should be discussed.

Weight loss diets: In overweight people, the lifestyle advice given above may gradually succeed. In obese patients, more active intervention is usually required. Weight loss diets require a reduction in daily total energy intake of around 2.5 MJ (600 kcal) from the patient's normal consumption. The goal is to lose around 0.5 kg per week. Patient adherence is the major determinant of success. In some patients, more rapid weight loss is required, for example, in preparation for surgery. There is no role for starvation diets, which carry a risk of sudden death from heart disease. Very low-calorie diets produce weight loss of 1.5 to 2.5 kg per week, but require the supervision of a physician and nutritionist.

Drugs: Drug therapy is usually reserved for obese patients with a high risk of complications. Patients who continue to take antiobesity drugs tend to regain weight with time. This has led to the recommendation that antiobesity drugs are used short-term to maximise weight loss in patients who are demonstrating their adherence to a low-calorie diet by current weight loss. Orlistat, which has been licensed for several years, inhibits pancreatic and gastric lipases, reducing dietary fat absorption by around 30%. Side effects relate to the resultant fat malabsorption: namely, loose stools, oily spotting, faecal urgency, flatus and malabsorption of fat-soluble vitamins. More recently, combination therapies such as phenteramine/topiramate and naltrexone/bupropion have been licensed for use in the United States. If unsuccessful, drug therapy should be discontinued.

Surgery: 'Bariatric' surgery to reduce the size of the stomach is the most effective long-term treatment for obesity. It should be contemplated in motivated patients with severe obesity (BMI ≥40) and a very high risk of developing the complications of obesity, in whom dietary and drug therapy has been ineffective. The mechanism of weight loss may not relate to limiting the stomach capacity per se, but rather in disrupting the release of ghrelin from the stomach, which signals hunger in the hypothalamus. Mortality is low in experienced centres, but postoperative complications are common.

Under-nutrition

Starvation and famine

There remain regions of the world, particularly in Africa, where the prevalence of BMI less than 18.5 in adults remains as high as 20%. Chronic under-nutrition is responsible for more than half of all childhood deaths worldwide. In adults, the predominant form of protein–energy malnutrition is under-nutrition, that is, a sustained negative energy (calorie) balance caused by one of the following:

Decreased energy intake: Causes include:
• Famine. • Persistent regurgitation or vomiting. • Anorexia. • Malabsorption (e.g. small intestinal disease). • Maldigestion (e.g. pancreatic exocrine insufficiency).

Increased energy expenditure: Causes include:
• Increased basal metabolic rate (thyrotoxicosis, trauma, fever, cancer cachexia). • Excessive physical activity (e.g. marathon runners). • Energy loss (e.g. glycosuria in diabetes). • Impaired energy storage (e.g. Addison's disease, phaeochromocytoma).

Clinical features

The severity of malnutrition can be assessed by measurements of BMI, mid-arm circumference and skinfold thickness. The clinical features of severe under-nutrition in adults include:
• Weight loss. • Thirst, weakness, feeling cold, nocturia, amenorrhoea, impotence. • Lax, pale, dry skin. • Hair thinning/loss. • Cold, cyanosed extremities, pressure sores. • Muscle wasting. • Loss of subcutaneous fat. • Oedema (even without hypoalbuminaemia). • Subnormal temperature, slow pulse, low BP. • Distended abdomen, with diarrhoea. • Diminished tendon jerks. • Apathy, loss of initiative, depression, introversion, aggression if food is nearby. • Susceptibility to infections.

Under-nutrition often leads to vitamin deficiencies, especially of thiamin, folate and vitamin C. Diarrhoea causes sodium, potassium and magnesium depletion. The high mortality is often because of infections, for example, typhus or cholera, but the usual signs may not appear. In advanced starvation, patients become completely inactive and may assume a flexed, fetal position; death comes quietly and often quite suddenly.

Investigations

Plasma free fatty acids are increased, with ketosis and a mild metabolic acidosis. Plasma glucose is low but albumin is often maintained. Insulin secretion is diminished, glucagon and cortisol increase and reverse T_3 replaces normal triiodothyronine. Resting metabolic rate falls, because of reduced lean body mass and hypothalamic compensation. There may be mild anaemia, leucopenia and thrombocytopenia.

Management

Patients should be graded according to BMI. Those with moderate starvation need extra feeding, whereas those who are severely underweight need hospital care. In severe starvation there is atrophy of the intestinal epithelium and the exocrine pancreas.

Small amounts of food should be given at first; it should be palatable and similar to the usual staple meal, for example, cereal with some sugar, milk powder and oil. Salt should be restricted, and micronutrient supplements (e.g. potassium, magnesium, zinc and multivitamins) may be essential. Between 6.3 and 8.4 MJ/day (1500–2000 kcal/day) will prevent deterioration, but additional calories are required for regain of weight. During refeeding, a gain of 5% body weight per month indicates satisfactory progress. Other measures are supportive, and include care for the skin, adequate hydration, treatment of infections and careful monitoring of body temperature, because thermoregulation may be impaired.

Under-nutrition in hospital

One-third of hospital patients in the UK (particularly the elderly) are affected by moderate or severe under-nutrition on admission. Once in hospital, many lose weight because of poor appetite, concurrent illness and being kept 'nil by mouth' for investigations. Under-nutrition leads to impaired immunity and muscle weakness, and to increased morbidity, mortality and length of stay.

Social issues affect food choices and may cause or exacerbate disease. Social isolation, low levels of disposable income and a lack of knowledge or interest in healthy eating may increase reliance on calorie-dense convenience foods of poor nutritional quality. The nonspecific effects of chronic inflammation, infection or malignancy, as well as specific gastrointestinal disorders, may adversely affect appetite, reducing food intake.

Nutritional support of the hospital patient

Enteral feeding is preferred to parenteral, provided the intestine is accessible and functioning.

Normal diet: Firstly address eating problems such as missing or poorly fitting dentures, difficulty with hand dexterity (arthritis, stroke) or immobility in bed. Food intake should be charted, and ample palatable food provided.

Oral nutritional supplements: Liquid dietary supplements with high energy and protein content should be used to supplement oral food intake.

Enteral tube feeding: Patients who cannot swallow may require artificial nutritional support. The enteral route should be used if possible, as this preserves the integrity of the mucosal barrier, prevents bacteraemia and, in intensive care patients, reduces the risk of multi-organ failure. For short-term support, liquid feeds are given by fine-bore nasogastric tube. Tube position should be checked before use; gastric aspirate has a pH less than 5. A CXR can confirm tube position if in doubt. A nasojejunal tube can be placed in cases of gastric stasis or outlet obstruction. For long-term enteral feeding, a PEG is more comfortable and less likely to become displaced. However, inserting a gastrostomy is an invasive procedure, and complications include local infection (30%) and perforation of intra-abdominal organs.

Parenteral nutrition: Feeding by direct infusion into a central vein via a wide-bore catheter may be indicated for malnourished patients who have inadequate or unsafe oral intake and an intestine that is inaccessible to tube feeding or is nonfunctioning. It is associated with many infective and metabolic complications (disturbances of electrolytes, hyperglycaemia). Strict aseptic practice in handling catheters and careful clinical and bio-chemical monitoring are necessary to minimise risk. In practice, it is most often required in acutely ill patients with multi-organ failure or in severely under-nourished patients undergoing surgery. Parenteral nutrition following surgery should be reserved for when enteral nutrition is not tolerated or feasible or where complications (especially sepsis) impair gastrointestinal function, such that oral or enteral feeding is not possible for at least 7 days.

Refeeding syndrome

When nutritional support is given to a malnourished patient, insulin is released, causing cellular uptake of phosphate, potassium and magnesium. Falling lev-els can have serious consequences, such as cardiac arrhythmias, muscle weakness and seizures. Electrolyte levels should be corrected before refeed-ing is commenced. Rapid depletion of thiamin exacerbates the condition. Restitution of feeding should always be done slowly, with careful monitoring of serum potassium, phosphate and magnesium in the first 3 to 5 days.

Ethical aspects

In severe or terminal disease, the patient and family should be involved in decisions about the extent of invasive nutritional support. Tube feeding is regarded as a medical treatment, and all invasive feeding procedures require consent where this is possible, or action in the best interests of the patient where consent is not possible. Teams should formulate, with the patient and family, an agreed nutritional plan for each patient individually.

Intestinal failure ('short bowel syndrome')

Intestinal failure (IF) means a reduction in the function of the gut below the minimum necessary for the absorption of macronutrients and/or water and electrolytes such that intravenous supplementation is required to support health and/or growth.

Management

IF is a complex clinical problem, best cared for by a dedicated multidisci-plinary team. Most cases result from short bowel syndrome with chronic intestinal dysmotility and chronic intestinal pseudo-obstruction accounting for the remainder. The severity of physiological derangement correlates with how much functioning intestine remains (rather than how much has been removed). The aims of treatment are to:

- provide nutrition, water and electrolytes to maintain health with normal body weight
- utilise the enteral or oral routes as much as possible
- minimise the burden of the underlying disease, as well as the IF and its treatment
- promote good quality of life.

If the ileum remains intact, long-term nutritional support can usually be avoided. Unlike the jejunum, the ileum can adapt to increase absorption of water and electrolytes over time. The presence of part or all of the colon further improves fluid absorption and can generate energy through production of short-chain fatty acids.

Vitamin deficiency

Vitamins are categorised as fat-soluble or water-soluble. Deficiency of fat-soluble vitamins occurs in fat malabsorption.

Vitamin deficiency diseases are most prevalent in developing countries, but still occur in developed countries, particularly in older people and alcoholics.

Box 12.6 summarises the sources of vitamins and their deficiency states.

Diseases of the mouth and salivary glands

Aphthous ulceration: Common, superficial, painful and idiopathic. In severe cases, causes such as infection, drug reaction or Behçet's syndrome must be considered. Topical triamcinolone in Orabase or choline salicylate gel can relieve symptoms.

Oral cancer: Squamous carcinoma of the oral cavity is common worldwide and increasing in the UK. Mortality is around 50%, largely because of late diagnosis. Poor diet, alcohol, smoking or chewing tobacco or areca nuts in betel leaves ('betel nuts') are traditional risk factors, but human papillomaviruses 16 and 18 are also implicated. Suspicious lesions should be biopsied if treatment for local trauma or infection fails to produce improvement after 2 weeks. Treatment is by resection, radiotherapy or photodynamic therapy.

Candidiasis: Caused by *Candida albicans*, a normal mouth commensal that proliferates to cause thrush in babies, people receiving glucocorticoids, antibiotics or cytotoxic therapy and patients with diabetes or HIV. White patches are seen on the tongue and buccal mucosa. Dysphagia suggests pharyngeal and oesophageal candidiasis. A clinical diagnosis is sufficient to instigate therapy, using nystatin or amphotericin suspensions or lozenges. Oral fluconazole is used in resistant cases.

Parotitis: Caused by viral or bacterial infection. Mumps causes a self-limiting acute parotitis. Bacterial parotitis usually occurs as a complication of major surgery and can be avoided by good postoperative care. Broad-spectrum antibiotics are required, whereas surgical drainage is necessary if abscesses are present.

Diseases of the oesophagus

Gastro-oesophageal reflux disease

Gastro-oesophageal reflux resulting in heartburn affects around 30% of the general population.

Gastro-oesophageal reflux disease (GORD) develops when the oesophageal mucosa is exposed to gastric contents for prolonged periods, resulting in symptoms and, in a proportion of cases, oesophagitis. Reflux may

	12.6 Clinically important vitamins and vitamin deficiency states		
Name	**Sources**	**Deficiency**	**Investigations**
Fat-soluble			
Vitamin A	Liver, milk, butter, fish oils	Xerophthalmia, night blindness, keratomalacia, follicular hyperkeratosis	Serum retinol
Vitamin D	Sun on skin, eggs, dairy food	Rickets, osteomalacia	Plasma 25(OH)D/1,25(OH)$_2$D
Vitamin E	Vegetables, seed oils	Haemolytic anaemia, ataxia	Plasma vitamin E
Vitamin K	Green vegetables	Coagulation disorder	Coagulation assay $\pm$ plasma vitamin K
Water-soluble			
Thiamin (B$_1$)	Cereals, grains, beans, pork	Beri-beri, Wernicke–Korsakoff syndrome	RBC transketolase, whole-blood vitamin B$_1$
Riboflavin (B$_2$)	Milk, cereals	Glossitis, stomatitis	RBC glutathione reductase, whole-blood B$_2$
Niacin (B$_3$)	Meat, cereals	Pellagra	Urinary metabolites
Pyridoxine (B$_6$)	Meat, fish, potatoes, bananas	Polyneuropathy	Plasma pyridoxal phosphate or RBC transaminase activation coefficient
Biotin	Liver, egg yolk, cereals	Dermatitis, alopecia, paraesthesiae	Whole-blood or urine biotin
Folate	Liver, milk	Anaemia, neural tube defects during gestation	RBC folate
Vitamin B$_{12}$	Animal products	Anaemia, neurological degeneration	Plasma B$_{12}$
Vitamin C	Citrus fruit, vegetables	Scurvy	Ascorbic acid (plasma: daily intake; leucocyte: tissue stores)

12

occur if there is reduced oesophageal sphincter tone or frequent inappropriate sphincter relaxation. Herniation of the stomach through the diaphragm (hiatus hernia) occurs in 30% of the population over 50 years of age and is often asymptomatic. It causes reflux because of loss of the oblique angle between the cardia and oesophagus. Almost all patients who develop oesophagitis, Barrett's oesophagus or peptic strictures have a hiatus hernia. Defective oesophageal peristaltic activity is common in patients with oesophagitis and persists after oesophagitis has been healed by acid-suppressing drugs.

Gastric acid is the most important oesophageal irritant, and there is a close relationship between acid exposure time and symptoms. Gastric emptying is delayed in patients with GORD. Increased intra-abdominal pressure because of pregnancy and obesity may contribute. Weight loss may improve symptoms. Dietary fat, chocolate, alcohol and coffee relax the lower oesophageal sphincter and may provoke symptoms.

Clinical features

The major symptoms are heartburn and regurgitation, often provoked by bending, straining or lying down. 'Waterbrash', reflex salivation on acid reflux, is often present. Recent weight gain is common. Some patients are woken at night by choking as refluxed fluid irritates the larynx. Others develop odynophagia, dysphagia, chronic cough or atypical chest pain that may mimic angina and is probably caused by reflux-induced oesophageal spasm.

Complications

Oesophagitis: Endoscopic findings range from normal through mild redness to severe, bleeding ulceration with stricture formation, with a poor correlation between symptoms and appearances. Normal endoscopy and histology do not exclude significant reflux disease.

Barrett's oesophagus (CLO): This is a premalignant condition in which the squamous lining of the lower oesophagus is replaced by columnar mucosa with areas of metaplasia. It occurs in response to chronic reflux and is seen in 10% of endoscopies for reflux. Epidemiology suggests a true prevalence of between 1.5% and 5% of the population because it is often asymptomatic or first discovered when the patient develops oesophageal cancer. The relative risk of oesophageal cancer is increased 40- to 120-fold, but the absolute risk is low (0.1%–0.5% per year). Prevalence is increasing, particularly in white men aged over 50 years. Other risk factors include obesity and smoking but not alcohol. Duodenogastro-oesophageal reflux, containing bile, pancreatic enzymes and pepsin in addition to acid, may be important. Diagnosis requires multiple biopsies to detect intestinal metaplasia and/or dysplasia. Neither acid suppression nor antireflux surgery stops progression of Barrett's oesophagus, and treatment is only indicated for symptoms of reflux or complications such as stricture. Endoscopic ablation or photodynamic therapy can induce regression, but islands of glandular mucosa remain, and cancer risk is not eliminated. Regular endoscopic surveillance is controversial; it can detect dysplasia and early malignancy but, because most Barrett's oesophagus is undetected until cancer develops, will not reduce overall oesophageal cancer mortality. Those known to have Barrett's oesophagus are recommended to have surveillance endoscopy 3- to 5-yearly, more often if dysplasia is present.

Those with high-grade dysplasia require intense follow-up in specialist centres; treatment options include endoscopic resection or ablation, or oesophagectomy.

Iron deficiency anaemia: This occurs as a consequence of occult blood loss from oesophagitis. Many such patients have bleeding from erosions in a hiatus hernia. Nevertheless, hiatus hernia is very common, and other causes of blood loss, particularly colorectal cancer, must be considered, even when endoscopy reveals oesophagitis and a hiatus hernia.

Benign oesophageal stricture: This develops as a consequence of long-standing oesophagitis, usually in elderly patients presenting with dysphagia for solids. A history of heartburn is common but not invariable in the elderly. Diagnosis is by endoscopy, when biopsies can be taken to exclude malignancy. Endoscopic balloon dilatation or bouginage is helpful, followed by long-term therapy with a PPI, to reduce the risk of recurrence. Dentition should be checked, and the patient advised to chew food thoroughly.

Gastric volvulus: Occasionally a massive intrathoracic hiatus hernia twists on itself (gastric volvulus), causing complete obstruction, severe chest pain, vomiting and dysphagia. The diagnosis is made by CXR and barium swallow. Most resolve spontaneously but then recur, and so elective preventive surgery is usually advised.

Investigations

Young patients with typical symptoms of GORD can be treated empirically without investigation.

Endoscopy: Advisable if patients present over the age of 50 years, if symptoms are atypical or if complications are suspected. A normal endoscopy in a patient with typical symptoms should not preclude treatment for reflux.

24-hour pH monitoring: If the diagnosis is unclear after endoscopy or if surgery is considered. Intraluminal pH and symptoms are recorded during normal activities. A pH of less than 4 for more than 6% to 7% of the study is diagnostic of reflux.

Management

Lifestyle advice should cover weight loss, avoidance of dietary triggers, elevation of the bed head, avoidance of late meals and giving up smoking. Antacids, alginates and H_2-receptor antagonists relieve symptoms without healing, whereas PPIs also heal oesophagitis in the majority, and are the treatment of choice for severe reflux disease. Recurrence is common, and some patients require lifelong treatment. Long-term PPI treatment increases the risk of enteric infections and of *H. pylori*-associated gastric mucosal atrophy. Laparoscopic fundoplication is reserved for patients who fail to respond or decline to take long-term PPIs, after continued regurgitation is confirmed by pH monitoring. Although heartburn and regurgitation are alleviated in most patients, a few develop complications.

Other causes of oesophagitis

Infection: Oesophageal candidiasis may complicate HIV infection (p. 464).

Corrosives: Suicide attempt by bleach or acid ingestion causes painful burns of the mouth and pharynx and erosive oesophagitis. Complications include perforation, mediastinitis and stricture. Early treatment is conservative (analgesia and nutritional support); vomiting and endoscopy are avoided to prevent perforation. Later, endoscopic dilatation of strictures is usually necessary, although hazardous.

Drugs: Potassium supplements and NSAIDs may cause oesophageal ulcers if tablets are trapped above a stricture. Bisphosphonates cause oesophageal ulceration and should be used with caution in patients with oesophageal disorders.

Eosinophilic oesophagitis: This may cause dysphagia in children and young adults and responds to topical glucocorticoids.

Motility disorders

Pharyngeal pouch

Incoordination of swallowing leads to herniation of a pouch through the cricopharyngeus muscle. Most patients are elderly and asymptomatic, but regurgitation, halitosis and dysphagia can occur. A barium swallow demonstrates the pouch and may show pulmonary aspiration. Endoscopy may perforate the pouch. Surgery is indicated in symptomatic patients.

Achalasia of the oesophagus

Achalasia is characterised by a hypertonic lower oesophageal sphincter that fails to relax during swallowing and by failure of propagated oesophageal contraction, with progressive dilatation. The cause is unknown, although failure of the local nerve supply is implicated. Chagas' disease (infestation with *Trypanosoma cruzi*) is endemic in South America and causes an indistinguishable clinical syndrome (p. 153).

Clinical features and investigations

Achalasia usually develops slowly in middle age with intermittent dysphagia for solids, which is eased by drinking, standing and moving around. Heartburn is absent, but some patients experience severe chest pain caused by oesophageal spasm. As dysphagia progresses, nocturnal pulmonary aspiration develops. Achalasia predisposes to squamous carcinoma of the oesophagus.

Endoscopy is essential to rule out carcinoma. Barium swallow (Fig. 12.2) shows tapered narrowing of the lower oesophagus and a dilated, aperistaltic and food-filled oesophageal body. Manometry confirms the nonrelaxing lower oesophageal sphincter and poor contractility of the oesophageal body. CXR may show widening of the mediastinum and features of aspiration.

Management

Endoscopic dilatation: Dilatation of the oesophageal sphincter using a fluoroscopically positioned balloon improves symptoms in 80% of patients. Some require repeat dilatation, but frequent recurrence is best treated surgically. Endoscopic injection of botulinum toxin into the sphincter induces

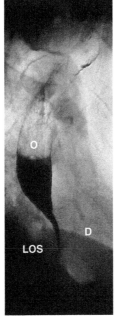

Fig. 12.2 Achalasia. X-ray showing a dilated, barium-filled oesophagus (O), with fluid level and distal tapering, and a closed lower oesophageal sphincter (LOS). *D*, Diaphragm.

remission but relapse is common. Endoscopic myotomy procedures may offer benefit in specialist centres.

Surgical myotomy: Performed either laparoscopically or as an open operation, this is extremely effective. Both dilatation and myotomy may be complicated by gastro-oesophageal reflux, and for this reason myotomy is often augmented by an antireflux procedure, and a PPI is given.

Other oesophageal motility disorders

Oesophageal spasm or abnormally forceful peristaltic activity: May lead to episodic chest pain mimicking angina. Use of oral or sublingual nitrates or nifedipine is sometimes beneficial.

Systemic sclerosis: In systemic sclerosis or CREST syndrome (p. 352), the muscle of the oesophagus is replaced by fibrous tissue, with failure of peristalsis leading to heartburn and dysphagia. Oesophagitis is often severe, and benign fibrous strictures occur. These patients require long-term PPIs. Dermatomyositis, rheumatoid arthritis and myasthenia gravis may also cause dysphagia.

Benign strictures: These usually occur in elderly patients as a conse-quence of GORD. Rings of submucosal fibrosis develop at the oesophago-gastric junction, causing intermittent dysphagia.

A postcricoid web is a rare complication of iron deficiency anaemia, which predisposes to squamous carcinoma. Benign strictures can be treated by endoscopic dilatation using wire-guided bougies or balloons.

Tumours of the oesophagus

Carcinoma of the oesophagus

Almost all are squamous cancers or adenocarcinomas. Small cell cancer is a rare third type.

Squamous cancer: Rare in Caucasians (~4:100 000) but common in Iran, parts of Africa and China (200:100 000). Squamous cancer can arise anywhere in the oesophagus, but almost all tumours in the upper oesophagus are squamous.

Adenocarcinoma: Arises in the lower third of the oesophagus from Barrett's oesophagus or from the cardia of the stomach. Incidence is increasing in the UK (~5:100 000).

Clinical features and investigations

There is progressive, painless dysphagia for solids. Food bolus obstruction may occur acutely. Chest pain or hoarseness suggests mediastinal invasion. Weight loss is common. Fistulation between the oesophagus and the airway leads to coughing after swallowing, pneumonia and pleural effusion. Physical signs include cachexia and cervical lymphadenopathy, but these may be absent.

Endoscopy with biopsy is the investigation of choice. Subsequent investigations are performed to classify the tumour using TNM staging and define operability. EUS permits nodal sampling and assessment of the depth of tumour penetration. Thoracic and abdominal CT, often combined with PET, defines metastatic spread and local invasion, which may preclude surgery.

Management and prognosis

Approximately 70% of patients have extensive disease at presentation. In these, treatment is palliative and based upon relief of dysphagia and pain. Endoscopic laser ablation or stenting may improve swallowing, whereas palliative radiotherapy may shrink both squamous cancers and adenocarcinomas. In high incidence areas, early superficial tumours are treated by endoscopic submucosal dissection.

Despite treatment, tumours that have breached the oesophageal wall or involve lymph nodes (T3, N1) have a 5-year survival of around 10% after surgery. This figure improves significantly for less extensive disease. Five-year survival following 'potentially curative' surgery (all visible tumour removed) is 30%, and this may be further improved by preoperative chemotherapy. Although squamous carcinomas are radiosensitive, radiotherapy alone is associated with a 5-year survival of only 5%; with chemoradiotherapy, this can rise to 25% to 30%.

Perforation of the oesophagus

The most common cause is endoscopic perforation complicating dilatation or intubation. A perforated peptic stricture is usually managed conservatively using broad-spectrum antibiotics and parenteral nutrition; most heal within days. Malignant, caustic and radiotherapy stricture perforations require surgery.

Spontaneous oesophageal perforation results from forceful vomiting. Patients present with severe chest pain, shock, subcutaneous emphysema, pleural effusions and pneumothorax. The diagnosis is made using a water-soluble contrast swallow. Treatment is surgical, and mortality is high.

Diseases of the stomach and duodenum

Gastritis

Acute gastritis: Most commonly results from alcohol, aspirin or NSAID ingestion. It is often asymptomatic and self-limiting, but may cause dyspepsia, anorexia, nausea, vomiting, haematemesis or melaena. In persistent cases, endoscopy is necessary to exclude peptic ulcer or cancer. Treatment involves avoiding the cause; symptomatic therapy with antacids and acid suppression using PPIs or antiemetics may also be necessary.

Chronic gastritis: Most commonly caused by *H. pylori* infection. Correlation between symptoms and endoscopic and pathological findings is poor. Most patients are asymptomatic and do not require treatment, but patients with dyspepsia may benefit from *H. pylori* eradication.

Autoimmune chronic gastritis: Usually asymptomatic and results from autoimmune activity against parietal cells in the body of the stomach. Circulating parietal cell and intrinsic factor antibodies may be present. In some patients, gastric atrophy leads to loss of intrinsic factor secretion and pernicious anaemia. Other autoimmune conditions, particularly thyroid disease, may be present. Long term, there is a two- to threefold increase in gastric cancer.

Peptic ulcer disease

Peptic ulcer means an ulcer in the lower oesophagus, stomach or duodenum, in the jejunum after gastrojejunostomy or, rarely, in the ileum adjacent to a Meckel's diverticulum. Ulcers in the stomach or duodenum may be acute or chronic; both penetrate the muscularis mucosae, but acute ulcers show no evidence of fibrosis. Erosions do not penetrate the muscularis mucosae.

Gastric and duodenal ulcer

The prevalence of peptic ulcer is decreasing in many Western communities as a result of *H. pylori* eradication therapy, but it remains high in developing countries. The male to female ratio for duodenal ulcer varies from 5:1 to 2:1, whereas that for gastric ulcer is 2 (or less):1. Chronic gastric ulcer is usually single; most are situated on the lesser curve within the antrum. Duodenal ulcer usually occurs in the first part of the duodenum just distal to the junction of pyloric and duodenal mucosa. Gastric and duodenal ulcers coexist in 10% of patients, and multiple ulcers occur in 10% to 15%.

Pathophysiology

H. pylori: In the UK, the prevalence of *H. pylori* infection rises with age (reaching 50% in those aged over 50 years); in the developing world, it affects up to 90%. Infections are probably acquired in childhood by person-to-person contact. Most colonised people remain healthy and asymptomatic. Around 90% of duodenal ulcer patients and 70% of gastric ulcer patients are infected with *H. pylori*; the remaining 30% of gastric ulcers are caused by NSAIDs.

H. pylori is a motile Gram-negative organism that uses multiple flagellae to burrow beneath the epithelial mucus layer. Here the pH is nearly neutral, and any acidity is buffered by the organism's production of ammonia from urea. *H. pylori* exclusively colonises gastric-type epithelium, and is found in the duodenum only at patches of gastric metaplasia. It stimulates chronic gastritis by provoking an inflammatory response in the epithelium. In most people, *H. pylori* causes antral gastritis with depletion of somatostatin. The subsequent hypergastrinaemia stimulates parietal cell acid production, but usually without clinical consequences. In a minority, infection causes antral-predominant gastritis with hypergastrinaemia and excessive parietal cell acid production, leading to duodenal ulceration. The pathogenesis of gastric ulcer is less clear, but *H. pylori* probably acts by reducing gastric mucosal resistance to acid and pepsin. Occasionally, *H. pylori* causes a pan-gastritis, leading to gastric atrophy and hypochlorhydria, with bacterial proliferation in the stomach, predisposing to gastric cancer.

NSAIDs: Treatment is associated with peptic ulcers caused by impairment of mucosal defences.

Smoking: This increases the risk of gastric and, to a lesser extent, duodenal ulcer. Once the ulcer has formed, it is more likely to cause complications and less likely to heal if the patient smokes.

Clinical features and investigations

Peptic ulcer disease is a chronic condition with spontaneous relapse and remission extending over decades. Duodenal and gastric ulcers share common symptoms:

• Recurrent episodes of epigastric pain in relation to meals.• Occasionally, vomiting; persistent daily vomiting suggests gastric outlet obstruction.

In one-third of patients, especially elderly subjects taking NSAIDs, the history is less characteristic; pain may be absent or experienced only as vague epigastric unease. Occasionally, the only symptoms are anorexia and nausea, or a sense of undue repletion after meals. The ulcer may even be 'silent', presenting with anaemia from chronic undetected blood loss, haematemesis or acute perforation. The diagnostic value of individual symptoms of ulcer disease is poor.

Endoscopy is the preferred investigation. Gastric ulcers may occasionally be malignant, and therefore must always be biopsied and followed up to ensure healing.

Patients should be screened for *H. pylori* infection (Box 12.7). Some tests require endoscopy; others are noninvasive. Overall, breath or faecal antigen tests are best because of their accuracy, simplicity and noninvasiveness.

Management

The aims of management are to relieve symptoms, induce healing and prevent recurrence.

	12.7 Methods for the diagnosis of *H. pylori* infection	
Test	Advantages	Disadvantages
Noninvasive		
Serology	Rapid office kits available; good for population studies	Lacks sensitivity and specificity; cannot differentiate current from past infection
^{13}C urea breath tests	High sensitivity and specificity	Requires expensive mass spectrometer
Faecal antigen test	Cheap, >95% specificity	Acceptability
Invasive (antral biopsy)		
Histology	Sensitivity and specificity	False negatives occur; takes several days to process
Rapid urease tests	Cheap, quick; >95% specificity	85% sensitivity
Microbiological culture	'Gold standard'; defines antibiotic sensitivity	Slow and laborious; lacks sensitivity

H. pylori **eradication:** All patients with proven ulcers who are *H. pylori*-positive should receive eradication therapy. This heals ulcers, prevents relapse and eliminates the need for long-term treatment in more than 90% of patients. A PPI is taken with two antibiotics (from amoxicillin, clarithromycin and metronidazole) for at least 7 days. First-line therapy is a PPI (twice daily), clarithromycin 500 mg twice daily and amoxicillin 1 g twice daily or metronidazole 400 mg twice daily, for 7 days. Adherence, side effects (usually diarrhoea, nausea, vomiting) and metronidazole resistance influence success rates.Patients who remain infected after initial therapy and those with resistant infections should be offered second-line therapy with omeprazole, bismuth subcitrate, metronidazole and tetracycline. For those who are still colonised after two treatments, the choice lies between a third attempt (guided by antibiotic sensitivity testing) and long-term acid suppression.

H. pylori and NSAIDs are independent risk factors for ulcers, and patients requiring long-term NSAID therapy should first undergo eradication therapy to reduce ulcer risk. Subsequent co-prescription of a PPI with the NSAID is advised but is not always necessary for patients being given low-dose aspirin.

General measures: Cigarette smoking, aspirin and NSAIDs should be avoided. Alcohol in moderation is not harmful, and no special dietary advice is required.

Maintenance treatment: This should not be necessary after successful *H. pylori* eradication.

Surgical treatment: Surgery is now rarely required for peptic ulcer, unless there is perforation, haemorrhage, gastric outflow obstruction or persisting or recurrent ulcer after medical treatment. Nonhealing gastric ulcer is treated by partial gastrectomy, in which the ulcer and the ulcer-bearing area of the stomach are resected to exclude an underlying cancer. In the emergency situation, biopsies are taken, and then 'under-running' the ulcer for bleeding or 'oversewing' (patch repair) for perforation is sufficient.

Complications of gastric resection or vagotomy

Although ulcer surgery is now uncommon, many patients underwent operations in the pre-*H. pylori* era, and some degree of disability is seen in up to 50% of these.

Dumping: Rapid gastric emptying leads to distension of the proximal small intestine as the hypertonic contents draw fluid into the lumen. This causes abdominal discomfort, flushing, palpitations, sweating, tachycardia, hypotension and diarrhoea after eating. Patients should avoid large meals with high carbohydrate content.

Bile reflux gastropathy: Duodenogastric bile reflux leads to chronic gastropathy, which can cause dyspepsia. Symptomatic treatment with aluminium-containing antacids or sucralfate may be effective. A few patients require revisional surgery.

Diarrhoea and maldigestion: Diarrhoea 1 to 2 hours after eating may develop after any peptic ulcer operation. Rapid stomach emptying, inadequate mixing with pancreaticobiliary secretions, rapid transit times and bacterial overgrowth may lead to malabsorption. Dietary advice should be given to eat small, dry meals with reduced refined carbohydrates. Drugs such as codeine phosphate or loperamide may also help.

Weight loss: Most patients lose weight after surgery, and 30% to 40% are unable to regain all the lost weight. The usual cause is reduced intake because of a small gastric remnant, but diarrhoea and mild steatorrhoea also contribute.

Anaemia: This is common many years after subtotal gastrectomy. Iron deficiency is the most common cause; folic acid and vitamin B_{12} deficiency are much less frequent. Inadequate dietary iron and folate, lack of acid and intrinsic factor secretion, mild chronic low-grade blood loss from the gastric remnant and recurrent ulceration are responsible.

Metabolic bone disease: Both osteoporosis and osteomalacia occur as a consequence of calcium and vitamin D malabsorption.

Gastric cancer: An increased risk of gastric cancer has been reported. The risk is highest in those with hypochlorhydria, duodenogastric reflux of bile, smoking and *H. pylori* infection. Although the relative risk is increased, the absolute risk of cancer remains low, and endoscopic surveillance is not indicated following gastric surgery.

Complications of peptic ulcer

Perforation: This allows stomach contents to escape into the peritoneum, causing peritonitis. It is more common in duodenal than in gastric ulcers. About one-quarter of cases occur in acute ulcers, often with NSAIDs. It causes:

• Sudden, severe pain, often the first sign of ulcer, starting in the upper abdomen and becoming generalised. Shoulder tip pain as a result of diaphragmatic irritation, shallow respiration caused by pain, and shock are common. • Generalised rigidity. • Absent bowel sounds. • Loss of liver dullness caused by gas under the diaphragm.

Rigidity persists, and although pain may temporarily improve, the patient's condition later deteriorates with general peritonitis. In at least 50% of cases, an erect CXR shows free air beneath the diaphragm. If not, a water-soluble contrast swallow will confirm perforation.

After resuscitation, the acute perforation is closed surgically. Following surgery, *H. pylori* should be treated (if present) and NSAIDs avoided. The mortality from perforation is 25%, reflecting the age and comorbidity of the population affected.

Gastric outlet obstruction: The most common cause is an ulcer near the pylorus, but occasional cases are caused by antral cancer or adult hypertrophic pyloric stenosis.

Clinical features:

• Nausea. • Vomiting of large quantities of gastric content. • Abdominal distension. • Examination reveals wasting, dehydration and a succussion splash persisting 4 hours or more after the last meal. Visible gastric peristalsis is diagnostic.

Loss of acidic gastric contents leads to alkalosis, dehydration, low serum chloride and potassium and raised serum bicarbonate and urea (hypochloraemic metabolic alkalosis). Paradoxical aciduria occurs because of enhanced renal sodium absorption in exchange for hydrogen. Endoscopy should be performed after the stomach has been emptied by wide-bore nasogastric tube.

Management:

• Nasogastric suction and the administration of large volumes of IV isotonic saline with potassium. • PPIs: may heal ulcers, relieve pyloric oedema and overcome the need for surgery. • Balloon dilatation of benign stenosis: may be possible. • Partial gastrectomy after a 7-day period of nasogastric aspiration may be necessary in some patients.

Bleeding: See p. 472.

Zollinger–Ellison syndrome

This rare disorder (0.1% of duodenal ulcers) is characterised by the triad of severe peptic ulceration, gastric acid hypersecretion and a neuro-endocrine tumour of the pancreas or duodenum ('gastrinoma'). It is most common between 30 and 50 years of age. The gastrinoma secretes gastrin, which maximally stimulates acid production and increases the parietal cell mass. Pancreatic lipase is inactivated, and bile acids are precipitated. Diarrhoea and steatorrhoea result. Around 90% of tumours occur in the proximal duodenal wall or the pancreatic head. Half are multiple, and over half are malignant but slow growing. MEN type 1 (p. 417) is present in 20% to 60%.

Patients present with multiple, severe peptic ulcers unresponsive to standard therapy. The history is usually short; bleeding and perforations are common. Diarrhoea occurs in one-third of patients and can be the presenting feature.

Hypersecretion of acid under basal conditions, with little increase following pentagastrin, may be confirmed by gastric aspiration. Serum gastrin is grossly elevated (10- to 1000-fold). Tumour localisation is by EUS, radio-labelled somatostatin receptor scintigraphy and ^{68}gallium dotatate PET scanning.

Approximately 30% of small and single tumours can be localised and resected. In those with multifocal or metastatic disease, continuous therapy with high-dose omeprazole heals ulcers and alleviates diarrhoea. Subcutaneous octreotide reduces gastrin secretion and may be of value. All patients should undergo genetic screening for MEN 1.

Functional disorders

Functional dyspepsia

This is defined as chronic dyspepsia in the absence of organic disease. Other commonly reported symptoms include fullness, bloating and nausea. The aetiology covers a spectrum of mucosal, motility and psychiatric disorders.

Clinical features and investigations

Patients are usually young (<40 years), and women are affected twice as commonly as men. Abdominal pain is associated with a combination of other 'dyspeptic' symptoms, the most common being nausea, early satiety and bloating after meals. Pain or nausea on waking is characteristic, and direct enquiry may elicit symptoms of irritable bowel syndrome. Peptic ulcer disease and intra-abdominal malignancy must be considered. Patients often appear anxious, but there are no diagnostic signs and no weight loss. A drug history should be taken, depression considered and pregnancy excluded. Alcohol misuse should be suspected when early morning nausea and retching are prominent.

The history will often suggest the diagnosis, but in patients over 55 years of age, an endoscopy is necessary to exclude mucosal disease.

Management

The most important elements are explanation and reassurance. Possible psychological factors should be explored, and the concept of psychological influences on gut function explained. Idiosyncratic diets are of little benefit, but fat restriction may help.

Drug treatment is not especially successful, but trials of antacids, metoclopramide, domperidone or H_2-receptor antagonists may be useful, according to symptoms. Low-dose amitriptyline sometimes helps. *H. pylori* eradication should be offered to infected patients. Counselling or psychotherapy may be of value in those with major stress.

Functional vomiting

This disorder typically occurs on wakening or immediately after breakfast and is probably a reaction to facing up to everyday worries; in the young it can be attributed to school phobia. Early morning vomiting also occurs in pregnancy, alcohol misuse and depression. Cyclical bouts of vomiting are often idiopathic or associated with cannabis use. There is little or no weight loss.

In all patients it is essential to exclude other common causes. Tranquillisers and antiemetic drugs have only a secondary place in management. Antidepressants may be effective.

Gastroparesis

Defective gastric emptying without obstruction can be caused by inherited or acquired disorders of the gastric pacemaker, autonomic disorders (particularly diabetic neuropathy), disease of the gastroduodenal musculature (e.g. systemic sclerosis and amyloidosis) or drugs (e.g. opiates or anticholinergics). Early satiety and vomiting are typical symptoms; abdominal fullness and a succussion splash may be present on examination. Treatment is with metoclopramide and domperidone.

Tumours of the stomach

Gastric carcinoma

Gastric cancer is extremely common in China, Japan and parts of South America, less common in the UK and uncommon in the United States. Studies of Japanese migrants to the United States show a much lower incidence in the second generation, confirming the importance of environmental factors. Gastric cancer is more common in men, and the incidence rises after 50 years of age.

H. pylori infection is associated with gastric cancer and may contribute to 60% to 70% of cases. Infection at an early age may be important. A few *H. pylori*-infected individuals become hypo- or achlorhydric, and these people are thought to be at greatest risk.

Diets rich in salted, smoked or pickled foods and lacking in fresh fruit and vegetables, as well as vitamins C and A, may predispose. Carcinogenic compounds formed by nitrite-reducing bacteria that colonise the achlorhydric stomach may also contribute. No predominant genetic abnormality has been identified, although cancer risk is increased two- to threefold in first-degree relatives of patients.

Virtually all tumours are adenocarcinomas arising from mucus-secreting cells in the base of the gastric crypts. In the developing world, 50% of gastric cancers develop in the antrum, 20% to 30% in the gastric body and 20% in the cardia. In Western populations, however, proximal gastric tumours are becoming more common than those arising in the body and distal stomach. This may reflect changes in lifestyle or the decreasing prevalence of *H. pylori* in the West. Diffuse submucosal infiltration by a scirrhous cancer (linitis plastica) is uncommon. Early gastric cancer is defined as cancer confined to the mucosa or submucosa, regardless of lymph node involvement. It is common in Japan, where widespread screening is practised. Over 80% of patients in the West present with advanced gastric cancer.

Clinical features

Early gastric cancer is usually asymptomatic but may be discovered during endoscopy for dyspepsia. Weight loss occurs in two-thirds of patients with advanced cancers. Ulcer-like pain occurs in 50%. Anaemia from occult bleeding is also common. Anorexia and nausea occur in one-third.

Early satiety, haematemesis, melaena and dyspepsia are less common features. Dysphagia occurs in tumours that obstruct the gastro-oesophageal junction.

Examination may reveal no abnormalities, but signs of weight loss, anaemia or a palpable epigastric mass are not infrequent. Jaundice or ascites may signify metastatic spread. Occasionally, tumour spread occurs to the supraclavicular lymph nodes, umbilicus or ovaries. Paraneoplastic phenomena, such as acanthosis nigricans, thrombophlebitis and dermatomyositis, occur rarely. Metastases occur most commonly in the liver, lungs, peritoneum and bone marrow.

Investigations

For diagnosis and staging, endoscopy is the investigation of choice and should be performed promptly in any dyspeptic patient with 'alarm features' (see Box 12.2). Multiple biopsies from the edge and base of a gastric ulcer are required. Once the diagnosis is made, CT is necessary for accurate staging and assessment of resectability but may miss small involved lymph nodes. Even with these techniques, laparoscopy is required to determine whether the tumour is resectable.

Management and prognosis

Surgery: Resection offers the only hope of cure, which can be achieved in 90% of patients with early gastric cancer. Extensive lymph node resection may increase survival rates but carries greater morbidity. Even for those who cannot be cured, palliative resection may be necessary when presentation is with bleeding or gastric outflow obstruction. Complete removal of all macroscopic tumour, combined with lymphadenectomy, will achieve a 50% to 60% 5-year survival. Perioperative chemotherapy with epirubicin, cisplatin and fluorouracil improves survival rates.

Inoperable tumours: Survival can be improved and palliation of symptoms achieved with chemotherapy. The biological agent trastuzumab may benefit patients whose tumours over-express HER2. Endoscopic insertion of stents or laser ablation of tumour for control of dysphagia or bleeding benefits some patients.

▌Gastric lymphoma

Primary gastric lymphoma accounts for less than 5% of all gastric malignancies, but 60% of primary GI lymphomas occur at this site. Lymphoid tissue is not found in the normal stomach, but lymphoid aggregates develop in the presence of *H. pylori* infection. Indeed, *H. pylori* infection is associated with development of a particular low-grade lymphoma (extranodal marginal-zone lymphoma of MALT type).

The clinical presentation is similar to that of gastric cancer and, endoscopically, the tumour appears as a polypoid or ulcerating mass. High-grade B-cell lymphomas are treated by a combination of rituximab, chemotherapy, surgery and radiotherapy. The prognosis depends on the stage at diagnosis. Features predicting a favourable prognosis are:
• Stage I or II disease. • Small, resectable tumours. • Tumours with low-grade histology. • Age under 60 years.

> **i** 12.8 Disease associations of coeliac disease
>
> - Insulin-dependent diabetes mellitus (2%–8%)
> - Thyroid disease (5%)
> - Primary biliary cirrhosis (3%)
> - Sjögren's syndrome (3%)
> - IgA deficiency (2%)
> - Pernicious anaemia
> - Inflammatory bowel disease
> - Sarcoidosis
> - Neurological complications: encephalopathy, cerebellar atrophy, peripheral neuropathy, epilepsy
> - Myasthenia gravis
> - Dermatitis herpetiformis
> - Down's syndrome
> - Enteropathy-associated T-cell lymphoma
> - Small bowel carcinoma
> - Squamous carcinoma of oesophagus
> - Ulcerative jejunitis
> - Pancreatic insufficiency
> - Microscopic colitis
> - Splenic atrophy

12

Diseases of the small intestine

Disorders causing malabsorption

Coeliac disease

Coeliac disease is an immunologically mediated inflammatory disorder of the small bowel occurring in genetically susceptible individuals. It is caused by intolerance to wheat gluten and similar proteins in rye, barley and oats. It can result in malabsorption and responds to a gluten-free diet. The condition occurs worldwide but is more common in northern Europe (prevalence in UK is 1%).

The pathogenesis is unclear, but immunological responses to gluten play a key role. There is a strong genetic component, with strong concordance in monozygotic twins and an association with HLA-DQ2/DQ8. Dysbiosis of the intestinal microbiota occurs, but it is unclear if this is pathological or secondary to the mucosal changes. There are many disease associations (Box 12.8).

Clinical features

• Infants: failure to thrive, malabsorption. • Older children: delayed growth and puberty, malnutrition, mild abdominal distension. • Adults: presents in third or fourth decade; 2:1 female predominance. • Florid malabsorption in some; others present with tiredness, weight loss, iron or folate deficiency. • Oral ulceration, dyspepsia and bloating.

12.9 Important causes of subtotal villous atrophy

- Coeliac disease
- Tropical sprue
- Dermatitis herpetiformis
- Lymphoma
- AIDS enteropathy
- Giardiasis
- Hypogammaglobulinaemia
- Radiation
- Whipple's disease
- Zollinger–Ellison syndrome

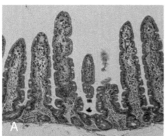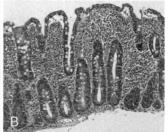

Fig. 12.3 Jejunal mucosa. (A) Normal. **(B)** Jejunum in coeliac disease, showing subtotal villous atrophy and marked inflammatory infiltrate.

Investigations

Duodenal biopsy: The mucosa may appear macroscopically normal, but multiple biopsies should be taken. Villous atrophy is characteristic but other causes should also be considered (Box 12.9 and Fig. 12.3).

Antibodies: These are a valuable screening tool in patients with suggestive symptoms but are not a substitute for duodenal biopsy. IgA antiendomysial antibodies are detectable in most untreated cases and are sensitive and specific. IgG antibodies must be analysed in patients with coexisting IgA deficiency. Tissue transglutaminase (tTG) assays are easier to perform, semi-quantitative and more accurate in patients with IgA deficiency.

Haematology and biochemistry: There is microcytic or macrocytic anaemia from iron or folate deficiency. Target cells, spherocytes and Howell–Jolly bodies are attributed to hyposplenism. Calcium, magnesium, total protein, albumin and vitamin D are reduced.

Measurement of bone density by DEXA scanning: Osteoporosis is common in older women.

Management

• Lifelong gluten-free diet aids mucosal healing. • Correction of deficiencies of iron, folate, calcium and vitamin D. • Regular monitoring of symptoms, weight and nutrition. • Repeat small bowel biopsies: reserved for patients who do not symptomatically improve or whose tTG antibodies remain high.

Dietary adherence should be carefully assessed, but if this is satisfactory, other conditions such as pancreatic insufficiency or microscopic colitis should be sought, as should complications of coeliac disease such as ulcerative jejunitis or enteropathy-associated T-cell lymphoma. Rarely, patients are 'refractory' and require glucocorticoids or immunosuppressive drugs to induce remission.

Complications

There is an increased risk of malignancy, particularly of enteropathy-associated T-cell lymphoma, small bowel carcinoma and squamous carcinoma of the oesophagus.

Ulcerative jejunoileitis may occur; fever, pain, obstruction or perforation may then supervene. The diagnosis is made by barium studies or endoscopy; laparotomy and full-thickness biopsy are occasionally needed. Glucocorticoids are used with mixed success, and some patients require surgical resection and parenteral nutrition.

Osteoporosis and osteomalacia occur but are less common in patients who adhere strictly to a gluten-free diet.

Dermatitis herpetiformis

This is characterised by crops of intensely itchy blisters over the elbows, knees, back and buttocks. Almost all patients have partial villous atrophy on jejunal biopsy, even though they usually have no GI symptoms. The rash usually responds to a gluten-free diet, but some patients require additional treatment with dapsone.

Tropical sprue

Tropical sprue is a chronic, progressive malabsorption with abnormalities of small intestinal structure and function occurring in patients in or from the tropics. The disease occurs mainly in the West Indies and in Asia, including southern India, Malaysia and Indonesia. It often begins after an acute diarrhoeal illness. Small bowel bacterial overgrowth with *Escherichia coli*, *Enterobacter* and *Klebsiella* is frequently seen. Mucosal pathology closely resembles that of coeliac disease.

Clinical features include:
• Diarrhoea, abdominal distension, anorexia, fatigue and weight loss.
• Sudden onset of severe diarrhoea with fever in travellers to the tropics.
When chronic:
• Megaloblastic anaemia (folic acid malabsorption). • Ankle oedema, glossitis and stomatitis are common.• Remissions and relapses may occur.

The differential diagnosis is infective diarrhoea, including giardiasis (p. 160).

Tetracycline (250 mg four times daily for 28 days) brings about long-term remission or cure. Folic acid (5 mg daily) improves symptoms and jejunal morphology.

Small bowel bacterial overgrowth ('blind loop syndrome')

The normal duodenum and jejunum contain coliform organisms, but numbers never exceed 10^3/mL. In bacterial overgrowth, there may be 10^8 to 10^{10}/mL organisms, most of which are normally found only in the colon. Disorders that predispose to bacterial overgrowth include hypochlorhydria, impaired motility (e.g. systemic sclerosis, diabetes), surgical resection, fistulae and hypogammaglobulinaemia.

Clinical features include:

• Watery diarrhoea and/or steatorrhoea.• Anaemia because of vitamin B_{12} deficiency.

There may also be symptoms from the underlying intestinal cause.

Investigations are as follows:

• Barium small bowel follow-through or small bowel MRI enterography may reveal blind loops or fistulae.• Endoscopic duodenal biopsies: exclude mucosal disease such as coeliac disease.• Endoscopic aspiration of jejunal contents: for anaerobic and aerobic culture.• Hydrogen breath test: serial breath samples are measured after oral ingestion of glucose or lactulose. Bacteria in the small bowel cause an early rise in breath hydrogen.

• Serum vitamin B_{12} concentration is low; folate levels are normal or elevated.• Immunoglobulin levels: may exclude hypogammaglobulinaemia.

Management is of the underlying cause. Tetracycline is the treatment of choice, although up to 50% of patients do not respond. Metronidazole or ciprofloxacin are alternatives. Some patients require up to 4 weeks of treatment, and a few cases become chronic. IM vitamin B_{12} supplementation is needed in the latter.

Whipple's disease

This rare condition is characterised by infiltration of small intestinal mucosa by 'foamy' macrophages, which stain positive with PAS reagent. The cause is infection of macrophages by Gram-positive bacilli (*Tropheryma whipplei*), detectable in biopsies by PCR.

This is a multisystem disease (Box 12.10). Middle-aged men are most commonly affected, and the presentation depends on the pattern of organ involvement. Low-grade fever is common.

Whipple's disease is often fatal if untreated but responds well to 2 weeks of IV ceftriaxone followed by co-trimoxazole for at least a year. Relapse occurs in up to one-third of patients, often within the CNS, requiring further prolonged antibiotic treatment.

Bile acid diarrhoea

This can occur idiopathically, after small bowel resection or cholecystectomy, or in association with microscopic colitis, chronic pancreatitis, coeliac disease, small intestinal bacterial overgrowth or diabetes mellitus. Most commonly, ileal resection is performed for Crohn's disease. The long-term effects depend on the site and the length of intestine resected and vary from trivial to life-threatening.

i	**12.10 Clinical features of Whipple's disease**
GI	Diarrhoea, steatorrhoea, protein-losing enteropathy
Musculoskeletal	Seronegative large joint arthritis, sacroiliitis
Cardiac	Pericarditis, myocarditis, endocarditis
Pulmonary	Pleurisy, cough, infiltrates
Haematological	Anaemia, lymphadenopathy
Neurological	Apathy, fits, dementia, myoclonus
Other	Fever, pigmentation

12.11 Clinical features of neuroendocrine tumours

- Small bowel obstruction caused by the tumour mass
- Intestinal ischaemia (caused by mesenteric infiltration or vasospasm)
- Hepatic metastases causing pain, hepatomegaly and jaundice
- Flushing and wheezing
- Diarrhoea
- Cardiac involvement (tricuspid regurgitation, pulmonary stenosis, right ventricular endocardial plaques) leading to heart failure
- Facial telangiectasia
- The diagnosis is made by detecting excess levels of the 5-HT metabolite, 5-HIAA, in a 24-hour urine collection.

Clinical features include:
• Diarrhoea.• Fat malabsorption because of loss of bile salts.• Gallstones because of lithogenic bile.• Oxalate renal calculi.• Vitamin B_{12} deficiency.

Contrast studies of the small bowel and tests of vitamin B_{12} and bile acid absorption are useful.

Diarrhoea usually responds well to colestyramine or aluminium hydroxide therapy.

Short bowel syndrome

See p. 463.

Radiation enteritis and proctocolitis

Intestinal damage occurs in 10% to 15% of patients undergoing radio-therapy for abdominal or pelvic malignancy. The risk varies with total dose, dosing schedule and the use of concomitant chemotherapy.

Acutely, there is nausea, vomiting, cramping abdominal pain and diarrhoea. When the rectum and colon are involved, mucus, bleeding and tenesmus occur. The chronic phase develops after 5–10 years in some patients, and may feature bleeding from telangiectasis, fistulae, adhesions, strictures or malabsorption.

Sigmoidoscopy appearances resemble ulcerative proctitis. Colonoscopy shows the extent of the lesion. Barium follow-through or MRI enterography shows small bowel strictures, ulcers and fistulae.

Management

• Diarrhoea: codeine, diphenoxylate or loperamide. • Antibiotics for bacterial overgrowth. • Nutritional supplements for malabsorption • Colestyramine for bile acid diarrhoea. • Surgery should be avoided, because the injured intestine is difficult to resect and anastomose, but may be necessary for obstruction, perforation or fistula. • Endoscopic argon plasma coagulation therapy is of limited benefit and can cause fistulas.

Miscellaneous disorders of the small intestine

Protein-losing enteropathy

Defined as excessive loss of protein into the gut lumen, sufficient to cause hypoproteinaemia, protein-losing enteropathy occurs in a variety of inflammatory and neoplastic gut disorders, but is most common in ulcerating conditions. In other disorders, protein loss results from increased mucosal permeability or obstruction of intestinal lymphatic vessels.

Patients present with peripheral oedema and hypoproteinaemia in the presence of normal liver function and without proteinuria. The diagnosis is confirmed by measurement of faecal clearance of α_1-antitrypsin or ^{51}Cr-labelled albumin after IV injection. Treatment is that of the underlying disorder, with nutritional support and measures to control peripheral oedema.

Meckel's diverticulum

This is the most common congenital anomaly of the GI tract and occurs in 0.3% to 3% of people. Most patients are asymptomatic. The diverticulum results from failure of closure of the vitelline duct, with persistence of a blind-ending sac, usually within 100 cm of the ileocaecal valve and up to 5 cm long. Approximately 50% contain ectopic gastric mucosa.

Complications usually occur in the first 2 years of life, but occasionally in young adults. Bleeding results from ulceration of ileal mucosa adjacent to the ectopic parietal cells, and presents as recurrent melaena or altered blood per rectum. Diagnosis can be made by gamma scanning following IV ^{99m}Tc-pertechnate, which is concentrated by ectopic parietal cells. Other complications include intestinal obstruction, diverticulitis, intussusception and perforation. Surgery is unnecessary unless complications occur.

Infections of the small intestine

Travellers' diarrhoea, giardiasis and amoebiasis

See pp. 138, 160.

Abdominal tuberculosis

Mycobacterium tuberculosis rarely causes abdominal disease in Caucasians but must be considered in the developing world and in AIDS patients. Gut infection usually results from human *M. tuberculosis* that is swallowed after coughing. Many patients have no pulmonary symptoms and a normal CXR. Infection most commonly affects the ileocaecal region; presentation and radiological findings may resemble those of Crohn's disease. Abdominal pain can be acute or chronic, but diarrhoea is less common in TB than in Crohn's disease. Low-grade fever is common. TB can affect any part of the GI tract, including perianal disease with fistula. Peritoneal TB may result in peritonitis with exudative ascites, abdominal pain and fever. Granulomatous hepatitis also occurs.

Investigations and management

• ESR: elevated.• Alkaline phosphatase: if raised, suggests hepatic involvement.• Endoscopy, laparoscopy or liver biopsy for histological confirmation.• Culture of biopsies may take 6 weeks, but faster diagnosis is now possible using rapid PCR techniques.

When the presentation is very suggestive of abdominal TB, standard antimycobacterial therapy should be started (modified if resistance is present), even if bacteriological or histological proof is lacking.

Tumours of the small intestine

The small intestine is rarely affected by neoplasia and less than 5% of all GI tumours occur here.

Benign tumours

The most common are periampullary adenomas, GIST, lipomas and hamartomas. Multiple adenomas are common in the duodenum of patients with familial adenomatous polyposis who merit regular endoscopic surveillance. Hamartomatous polyps with almost no malignant potential occur in Peutz–Jeghers syndrome (p. 495).

Malignant tumours

These are rare and include adenocarcinoma, neuro endocrine tumours, malignant GIST and lymphoma. The majority occur in middle age or later. Kaposi's sarcoma is seen in patients with AIDS.

Adenocarcinomas

Adenocarcinomas occur with increased frequency in patients with FAP, coeliac disease and Peutz–Jeghers syndrome. Barium follow-through examination or small bowel enema studies will demonstrate most lesions. Enteroscopy, capsule endoscopy, mesenteric angiography and CT are also used. Treatment is by surgical resection.

Neuro endocrine tumours

Neuroendocrine tumours (NETs) in the small intestine can cause a variety of symptoms (Box 12.11). Their investigation and treatment are described on p. 409.

Lymphoma

Non-Hodgkin lymphoma may involve the GI tract as part of generalised disease or may rarely arise in the gut, most commonly in the small intestine.

12

Lymphomas are more common in patients with coeliac disease, AIDS and other immunodeficiencies.

Colicky abdominal pain, obstruction and weight loss are the usual presenting features, and diagnosis is by small bowel biopsy, contrast studies and CT. After staging, surgical resection is performed where possible, with radiotherapy and chemotherapy reserved for advanced disease.

Inflammatory bowel disease

Ulcerative colitis and Crohn's disease are chronic inflammatory bowel diseases that relapse and remit over years. The diseases have many similarities, and it is sometimes impossible to distinguish them (Box 12.12).

i	12.12 Comparison of ulcerative colitis and Crohn's disease	
	Ulcerative colitis	**Crohn's disease**
Age group	Any	Any
Gender	M = F	Slight female preponderance
Ethnic group	Any	Any; more common in Ashkenazi Jews
Genetic factors	*HLA-DR*103* associated with severe disease	Defective innate immunity: *NOD2* mutations predispose
Risk factors	More common in non/exsmokers; appendicectomy protects	More common in smokers
Anatomical distribution	Colon only; begins at anorectal margin with variable proximal extension	Any part of GI tract; perianal disease common; patchy distribution–'skip lesions'
Extra-intestinal manifestations	Common	Common
Presentation	Bloody diarrhoea	Variable; pain, diarrhoea, weight loss all common
Histology	Inflammation limited to mucosa; crypt distortion, cryptitis, crypt abscesses, loss of goblet cells	Submucosal or transmural inflammation common; deep fissuring ulcers, fistulae; patchy changes; granulomas
Management	5-ASA; glucocorticoids; azathioprine; anti-TNF; colectomy is curative	Glucocorticoids; azathioprine; methotrexate; anti-TNF; nutritional therapy; surgery is not curative; 5-ASA ineffective

However, ulcerative colitis only involves the colon, whereas Crohn's disease can involve any part of the GI tract.

The incidence of IBD varies widely between populations. The incidence of both ulcerative colitis and Crohn's disease increased markedly in the Western world from the mid-20th century, coinciding with the advent of a more 'hygienic' environment, refrigeration and widespread antibiotic use. The developing world experiences similar patterns where a Westernised lifestyle is adopted. Ulcerative colitis has a prevalence of 100 to 200 per 100 000, compared with 50 to 100 per 100 000 for Crohn's disease. Both diseases present most commonly in the second and third decades.

It is thought that IBD develops because genetically susceptible individuals mount an abnormal inflammatory response to environmental triggers, such as intestinal bacteria. There is emerging evidence that microbial dysbiosis, the virome and the mycobiome (fungal species) may be important in the development of IBD.

Clinical features

Ulcerative colitis: The cardinal symptoms are rectal bleeding with passage of mucus and bloody diarrhoea. Findings vary with the site and activity of the disease (Box 12.13):

Proctitis: Rectal bleeding and mucus discharge, sometimes with tenesmus. Some pass frequent, small-volume fluid stools, while others are constipated. Constitutional symptoms do not occur.

Extensive colitis: Bloody diarrhoea with mucus, anorexia, malaise, weight loss and abdominal pain. The patient is toxic, with fever, tachycardia and peritoneal inflammation. The first attack is usually the most severe and

12

12.13 Assessment of disease severity in ulcerative colitis		
	Mild	Severe
Daily bowel frequency	<4	≥6
Blood in stools	±	+++
Stool volume (g/24 hours)	<200	>400
Pulse (beats/min)	<90	≥90
Temperature (°C)	Normal	>37.8°C
Hb (g/L)	Normal	<100
ESR (mm/hour)	Normal	>30
Serum albumin (g/L)	>35	<30
AXR	Normal	Dilated bowel and/or mucosal islands
Sigmoidoscopy	Normal or granular mucosa	Blood in lumen

is followed by relapses and remissions; a few have unremitting symptoms. Stress, intercurrent infection, gastroenteritis, antibiotics or NSAIDs may provoke relapse.

Crohn's disease

The major symptoms are abdominal pain, diarrhoea and weight loss.

Ileal Crohn's disease: Presents with abdominal pain caused by sub-acute intestinal obstruction, an inflammatory mass, intra-abdominal abscess or acute obstruction. Diarrhoea is watery without blood or mucus. Weight loss is as a result of anorexia or malabsorption with fat, protein or vitamin deficiencies.

Crohn's colitis: Presents exactly like ulcerative colitis, with bloody diarrhoea, mucus, lethargy, malaise, anorexia and weight loss. Rectal sparing and perianal disease suggest Crohn's disease rather than ulcerative colitis.

Many patients present with both small bowel and colonic disease. A few have isolated perianal disease, vomiting from jejunal strictures or severe oral ulceration.

Physical examination reveals:

• Weight loss, anaemia, glossitis and angular stomatitis.• Abdominal tenderness, most marked over the inflamed area.• Abdominal mass as a result of matted loops of thickened bowel or an intra-abdominal abscess.
• Perianal skin tags, fissures or fistulae in at least 50% of patients.

Complications

Life-threatening colonic inflammation: This occurs in both ulcerative colitis and Crohn's disease. In extreme cases, the colon dilates (toxic megacolon), and bacterial toxins cross the diseased mucosa into the circulation. This occurs most commonly during the first attack of colitis and is associated with the severity indicators in Box 12.13—it is an emergency usually requiring colectomy. If an AXR shows the transverse colon is dilated to more than 6 cm, there is a high risk of perforation, although perforation can also occur in the absence of toxic megacolon.

Haemorrhage: Due to erosion of a major artery, occurs rarely.

Fistulae: These occur only in Crohn's disease. Enteroenteric fistulae cause diarrhoea and malabsorption. Enterovesical fistulation causes recurrent urinary infections and pneumaturia. Enterovaginal fistula causes faeculent vaginal discharge. Fistulation from the bowel may also cause perianal or ischiorectal abscesses, and fissures.

Cancer: Extensive, long-lasting colitis increases the risk of cancer. The cumulative risk for ulcerative colitis reaches 20% after 30 years but is lower for Crohn's colitis. Small bowel adenocarcinoma occasionally complicates long-standing small bowel Crohn's disease. Patients with chronic colitis should start surveillance colonoscopy 10 years after diagnosis, with targeted biopsy of areas showing abnormal dye staining (pancolonic chromo-endoscopy). Those with high-grade dysplasia should be considered for panproctocolectomy to prevent cancer.

	12.14 Systemic manifestations of inflammatory bowel disease	
	When IBD active	**Unrelated to IBD activity**
Eyes	Conjunctivitis, iritis, episcleritis	
Mouth	Ulcers	
Liver	Abscess, portal pyaemia, fatty change	Autoimmune hepatitis, gallstones, sclerosing cholangitis
Vascular	Mesenteric, portal or deep vein thrombosis	
Skin	Erythema nodosum, pyoderma gangrenosum	
Bone/joint	Large joint arthritis	Metabolic bone disease, sacroiliitis

Extra-intestinal complications: IBD can be considered as a systemic illness, and in some patients extra-intestinal complications dominate the clinical picture. Some of these occur during relapse of intestinal disease; others appear unrelated to intestinal disease activity (Box 12.14).

The differential diagnosis is shown in Boxes 12.15 and 12.16.

Investigations

FBC: May show anaemia from bleeding or malabsorption of iron, folic acid or vitamin B_{12}. Serum albumin is low because of protein-losing enteropathy or poor nutrition.

ESR: Raised in exacerbations or abscess.

CRP: Helpful in monitoring Crohn's disease activity.

Faecal calprotectin: Sensitive; useful to distinguish from irritable bowel syndrome and for monitoring activity.

Stool cultures: Help to exclude superimposed enteric infection in exacerbations.

Blood cultures: Advisable in febrile patients with known colitis or Crohn's disease.

	12.15 Conditions mimicking ulcerative or Crohn's colitis
Infective	For example, *Salmonella*, *Shigella*, *Campylobacter*, *E. coli* O157, herpes simplex, amoebiasis
Vascular	Radiation proctitis, ischaemic colitis
Neoplastic	Colonic carcinoma
Inflammatory	Behçet's disease
Drugs	NSAIDs

12.16 Differential diagnosis of small bowel Crohn's disease

- Other causes of right iliac fossa mass: caecal carcinoma[a], appendix abscess[a]
- Infection (TB, *Yersinia*, actinomycosis)
- Mesenteric adenitis
- Pelvic inflammatory disease
- Lymphoma

[a]*Common; other causes are rare.*

Endoscopy: Ileocolonoscopy should be performed in those with diarrhoea and raised inflammatory markers. In ulcerative colitis, there is loss of vascular pattern, granularity, friability and ulceration. In Crohn's disease, patchy inflammation is seen with discrete, deep ulcers, perianal disease or rectal sparing. Biopsies are taken to define disease extent and to seek dysplasia in long-standing colitis. In ulcerative colitis, the abnormalities are confluent and most severe in the distal colon and rectum. Stricture formation does not occur in the absence of a carcinoma. In Crohn's colitis, the endoscopic abnormalities are patchy, with intervening normal mucosa, and ulcers and strictures are common. Enteroscopy and upper GI endoscopy may be required for complete evaluation of Crohn's disease.

Radiology: Barium enema can show ulcers or strictures but is less sensitive than colonoscopy. If colonoscopy is incomplete, CT colonogram is preferred. Small bowel imaging is essential for staging Crohn's disease, and MRI enterography has replaced barium follow-through, as it can also show extra-intestinal and pelvic manifestations. It can also distinguish inflammatory from fibrotic strictures; the former respond to antiinflammatory treatment, but the latter require surgery or balloon dilatation. Abdominal X-ray is useful in active disease to show dilatation of the colon, mucosal oedema or evidence of perforation. In small bowel Crohn's disease, there may be intestinal obstruction or displacement of bowel loops by a mass.

USS: May identify thickened small bowel and stricture in Crohn's disease.

Management

Multidisciplinary management by physicians, surgeons, radiologists and dietitians is advantageous. Ulcerative colitis and Crohn's disease are lifelong conditions, and counsellors and patient support groups have important roles. The key aims are to:

• Treat acute attacks.• Prevent bowel damage and relapses.• Detect carcinoma early.• Select patients for surgery.

Ulcerative colitis

Active proctitis: In mild to moderate disease, mesalazine enemas or suppositories, combined with oral mesalazine, are effective. Topical glucocorticoids are less effective and are reserved for patients intolerant of topical mesalazine. Patients with resistant disease are treated with oral prednisolone.

Active left-sided or extensive ulcerative colitis: In mild cases, high-dose oral 5-ASAs, combined with topical 5-ASA foam enemas, are effective. Oral prednisolone is indicated for severe or unresponsive cases.

Severe ulcerative colitis: Patients with severe colitis (see Box 12.13) unresponsive to maximal oral therapy should be monitored in hospital:

Clinically: Abdominal pain, temperature, pulse, stool blood and frequency

By lab testing: Hb, WCC, albumen, electrolytes, ESR, CRP, stool culture

Radiologically: For colonic dilatation on AXR.

IV fluids and enteral nutritional support are often needed. IV gluco-corticoids are given as a bolus or infusion. Topical and oral aminosalicy-lates have no role in the acute severe attack. In patients unresponsive to glucocorticoids over 3 days, rescue therapy with IV ciclosporin or infliximab avoids the need for colectomy in 60%. Patients who deteriorate, despite 7 to 10 days' maximal medical therapy, and those with colonic dilatation (>6 cm) require urgentcolectomy.

Maintenance of remission: Lifelong maintenance therapy is recommended for all patients with extensive disease but is not necessary in those with proctitis. 5-aminosalicylates, for example mesalazine, are first-line agents. Patients who relapse frequently despite 5-ASAs are treated with thiopurines, for example, azathioprine or biologic therapies such as infliximab.

Crohn's disease

Crohn's is a progressive disease with fistula and stricture formation if sub-optimally managed. The goal is induction of remission, then maintenance with minimum glucocorticoid use.

Induction of remission: Ileal disease is treated with budesonide, which minimises side effects. Colitis or resistant ileal disease is treated with oral prednisolone. Patients on glucocorticoids should also receive calcium and vitamin D. Nutritional therapy using polymeric or elemental diets can induce remission without glucocorticoids and is a useful option in children and in extensive ileal disease.

Severe colonic disease is treated with IV glucocorticoids. Severe ileal or panenteric disease requires anti-TNF therapy (infliximab or adalimubab) with a thiopurine. These are used to induce remission, provided abscess and perforation have been excluded.

Maintenance of remission: A thiopurine (azathioprine or mercaptopu-rine) or methotrexate is widely used for maintenance. Patients with unresponsive disease are managed with both immunomodulating agents and anti-TNF therapy. Smoking cessation is important, as continued smoking predicts relapse.

Fistulating and perianal disease: The site of fistulation is defined using imaging, usually pelvic MRI. Examination under anaesthetic and surgical intervention are usually required, and nutritional support is also frequently necessary. For simple perianal disease, metronidazole and/or ciprofloxacin can aid healing. Thiopurines are given in chronic disease. Anti-TNF therapy helps to heal enterocutaneous fistulae and perianal disease.

Surgical treatment

Ulcerative colitis

Up to 60% of patients with extensive ulcerative colitis eventually require surgery. Indications include impaired quality of life, failure of medical therapy, fulminant colitis, cancer or severe dysplasia. Panproctocolectomy with ileostomy or proctocolectomy with ileal–anal pouch anastomosis cures the patient. Before surgery, patients must be counselled both by staff and by patients who have had surgery.

Crohn's disease

The indications for surgery are similar to those for ulcerative colitis. Operations are often necessary to deal with fistulae, abscesses and perianal disease, or to relieve small or large bowel obstruction. In contrast to ulcerative colitis, surgery is not curative, and disease recurrence is the rule, so a conservative approach is used. Those with extensive colitis require total colectomy, but ileal–anal pouch formation should be avoided because of the high risk of recurrence within the pouch with fistulae, abscess formation and pouch failure.

Microscopic colitis

This comprises two related conditions: lymphocytic and collagenous colitis, and has no known cause. The presentation is with watery diarrhoea, with normal colonoscopic appearances; however, histology shows a submucosal band of collagen with a chronic inflammatory infiltrate. The disease is commoner in women and is associated with rheumatoid arthritis, diabetes, coeliac disease and drugs such as NSAIDs or PPIs. Treatment with budesonide or 5-ASAs is usually effective, but the condition often recurs on discontinuation.

Irritable bowel syndrome

IBS is a common functional bowel disorder in which abdominal pain is associated with defecation or a change in bowel habit in the absence of structural pathology.

Approximately 10% to 15% of the general population are affected, but only 10% of these consult their doctors with symptoms. IBS is the most common cause of GI referral, and causes frequent absence from work and impaired quality of life. Young women are affected 2 to 3 times more often than men. There is wide overlap with nonulcer dyspepsia, chronic fatigue syndrome, dysmenorrhoea and urinary frequency. IBS is sometimes associated with a history of physical or sexual abuse, and this is an important aspect of the history because these patients benefit from psychologically based therapy.

Most patients seen in general practice do not have psychological problems, but around 50% of patients referred to hospital have significant anxiety, depression, somatisation, panic attacks and neurosis. Acute psychological stress and overt psychiatric disease alter visceral perception and GI motility. These factors, coupled with abnormal illness behaviour, contribute to but do not cause IBS.

A range of motility disorders from diarrhoea to constipation is found, but none is diagnostic. IBS is associated with altered 5-HT release, which is increased in diarrhoea-predominant disease and reduced when constipation occurs.

Some patients develop IBS following an episode of gastroenteritis, more commonly young women and those with existing background psychological problems. Others may be intolerant of specific dietary components, particularly lactose and wheat.

Clinical features and investigations

Recurrent colicky pain in the lower abdomen is relieved by defecation. Abdominal bloating worsens throughout the day; the cause is unknown but it is not excessive intestinal gas. Patients have an abnormal bowel habit. It is useful to classify these as having predominantly constipation or predominantly diarrhoea. The constipated type tends to pass infrequent pellety stools, usually with abdominal pain or proctalgia. Those with diarrhoea have frequent defecation but produce low-volume stools and rarely have nocturnal symptoms. Passage of mucus is common, but rectal bleeding does not occur.

Patients do not lose weight and are constitutionally well. Examination does not reveal any abnormalities, although bloating and tenderness to palpation are common.

Investigations are normal. FBC, faecal calprotectin and sigmoidoscopy are usually done routinely, but colonoscopy should only be undertaken in older patients and those with rectal bleeding to exclude colorectal cancer and IBD. Atypical presentations require investigations to exclude organic GI disease. In diarrhoea-predominant cases, coeliac disease, lactose intolerance, thyrotoxicosis and parasitic infection should be excluded.

Management

Many patients are concerned that they have developed cancer, and a cycle of anxiety leading to colonic symptoms, which further heighten anxiety, can be broken by explanation that symptoms are not because of organic disease, but are the result of altered bowel motility and sensation. In patients who fail to respond to reassurance, symptomatic treatment should be tried. Some benefit from exclusion of wheat, lactose, excess caffeine or artificial sweeteners. A more restrictive, 'low-FODMAP' diet, supervised by a dietitian, with gradual re-introduction of different food groups, may help some patients, as may a trial of a gluten-free diet. Probiotics can be effective in some.

Patients with intractable symptoms sometimes benefit from several months of therapy with low-dose amitriptyline. Anxiety or affective disorders should be separately treated. Psychological interventions, such as cognitive behavioural therapy, relaxation and gut-directed hypnotherapy, are reserved for the most difficult cases. Most patients have a relapsing and remitting course.

Ischaemic gut injury

Ischaemic gut injury is usually the result of arterial occlusion. The presentation is variable, and the diagnosis is difficult.

Acute small bowel ischaemia

Superior mesenteric blood flow may be compromised by embolism from the heart or aorta (40%–50%), thrombosis on underlying atheroma (25%) or hypotension (25%). Vasculitis and venous occlusion are rare causes. Patients usually have evidence of cardiac disease and arrhythmia.

Abdominal pain develops, which is more impressive than the physical findings. In the early stages, the abdomen may be distended, with absent or diminished bowel sounds, and peritonitis is a later feature.

Investigations reveal:
• Leucocytosis.• Metabolic acidosis.• Raised phosphate and amylase. • 'Thumb-printing' on AXR because of mucosal oedema.• An occluded or narrowed major artery on mesenteric or CT angiography.

Management

Resuscitation, management of cardiac disease and IV antibiotic therapy should be followed by laparotomy, embolectomy and vascular reconstruction. In patients at high surgical risk, thrombolysis may sometimes be effective. Survivors often develop short bowel syndrome requiring nutritional support, sometimes including home parenteral nutrition, as well as anticoagulation. Small bowel transplantation can be considered in selected patients.

Acute colonic ischaemia

The splenic flexure and descending colon lie in 'watershed' areas of arterial supply. Arterial thromboembolism is usually responsible, but colonic ischaemia can also follow severe hypotension, colonic volvulus, strangulated hernia, systemic vasculitis, aortic aneurysm surgery or hypercoagulable states. The patient is usually elderly and presents with sudden cramping left-sided lower abdominal pain and rectal bleeding. The diagnosis is established by colonoscopy within 48 hours of onset. Symptoms usually resolve spontaneously over 24 to 48 hours, and healing occurs within 2 weeks. Some have a residual fibrous stricture or segment of colitis.

Chronic mesenteric ischaemia

This results from atherosclerotic stenosis affecting at least two of the coeliac axis, superior mesenteric and inferior mesenteric arteries. Patients present with dull but severe mid- or upper abdominal pain around 30 minutes after eating, with weight loss and sometimes with diarrhoea. Examination reveals generalised arterial disease and sometimes an audible abdominal bruit. Mesenteric angiography confirms at least two affected arteries. Vascular reconstruction or percutaneous angioplasty is sometimes possible. Left untreated, many patients develop intestinal infarction.

Disorders of the colon and rectum

Tumours of the colon and rectum

Polyps and polyposis syndromes

Polyps may be neoplastic or nonneoplastic, single or multiple, and vary from a few mm to several cm in size.

Colorectal adenomas: Extremely common in the Western world; 50% of people older than 60 years of age have adenomas, usually in the rectum and distal colon. Nearly all colorectal carcinomas develop from adenomatous polyps. Large, multiple, villous or dysplastic polyps carry a higher risk of malignancy. Adenomas are usually asymptomatic and discovered incidentally. Occasionally, they cause bleeding and anaemia. Villous adenomas sometimes secrete large amounts of mucus, leading to diarrhoea and hypokalaemia.

Discovery of a polyp at sigmoidoscopy is an indication for colonoscopy and polypectomy, which considerably reduce subsequent cancer risk. Very large or sessile polyps sometimes require surgery. Once all polyps have been removed, patients under 75 years of age should undergo surveillance colonoscopy at 3- to 5-year intervals because new polyps develop in 50%.

Between 10% and 20% of polyps show evidence of malignancy. When cancer cells are found within 2 mm of the resection margin, and when the polyp cancer is poorly differentiated or invading lymphatics, segmental colonic resection is recommended. Others can be followed up by surveillance colonoscopy.

The polyposis syndromes are classified by histopathology. They include neoplastic familial adenomatous polyposis and several nonneoplastic syndromes, including Peutz–Jeghers syndrome.

Familial adenomatous polyposis: An uncommon (1 in 13 000) autosomal dominant disorder. Around 20% are new mutations with no family history. By age 15, 80% of patients will develop up to several thousand adenomatous colonic polyps, with symptoms such as rectal bleeding beginning a few years later. Within 10 to 15 years of the appearance of adenomas, colorectal cancer will develop, affecting 90% by the age of 50 years. Malignant transformation of duodenal adenomas occurs in 10% and is the leading cause of death after prophylactic colectomy. Extra-intestinal features include subcutaneous epidermoid cysts, benign osteomas, dental abnormalities and lipomas. Dark, round, pigmented retinal lesions (congenital hypertrophy of the retinal pigment epithelium) occur in some patients; in at-risk individuals, these are 100% predictive of FAP.

Early identification is essential. Sigmoidoscopy, if normal, excludes the diagnosis. Genetic testing confirms the diagnosis, and first-degree relatives should also be tested. Children of FAP families should undergo mutation testing at 13 to 14 years of age, followed by regular sigmoidoscopy in those carrying the mutation. Affected individuals should undergo colectomy on leaving school or college. Periodic upper GI endoscopy is recommended to detect duodenal adenomas.

Peutz–Jeghers syndrome: Comprises multiple hamartomatous polyps in the small intestine and colon, and melanin pigmentation of the lips, mouth and digits, and is usually asymptomatic. There is a small but significant risk of small bowel or colonic adenocarcinoma and of cancer of the pancreas, lung, testis, ovary, breast and endometrium. Patients should undergo regular upper endoscopy and colonoscopy (with removal of polyps >1cm) and small bowel and pancreatic imaging.

Colorectal cancer

Although relatively rare in the developing world, colorectal cancer is the second most common malignancy and the second leading cause of cancer deaths in Western countries. In the UK the incidence is 50 to 60 per 100 000/year. It becomes increasingly common over the age of 50 years.

Both genetic and environmental factors are important. Around 70% are associated with multiple somatic mutations, 25% with multiple susceptibility genes and 5% with inherited single gene mutations. Environmental factors account for the wide geographical variation in incidence and the decrease in risk seen when migrants move from high- to low-risk countries. Dietary factors increasing risk are red meat and saturated fat, whereas fibre, fruit, vegetables, folic acid and calcium appear to protect.

Hereditary nonpolyposis colon cancer occurs in patients with history of relatives who were affected at a young age. The lifetime risk of colorectal cancer in affected individuals is 80%. Those who fulfil the criteria for diagnosis should be referred for pedigree assessment, genetic testing and colonoscopy, which needs to be repeated every 1 to 2 years, despite which interval cancers still occur.

The lifetime risk of colon cancer in the 20% of patients with a family history, when one or two first-degree relatives are affected is 1 in 12 and 1 in 6, respectively.

Most tumours arise from malignant transformation of a benign adenomatous polyp. Over 65% occur in the rectosigmoid, and a further 15% recur in the caecum or ascending colon. Rectal cancers may invade the pelvic viscera and side walls. Lymphatic invasion is common at presentation, as is hepatic spread. Tumour stage at diagnosis determines prognosis.

Clinical features

In tumours of the left colon, fresh rectal bleeding is common, and obstruction occurs early. Tumours of the right colon present with anaemia from occult bleeding or with altered bowel habit, but obstruction is a late feature. Colicky lower abdominal pain is present in two-thirds of patients, and rectal bleeding occurs in 50%. A minority present with either obstruction or perforation. Carcinoma of the rectum usually causes early bleeding, mucus discharge or a feeling of incomplete emptying.

On examination there may be a palpable mass, signs of anaemia or hepatomegaly from metastases. Low rectal tumours may be palpable on digital examination.

Investigations and management

- Colonoscopy: more sensitive and specific than barium enema and permits biopsy Fig. 12.4.
- CT colonography: detects tumours and polyps larger than 6 mm diameter and can be used if colonoscopy is incomplete or high risk.
- CT: valuable for detecting hepatic metastases.
- Pelvic MRI or endoanal USS: to stage rectal tumours.
- Carcinoembryonic antigen: normal in many patients and so of little use in diagnosis, but serial carcinoembryonic antigen can help to detect early recurrence during follow-up.

Treatment should be discussed and planned at a multidisciplinary meeting.

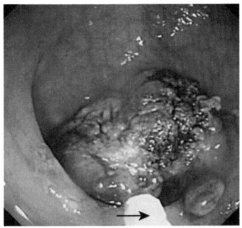

Fig. 12.4 Colonoscopic view of a polypoid rectal carcinoma undergoing laser therapy (arrow) in a patient unfit for surgery.

Neo-adjuvant therapy: Preoperative radiotherapy or chemoradiotherapy is used to 'down-stage' large rectal cancers, making them resectable.

Surgery: The tumour is removed, along with pericolic lymph nodes. Direct anastomosis is performed wherever possible, or colostomy if not. Solitary hepatic or lung metastases are sometimes resected at a later stage. Postoperatively, patients should undergo colonoscopy after 6 to 12 months and periodically thereafter to search for local recurrence or development of new 'metachronous' lesions, which occur in 6% of cases.

Adjuvant therapy: Some 30% to 40% of patients have lymph node spread at presentation and are, therefore, at risk of recurrence (Box 12.17). Most recurrences are within 3 years, either at the site of resection

	12.17 **Staging and survival in colorectal cancer**			
	\multicolumn{4}{c}{**Dukes stage**}			
	A	**B**	**C**	**D**
Definition	Tumour confined within bowel wall	Extension through bowel wall	Tumour involving lymph nodes	Distant metastases
Prevalence at diagnosis (%)	10	35	30	25
5-year survival rate (%)	>90	65	30–35	<5

or in lymph nodes, liver or peritoneum. Adjuvant chemotherapy reduces recurrence risk in patients with Dukes C colon cancer and some Dukes B tumours. Postoperative radiotherapy is used to reduce the risk of local recurrence if resection margins are involved.

Palliation: Surgical resection of the primary tumour is appropriate for some patients with metastases to treat obstruction, bleeding or pain. Palliative chemotherapy with 5-fluorouracil/folinic acid, oxaliplatin or irinotecan improves survival. Pelvic radiotherapy is sometimes useful for rectal pain, bleeding or severe tenesmus. Endoscopic laser therapy or insertion of an expandable metal stent can be used to relieve obstruction.

Prevention and screening: This aims to detect and remove lesions at an early or premalignant stage. Several potential methods exist. Population screening by regular FOB testing in those over 50 years of age increases early detection and reduces colorectal cancer mortality, and has been adopted in a number of countries. Colonoscopy remains the gold standard, but requires expertise, is expensive and carries risks. Flexible sigmoidoscopy has been shown to reduce overall colorectal cancer mortality by around 35% (70% for cases arising in the rectosigmoid). It is recommended in the United States every 5 years in all persons over the age of 50 years.

Diverticulosis

Asymptomatic diverticula ('diverticulosis') occur in the sigmoid and descending colon in more than 50% of people over 70 years of age. Symptomatic diverticular disease occurs in 10% to 25% of cases, whereas complicated diverticulosis (acute diverticulitis, pericolic abscess, bleeding, perforation or stricture) is uncommon.

Dietary fibre deficiency is thought to be responsible, and diverticulosis is rare in populations with a high dietary fibre. Small-volume stools require high intracolonic pressures for propulsion, leading to herniation of mucosa.

Diverticula are protrusions of mucosa covered by peritoneum, which become impacted with faecoliths, then inflamed. This may resolve or progress with haemorrhage, perforation, abscess formation, fistula and peritonitis. Repeated attacks may lead to fibrotic strictures.

Clinical features

• Colicky pain in the suprapubic area or left iliac fossa from associated constipation or spasm.• Palpable sigmoid colon or iliac fossa mass.• Local tenderness, guarding, rigidity ('left-sided appendicitis') with diverticulitis. • Diarrhoea, rectal bleeding or fever.• Complications occur in around 5%; they are more common in patients who take NSAIDs or aspirin.

Investigations and management

• CT colonography or barium enema: shows diverticula, strictures and fistulae. CT can also show complications such as perforation or pericolic abscess.• Colonoscopy: requires experience to avoid risk of perforation.

Asymptomatic diverticulosis requires no treatment. Constipation is relieved by a high-fibre diet with or without a bulking laxative and plenty of fluids. Stimulants should be avoided, but antispasmodics sometimes help.

Acute diverticulitis can be treated with antibiotics against Gram-negative and anaerobic bacteria. Trials show no benefit from acute resection compared with conservative management, except with severe haemorrhage or perforation. Percutaneous drainage of paracolic abscesses can be effective. Elective resection of the affected segment with primary anastomosis is indicated after repeated acute obstruction.

Constipation and disorders of defecation

Simple constipation: Constipation is extremely common, and usually responds to increased dietary fibre or bulking agents with an adequate fluid intake.

Severe idiopathic constipation: This occurs almost exclusively in young women, and often begins in childhood or adolescence. The cause is unknown, and the condition is often resistant to treatment. Bulking agents may exacerbate symptoms, but prokinetic agents or balanced solutions of polyethylene glycol 3350 benefit some patients with slow transit.

Faecal impaction: Impaction tends to occur in frail, disabled, immobile or institutionalised patients. Drugs, autonomic neuropathy and painful anal conditions also contribute. Obstruction, perforation and bleeding may supervene. Treatment involves softening the stool with arachis oil enemas, hydration and careful digital disimpaction.

Melanosis coli and laxative misuse syndromes: Long-term stimulant laxative use causes brown discoloration of the colonic mucosa ('tiger skin'), which is benign and resolves with laxative withdrawal. Surreptitious laxative misuse is a psychiatric condition seen in young women, who may have a history of bulimia or anorexia nervosa. They complain of refractory watery diarrhoea and deny laxative use. Screening of urine for laxatives may be helpful.

Hirschsprung's disease: Congenital absence of ganglion cells causes the internal anal sphincter to fail to relax, leading to constipation and colonic dilatation (megacolon). Constipation, abdominal distension and vomiting usually develop immediately after birth, but occasionally in childhood or adolescence. A family history is present in one-third. The rectum is empty on digital examination. Barium enema shows a small rectum and colonic dilatation above the narrowed segment. Full-thickness biopsies confirm the absence of ganglion cells. Treatment involves resection of the affected segment.

Acquired megacolon: In childhood, this is a result of voluntary withholding of stool during toilet training. It presents after the first year and is distinguished from Hirschsprung's disease by the urge to defecate and the presence of stool in the rectum. It usually responds to osmotic laxatives. In adults, acquired megacolon may occur in patients with depression or dementia, either as part of the condition or as a side effect of antidepressant drugs. Prolonged misuse of stimulant laxatives may cause megacolon, as may neurological disorders, systemic sclerosis, hypothyroidism and opioid abuse. Patients are managed by treating the underlying cause, and with high-residue diets, laxatives and enemas.

Acute colonic pseudo-obstruction (Ogilvie's syndrome): This can be caused by trauma, surgery, respiratory or renal failure, or diabetes mellitus. There is sudden, painless, massive enlargement of the proximal colon without features of mechanical obstruction. Bowel sounds are normal or

12

high-pitched rather than absent. The condition may progress to perforation and peritonitis. X-rays show colonic dilatation with air extending to the rectum. A caecal diameter greater than 10 to 12 cm is associated with a high risk of perforation. Barium enemas demonstrate the absence of mechanical obstruction. Management consists of treating the underlying disorder and correcting any biochemical abnormalities. Neostigmine is used to enhance gut motility. Decompression either with a rectal tube or by careful colonoscopy may be effective.

Anorectal disorders

Faecal incontinence

Common causes include severe diarrhoea, impaction, anorectal or neurological disease and obstetric trauma. A careful history and examination, especially of the anorectum and perineum, may help to establish the underlying cause. Endoanal USS is valuable for defining the integrity of the anal sphincters, while magnetic resonance proctography, manometry and electrophysiology are also useful.

Management involves treating underlying disorders. Pelvic floor exercises, biofeedback techniques and sphincter repair operations help some patients.

Haemorrhoids ('piles')

Haemorrhoids are extremely common and arise from congestion of the venous plexuses around the anal canal. They are associated with constipation and straining and may develop during pregnancy. First-degree piles bleed, second-degree piles prolapse but retract spontaneously and third-degree piles require manual replacement. Symptoms include bright red bleeding after defecation, pain, pruritus ani and mucus discharge. Treatment involves prevention of constipation, injection sclerotherapy or band ligation. A minority require haemorrhoidectomy, which is usually curative. Haemorrhoidal artery ligation is promising and may replace surgery.

Pruritus ani

This is common, and causes include infections, skin disorders and anal disorders such as haemorrhoids or fissures. These result in contamination of the perianal skin with faecal contents, leading to an itch–scratch–itch cycle that exacerbates the problem. Good personal hygiene is essential, with careful washing after defecation. The perineal area must be kept dry and clean.

Solitary rectal ulcer syndrome

This occurs in young adults who develop an ulcer with mucosal prolapse on the anterior rectal wall. Symptoms include minor bleeding and mucus per rectum, tenesmus and perineal pain. Treatment is often difficult, but avoidance of straining at defecation is important.

Anal fissure

This is a superficial tear in the anal mucosa, most commonly in the midline posteriorly, with spasm of the internal anal sphincter. Severe pain occurs on defecation, with minor bleeding, mucus discharge and pruritus. The skin may be indurated, and an oedematous skin tag, or 'sentinel pile', is common.

Avoidance of constipation with bulk-forming laxatives and increased fluid intake is important. Relaxation of the internal sphincter using glyceryl trinitrate is effective in 60% to 80% of patients; diltiazem cream is an alternative. Resistant cases may respond to injection of botulinum toxin into the internal anal sphincter to induce sphincter relaxation. Manual dilatation under anaesthesia leads to long-term incontinence and should not be considered.

Anorectal abscesses and fistulae

Perianal abscesses develop between the anal sphincters and may point at the perianal skin. Ischiorectal abscesses occur in the ischiorectal fossa. Crohn's disease is sometimes responsible.

Patients complain of extreme perianal pain, fever and/or discharge of pus. Spontaneous rupture may also lead to the development of fistulae. Abscesses and fistulae are treated surgically.

Diseases of the peritoneal cavity

Peritonitis

Peritonitis usually occurs as the result of a ruptured viscus but may also complicate ascites or occur in children without ascites, because of pneumococcal or streptococcal infection. Chlamydial peritonitis is a complication of pelvic inflammatory disease, and presents with right upper quadrant pain, pyrexia and a hepatic rub. TB may cause peritonitis and ascites.

Tumours

The most common is secondary adenocarcinoma from the ovary or GI tract. Mesothelioma is a rare tumour complicating asbestos exposure. The prognosis is extremely poor.

Endometriosis

Ectopic endometrial tissue can become embedded on the serosal aspect of the sigmoid and rectum. Cyclical engorgement and inflammation cause low backache, bleeding, diarrhoea, constipation, adhesions or obstruction. It usually affects nulliparous women between 20 and 45 years of age. Bimanual examination may reveal tender nodules in the pouch of Douglas. Sigmoidoscopy during menstruation reveals a bluish mass with intact overlying mucosa. Treatment options include laparoscopic diathermy and hormonal therapy with progestogens.

Diseases of the pancreas

Acute pancreatitis

Acute pancreatitis accounts for 3% of all cases of abdominal pain admitted to hospital. It affects 2 to 28 per 100 000 of the population and is increasing in incidence.

12.18 Causes of acute pancreatitis

Common (90% of cases)

- Gallstones
- Alcohol
- Idiopathic
- Post-ERCP

Rare

- Postsurgical
- Trauma
- Drugs (e.g. azathioprine)
- Infection (e.g. mumps)
- Renal failure
- Hypothermia
- Sphincter of Oddi dysfunction
- Petrochemical exposure

The condition results from premature activation of intracellular trypsinogen, releasing proteases that digest the pancreas and surrounding tissue. Causes of acute pancreatitis are given in Box 12.18. It is usually mild and self-limiting, with minimal organ dysfunction and uneventful recovery. In around 20% of patients it is severe, with complications such as necrosis, pseudocyst or abscess and multiorgan failure.

Clinical features and complications

Severe, constant upper abdominal pain builds up over 15 to 60 minutes, radiating to the back. There is nausea, vomiting and epigastric tenderness, but, in the early stages, guarding and rebound tenderness are absent because inflammation is mainly retroperitoneal. Bowel sounds become quiet or absent as paralytic ileus develops. There is hypoxia and hypovolaemic shock with oliguria in severe cases. Discoloration of the flanks (Grey Turner's sign) or the periumbilical region (Cullen's sign) is a feature of severe pancreatitis with haemorrhage.

Complications are listed in Box 12.19.

Investigations

The diagnosis is based on raised serum amylase or lipase (although amylase may return to normal in 24–48 hours) and ultrasound or CT evidence of pancreatic swelling. Amylase is also elevated (but less so) in intestinal ischaemia, perforated ulcer and ruptured ovarian cyst, whereas salivary amylase is elevated in parotitis. Persistently elevated serum amylase suggests pseudocyst formation. Peritoneal amylase is massively elevated in pancreatic ascites. Serum lipase, if available, has greater diagnostic accuracy for acute pancreatitis than amylase. USS may reveal pancreatic swelling, gallstones, biliary obstruction or pseudocyst formation. Plain X-rays help to exclude perforation, obstruction and pulmonary complications. CT 6 to 10 days after onset helps to define the viability of the pancreas; decreased contrast enhancement indicates necrotising pancreatitis. Gas

i 12.19 Complications of acute pancreatitis	
Complication	**Cause**
Systemic	
Systemic inflammatory response syndrome	Increased vascular permeability from cytokine, platelet aggregating factor and kinin release
Hypoxia	ARDS caused by microthrombi in pulmonary vessels
Hyperglycaemia	Disruption of islets of Langerhans with altered insulin/glucagon release
Hypocalcaemia	Sequestration of calcium in fat necrosis, fall in ionised calcium
Reduced serum albumin	Increased capillary permeability
Pancreatic	
Necrosis	Nonviable pancreatic tissue and peripancreatic tissue death; frequently infected
Abscess	Circumscribed collection of pus close to the pancreas and containing little or no pancreatic necrotic tissue
Pseudocyst	Disruption of pancreatic ducts
Pancreatic ascites or pleural effusion	Disruption of pancreatic ducts
GI	
Upper GI bleeding	Gastric or duodenal erosions
Variceal haemorrhage	Splenic or portal vein thrombosis
Erosion into colon	Erosion by pancreatic pseudocyst
Duodenal obstruction	Compression by pancreatic mass
Obstructive jaundice	Compression of common bile duct

12

pockets suggest infection and impending abscess formation, in which case percutaneous aspiration for bacterial culture and appropriate antibiotics are required. CT also reveals involvement of the colon, blood vessels and surrounding structures by the inflammatory process.

Management and prognosis

Adverse prognostic factors are shown in Box 12.20. Serial CRP is a useful indicator of progress. A peak CRP greater than 210 mg/L in the first 4 days predicts severe acute pancreatitis with 80% accuracy. Serum amylase has no prognostic value. Mortality is around 10%. About 80% of all cases are mild with a good prognosis; 98% of deaths occur in the 20% of severe cases. One-third occur within the first week, usually from multiorgan failure.

> **i** | **12.20 Adverse prognostic factors in acute pancreatitis (Glasgow criteria)[a]**
>
> - Age >55 years
> - PO_2 <8 kPa (60 mmHg)
> - WBC >15 × 10^9/L
> - Albumin <32 g/L (3.2 g/dL)
> - Serum calcium <2 mmol/L (8 mg/dL) (corrected)
> - Glucose >10 mmol/L (180 mg/dL)
> - Urea >16 mmol/L (45 mg/dL) (after rehydration)
> - ALT >200 U/L
> - LDH >600 U/L
>
> [a]*Severity and prognosis worsen as the number of these factors increases; >3 implies severe disease.*

Management comprises diagnosis, resuscitation, detection and treatment of complications, as well as treatment of the underlying cause—specifically, gallstones.

All severe cases should be managed in HDU/ICU. A central venous catheter and urinary catheter are used to monitor patients with shock. Treatment includes:

• Analgesia using opiates.• Correction of hypovolaemia using normal saline or other crystalloids.• Nasogastric aspiration: only necessary if paralytic ileus is present.• Enteral feeding via a nasogastric tube: should be started early. It decreases endotoxaemia and thereby systemic complications. • Insulin to correct hyperglycaemia.• Oxygen for hypoxic patients; those with SIRS may require ventilatory support.• Calcium: only needed if hypocalcaemic tetany occurs.• Prophylaxis of thromboembolism with low-dose SC heparin: advisable.• Broad-spectrum IV antibiotics such as imipenem or cefuroxime: may improve outcome in infected necrosis.

Patients with cholangitis or jaundice in association with severe acute pancreatitis should undergo urgent ERCP to diagnose and treat choledocholithiasis. In less severe cases of gallstone pancreatitis, biliary imaging (using MRCP) can be carried out after the acute phase has resolved. Cholecystectomy with an on-table cholangiogram should be undertaken within 2 weeks of resolution of pancreatitis to prevent further potentially fatal attacks.

Patients with necrotising pancreatitis or pancreatic abscess require urgent endoscopic or minimally invasive debridement of all cavities to remove necrotic material. Pancreatic pseudocysts are treated by delayed drainage into the stomach, duodenum or jejunum.

Chronic pancreatitis

Chronic pancreatitis is a chronic inflammatory disease characterised by fibrosis and destruction of exocrine pancreatic tissue. Diabetes mellitus occurs in advanced cases because the islets of Langerhans are involved. Around 80% of cases in Western countries result from alcohol misuse. Other causes include malnutrition, cassava consumption and recurrent acute pancreatitis, although some cases are idiopathic. Cystic fibrosis causes painless chronic pancreatic destruction (see p. 331). Chronic pancreatitis predominantly affects middle-aged alcoholic men.

Clinical features and complications

• Abdominal pain: in 50% this occurs as episodes of 'acute pancreatitis', although each attack results in further pancreatic damage. Relentless, slowly progressive pain without acute exacerbations affects 35% of patients. Pain may be relieved by leaning forwards or by alcohol.• Diarrhoea without pain: an uncommon presentation.• Weight loss.• Steatorrhoea: indicates that more than 90% of the exocrine tissue has been destroyed; protein malabsorption develops in the most advanced cases.• Diabetes mellitus in 30%, rising to 70% in those with chronic calcific pancreatitis. • Epigastric tenderness, sometimes with erythema ab igne over the abdomen and back caused by chronic use of a hot water bottle.• Features of other alcohol- and smoking-related diseases.

Investigations

Investigations are shown in Box 12.21 and Fig. 12.5.

Complications include:

• Pseudocysts and pancreatic ascites: occur in both acute and chronic pancreatitis.• Extrahepatic obstructive jaundice: caused by a benign stricture of the common bile duct as it passes through the diseased pancreas. • Duodenal stenosis.• Portal or splenic vein thrombosis leading to segmental portal hypertension and gastric varices.• Peptic ulcer.

Management

Alcohol avoidance: This is crucial in halting disease progression and reducing pain, but advice is frequently ignored.

Pain relief: NSAIDs are valuable, but the severe, unremitting pain often leads to opiate use with risk of addiction. Oral pancreatic enzyme supplements suppress pancreatic secretion and reduce analgesic requirement in some patients.

  12.21 Investigations in chronic pancreatitis

Tests to establish the diagnosis

- USS
- CT (may show atrophy, calcification or ductal dilatation)
- AXR (may show calcification)
- MRCP
- EUS

Tests of pancreatic function

- Collection of pure pancreatic juice after secretin injection (gold standard, but invasive and seldom used)
- Pancreolauryl or PABA test
- Faecal pancreatic elastase

Tests of anatomy before surgery

- MRCP

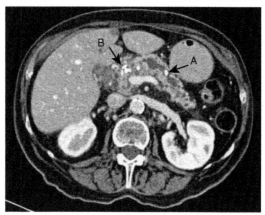

Fig. 12.5 Imaging in chronic pancreatitis. CT scan showing a grossly dilated and irregular duct with a calcified stone (arrow A). Note the calcification in the head of the gland (arrow B).

Surgery/endoscopy: Abstinent patients with severe chronic pain resistant to conservative measures may respond to surgical or endoscopic treatment of strictures, calculi and pseudocysts or coeliac plexus neurolysis. Patients without such correctable abnormalities require total pancreatectomy. Unfortunately, even after this, some patients continue to experience pain. Moreover, the procedure causes diabetes, which may be difficult to control.

Fat restriction and oral pancreatic enzyme supplements: These are used to treat steatorrhoea. A PPI is added to optimise duodenal pH for pancreatic enzyme activity.

Congenital abnormalities of the pancreas

Annular pancreas

In this congenital anomaly, the pancreas encircles the second/third part of the duodenum, leading to gastric outlet obstruction.

Cystic fibrosis

See p. 331.

Tumours of the pancreas

Pancreatic carcinoma affects 10 to 15 per 100 000 in Western populations, rising to 100 per 100 000 in those over the age of 70 years. Men are affected twice as often as women. The disease is associated with smoking and chronic pancreatitis. Between 5% and 10% of patients have a genetic predisposition.

Approximately 90% of pancreatic neoplasms are adenocarcinomas, which arise from the pancreatic ducts and spread early to involve local structures and regional lymph nodes.

Clinical features

• Pain: incessant, boring, with radiation to the back; may be eased by bending forward.• Weight loss caused by anorexia, steatorrhoea and metabolic effects of the tumour.• Obstructive jaundice: 60% of tumours arise from the head of the pancreas, with obstruction of the common bile duct and associated severe pruritus.• Less common: diarrhoea, vomiting from duodenal obstruction, diabetes mellitus, recurrent venous thrombosis, acute pancreatitis or depression.

Examination reveals evidence of weight loss, abdominal mass caused by the tumour itself, a palpable gallbladder or hepatic metastasis. A palpable gallbladder in a jaundiced patient is usually attributed to biliary obstruction by a pancreatic cancer.

Investigations

• USS and CT: demonstrate a pancreatic mass.• LFTs: for cholestatic jaundice. • Staging to define operability: entails laparoscopy with laparoscopic EUS to define tumour size, involvement of blood vessels and metastatic spread.• MRCP or ERCP: when diagnosis is in doubt.

In patients unsuitable for surgery because of advanced disease, frailty or comorbidity, USS- or CT-guided cytology or biopsy can be used. EUS with fine needle aspiration is used to define vascular invasion and obtain cytological proof of diagnosis.

Management

Surgical resection: The only curative treatment; 5-year survival after complete resection is around 20%. Survival may be improved with adjuvant chemotherapy. Only 15% of tumours are amenable to curative resection because most are locally advanced at diagnosis. For the great majority, therapy is based on palliation. Chemotherapy with FOLFIRINOX (5-fluorouracil, leucovorin, irinotecan and oxaliplatin) improves median survival to 11 months.

Pain relief: Analgesics with or without coeliac plexus neurolysis by a percutaneous or EUS-guided alcohol injection.

Jaundice: Choledochojejunostomy in fit patients; percutaneous or endoscopic stenting of the common bile duct is useful palliation in the elderly or those with very advanced disease.

Overall survival is only 3% to 5%; median survival is 3 to 10 months, depending on stage.

Pancreatic neuro endocrine tumours

These may occur in association with parathyroid and pituitary adenomas (p. 409). The majority of endocrine tumours are nonsecretory and, although malignant, grow slowly and metastasise late. Other tumours secrete hormones and present because of their endocrine effects.

Hepatology

The liver weighs 1 to 1.8 kg and performs many important functions (Fig. 13.1). In the developed world, the most common cause of liver disease is alcohol abuse, and cirrhosis causes many deaths. In contrast, in the developing world, infections caused by hepatitis viruses and parasites are responsible for most chronic liver disease and hepatobiliary cancer. Clinically silent chronic liver disease frequently presents with abnormalities on routine blood tests or when events such as intercurrent infection or surgery cause decompensation.

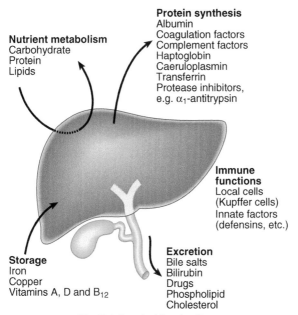

Nutrient metabolism
Carbohydrate
Protein
Lipids

Protein synthesis
Albumin
Coagulation factors
Complement factors
Haptoglobin
Caeruloplasmin
Transferrin
Protease inhibitors,
e.g. α_1-antitrypsin

Immune functions
Local cells
(Kupffer cells)
Innate factors
(defensins, etc.)

Storage
Iron
Copper
Vitamins A, D and B_{12}

Excretion
Bile salts
Bilirubin
Drugs
Phospholipid
Cholesterol

Fig. 13.1 Important liver functions.

Clinical examination of the abdomen for liver and biliary disease

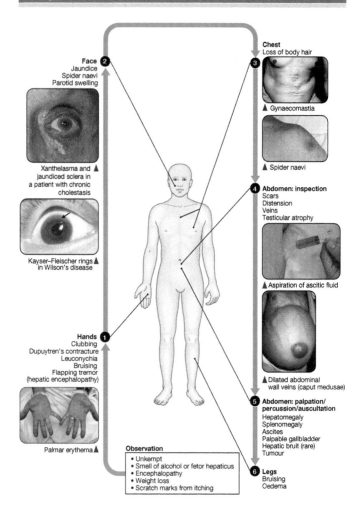

Face ❷
Jaundice
Spider naevi
Parotid swelling

Xanthelasma and ▲
jaundiced sclera in
a patient with chronic
cholestasis

Kayser–Fleischer rings ▲
in Wilson's disease

Chest ❸
Loss of body hair

▲ Gynaecomastia

▲ Spider naevi

Abdomen: inspection ❹
Scars
Distension
Veins
Testicular atrophy

▲ Aspiration of ascitic fluid

▲ Dilated abdominal
wall veins (caput medusae)

Abdomen: palpation/ ❺
percussion/auscultation
Hepatomegaly
Splenomegaly
Ascites
Palpable gallbladder
Hepatic bruit (rare)
Tumour

Hands ❶
Clubbing
Dupuytren's contracture
Leuconychia
Bruising
Flapping tremor
(hepatic encephalopathy)

Palmar erythema ▲

Observation
• Unkempt
• Smell of alcohol or fetor hepaticus
• Encephalopathy
• Weight loss
• Scratch marks from itching

Legs ❻
Bruising
Oedema

Presenting problems in liver disease

Acute liver failure

Acute liver failure is an uncommon syndrome in which hepatic encephalopathy, characterised by mental changes progressing from delirium to stupor and coma, results from a sudden severe impairment of hepatic function (Box 13.1). In a patient whose liver was previously normal, the level of injury needed to cause liver failure is very high, whereas in those with preexisting chronic liver disease, minor additional insults can precipitate acute liver failure. Although liver biopsy is often necessary, it is the presence or absence of the clinical features suggesting chronicity that guides the clinician.

Acute viral hepatitis is the most common cause worldwide, whereas paracetamol toxicity (p. 43) is the most frequent cause in the UK. Acute liver failure occurs occasionally with other drugs, or from *Amanita phalloides* (mushroom) poisoning, in pregnancy, in Wilson's disease or following shock. The cause remains unknown in others; these patients are often labelled as having non-A–E viral hepatitis or cryptogenic acute liver failure.

Clinical assessment

Cerebral disturbance (hepatic encephalopathy) is the cardinal manifestation of acute liver failure, starting with mild, episodic reduced concentration and alertness, progressing through restlessness and aggressive outbursts to drowsiness and coma. Cerebral oedema may cause increased intracranial pressure, leading to unequal, abnormally reacting or fixed pupils, hypertensive episodes, bradycardia, hyperventilation, profuse sweating, local or general myoclonus, focal fits or decerebrate posturing. Papilloedema occurs rarely as a late sign. More general symptoms include weakness, nausea, vomiting and right hypochondrial discomfort.

Examination shows jaundice, which develops rapidly and is usually deep in subsequently fatal cases. However, jaundice is absent in Reye's syndrome, and death occasionally occurs in fulminant acute liver failure before jaundice develops. Hepatomegaly is unusual; if found with sudden-onset ascites, it suggests venous outflow obstruction (Budd–Chiari syndrome). Splenomegaly is uncommon and never prominent. Ascites and oedema are late developments and may be a consequence of fluid therapy.

13

	13.1 Classification of acute liver failure		
Type	**Time: jaundice to encephalopathy**	**Cerebral oedema**	**Common causes**
Hyperacute	<7 days	Common	Viral, paracetamol
Acute	8–28 days	Common	Cryptogenic, drugs
Subacute	29 days to 12 weeks	Uncommon	Cryptogenic, drugs

13.2 Investigations to determine the cause of acute liver failure

- Toxicology screen of blood and urine
- IgM anti-HBc, HBsAg
- IgM anti-HAV
- Anti-HEV, HCV, cytomegalovirus, herpes simplex, Epstein–Barr virus
- Caeruloplasmin, serum copper, urinary copper, slit-lamp eye examination
- Autoantibodies: ANF, ASMA, LKM, SLA
- Immunoglobulins
- USS of liver and Doppler of hepatic veins

13.3 Adverse prognostic criteria in acute liver failure[a]

Paracetamol overdose

- H+ >50 nmol/L (pH <7.3) at or beyond 24 hours following the overdose
  or
- Serum creatinine >300 μmol/L (3.38 mg/dL) + prothrombin time >100 seconds + encephalopathy grade 3 or 4

Nonparacetamol cases

- Prothrombin time >100 seconds
  or
- Any three of the following: jaundice to encephalopathy time >7 days; age <10 or >40 years; indeterminate or drug-induced causes; bilirubin >300 μmol/L (17.6 mg/dL); prothrombin time >50 seconds
  or
- Factor V level <15% and encephalopathy grade 3 or 4

[a]Predict a mortality rate of ≥90%.

Investigations

Investigations help to define the cause of the liver failure (Box 13.2) and the prognosis (Box 13.3). The prothrombin time rapidly becomes prolonged as coagulation factor synthesis fails; this test is of great prognostic value and should be performed twice daily. Plasma aminotransferase activity rises to 100 to 500 times normal after paracetamol overdose, but falls as liver damage progresses and is not helpful in determining prognosis.

Management

A patient with acute hepatic damage should be treated in an HDU or ICU as soon as progressive prolongation of the prothrombin time or hepatic encephalopathy is identified, to facilitate prompt treatment of complications (hypoglycaemia, infections, renal failure, metabolic acidosis). Treatment is supportive in the hope that hepatic regeneration will occur. *N*-acetylcysteine therapy may improve outcome, particularly following paracetamol poisoning. Artificial liver support systems are being developed but are not yet routinely available. Liver transplantation is an important treatment option, so wherever possible, patients should be transferred to a transplant centre early to allow full assessment and to maximise the time for a donor liver to become available. Survival following liver transplantation for acute liver failure is improving, and 1-year survival rates of around 60% can be expected.

Abnormal liver function tests

Abnormal LFTs are frequently detected on routine testing (e.g. 3.5% of patients measured routinely before elective surgery). Most patients with persistently abnormal LFTs have significant liver disease. The most common abnormality is alcoholic liver disease or NAFLD (p. 536). An algorithm for investigating abnormal LFTs is shown in Fig. 13.2. A full history must include alcohol and drug use (prescribed and otherwise), autoimmune disease, family history, diabetes and features of the metabolic syndrome (p. 425). The presence or absence of stigmata of chronic liver disease (p. 537) does not reliably identify patients with significant chronic liver disease. Also, normal LFTs do not exclude significant chronic liver disease, which might progress to cirrhosis, for example, primary sclerosing cholangitis, haemochromatosis and chronic hepatitis C.

The pattern of abnormal LFTs (hepatitic or obstructive) indicates the likely causes (Box 13.4).

Jaundice

Jaundice is usually detectable clinically when the plasma bilirubin exceeds 40 μmol/L (~2.5 mg/dL).

Bilirubin metabolism

Bilirubin in the blood is normally almost all unconjugated and, because it is not water-soluble, it is bound to albumin and does not enter the urine. Unconjugated bilirubin is conjugated by glucuronyl transferase into water-soluble conjugates, which are exported into the bile. Bilirubin excretion pathways are shown in Fig. 13.3.

Prehepatic jaundice

This is caused either by haemolysis or by congenital hyperbilirubinaemia, and is characterised by an isolated raised bilirubin level.

In haemolysis, destruction of red blood cells or their marrow precursors causes increased bilirubin production. Jaundice because of haemolysis is usually mild because a healthy liver can excrete a bilirubin load six times greater than normal before unconjugated bilirubin accumulates in the plasma. This does not apply to newborns, who have less capacity to metabolise bilirubin.

The only common form of nonhaemolytic hyperbilirubinaemia is Gilbert's syndrome, an inherited condition causing decreased bilirubin conjugation, with accumulation of unconjugated bilirubin in the blood. It has an excellent prognosis and needs no treatment. Other inherited disorders of bilirubin metabolism are very rare.

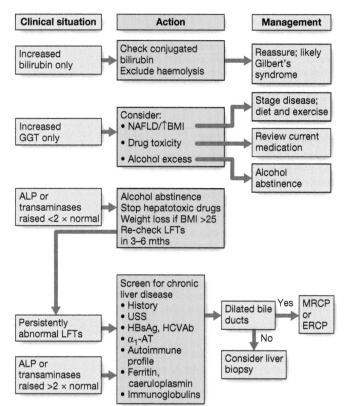

Fig. 13.2 Suggested management of abnormal LFTs in asymptomatic patients.
α_1-AT, Alpha$_1$-antitrypsin; ALP, alkaline phosphatase; ERCP, endoscopic retrograde cholangiopancreatography; GGT, γ-glutamyl transferase; HBsAg, hepatitis B surface antigen; HCVAb, antibody to hepatitis C virus; MRCP, magnetic resonance cholangiopancreatography; NAFLD, nonalcoholic fatty liver disease.

i	13.4 Causes of hepatitic and obstructive abnormal liver function	
Hepatitic pattern–disproportionately elevated transaminases		
Minor (<100 U/L)	Hepatitis C	
	Chronic hepatitis B	
	Haemochromatosis	
	Fatty liver disease	
Moderate (100–300 U/L)	Alcoholic hepatitis	
	Nonalcoholic steatohepatitis	
	Autoimmune hepatitis	
	Wilson's disease	

i	**13.4 Causes of hepatitic and obstructive abnormal liver function—cont'd**	

Major (>300 U/L)	Drugs (e.g. paracetamol)
	Acute viral hepatitis
	Autoimmune liver disease
	Ischaemic liver
	Toxins (e.g. *Amanita phalloides* poisoning)
	Flare of chronic hepatitis B

Obstructive pattern–disproportionately elevated alkaline phosphatase

Intrahepatic	Primary biliary cholangitis
	Primary sclerosing cholangitis
	Alcohol
	Drugs
	Hepatic infiltrations (lymphoma, granuloma, amyloid, metastases)
	Cystic fibrosis
	Severe bacterial infections
	Pregnancy
	Inherited cholestatic liver disease, e.g. benign recurrent intrahepatic cholestasis
	Chronic right heart failure
Extrahepatic	Carcinoma: ampullary, pancreatic, bile duct (cholangiocarcinoma), liver metastases
	Choledocholithiasis
	Parasitic infection
	Traumatic biliary strictures
	Chronic pancreatitis

13

Hepatocellular jaundice

Hepatocellular jaundice results from an inability of the liver to transport bilirubin into the bile, as a consequence of parenchymal liver disease. In hepatocellular jaundice, the concentrations of both unconjugated and conjugated bilirubin in the blood increase, perhaps because of the variable way in which bilirubin transport is disturbed.

Parenchymal disease causing jaundice usually also elevates transaminase levels. Acute jaundice with an alanine aminotransferase (ALT) greater than 1000 U/L suggests hepatitis A or B, drug toxicity (e.g. paracetamol) or hepatic ischaemia. Imaging and biopsy are frequently needed for precise diagnosis.

Obstructive (cholestatic) jaundice

Cholestatic jaundice may be caused by:
- Failure of hepatocytes to initiate bile flow.
- Obstruction of the bile ducts or portal tracts.
- Obstruction of bile flow in the extrahepatic bile ducts between the porta hepatis and the ampulla of Vater.

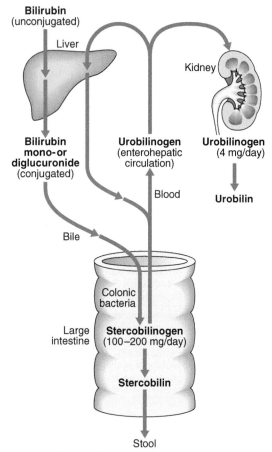

Fig. 13.3 Pathway of bilirubin excretion.

Without treatment, cholestatic jaundice tends to progress because conjugated bilirubin is unable to enter the bile canaliculi and passes back into the blood, and also because there is a failure of clearance of unconjugated bilirubin arriving at the liver cells. Cholestatic jaundice causes an obstructive pattern of liver function tests; the causes are listed in Box 13.4. Those confined to the extrahepatic bile ducts may be amenable to surgical or endoscopic correction.

Clinical assessment

Abdominal pain suggests choledocholithiasis, pancreatitis or choledochal cyst. Jaundice is progressive in cancer, and fluctuating in sclerosing cholangitis, pancreatitis and stricture. Abdominal examination may reveal irregular

> ### 13.5 Causes of ascites
>
> **Common causes**
> - Malignant disease: hepatic, peritoneal
> - Cardiac failure
> - Hepatic cirrhosis
>
> **Other causes**
> - Hypoproteinaemia: nephrotic syndrome, protein-losing enteropathy, malnutrition
> - Pancreatitis
> - Lymphatic obstruction
> - Infection: TB
> - Hepatic venous occlusion: Budd–Chiari syndrome, veno-occlusive disease
> - Rare: Meigs' syndrome, hypothyroidism

hepatomegaly or masses in carcinoma. If the gallbladder is palpable, the jaundice is unlikely to be caused by gallstones, because a chronically inflamed, stone-containing gallbladder cannot readily dilate. Cholangitis is characterised by jaundice, right upper quadrant pain and fever.

Hepatomegaly

In Western countries, the most common malignant cause is liver metastasis, whereas primary liver cancer complicating chronic viral hepatitis is more common in the Far East. Cirrhosis can be associated with either hepatomegaly (particularly if caused by alcohol or haemochromatosis) or reduced liver size in advanced disease.

13

Ascites

Ascites means the accumulation of free fluid in the peritoneal cavity and is usually because of malignant disease, cirrhosis or heart failure; however, primary disorders of the peritoneum and visceral organs can produce ascites, even in a patient with chronic liver disease (Box 13.5).

Pathophysiology

Splanchnic vasodilatation, mediated mainly by nitric oxide, causes a fall in systemic arterial pressure as cirrhosis advances. This leads to activation of the renin–angiotensin system, secondary aldosteronism, increased sympathetic nervous activity, increased atrial natriuretic hormone secretion and altered activity of the kallikrein–kinin system (Fig. 13.4). These systems tend to normalise arterial pressure but produce salt and water retention. The combination of splanchnic vasodilatation and portal hypertension alter intestinal capillary permeability, promoting fluid accumulation within the peritoneum.

Clinical assessment

Small volumes are asymptomatic, but ascites greater than 1 L causes abdominal distension, fullness in the flanks, shifting dullness on

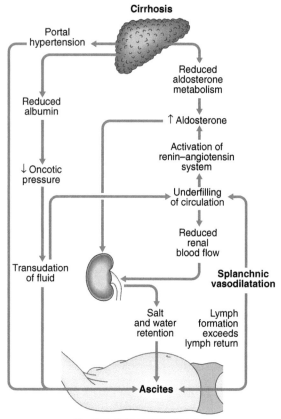

Fig. 13.4 Pathogenesis of ascites.

percussion and a fluid thrill. Other signs include everted umbilicus, divarication of the recti, scrotal oedema and dilated abdominal veins (with portal hypertension).

Investigations

Ultrasound is the best means of detecting ascites. Paracentesis may point to the underlying cause (Box 13.6). Measurement of total protein and serum–ascites albumin gradient (SAAG = serum albumin – ascites albumin) distinguishes transudate from exudate. Cirrhosis typically causes a transudate (total protein <25 g/L with few cells). A SAAG greater than 11 g/L is 96% predictive that ascites is because of portal hypertension. Venous outflow obstruction because of cardiac failure or hepatic venous obstruction can also cause transudative ascites (SAAG >11 g/L) but, unlike in cirrhosis, total protein is usually greater than 25 g/L. Exudative ascites (protein >25 g/L or SAAG <11 g/L) suggests infection (especially TB), malignancy,

13.6 Ascitic fluid: appearance and analysis

Cause/appearance

- Cirrhosis: clear, straw-coloured or light green
- Malignant disease: bloody
- Infection: cloudy
- Biliary communication: heavy bile staining
- Lymphatic obstruction: milky-white (chylous)

Useful investigations

- Total albumin (plus serum albumin)
- Amylase
- WCC
- Cytology
- Microscopy and culture

pancreatic ascites or hypothyroidism. Ascites amylase more than 1000 U/L identifies pancreatic ascites, whereas low ascites glucose suggests malignancy or TB. Cytology may reveal malignant cells (one-third of cirrhotic patients with a bloody tap have a hepatoma). Polymorphonuclear leucocyte counts greater than 250×10^6/L strongly suggest spontaneous bacterial peritonitis. Triglyceride levels greater than 1.1 g/L are diagnostic of chylous ascites, which is milky-white in appearance.

Management

Treatment of ascites relieves discomfort but does not prolong life. Removal of more than 1 L per day can produce serious disorders of fluid and electrolyte balance, and may precipitate hepatic encephalopathy (p. 511).

Sodium restriction: Restriction to 100 mmol/day ('no added salt diet') is normally adequate. Avoid sodium-rich drugs (e.g. many antibiotics, antacids) and those promoting sodium retention (e.g. steroids, NSAIDs).

Diuretics: Usually required in addition to sodium restriction. Spironolactone (100–400 mg/day) is the drug of choice but may cause gynaecomastia. Some patients also require loop diuretics, for example, furosemide.

Paracentesis: Large-volume paracentesis with IV albumin can be used as first-line treatment of refractory ascites or when other treatments fail.

Transjugular intrahepatic portosystemic stent shunt (TIPSS, p. 525): TIPSS can relieve resistant ascites but does not prolong life and may aggravate encephalopathy.

Hepatorenal syndrome

Around 10% of patients with advanced cirrhosis and ascites develop the hepatorenal syndrome, which is mediated by severe renal vasoconstriction because of under-filling of the arterial circulation.

Type 1 hepatorenal syndrome: Characterised by progressive oliguria, a rapid rise of the serum creatinine and a very poor prognosis. There is usually no proteinuria, urine sodium excretion is less than 10 mmol/day,

13

and urine/plasma osmolarity ratio is greater than 1.5. Treatment consists of albumin infusions in combination with terlipressin or octreotide and is effective in about two-thirds of patients. Haemodialysis should not be used routinely, because it does not improve the outcome.

Type 2 hepatorenal syndrome: Usually occurs in patients with refractory ascites, is characterised by a moderate and stable increase in serum creatinine and has a better prognosis.

Spontaneous bacterial peritonitis

SBP may present with abdominal pain, rebound tenderness, absent bowel sounds and fever in a patient with obvious cirrhosis and ascites. Abdominal signs are mild or absent in about one-third of patients, in whom hepatic encephalopathy and fever dominate. Paracentesis shows cloudy fluid, with a neutrophil count greater than 250×10^6/L. The source of infection is often unclear, but enteric organisms such as *Escherichia coli* are frequently found in ascitic fluid or blood cultures. SBP needs to be differentiated from other intra-abdominal emergencies; the finding of multiple organisms on culture suggests a perforated viscus.

Treatment should be started immediately with broad-spectrum antibiotics like cefotaxime. Recurrence is common and may be reduced by prophylactic quinolones such as norfloxacin (400 mg daily) or ciprofloxacin (250 mg daily).

Hepatic encephalopathy

Hepatic encephalopathy is a neuropsychiatric syndrome caused by liver disease that progresses from delirium to coma. Simple delirium needs to be differentiated from delirium tremens and Wernicke's encephalopathy, and coma from subdural haematoma, which can occur in alcoholics after a fall. Liver failure and portosystemic shunting of blood are two important factors underlying hepatic encephalopathy, and the balance between these varies in different patients. The 'neurotoxins' causing the encephalopathy are mainly nitrogenous substances produced by bacteria in the gut, which are normally metabolised by the healthy liver and excluded from the systemic circulation. Ammonia has long been considered an important factor, but much interest has centred recently on γ-aminobutyric acid.

Clinical assessment

The earliest features are mild and easily overlooked, but mental impairment increases as the condition becomes more severe (Box 13.7). Precipitating causes include drugs, dehydration, infection, protein load (including GI bleeding) and constipation. Convulsions sometimes occur. Examination usually shows:

*   A flapping tremor (asterixis).
*   Inability to perform simple mental arithmetic.
*   Inability to draw objects such as a star (constructional apraxia).
*   Hyper-reflexia.
*   Bilateral extensor plantar responses.

An EEG shows diffuse slowing of the normal alpha waves with eventual development of delta waves.

13.7 Clinical grading of hepatic encephalopathy	
Clinical grade	Clinical signs
Grade 1	Poor concentration, slurred speech, slow mentation, disordered sleep rhythm
Grade 2	Drowsy but easily rousable, occasional aggressive behaviour, lethargic
Grade 3	Marked delirium, drowsy, sleepy but responds to pain and voice, gross disorientation
Grade 4	Unresponsive to voice, may or may not respond to painful stimuli, unconscious

13.8 Causes of cirrhosis

- Alcohol
- Chronic viral hepatitis (B or C)
- Nonalcoholic fatty liver disease
- Immune: primary sclerosing cholangitis, autoimmune liver disease
- Biliary: primary biliary cholangitis, secondary biliary cirrhosis, cystic fibrosis
- Genetic: haemochromatosis, α_1-antitrypsin deficiency, Wilson's disease
- Chronic venous outflow obstruction
- Cryptogenic (unknown)

13

Management

The principles are to treat or remove precipitating causes and to suppress production of neurotoxins by bowel bacteria. Lactulose (15–30 mL three times daily) produces an osmotic laxative effect, reduces the colonic pH (thereby limiting colonic ammonia absorption) and promotes the incorporation of nitrogen into bacteria. Rifaximin (400 mg three times daily) is a nonabsorbed antibiotic that acts by reducing the bacterial content of the bowel. Dietary protein restriction is no longer recommended and can lead to worsening nutritional state in already malnourished patients.

Cirrhosis

Cirrhosis is characterised by diffuse hepatic fibrosis and nodule formation and is an important cause of morbidity and premature death. Worldwide, the most common causes are viral hepatitis, alcohol and NAFLD. Cirrhosis is the most common cause of portal hypertension and its complications.

Any condition leading to persistent or recurrent hepatocyte death may result in cirrhosis. The causes of cirrhosis are listed in Box 13.8. It may also occur in prolonged biliary damage or obstruction, as in primary biliary cholangitis, primary sclerosing cholangitis and postsurgical biliary strictures. Persistent blockage of venous return from the liver, such as occurs in veno-occlusive disease and Budd–Chiari syndrome, can also cause cirrhosis.

Clinical features

Cirrhosis may be entirely asymptomatic; often the diagnosis is made incidentally at ultrasound or at surgery. Other patients present with isolated hepatomegaly, splenomegaly, portal hypertension or hepatic insufficiency. When symptoms are present, they are often nonspecific, for example, weakness, fatigue, muscle cramps, weight loss, anorexia, nausea, vomiting and upper abdominal discomfort.

Hepatomegaly is common in alcoholic liver disease or haemochromatosis. In other causes of cirrhosis (e.g. viral hepatitis or autoimmune liver disease), progressive hepatocyte destruction and fibrosis gradually reduce liver size. The liver is often hard, irregular and nontender. Jaundice is mild when it first appears and is due primarily to a failure to excrete bilirubin. Palmar erythema can be seen early in the disease, but also occurs in many other conditions and in some healthy people. One or two small spider telangiectasia are found in around 2% of healthy people, and greater numbers occur transiently in the third trimester of pregnancy, but otherwise they are a strong indicator of liver disease. Endocrine changes are noticed more readily in men, who show loss of male hair distribution and testicular atrophy. Gynaecomastia is common but may also be attributed to spironolactone. Easy bruising becomes more frequent as cirrhosis advances. Splenomegaly and collateral vessel formation are features of portal hypertension, which occurs in more advanced disease. Ascites and hepatic encephalopathy also become increasingly common with advancing disease. Nonspecific features include finger and toe clubbing. Dupuytren's contracture is traditionally regarded as being associated with cirrhosis, but the evidence for this association is weak.

Chronic liver failure develops when the metabolic capacity of the liver is exceeded. It is characterised by the presence of encephalopathy and/or ascites. The term 'hepatic decompensation' or 'decompensated liver disease' is often used at this stage.

Management and prognosis

Management of cirrhosis is by treatment of the underlying cause and its complications, or by liver transplantation in selected cases of advanced cirrhosis. Surveillance should include endoscopy to screen for oesophageal varices every 2 years, and ultrasound to detect hepatocellular carcinoma. Prognosis is linked to severity (Box 13.9).

Portal hypertension

Portal hypertension is characterised by prolonged elevation of the hepatic venous pressure gradient (normally 5–6 mmHg). Clinically significant portal hypertension is present when the gradient exceeds 10 mmHg and risk of variceal bleeding increases over 12 mmHg.

Extrahepatic portal vein obstruction is the usual cause of portal hypertension in childhood and adolescence, whereas cirrhosis causes over 90% of portal hypertension in adults in developed countries. Schistosomiasis is a common cause of portal hypertension worldwide but is infrequent outside endemic areas. Causes classified by site of obstruction are shown in Fig. 13.5. Increased portal vascular resistance leads to a gradual reduction

13.9 Child–Pugh classification of prognosis in cirrhosis			
Score	1	2	3
Encephalopathy	None	Mild	Marked
Bilirubin (µmol/L)*			
Primary biliary cholangitis/sclerosing cholangitis	<68	68–170	>170
Other causes of cirrhosis	<34	34–50	>50
Albumin (g/L)	>35	28–35	<28
Prothrombin time (secs prolonged)	<4	4–6	>6
Ascites	None	Mild	Marked
Add the individual scores: <7 = Child's A; 1-year survival 82% 7–9 = Child's B; 1-year survival 62% >9 = Child's C; 1-year survival 42%			
*To convert bilirubin in mol/L to mg/dL, divide by 17.			

in the flow of portal blood to the liver and simultaneously to the development of collateral vessels, allowing half or more of the portal blood to bypass the liver and enter the systemic circulation directly.

Clinical features

Splenomegaly is a cardinal finding, and a diagnosis of portal hypertension is unlikely when splenomegaly cannot be detected clinically or by ultrasound. The spleen is rarely enlarged more than 5 cm below the left costal margin in adults. Collateral vessels may be visible on the anterior abdominal wall, and occasionally several radiate from the umbilicus to form a 'caput medusae'. The most important collateral vessels occur in the oesophagus and stomach, where they can cause severe bleeding. Rectal varices also lead to bleeding and are often mistaken for haemorrhoids. Fetor hepaticus results from portosystemic shunting of blood, which allows mercaptans to pass directly to the lungs. Ascites occurs because of renal sodium retention (p. 518). Bleeding from oesophageal or gastric varices is the most important consequence of portal hypertension.

Investigations

- Endoscopic examination of the upper GI tract: used to detect and to check periodically for varices.
- Ultrasound: can show splenomegaly and collateral vessels, and may reveal the cause, such as liver disease or portal vein thrombosis.
- CT and MRI angiography: can identify portal vein clot and hepatic vein patency.
- Thrombocytopenia: common because hypersplenism–platelet counts are usually around 100×10^9/L. Leucopenia occurs occasionally, but anaemia is more likely to be caused by bleeding than hypersplenism.
- Portal venous pressure measurements: not routinely needed but can distinguish sinusoidal from presinusoidal forms.

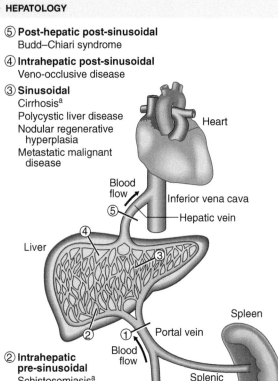

⑤ **Post-hepatic post-sinusoidal**
Budd–Chiari syndrome

④ **Intrahepatic post-sinusoidal**
Veno-occlusive disease

③ **Sinusoidal**
Cirrhosis[a]
Polycystic liver disease
Nodular regenerative
hyperplasia
Metastatic malignant
disease

② **Intrahepatic
pre-sinusoidal**
Schistosomiasis[a]
Congenital hepatic
fibrosis
Drugs
Vinyl chloride
Sarcoidosis

① **Prehepatic pre-sinusoidal**
Portal vein thrombosis due to sepsis (umbilical,
portal pyaemia) or procoagulopathy or secondary
to cirrhosis
Abdominal trauma including surgery

Fig. 13.5 Classification of portal hypertension according to site of vascular obstruction. [a]Most common cause. Note that splenic vein occlusion can also follow pancreatitis, leading to gastric varices.

Management

Management of portal hypertension centres on the prevention and/or control of variceal haemorrhage. Bleeding usually occurs from varices near the gastro-oesophageal junction or in the stomach. Risk of bleeding within 2 years varies from 7% for small varices to 30% for large varices. It is often severe and recurs if preventative treatment is not given. The overall mortality from bleeding oesophageal varices has improved to around 15% but remains about 45% in those with advanced liver disease.

Primary prevention of variceal bleeding

If nonbleeding varices are identified at endoscopy, β-blocker therapy with propranolol (80–160 mg/day) or nadolol is effective in reducing portal venous pressure and preventing bleeding. Prophylactic banding is also effective in patients unable to tolerate β-blockers.

Management of acute variceal bleeding

See also acute upper GI haemorrhage (p. 452).

The priority in acute bleeding is to restore the circulation with blood and plasma. All patients with cirrhosis and GI bleeding should receive prophylactic broad-spectrum antibiotics such as ciprofloxacin because sepsis is common.

Pharmacological reduction of portal venous pressure: Terlipressin is a synthetic vasopressin analogue given by intermittent injection that lowers portal pressure. It lowers mortality in variceal bleeding, but should be used with caution in ischaemic heart disease.

Variceal ligation ('banding') and sclerotherapy: This is the most widely used initial treatment, and should ideally be undertaken during diagnostic endoscopy. It stops variceal bleeding in 80% of patients and can be repeated if bleeding recurs. Banding has largely replaced sclerotherapy, as it is less likely to cause perforation and stricture. Banding is less effective for gastric fundal varices, which are treated by endoscopic injection of thrombin or cyanoacrylate glue to induce thrombosis. Active bleeding may make endoscopic therapy difficult, and endotracheal intubation may be required to protect the airway.

Balloon tamponade: This technique employs a Sengstaken–Blakemore tube with two balloons that exert pressure in the fundus of the stomach and in the lower oesophagus, respectively. Additional lumens allow aspiration from the stomach and from above the oesophageal balloon. Endotracheal intubation before tube insertion reduces the risk of aspiration. Gentle traction is essential to maintain pressure on the varices. Initially, only the gastric balloon should be inflated with 200 to 250 mL of air because this will usually control bleeding. Inadvertent inflation of the gastric balloon in the oesophagus causes pain and can cause rupture. If the oesophageal balloon needs to be used because of continued bleeding, it should be deflated for 10 minutes every 3 hours to avoid oesophageal mucosal damage. Pressure in the oesophageal balloon is maintained at less than 40 mmHg using a sphygmomanometer. Balloon tamponade will almost always stop variceal bleeding, but only creates time for the use of definitive therapy.

Transjugular intrahepatic portosystemic stent shunt (TIPSS): This technique uses a stent placed between the portal and hepatic veins within the liver to provide a portosystemic shunt and reduce portal pressure. It is carried out under radiological control via the internal jugular vein. Prior patency of the portal vein must be determined angiographically, coagulation deficiencies may require correction with fresh frozen plasma, and antibiotic cover is provided. Successful shunt placement stops and prevents variceal bleeding. Further bleeding necessitates investigation and treatment (e.g. angioplasty) because it is usually associated with shunt narrowing or occlusion. Hepatic encephalopathy may occur following TIPSS and is managed by reducing the shunt diameter. Although TIPSS is associated with less rebleeding than endoscopic therapy, survival is not improved.

Portosystemic shunt surgery: Surgery prevents recurrent bleeding but carries a high mortality and often leads to encephalopathy. In practice, portosystemic shunts are now reserved for patients with good liver function in whom other treatments have failed.

Oesophageal transection: Rarely, surgical transection of the varices may be performed as a last resort when bleeding cannot otherwise be controlled, but operative mortality is high.

Secondary prevention of variceal bleeding

β-Blockers are used to prevent recurrent variceal bleeding. Following successful endoscopic therapy, patients should be entered into an oesophageal banding programme with repeated sessions of therapy at 12- to 24-week intervals until the varices are obliterated. In selected individuals, TIPSS may also be considered in this setting.

Congestive 'portal hypertensive' gastropathy

Long-standing portal hypertension causes chronic gastric congestion, recognisable at endoscopy as multiple areas of punctate erythema. These areas may become eroded, causing bleeding from multiple sites. Acute bleeding can occur, but repeated minor bleeding causing iron-deficiency anaemia is more common. Reduction of the portal pressure using propranolol is the best treatment. If this is ineffective, TIPSS can be undertaken.

Infections and the liver

Viral hepatitis

This must be considered in anyone presenting with hepatitic liver blood tests (high transaminases). Hepatitis viruses are the most common cause, with cytomegalovirus, Epstein–Barr, herpes simplex and yellow fever causing occasional cases (Box 13.10). All these viruses cause illnesses with similar clinical and pathological features, which are frequently anicteric or even asymptomatic. The viruses differ in their tendency to cause acute and chronic infections.

Clinical features of acute infection

Prodromal symptoms (headache, myalgia, arthralgia, nausea and anorexia) usually precede jaundice by a few days to 2 weeks. Vomiting and diarrhoea may follow, and abdominal discomfort is common. Dark urine and pale stools may precede jaundice. There are usually few physical signs. The liver is often tender, but only minimally enlarged. Occasionally, mild splenomegaly and cervical lymphadenopathy are seen. Jaundice may be mild, and the diagnosis may be suspected only after finding abnormal liver blood tests in the setting of nonspecific symptoms. Symptoms rarely last longer than 3 to 6weeks, and complications such as liver failure or chronic liver disease are rare.

	13.10 Features of the main hepatitis viruses				
	Hepatitis A	**Hepatitis B**	**Hepatitis C**	**Hepatitis D**	**Hepatitis E**
Virus					
Group	Enterovirus	Hepadna virus	Flavivirus	Incomplete virus	Calicivirus
Nucleic acid	RNA	DNA	RNA	RNA	RNA
Size (diameter)	27 nm	42 nm	30–38 nm	35 nm	27 nm
Incubation (weeks)	2–4	4–20	2–26	6–9	3–8
Spread[a]					
Faeces	Yes	No	No	No	Yes
Blood	Uncommon	Yes	Yes	Yes	No
Saliva	Yes	Yes	Yes	Unknown	Unknown
Sexual	Uncommon	Yes	Uncommon	Yes	Unknown
Vertical	No	Yes	Uncommon	Yes	No
Chronic infection	No	Yes	Yes	Yes	No[b]
Prevention					
Active	Vaccine	Vaccine	No	Prevented by hepatitis B vaccination	No
Passive	Immune serum globulin	Hyperimmune serum globulin	No		No

[a]All body fluids are potentially infectious, although some (e.g. urine) are less infectious than others.
[b]except in immunosuppressed

13

Investigations

- LFTs: a hepatitic pattern, with serum transaminases typically between 200 and 2000 U/L.
- Plasma bilirubin: reflects the degree of liver damage.
- ALP: rarely exceeds twice the upper limit of normal.
- Prolongation of the prothrombin time: indicates the severity of the hepatitis, but rarely exceeds 25 seconds.
- WCC: usually normal, with a relative lymphocytosis.
- Serological tests: confirm the aetiology of the infection.

Management

Most individuals do not need hospital care. Drugs that are metabolised in the liver, such as sedatives and narcotics, should be avoided. Dietary modifications are not needed, but alcohol should be avoided during the acute illness. Elective surgery should be avoided during acute viral hepatitis, as there is a risk of postoperative liver failure.

Hepatitis A

Hepatitis A virus is highly infectious and is spread by the faecal–oral route. Infection is common in children but often asymptomatic, so up to 30% of adults will be seropositive despite no history of jaundice. Infection is increased by overcrowding and poor sanitation. In occasional outbreaks, water and shellfish have been the vehicles of transmission. A chronic carrier state does not occur.

Investigations

Anti-HAV IgM antibodies are diagnostic of acute HAV infection and are present from the onset of symptoms until up to 3 months after recovery.

Management

Infection in the community is best prevented by improving overcrowding and poor sanitation. Individuals can be protected by active immunisation with an inactivated virus vaccine. Immunisation should be considered for individuals with chronic hepatitis B or C infections and for close contacts, the elderly, those with other major disease, people travelling to endemic areas and perhaps pregnant women. Immediate protection can be provided by immune serum globulin if given soon after exposure to the virus.

Acute liver failure is rare in hepatitis A (0.1%); however, HAV infection in patients with chronic liver disease may cause serious or life-threatening disease.

Hepatitis B

Hepatitis B virus consists of a core surrounded by surface protein. The virus and an excess of its surface protein (known as HBsAg) circulate in the blood. Humans are the only source of infection. Approximately one-third of the world's population have serology indicating past or current HBV infection. It is a common cause of chronic liver disease and hepatocellular carcinoma worldwide. The natural history of HBV infection is shown in Fig. 13.6. Hepatitis B may cause an acute hepatitis, but infection is frequently asymptomatic, particularly neonatal infection. The risk of progression to chronic disease depends on the source and timing of infection and is greatest with vertical transmission from mother to child. Chronic hepatitis may lead to cirrhosis or hepatocellular carcinoma after many decades.

Investigations

Serology: In acute infection, HBsAg is a reliable marker of infection (Fig. 13.7). Anti-HBs antibodies appear after 3 to 6 months and persist for years or even permanently. Anti-HBs imply either a previous infection, in which case antibody to core antigen (anti-HBc, see later) is usually also present; or previous vaccination, when anti-HBc is absent.

HBcAg is not found in the blood, but anti-HBc appears early in the illness. Anti-HBc is initially of IgM type, with IgG antibody appearing later.

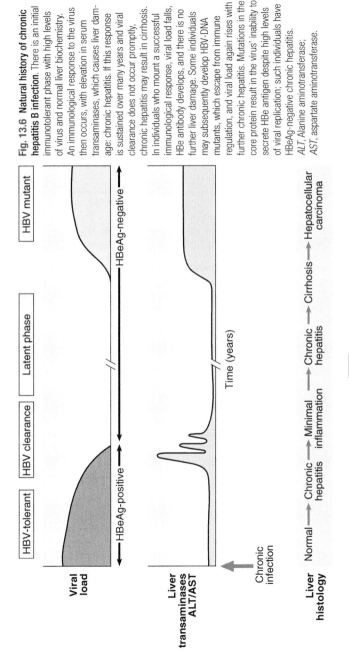

Fig. 13.6 Natural history of chronic hepatitis B infection. There is an initial immunotolerant phase with high levels of virus and normal liver biochemistry. An immunological response to the virus then occurs, with elevation in serum transaminases, which causes liver damage: chronic hepatitis. If this response is sustained over many years and viral clearance does not occur promptly, chronic hepatitis may result in cirrhosis. In individuals who mount a successful immunological response, viral load falls, HBe antibody develops, and there is no further liver damage. Some individuals may subsequently develop HBV-DNA mutants, which escape from immune regulation, and viral load again rises with further chronic hepatitis. Mutations in the core protein result in the virus' inability to secrete HBe antigen despite high levels of viral replication; such individuals have HBeAg-negative chronic hepatitis.

ALT, Alanine aminotransferase;
AST, aspartate aminotransferase.

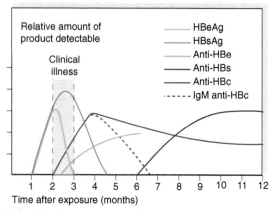

Fig. 13.7 Serological responses to hepatitis B virus infection. *HBsAg*, Hepatitis B surface antigen; *anti-HBs*, antibody to HBsAg; *HBeAg*, hepatitis B e antigen; *anti-HBe*, antibody to HBeAg; *anti-HBc*, antibody to hepatitis B core antigen.

HBeAg is an indicator of viral replication. It appears only transiently at the outset of the illness and is followed by the production of anti-HBe. Chronic HBV infection (see later) is marked by the persistence of HBsAg and anti-HBc (IgG) in the blood. Usually, HBeAg or anti-HBe is also present. Interpretation of serological tests is shown in Box 13.11.

Viral load: HBV-DNA can be measured by PCR in the blood. Viral loads are usually greater than 10^5 copies/mL in the presence of active viral replication, as indicated by the presence of e antigen. In contrast, in those with low viral replication, HBsAg- and anti-HBe-positive, viral loads are usually less than 10^5 copies/mL. High viral loads are also found in e antigen-negative chronic hepatitis, which occurs in the Far East and is caused by a mutation.

Management

Acute hepatitis B: Treatment is supportive, with monitoring for acute liver failure, which occurs in less than 1% of cases.

Chronic hepatitis B: This develops in 5% to 10% of acute cases and is lifelong. No drug is consistently able to render patients HBsAg-negative. Treatment is indicated for high viral load in the presence of active hepatitis, (elevated transaminases ± biopsy showing inflammation and fibrosis). Entecavir and tenofovir are both effective. Both have anti-HIV efficacy, so monotherapy should be avoided in HIV co-infected patients to prevent HIV antiviral drug resistance. Lamivudine is limited by the development of viral resistance. Interferon alfa is used in patients with low viral load and high transaminases, in whom it augments the native immune response. Interferon is contraindicated in cirrhosis, as it may precipitate liver failure. Longer-acting pegylated interferons, given

13.11 How to interpret the serological tests of acute hepatitis B virus infection

Interpretation	HBsAg	Anti-HBc IgM	Anti-HBc IgG	Anti-HBs
Incubation period	+	+	−	−
Acute hepatitis				
Early	+	+	−	−
Established	+	+	+	−
Established (occasional)	−	+	+	−
Convalescence				
(3–6 months)	−	±	+	±
(6–9 months)	−	−	+	+
Postinfection	−	−	+	±
Immunisation without infection	−	−	−	+

+, Positive: −; negative; ±, present at low titre or absent.

once weekly, have been evaluated in both HBeAg-positive and HBeAg-negative chronic hepatitis.

The use of post-liver transplant prophylaxis with antivirals and HBV immunoglobulins has reduced the re-infection rate to 10% and increased 5-year survival to 80%, making transplantation an acceptable treatment option.

Prevention

Individuals are most infectious when markers of continuing viral replication (HBeAg and high viral load) are present in the blood. HBV-DNA can be found in saliva, urine, semen and vaginal secretions. The virus is about ten times more infectious than hepatitis C, which itself is ten times more infectious than HIV. Recombinant hepatitis B vaccines containing HBsAg produce active immunisation in 95% of normal individuals. Infection can also be prevented or minimised by the IM injection of specific HBIg prepared from blood containing anti-HBs. This should be given within 48 hours, or at most a week, of significant exposure to infected blood (e.g. needlestick injury, contamination of cuts or mucous membranes).

Neonates born to HBV-infected mothers should be immunised at birth and given immunoglobulin.

Co-infection with HIV

Some 10-25% of the HIV-infected population has concurrent HBV. Specialist treatment with combinations of antivirals is required.

13

Hepatitis D (delta virus)

Hepatitis D virus is an RNA-defective virus that has no independent existence; it requires HBV for replication. It can infect individuals simultaneously with HBV or can superinfect existing chronic carriers of HBV. Simultaneous infections give rise to acute hepatitis, which is often severe but is limited by recovery from the HBV infection. Infections in chronic carriers of HBV can cause acute hepatitis with spontaneous recovery, and occasionally there is simultaneous cessation of the chronic HBV infection. Chronic infection with HBV and HDV can also occur, and this frequently causes rapidly progressive chronic hepatitis, and eventually cirrhosis.

HDV occurs worldwide; it is endemic in parts of the Mediterranean, Africa and South America, where transmission is mainly by close personal contact and occasionally by vertical transmission from mothers who also carry HBV. In nonendemic areas, transmission is associated with parenteral drug misuse.

HDV contains a single antigen to which infected individuals make an antibody (anti-HDV). Diagnosis depends on detecting anti-HDV. This antibody generally disappears within 2 months but persists in a few patients.

Hepatitis C

This is caused by an RNA flavivirus. Acute symptomatic infection with HCV is rare. Infection occurs with IV drug misuse (95% of new UK cases), needlestick injury, unscreened blood products, vertical transmission or through sharing toothbrushes or razors. In most individuals, initial infection is asymptomatic and only discovered if they have screening (because they have risk factors for infection), have abnormal liver blood tests or develop chronic liver disease. Some 80% of individuals exposed to the virus become chronically infected. About 20% of patients progress from chronic hepatitis to cirrhosis over 20 to 40 years. Risk factors for progression include male gender, immunosuppression, prothrombotic states and alcohol misuse. Cirrhosis is associated with:

- A risk of hepatocellular carcinoma of 2% to 5% per year.
- A 25% complication rate in 10 years.
- An 81% survival rate at 10 years.

Investigations

It may take 6 to 12 weeks for antibodies to appear in the blood following acute infection such as a needlestick injury. In these cases, hepatitis C RNA can be identified in the blood 2 to 4 weeks after infection. Active infection is confirmed by the presence of serum hepatitis C RNA in anyone who is antibody-positive. LFTs may be normal or show fluctuating serum transaminases with ALT between 50 and 200 U/L. Jaundice only usually appears in end-stage cirrhosis. Serum transaminase levels in hepatitis C are a poor predictor of the degree of liver fibrosis in chronic viral hepatitis, and so a liver biopsy is often required to stage the degree of liver damage.

Management

The aim of treatment is to eradicate infection. Recently, new antivirals have increased the chances of sustained virological response, which predicts cure, to nearly 100%, but the drugs are costly. These new direct-acting antiviral agents (DAAs) are targeted to disrupt specific steps in the HCV replication cycle. Initially, DAAs were added to older interferon-/ribavirin regimens; more recently, however, combinations of DAAs (e.g. sofosbuvir with velpatasvir) have increasingly been used in 'interferon-free' regimens, avoiding the side-effects of interferon. Liver transplantation should be considered when complications of cirrhosis occur. Modern antiviral therapy is required posttransplant to prevent infection in the transplanted liver.

Hepatitis E

Hepatitis E is caused by an RNA virus that is endemic in India and the Middle East and is increasingly prevalent in southern Europe. The clinical presentation is similar to hepatitis A. It is spread via the faecal–oral route or through contaminated food. It presents as a self-limiting acute hepatitis; chronic liver disease is unusual, but chronic infection occurs in the immunocompromised. It differs from hepatitis A in that infection during pregnancy is associated with the development of acute liver failure, which has a high mortality. In acute infection, IgM antibodies to HEV are positive.

Other forms of viral hepatitis

Cytomegalovirus and Epstein–Barr virus infection causes abnormal LFTs in most patients, and occasionally jaundice occurs. Herpes simplex occasionally causes hepatitis in immunocompromised adults. Abnormal LFTs are also common in chickenpox, measles, rubella and acute HIV infection.

HIV infection and the liver

This is covered on p. 175.

Liver abscesses

Liver abscesses can be classified as pyogenic, hydatid or amoebic.

Pyogenic liver abscess

Pyogenic liver abscesses are uncommon but important because they are potentially curable, carry significant risk if untreated and are easily overlooked.

Infection reaches the liver through the hepatic or portal circulation, up the biliary tree, via injury or by direct spread from adjacent organs. Abscesses most commonly occur in older patients through ascending infection because of biliary obstruction (cholangitis) or contiguous spread from an empyema of the gallbladder. Immunocompromised patients are particularly likely to develop liver abscesses. *E. coli* and various streptococci, particularly *Streptococcus milleri*, are the most common organisms; anaerobes, including streptococci and *Bacteroides*, may be found when infection has spread from large bowel pathology via the portal vein.

Clinical features

Patients are generally ill with fever, and sometimes exhibit rigours and weight loss. Abdominal pain in the right upper quadrant, sometimes radiating to the right shoulder, is the most common symptom. The pain may be pleuritic in nature. Hepatomegaly, often with tenderness to percussion, occurs in more than half of patients. Mild jaundice may be present but is severe only when large abscesses cause biliary obstruction. Atypical presentations are common, and a gradual onset of pyrexia of unknown origin without localising features may lead to the diagnosis being missed.

Investigations

- USS: reveals 90% or more of symptomatic abscesses and is also used to guide needle aspiration of pus for culture.
- Leucocytosis: frequently found.
- Plasma ALP activity: usually increased.
- Serum albumin: often low.
- CXR: may show a raised right diaphragm and lung collapse or an effusion at the base of the right lung.
- Blood cultures: positive in 50% to 80%.
- Colonic pathology: should be excluded.

Management and prognosis

Pending the culture results of blood and pus from the abscess, treatment with ampicillin, gentamicin and metronidazole should be commenced. Any biliary obstruction should be relieved endoscopically. Aspiration or drainage with a catheter placed in the abscess under ultrasound guidance is required if the abscess is large or does not respond to antibiotics. Surgical drainage is rarely required.

The mortality of liver abscesses is 20% to 40%; failure to make the diagnosis is the most common cause of death. Older patients and those with multiple abscesses also have a higher mortality.

Hydatid cysts and amoebic liver abscesses

These are covered elsewhere (p. 160).

Alcoholic liver disease

Alcoholic liver disease (ALD) is variable; not everyone who drinks heavily will develop it. A threshold of 14 U per week in women and 21 U per week in men is generally considered safe (1 unit = 8 g of ethanol); however, Public Health England recently adopted a threshold of 14 units per week for both men and women. The risk of ALD begins at around 30 g per day. There is no clear linear relationship between dose and liver damage.

Risk factors include:

- Drinking patterns: ALD occurs more in continuous rather than binge drinkers.
- Gender: women are at higher risk for a given intake because of their lower volume of distribution.

- Genetics: alcoholism is more common in monozygotic than dizygotic twins.
- Nutrition: obesity increases the incidence of liver-related death fivefold in heavy drinkers.

Clinical features

Three clinical syndromes occur, with some overlap:

- Alcoholic fatty liver: abnormal liver biochemistry and hepatomegaly. This has a good prognosis; steatosis usually disappears after 3 months of abstinence.
- Alcoholic hepatitis: jaundice, malnutrition, hepatomegaly, portal hypertension. The 5-year survival is 70% in those who abstain, and 34% in continued drinkers.
- Alcoholic cirrhosis: often presents with a serious complication, such as variceal haemorrhage or ascites, and only half of such patients will survive 5 years from presentation.

Investigations

A drinking history should be taken from the patient, relatives and friends. Macrocytosis without anaemia may suggest alcohol misuse. Raised GGT is not specific for alcohol misuse, and is also elevated in NAFLD; it may not return to normal with abstinence. Jaundice suggests alcoholic hepatitis. Prothrombin time and bilirubin can be used to give a 'discriminant function' (DF, Maddrey's score), which predicts prognosis in alcoholic hepatitis:

$$DF = [4.6 \times \text{Increase in PT (sec)}] + \text{bilirubin} \ (\text{mg/dL})$$

(PT=prothrombin time; divide bilirubin in μmol/L by 17 to convert to mg/dL). A value higher than 32 implies severe liver disease with a poor prognosis.

Management

Cessation of alcohol consumption is the most important treatment; without this, other therapies are of limited value. Abstinence is even effective at preventing progression of liver disease and death when cirrhosis is present. Good nutrition is very important, and enteral feeding via a fine-bore nasogastric tube may be needed in severely ill patients.

In severe alcoholic hepatitis (Maddrey's score >32), trials showed prednisolone (40 mg daily for 28 days) caused a modest reduction in short-term mortality, but no survival advantage at 90 days or 1 year. Existing sepsis and variceal haemorrhage are contraindications to glucocorticoids.

In many centres, alcoholic liver disease is a common indication for liver transplantation. The challenge is to identify patients with an unacceptable risk of returning to harmful alcohol consumption. Many programmes require 6 months of abstinence from alcohol before a patient is considered for transplantation. Although this relates poorly to the incidence of alcohol relapse after transplantation, liver function may improve to the extent that transplantation becomes unnecessary. Transplantation for alcoholic hepatitis has a poorer outcome and is seldom performed.

13

Non-alcoholic fatty liver disease

Sedentary lifestyles and changing dietary patterns have increased the prevalence of obesity and insulin resistance worldwide, and so fat in the liver is a common finding on imaging and biopsy. In the absence of alcohol excess this is called non-alcoholic fatty liver disease (NAFLD), and ranges from fatty infiltration alone (steatosis) to fatty infiltration with inflammation (non-alcoholic steatohepatitis, NASH). It may progress to cirrhosis and primary liver cancer. NAFLD may be considered as the hepatic manifestation of the 'metabolic syndrome' (p. 425), as is strongly associated with obesity, dyslipidaemia, type 2 diabetes and hypertension. Overall, NAFLD affects 20% to 30% of the population in Western countries and 5% to 18% in Asia, with about 1 in 10 NAFLD cases exhibiting NASH.

Clinical features

Most patients are asymptomatic with abnormal LFTs, particularly elevation of the transaminases or isolated elevation of the GGT. Occasionally, NASH presents with a complication of cirrhosis, such as variceal bleeding. Risk factors include:
• Age over 45 years.• Type 2 diabetes.• Obesity (BMI >30).• Hypertension.

Investigations

Alternative causes, including alcohol and viral hepatitis, should first be excluded.

LFTs: Unlike in alcoholic liver disease, ALT is normally higher than AST in the early stages, but this reverses with cirrhosis. It is important to differentiate simple fatty liver disease, which does not require follow-up, from NASH. Scores such as the FIB-4 Score, based on routine blood tests and anthropometrics, can be used to rule out advanced fibrosis in many NAFLD patients. Higher echogenicity on ultrasound indicates hepatic fat, but no routine imaging modality can accurately quantify hepatic fibrosis short of cirrhosis.

Liver biopsy: This remains the gold standard for assessing the degree of inflammation and the extent of liver fibrosis.

Management and prognosis

Treatment comprises lifestyle interventions to promote weight loss and improve insulin sensitivity through dietary changes and physical exercise. Sustained weight reduction of 7% to 10% causes significant biochemical and histological improvement in NASH.

No drugs are currently licensed specifically for NASH. Coexisting metabolic disorders, such as dyslipidaemia and hypertension, should be identified and treated. Specific insulin-sensitising agents, in particular glitazones, may help selected patients.

Autoimmune liver and biliary disease

Autoimmune hepatitis

Autoimmune hepatitis is a liver disease of unknown aetiology, characterised by autoantibodies, autoimmune T cells, hypergammaglobulinaemia and a strong association with other autoimmune diseases (Box 13.12). It occurs

13.12 Conditions associated with autoimmune hepatitis

- Migrating polyarthritis
- Urticarial rashes
- Lymphadenopathy
- Hashimoto's thyroiditis
- Thyrotoxicosis
- Myxoedema
- Ulcerative colitis
- Coombs-positive haemolytic anaemia
- Pleurisy
- Transient pulmonary infiltrates
- Glomerulonephritis
- Nephrotic syndrome

most often in women, particularly in the second and third decades of life, but may develop in either sex at any age.

Clinical features

The onset is usually insidious, with fatigue, anorexia and eventually jaundice. In about one-quarter of patients, the onset is acute, resembling viral hepatitis, but resolution does not occur. This acute presentation can lead to extensive liver necrosis and liver failure. Other features include fever, arthralgia, vitiligo, epistaxis and amenorrhoea. Jaundice is mild to moderate or occasionally absent, but signs of chronic liver disease, especially spider naevi and hepatosplenomegaly, may occur. Associated autoimmune disease is often present and can modulate the presentation.

Investigations

- Serology: often reveals autoantibodies (Box 13.13), but these are nonspecific and occur in health and other diseases. Antimicrosomal antibodies (anti-LKM) occur, particularly in children and adolescents.
- Elevated serum IgG: diagnostically helpful but may be absent.
- Liver biopsy: typically shows interface hepatitis, with or without cirrhosis.

Management

Treatment with glucocorticoids is life-saving in autoimmune hepatitis. Initially, prednisolone 40 mg/day is given orally; the dose is then gradually reduced as the patient and LFTs improve. Maintenance therapy of azathioprine, with or without low-dose prednisolone, is given once LFTs are normal. Exacerbations should be treated with glucocorticoids. Although treatment can significantly reduce the rate of progression to cirrhosis, end-stage disease can still occur despite treatment.

Primary biliary cholangitis

PBC is a chronic, progressive cholestatic liver disease of unknown cause, which predominantly affects women aged over 30. It is strongly associated with antimitochondrial antibodies (AMA), which are diagnostic.

13

	13.13 Frequency of autoantibodies in chronic nonviral liver diseases and in healthy people		
Disease	Antinuclear antibody (%)	Antismooth muscle antibody (%)	Antimitochondrial antibody[a]
Healthy controls	5	1.5	0.01
Autoimmune hepatitis	80	70	15
Primary biliary cirrhosis	25	35	95
Cryptogenic cirrhosis	40	30	15

[a]Patients with antimitochondrial antibody frequently have cholestatic LFTs and may have primary biliary cholangitis (see text).

Granulomatous inflammation of the portal tracts occurs, leading to progressive fibrosis and cirrhosis. It is associated with smoking and occurs in clusters, suggesting an environmental trigger in susceptible individuals.

Clinical features

Nonspecific symptoms, such as lethargy and arthralgia, are common and may precede diagnosis for years. Pruritus is the most common initial complaint and may precede jaundice by months or years. Bone pain or fractures can rarely result from osteomalacia (fat-soluble vitamin malabsorption) or from accelerated osteoporosis (hepatic osteodystrophy).

Initially patients are well nourished but considerable weight loss can occur as the disease progresses. Scratch marks may be found. Jaundice is a late feature but can become intense. Xanthomatous deposits occur in a minority, especially around the eyes, in the hand creases and over the elbows, knees and buttocks. Mild hepatomegaly is common, and splenomegaly becomes increasingly common as portal hypertension develops. Liver failure may supervene.

Autoimmune and connective tissue diseases occur with increased frequency in PBC, particularly sicca syndrome (p. 626), systemic sclerosis, coeliac disease (p. 479) and thyroid diseases.

Diagnosis and investigations

- LFTs: show the pattern of cholestasis.
- Hypercholesterolaemia: common but nonspecific.
- AMA: present in more than 95% of patients; when absent, the diagnosis should not be made without biopsy and cholangiography (MRCP) to exclude other biliary disease.
- Ultrasound shows no sign of biliary obstruction.

Management

The hydrophilic bile acid ursodeoxycholic acid (UDCA) improves bile flow, replaces toxic hydrophobic bile acids in the bile acid pool and reduces apoptosis of the biliary epithelium. It improves LFTs, may slow down histological and clinical progression, and has few side effects. Obeticholic acid can be tried if response to UDCA is inadequate.

> **i 13.14 Diseases associated with primary sclerosing cholangitis**
>
> - Ulcerative colitis
> - Crohn's colitis
> - Chronic pancreatitis
> - Retroperitoneal fibrosis
> - Riedel's thyroiditis
> - Retro-orbital tumour
> - Immune deficiency states
> - Sjögren's syndrome
> - Angio-immunoplastic lymphadenopathy
> - Histiocytosis X
> - Autoimmune haemolytic anaemia
> - Autoimmune pancreatitis

Liver transplantation should be considered once liver failure has developed and may be indicated for intractable pruritus. Transplantation is associated with an excellent 5-year survival of greater than 80%, although late recurrence can occur.

Pruritus: This is best treated with the anion-binding resin colestyramine, which probably acts by binding potential pruritogens in the intestine and increasing their excretion in the stool. Alternative treatments for pruritus include rifampicin, naltrexone (an opioid antagonist), plasmapheresis and a liver support device (e.g. a molecular adsorbent recirculating system (MARS)).

Fatigue: This affects about one-third of patients with PBC. Unfortunately, once depression and hypothyroidism have been excluded, there is no treatment.

Malabsorption: Cholestasis is associated with steatorrhoea and malabsorption of fat-soluble vitamins, which should be replaced as necessary.

Osteopenia and osteoporosis: These are common, and should be treated with replacement calcium and vitamin D_3. Bisphosphonates should be used if there is evidence of osteoporosis.

Primary sclerosing cholangitis

PSC is a cholestatic liver disease caused by diffuse inflammation and fibrosis that can involve the entire biliary tree. It leads to the gradual obliteration of intrahepatic and extrahepatic bile ducts, and ultimately biliary cirrhosis, portal hypertension and hepatic failure. Cholangiocarcinoma ultimately develops in around 10% to 30% of patients.

PSC is twice as common in young men. Most patients present at age 25 to 40 years. There is a close association with inflammatory bowel disease, particularly ulcerative colitis (Box 13.14).

The diagnostic criteria are:
- Generalised beading and stenosis of the biliary system on cholangiography.
- Absence of choledocholithiasis (or history of bile duct surgery).
- Exclusion of bile duct cancer, by prolonged follow-up.

Clinical features

The diagnosis is often made incidentally when persistently raised serum ALP is discovered in an individual with ulcerative colitis. Symptoms include fatigue, intermittent jaundice, weight loss, right upper quadrant pain and pruritus. Physical signs, most commonly jaundice and hepatomegaly/splenomegaly, are present in only 50% of symptomatic patients.

Investigations

Serum biochemical tests: These usually indicate cholestasis. However, ALP and bilirubin levels vary widely in individual patients during the course of the disease, sometimes spontaneously, sometimes with therapy. In addition to ANCA, low titres of serum ANA and antismooth muscle antibodies have been found in PSC but have no diagnostic significance.

Radiology: The key investigation is now MRCP, which is usually diagnostic, revealing multiple irregular stricturing and dilatation. ERCP should be reserved for when therapeutic intervention is likely to be necessary and should follow MRCP.

Histology: The characteristic early features of PSC are periductal 'onion-skin' fibrosis and inflammation.

Management and prognosis

There is no cure for PSC, but cholestasis and its complications should be treated. UDCA is widely used, although evidence of effect is limited.

The course of PSC is variable. In symptomatic patients, median survival from presentation to death or liver transplantation is around 12 years. About 75% of asymptomatic patients survive for more than 15 years. Most die from liver failure, around 30% from cholangiocarcinoma, and the remainder from colonic cancer or complications of colitis. Immunosuppressive agents (prednisolone, azathioprine, methotrexate, ciclosporin) have been tried, but are generally disappointing.

Pruritus is treated with colestyramine. Broad-spectrum antibiotics (e.g. ciprofloxacin) should be given for acute cholangitis but do not prevent attacks. If cholangiography shows a well-defined extrahepatic bile duct obstruction, and cholangiocarcinoma has been excluded, balloon dilatation or stenting at ERCP is indicated. Fat-soluble vitamin replacement is necessary in jaundiced patients. Metabolic bone disease (usually osteoporosis) should be treated (p. 539).

Surgical biliary reconstruction has a limited role in non-cirrhotic patients with dominant extrahepatic disease. Transplantation is the only surgical option in patients with advanced liver disease but is contraindicated if cholangiocarcinoma is present. Colon carcinoma is increased in patients following transplant because of immune suppression, and enhanced surveillance should be instituted.

Liver tumours

Primary malignant tumours

Hepatocellular carcinoma

HCC is the most common primary liver tumour. Cirrhosis is present in 75% to 90% of individuals with HCC and is an important risk factor. The risk is between 1% and 5% in cirrhosis caused by hepatitis B and C. Risk is also increased in cirrhosis because of haemochromatosis, alcohol, NASH and α_1-antitrypsin deficiency. In northern Europe, 90% of HCC patients have underlying cirrhosis, compared with 30% in Taiwan, where hepatitis B is the main cause.

Clinical features

Many tumours are asymptomatic and discovered on screening of high-risk patients. In patients with cirrhosis, HCC may cause variceal haemorrhage, increasing ascites or deterioration in jaundice and LFTs. Other symptoms include weight loss, anorexia and abdominal pain. Examination may reveal hepatomegaly or a right hypochondrial mass.

Investigations

Alpha-fetoprotein (AFP) is produced by 60% of hepatocellular carcinomas, but is also raised in active hepatitis B and C and in acute hepatic necrosis, for example, paracetamol toxicity. Combinations of ultrasound and CT or MRI are recommended for sizing and staging, as imaging is difficult in cirrhotic liver. Biopsy is advisable to confirm the diagnosis and exclude metastatic tumour in patients with large tumours who do not have cirrhosis or hepatitis B. Biopsy is avoided in patients eligible for transplantation or resection because of a small risk of tumour seeding along the needle tract.

High-risk patients, including those with chronic hepatitis B and with cirrhosis, should be screened 6-monthly with ultrasound and AFP to detect early HCC.

Management

Hepatic resection: This is the treatment of choice for noncirrhotic patients. The 5-year survival in this group is around 50%. However, there is a 50% recurrence rate at 5 years.

Liver transplantation: Transplantation has the benefit of curing underlying cirrhosis and removing the risk of a second de novo tumour.

Percutaneous ablation: Percutaneous ethanol injection into the tumour under ultrasound guidance is effective (80% cure rate) for tumours of 3 cm or less. Recurrence rates (50% at 3 years) are similar to those following surgical resection. Radiofrequency ablation is a useful alternative.

Trans-arterial chemo-embolisation: Hepatic artery embolisation with absorbable gelatin powder and doxorubicin yields survival rates of 60% in cirrhotic patients with unresectable HCC and good liver function (compared with 20% in untreated patients) at 2 years. Unfortunately, any survival benefit is lost at 4 years.

Chemotherapy: Sorafenib is under investigation for advanced disease.

Fibrolamellar hepatocellular carcinoma

This rare variant occurs in young adults, in the absence of hepatitis B infection and cirrhosis. The tumours are often large at presentation, and the AFP is usually normal. Treatment is by surgical resection.

Secondary malignant tumours

The primary neoplasm (most commonly of the lung, breast or abdomen) is asymptomatic in about half of patients with liver metastases. There is hepatomegaly and weight loss; jaundice may be present. Ascitic fluid, if present, has a high protein content and may be blood-stained; cytology sometimes reveals malignant cells. Hepatic resection can improve survival for slow-growing tumours such as colonic carcinomas.

Haemangiomas

These are the most common benign liver tumours and are present in 1% to 20% of the population. Most are smaller than 5 cm and rarely cause symptoms.

Cystic liver disease

Isolated or multiple simple liver cysts are a relatively frequent finding on ultrasound screening, sometimes associated with polycystic renal disease. They are benign and require no therapy.

Drugs and the liver

Types of liver injury

Cholestasis: Chlorpromazine, antibiotics (e.g. flucloxacillin) and anabolic glucocorticoids cause cholestatic hepatitis, with inflammation and cana-licular injury. Co-amoxiclav is the most common antibiotic to cause abnormal LFTs, but it may not produce symptoms until 10 to 42 days after it is stopped.

Hepatocyte necrosis: Paracetamol (p. 43) is the best-known cause. Inflammation is not always present but does accompany necrosis in liver injury because of diclofenac (an NSAID) and isoniazid. Acute hepatocellular necrosis has also been described following the use of cocaine, ecstasy and herbal remedies, including germander, comfrey and jin bu huan.

Steatosis: Tetracyclines and sodium valproate cause microvesicular steatosis; amiodarone toxicity can produce a similar histological picture to NASH.

Hepatic fibrosis: Most drugs cause reversible liver injury, and hepatic fibrosis is very uncommon. Methotrexate, however, as well as causing acute liver injury when it is started, can lead to cirrhosis when used in high doses over a long period of time.

Inherited liver diseases

Haemochromatosis

In haemochromatosis, total body iron is increased and excess iron is deposited in and damages several organs, including the liver. It may be primary, or secondary to iatrogenic or dietary iron overload or other rare diseases.

Hereditary haemochromatosis

HHC is an autosomal recessive condition that results in increased absorption of dietary iron, such that total body iron may reach 20 to 60 g (normally 4 g). Approximately 90% of patients have a single-point mutation (C282Y) in a protein (HFE). Iron loss in menstruation and pregnancy may delay the onset in females.

Clinical features

The important organs involved are the liver, pancreatic islets, endocrine glands, joints and heart. Symptomatic disease usually presents in men aged 40 years and older with features of cirrhosis (especially hepatomegaly), diabetes or heart failure. Fatigue and arthropathy are early symptoms. Leaden-grey skin pigmentation because of excess melanin occurs, especially in exposed parts, axillae, groins and genitalia: 'bronzed diabetes'. Impotence, loss of libido, testicular atrophy and arthritis are common. Cardiac failure or dysrhythmia may complicate heart muscle disease.

Investigations

- Serum ferritin: greatly increased.
- Plasma iron: also increased, with saturated plasma iron-binding capacity.
- Liver biopsy: used to confirm the diagnosis. The iron content of the liver can be measured directly.
- Genetic testing: identifies the common mutations.

Management and prognosis

Weekly venesection of 500 mL blood (250 mg iron) is performed until the serum iron is normal; this may take 2 years or more. Thereafter, venesection is continued as required to keep the serum ferritin below 50 µg/L. Liver and cardiac problems improve after iron removal, but diabetes does not resolve. First-degree relatives should be screened.

Precirrhotic patients with HHC have a normal life expectancy, and three-quarters of cirrhotic patients are alive 5 years after diagnosis. Screening for hepatocellular carcinoma (p. 522) is mandatory because this affects about one-third of patients with cirrhosis, irrespective of therapy.

Secondary haemochromatosis

13

Many conditions, including chronic haemolytic disorders, sideroblastic anaemia, other conditions requiring multiple blood transfusion (generally >50 L), porphyria cutanea tarda, dietary iron overload and occasionally alcoholic cirrhosis, are associated with widespread secondary siderosis.

Wilson's disease

Wilson's disease (hepatolenticular degeneration) is a rare but important autosomal recessive disorder of copper metabolism. Normally, dietary copper absorbed from the upper GI tract is stored in the liver incorporated into caeruloplasmin, which is secreted into the blood. Excessive copper accumulation in the body is prevented by its excretion, mainly in bile. Wilson's disease is usually caused by a failure of synthesis of caeruloplasmin. The amount of copper in the body at birth is normal, but thereafter it increases steadily; the organs most affected are the liver, basal ganglia of the brain, eyes, kidneys and skeleton.

Clinical features

Symptoms usually appear between the ages of 5 and 45 years. Acute hepatitis, sometimes recurrent, can occur, especially in children, and may progress to fulminant liver failure. Chronic hepatitis can develop insidiously and eventually present with established cirrhosis. Neurological effects include extrapyramidal features, particularly tremor, choreoathetosis, dystonia, parkinsonism and dementia (p. 683). Unusual clumsiness for age may be an early symptom. Kayser–Fleischer rings (greenish-brown discoloration of the corneal margin appearing first at the upper periphery, p. 717) are the most important single clinical clue to the diagnosis and are seen in 60% of adults with Wilson's disease. They disappear with treatment.

Investigations

- Low serum caeruloplasmin: the best single laboratory clue to the diagnosis.
- High free serum copper concentration.
- High urine copper excretion.
- Very high hepatic copper content.

Management

The copper-binding agent penicillamine is the drug of choice, given orally for life. Liver transplantation is indicated for fulminant liver failure or for advanced cirrhosis with liver failure. The prognosis is excellent, provided treatment is started before there is irreversible damage. Siblings of patients should be screened.

Alpha$_1$-antitrypsin deficiency

α_1-AT is a serine PI produced by the liver. The mutated PiZ protein cannot be secreted into the blood, so PiZZ homozygotes have low plasma α_1-AT concentrations and may develop hepatic and pulmonary disease (p. 514). Liver disease includes cholestatic jaundice in the neonatal period (neonatal hepatitis), which can resolve spontaneously; chronic hepatitis and cirrhosis in adults; and ultimately hepatocellular carcinoma. There are no clinical features to distinguish α_1-AT deficiency from other causes of liver disease, and the diagnosis is made from the low plasma α_1-AT concentration and the genotype. No specific treatment is available; the concurrent risk of severe early-onset emphysema means that all patients must stop smoking.

Gilbert's syndrome

This is covered on p. 513.

Cystic fibrosis

CF (p. 331) is sometimes associated with biliary cirrhosis, which can lead to portal hypertension and varices requiring banding. Liver failure is rare in CF but transplantation is occasionally required.

Vascular liver diseases

Hepatic arterial disease

Liver ischaemic injury is relatively common during hypotensive or hypoxic events and is under diagnosed. Hepatic artery occlusion may result from inadvertent injury during biliary surgery or may be caused by emboli, neoplasms, polyarteritis nodosa, blunt trauma or radiation. It usually causes severe upper abdominal pain with or without circulatory shock. LFTs show a high transaminase activity. Patients usually survive if the liver and portal blood supply are otherwise normal.

Portal venous disease

Portal venous thrombosis is rare, but can occur in prothrombotic conditions or complicating abdominal inflammation or malignancy. Acute portal venous thrombosis causes abdominal pain and diarrhoea, and may lead to bowel infarction, requiring surgery. Patients need anticoagulation and investigation for underlying thrombophilia. Subacute thrombosis can be asymptomatic but may lead to extrahepatic portal hypertension (p. 522).

Hepatopulmonary syndrome

In this condition, patients with cirrhosis and portal hypertension develop resistant hypoxaemia (PaO_2 <9.3 kPa [70 mmHg]) because of intrapulmonary shunting through direct arteriovenous communications. Clinical features include finger clubbing, spider naevi, cyanosis and a fall in SaO_2 on standing. It resolves following liver transplantation.

Portopulmonary hypertension

This is defined as pulmonary hypertension in a patient with portal hypertension. It is caused by vasoconstriction and obliteration of the pulmonary arterial system and presents with breathlessness and fatigue.

Hepatic venous disease

Obstruction to hepatic venous blood flow can occur in the small central hepatic veins, the large hepatic veins, the inferior vena cava or the heart.

Budd–Chiari syndrome

This uncommon condition is caused by thrombosis of the larger hepatic veins and sometimes the inferior vena cava. Some have haematological disorders such as myelofibrosis, primary polycythaemia, paroxysmal nocturnal haemoglobinuria and antithrombin III, protein C or protein S deficiencies (p. 521). The cause cannot be found in about half of patients. Hepatic congestion affecting the centrilobular areas is followed by centrilobular fibrosis, and eventually cirrhosis in those who survive long enough.

Clinical features

Acute venous occlusion causes the rapid development of upper abdominal pain, marked ascites and occasionally acute liver failure. More gradual occlusion causes gross ascites and often upper abdominal discomfort. Hepatomegaly, often with liver tenderness, is almost always present.

Investigations

- LFTs: vary depending on the presentation; can show features of acute hepatitis (p. 543) when the onset is rapid. Ascitic fluid analysis typically shows a protein concentration greater than 25 g/L (exudate) in the early stages.
- Doppler ultrasound, CT, MRI: may demonstrate occlusion of the hepatic veins and inferior vena cava.

Management

Where recent thrombosis is suspected, thrombolysis with streptokinase followed by heparin and oral anticoagulation should be considered. Short

13

hepatic venous strictures can be treated with angioplasty; more extensive hepatic vein occlusion can be managed by TIPSS.

Sinusoidal obstruction syndrome (veno-occlusive disease)

Widespread occlusion of central hepatic veins is the characteristic of this rare condition. Recognised causes include pyrrolizidine alkaloids in *Senecio* and *Heliotropium* plants used to make teas, cytotoxic drugs and hepatic irradiation. The clinical features are similar to those of the Budd–Chiari syndrome (see earlier).

Cardiac disease

Hepatic damage due primarily to congestion may develop in all forms of right heart failure; the clinical features are predominately cardiac. Very rarely, long-standing cardiac failure and hepatic congestion cause cardiac cirrhosis.

Nodular regenerative hyperplasia of the liver

This is the most common cause of noncirrhotic portal hypertension in developed countries. Small hepatocyte nodules form throughout the liver without fibrosis. It occurs in older people, associated with connective tissue disease, haematological diseases and immunosuppressive drugs. It is usually asymptomatic but can present with portal hypertension.

Pregnancy and the liver

Obstetric cholestasis

This usually occurs in the third trimester and is associated with intrauterine growth retardation and premature birth. Presentation is with itching and cholestatic or hepatitic LFTs. Ursodeoxycholic acid (250 mg twice daily) controls itch and prevents premature birth.

Acute fatty liver of pregnancy

This is more common in twin and first pregnancies. It typically presents in the third trimester with vomiting and abdominal pain followed by jaundice. Rarely, fulminant hepatic failure may occur. Diagnosis is from clinical features, LFTs and ultrasound. Management is with supportive care and delivery of the fetus.

Toxaemia of pregnancy and HELLP

HELLP syndrome (haemolysis, elevated liver enzymes and low platelets) is a variant of preeclampsia affecting mainly multiparous women. It presents with hypertension and proteinuria; complications include disseminated intravascular coagulation, hepatic infarction and rupture. Delivery leads to prompt resolution.

Liver transplantation

The outcome following liver transplantation has improved significantly over the last decade and it is now an effective treatment for end-stage liver disease.

Indications: Some 71% of surgery is performed for cirrhosis, 11% for hepatocellular carcinoma, 10% for acute liver failure and 6% for metabolic diseases.

Contraindications: The main contraindications to transplantation are sepsis, extrahepatic malignancy, active alcohol or other substance misuse, and marked cardiorespiratory dysfunction.

Complications: These include primary graft nonfunction, acute rejection, hepatic artery thrombosis, anastomotic biliary strictures and infections.

Outcomes: The outcome following transplantation for acute liver failure is worse than for chronic liver disease because most patients have coexisting multi-organ failure. The 1-year survival is 65%, falling to 59% at 5 years. The 1-year survival for patients with cirrhosis is greater than 90%, falling to 70% to 75% at 5 years.

Cholestatic and biliary disease

'Cholestasis' relates to a biochemical abnormality resulting from an abnormality in bile flow. 'Biliary disease' relates to pathology at any level from the small intrahepatic bile ducts to the sphincter of Oddi.

Cholestasis

Chemical cholestasis

This can occur as an inherited condition, as a consequence of sepsis, cholestatic drug reactions or during pregnancy.

Benign recurrent intrahepatic cholestasis

This rare condition usually presents with pruritis and painless jaundice in adolescence with recurrent episodes of cholestasis, lasting 1 to 6 months. The prognosis is good.

Intrahepatic biliary disease

Inflammatory and immune disease

Immune injury to the small intrahepatic bile ducts occurs in graft-versus-host disease, sarcoidosis, primary biliary cholangitis and during rejection following liver transplantation.

Congenital hepatic fibrosis

This inherited condition features broad bands of fibrous tissue linking the portal tracts, abnormalities of the bile ducts and portal venules. It causes portal hypertension and splenomegaly and is associated with cystic renal disease in adolescence or in early adult life.

Cystic fibrosis

CF (p. 331) is associated with biliary cirrhosis in about 5% of individuals and can cause portal hypertension with variceal bleeding. UDCA improves liver blood tests but may not prevent progression of liver disease. Fat-soluble

13

vitamin deficiency (A, D, E and K) is common because of coexistant biliary and pancreatic disease.

Extrahepatic biliary disease

This presents with impaired bile flow (obstructive jaundice and fat malabsorption). Obstruction is often caused by stricturing following gallstone passage or surgery. Cholangiocarcinoma or carcinoma of the head of pancreas should be considered in all patients with extrahepatic biliary obstruction.

Choledochal cysts

Cysts may occur at any part of the biliary tree. In adults, they may present with recurrent jaundice, abdominal pain and cholangitis. Liver abscess and biliary cirrhosis may develop and there is an increased incidence of cholangiocarcinoma. Cyst excision is the treatment of choice.

Secondary biliary cirrhosis

Secondary biliary cirrhosis develops after prolonged large duct biliary obstruction because of gallstones, benign bile duct strictures or sclerosing cholangitis. The clinical features of chronic cholestasis include ascending cholangitis or even liver abscess. Cirrhosis, ascites and portal hypertension are late features.

Gallstones

Gallstones are conveniently classified into cholesterol or pigment stones, although the majority are of mixed composition. In developed countries, gallstones occur in 7% of males and 15% of females aged 18 to 65 years, with an overall prevalence of 11%.

Cholesterol gallstones: Cholesterol is held in solution in bile by its association with bile acids and phospholipids in the form of micelles and vesicles. In gallstone disease, the liver produces bile that contains a relative excess of cholesterol ('lithogenic bile').

Pigment stones: Brown, crumbly pigment stones are almost always the consequence of bacterial or parasitic infection in the biliary tree. They are common in the Far East, where infection allows bacterial β-glucuronidase to hydrolyse conjugated bilirubin to its free form, which then precipitates as calcium bilirubinate. The mechanism of black pigment gallstone formation in developed countries is not satisfactorily explained, but haemolysis is important.

Clinical features

Only 10% of people with gallstones develop clinical disease. Symptomatic gallstones (Box 13.15) cause either biliary pain ('biliary colic') or cholecystitis (see later). Typically, the pain occurs suddenly and persists for about 2 hours; if it continues for more than 6 hours, a complication such as cholecystitis or pancreatitis may be present. Pain is usually felt in the epigastrium (70% of patients) or right upper quadrant (20%) and radiates to the interscapular region or the tip of the right scapula. Gallstones in the gallbladder (cholecystolithiasis) can migrate to the common bile

---

i | **13.15 Clinical features and complications of gallstones**

Clinical features

- Asymptomatic
- Biliary colic
- Acute cholecystitis
- Chronic cholecystitis

Complications

- Empyema of the gallbladder
- Porcelain gallbladder
- Choledocholithiasis
- Pancreatitis
- Fistulae between the gallbladder and duodenum or colon
- Pressure on/inflammation of the common bile duct by a gallstone in the cystic duct (Mirizzi's syndrome)
- Gallstone ileus
- Cancer of the gallbladder

---

duct (choledocholithiasis) and may result in jaundice, cholangitis or acute pancreatitis.

Investigations

- USS: the method of choice for diagnosing gallstones.
- CT, MRCP and endoscopic ultrasound: useful for detecting complications (distal bile duct stone or gallbladder empyema).

Management

Asymptomatic gallstones found incidentally should not be treated, because the majority remain asymptomatic. Symptomatic gallstones are best treated by laparoscopic cholecystectomy. Small radiolucent stones causing mild symptoms may alternatively be dissolved by oral administration of ursodeoxycholic acid. Bile duct stones can be treated by shock-wave lithotripsy, endoscopic sphincterotomy with balloon trawl or surgical exploration.

Cholecystitis

Acute cholecystitis

Acute cholecystitis is almost always associated with obstruction of the gallbladder neck or cystic duct by a gallstone. Occasionally, obstruction may be by mucus, parasitic worms or a tumour. Acalculous cholecystitis can occur in the intensive care setting.

Clinical features

The cardinal feature is severe and prolonged pain in the right upper quadrant, but also in the epigastrium, the right shoulder tip or interscapular region. There is usually fever and leucocytosis. Examination shows right hypochondrial tenderness, rigidity worse on inspiration (Murphy's sign) and sometimes a gallbladder mass (in 30%). Jaundice occurs in less than 10% of patients and is usually because of the passage of stones in the common bile duct.

Investigations

- Leucocytosis: common.
- Ultrasound: detects gallstones and gallbladder thickening because of cholecystitis.
- Plasma amylase: should be measured to detect acute pancreatitis (p. 501).
- Plain X-rays of the abdomen and chest: may show radio-opaque gallstones, and rarely intrabiliary gas because of fistulation of a gallstone into the intestine, and are important in excluding lower lobe pneumonia and a perforated viscus.

Management

Medical: This consists of bed rest, pain relief, antibiotics (e.g. cefuroxime and metronidazole) and maintenance of fluid balance.

Surgical: Urgent surgery is required when cholecystitis progresses in spite of medical therapy and when complications such as empyema or perforation develop. Operation should be carried out within 5 days of the onset of symptoms. Delayed surgery after 2 to 3 months is no longer favoured. Recurrent biliary colic or cholecystitis is frequent if the gallbladder is not removed.

Chronic cholecystitis

Chronic inflammation of the gallbladder is almost invariably associated with gallstones. The usual symptoms are those of recurrent attacks of upper abdominal pain, often at night and following a heavy meal. The clinical features are similar to those of acute calculous cholecystitis but milder. Patients who recover spontaneously or following analgesia and antibiotics are usually advised to undergo elective laparoscopic cholecystectomy.

Acute cholangitis

Acute cholangitis is caused by bacterial infection of bile ducts and occurs in patients with other biliary problems such as choledocholithiasis (see later), biliary strictures or tumours, or after ERCP. Jaundice, fever (with or without rigours) and right upper quadrant pain are the main presenting features. Treatment is with antibiotics and relief of biliary obstruction.

Choledocholithiasis

Stones in the common bile duct (choledocholithiasis) occur in 10% to 15% of patients with gallstones that have usually migrated from the gallbladder. In Far Eastern countries, primary common bile duct stones are found after bacterial infection secondary to parasitic infections with *Clonorchis sinensis*, *Ascaris lumbricoides* or *Fasciola hepatica* Chapter 5. Common bile duct stones can cause partial or complete bile duct obstruction and may be complicated by cholangitis because of secondary bacterial infection, sepsis, liver abscess and biliary stricture.

Clinical features

Choledocholithiasis may be asymptomatic, may be found incidentally by operative cholangiography at cholecystectomy or may present with recurrent abdominal pain with or without jaundice. The pain is usually in the right upper quadrant, and fever, pruritus and dark urine may be present. Rigours may be a feature; jaundice is common, usually with pain.

Investigations

- Transabdominal ultrasound: shows dilated extrahepatic and intrahepatic bile ducts, but endoscopic ultrasound may be needed to image distal bile duct stones.
- LFTs: show a cholestatic pattern with bilirubinuria.
- Cholangitis: if present, the patient usually has a leucocytosis.

Management

- Analgesia, IV fluids and broad-spectrum antibiotics, such as cefuroxime and metronidazole.
- Urgent ERCP with biliary sphincterotomy and stone extraction: the treatment of choice, successful in around 90% of patients.
- Cholangiography: to check clearance of all stones.
- Lithotripsy or percutaneous drainage: alternatives if ERCP fails.
- Surgery: performed less frequently than ERCP for choledocholithiasis because of higher morbidity and mortality.

Tumours of the gallbladder and bile duct

Carcinoma of the gallbladder

This is uncommon, occurring more often in females and usually encountered above the age of 70 years. More than 90% are adenocarcinomas; the remainder are anaplastic or, rarely, squamous tumours. Gallstones are usually present and are thought to be important in the aetiology of the tumour. Local invasion often precludes excision, and treatment is frequently palliative.

Cholangiocarcinoma

This uncommon tumour can arise anywhere in the biliary tree from the small intrahepatic bile ducts to the papilla of Vater. The cause is unknown, but the tumour is associated with gallstones, primary and secondary sclerosing cholangitis and choledochal cysts. In the Far East, chronic liver fluke infection is a major risk factor. The patient presents with obstructive jaundice. The diagnosis is made by a combination of CT and MRI but can be difficult to confirm in patients with sclerosing cholangitis. Surgery is possible in a minority, and endoscopic stenting is useful for palliation, but the prognosis is poor.

Carcinoma at the ampulla of vater

Nearly 40% of all adenocarcinomas of the small intestine arise in relationship to the ampulla of Vater, and present with pain, anaemia, vomiting and weight loss. Jaundice may be intermittent or persistent. Diagnosis is by duodenal endoscopy and biopsy, and staging by CT/MRI and EUS. Ampullary carcinoma must be differentiated from carcinoma of the head of the pancreas and cholangiocarcinoma because both have a worse prognosis. Pancreaticoduodenectomy can result in 50% 5-year survival.

13

Miscellaneous biliary disorders

Postcholecystectomy syndrome

Dyspeptic symptoms following cholecystectomy (postcholecystectomy syndrome) occur in around 30% of patients. The usual complaints include right upper quadrant abdominal pain, flatulence, fatty food intolerance and occasionally jaundice and cholangitis. Ultrasound is used to detect biliary obstruction, and EUS or MRCP to detect common bile duct stones. If retained bile duct stones are excluded, sphincter of Oddi dysfunction should be considered (see later).

Functional biliary sphincter disorders

The sphincter of Oddi is a small smooth muscle sphincter situated at the junction of the bile duct and pancreatic duct in the duodenum. Sphincter of Oddi dysfunction (SOD) is characterised by an increase in contractility that produces a benign noncalculous obstruction to the flow of bile or pancreatic juice. This may cause pancreaticobiliary pain, deranged LFTs or recurrent pancreatitis. Patients are predominantly female. Patients with biliary-type SOD experience recurrent episodic biliary-type pain. Patients with pancreatic SOD usually present with unexplained recurrent attacks of pancreatitis. The diagnosis is established by excluding gallstones and demonstrating a dilated or slowly draining bile duct.

Patients with organic stenosis are treated with endoscopic sphincterotomy. The results are good, but patients should be warned that there is a high risk of complications, particularly acute pancreatitis.

Haematology and transfusion medicine

Blood disease covers a wide spectrum of illnesses, from common anaemias to rare conditions such as leukaemias and congenital coagulation disorders. Haematological changes occur as a consequence of diseases affecting any system, and provide important information in the diagnosis and monitoring of many conditions.

Presenting problems in blood disease

Anaemia

Anaemia refers to a state in which the level of Hb in the blood is below the reference range for age and sex. Other factors, including pregnancy and altitude, also affect Hb levels. The clinical features of anaemia reflect diminished tissue oxygen supply. The symptoms of anaemia will be more severe if the onset is rapid or if there is coexisting cardiorespiratory disease. Many clinical features are nonspecific, but together they should raise suspicion of anaemia.

Symptoms include:

• Tiredness. • Lightheadedness. • Breathlessness. • Worsening of coexisting disease, for example, angina.

Signs include:

• Mucous membrane pallor. • Tachypnoea. • Raised JVP. • Flow murmurs. • Ankle oedema. • Postural hypotension. • Tachycardia.

The clinical assessment and investigation of anaemia should gauge its severity and define the underlying cause.

Clinical assessment

Iron deficiency anaemia: This is the most common type of anaemia worldwide. Seek symptoms indicating GI blood loss and menorrhagia in females.

Dietary history: This should assess the intake of iron and folate, which may become deficient in comparison to needs (e.g. in pregnancy or during periods of rapid growth).

Past medical history: The history may reveal disease known to be associated with anaemia (e.g. rheumatoid arthritis) or previous surgery (e.g. stomach or small bowel resection, which may lead to malabsorption of iron and/or vitamin B_{12}).

Family history: This may be relevant in haemolytic anaemias and pernicious anaemia.

Drug history: Many drugs can be associated with blood loss (e.g. NSAIDs) and others may cause haemolysis or aplasia.

These findings may be accompanied by specific findings related to the underlying aetiology. Examples include a right iliac fossa mass in a patient with caecal carcinoma; jaundice in haemolytic anaemia; and neurological signs, including peripheral neuropathy and subacute combined degeneration of the cord, in patients with vitamin B_{12} deficiency.

Investigations

The investigation of anaemias usually starts with the size of the red cells, indicated by the MCV in the FBC. Commonly:
• A normal MCV (normocytic anaemia) suggests acute blood loss or anaemia of chronic disease (ACD). • A low MCV (microcytic anaemia) suggests iron deficiency or thalassaemia. • A high MCV (macrocytic anaemia) suggests vitamin B_{12} or folate deficiency, or myelodysplasia. • A high MCV (in the absence of anaemia) may be caused by alcohol, liver disease, hypothyroidism, splenectomy, hyperlipidaemia or pregnancy.

Supplementary investigations are often required for precise diagnosis. A raised reticulocyte count in microcytic anaemia suggests bleeding or haemolysis. A low ferritin level indicates iron deficiency. In macrocytic anaemia, the blood film may show specific abnormalities, for example, a dimorphic picture in sideroblastic anaemia, target cells in liver disease or hypersegmented neutrophils caused by vitamin B_{12} or folate deficiency or drug toxicity.

High haemoglobin

Patients with a raised Hct (>0.52 males, >0.48 females) for more than 2 months should be investigated. 'True' polycythaemia (or absolute erythrocytosis) indicates an excess of red cells, whereas 'relative' (or 'low-volume') polycythaemia is caused by a decreased plasma volume. Causes are shown in Box 14.1.

Clinical assessment and investigations

Males and females with Hct values of greater than 0.60 and greater than 0.56, respectively, can be assumed to have an absolute erythrocytosis. History and examination will identify most patients with polycythaemia secondary to hypoxia. The presence of hypertension, smoking, excess alcohol consumption and/or diuretic use is consistent with low-volume polycythaemia (Gaisbock's syndrome). In polycythaemia rubra vera (PRV), a mutation in a kinase, JAK-2 V617F, is found in more than 90% of cases (p. 584). If the JAK-2 mutation is absent and there is no obvious secondary cause, a measurement of red cell mass is required to confirm an absolute erythrocytosis, followed by further investigations to exclude hypoxia and identify causes of inappropriate erythropoietin secretion.

i	**14.1 Causes of erythrocytosis**	

	Absolute erythrocytosis	Relative (low-volume) erythrocytosis
Haematocrit	High	High
Red cell mass	High	Normal
Plasma volume	Normal	Low
Causes	*Primary* Myeloproliferative disorder: poly- cythaemia rubra vera *Secondary* ↑Epo caused by tissue hypoxia: altitude, lung disease, cyanotic heart disease Inappropriately ↑Epo: renal disease (hydronephrosis, cysts, carcinoma), other tumours (hepatoma, bronchial carcinoma, fibroids, phaeochromocytoma, cerebellar haemangioblastoma) Exogenous Epo: drug-taking in athletes	Diuretics Smoking Obesity Alcohol excess Gaisbock's syndrome

Leucopenia (low white count)

Leucopenia may be caused by a reduction in all types of white cells or in individual cell types.

Neutropenia (neutrophil count $<1.5 \times 10^9$/L): Occurs with:
• Infection. • Connective tissue disease. • Alcohol. • Bone marrow infiltration (e.g. leukaemia, myelodysplasia).

A number of drugs can also result in neutropenia, for example:

• Antirheumatic drugs (e.g. gold, penicillamine). • Antithyroid drugs (e.g. carbimazole). • Anticonvulsants (e.g. phenytoin, sodium valproate). • Antibiotics (e.g. sulphonamides).

Clinical manifestations of neutropenia range from no symptoms to over-whelming sepsis. Risk increases with lower counts. Fever may be the only manifestation of infection, and immediate antibiotic therapy is required to prevent rapid development of septic shock.

Lymphopenia (lymphocytes $<1 \times 10^9$/L): Occurs in sarcoidosis, lymphoma, renal failure, connective tissue disease and HIV infection.

Leucocytosis (high white count)

Leucocytosis is usually caused by an increase in a specific type of white blood cell.

14

i	**14.2 Causes of lymphadenopathy**
Infective	Bacterial, e.g. streptococcal, TB
	Viral, e.g. Epstein–Barr, HIV
	Protozoal, e.g. toxoplasmosis
	Fungal, e.g. histoplasmosis
Neoplastic	Primary, e.g. lymphomas, leukaemias
	Secondary, e.g. lung, breast, thyroid, stomach
Inflammatory	Connective tissue disorders, e.g. rheumatoid arthritis, systemic lupus erythematosus
	Sarcoidosis
Miscellaneous	Amyloidosis

Neutrophilia (increased circulating neutrophils): Occurs with:
• Infection. • Trauma. • Myocardial infarction. • Inflammation.
• Malignancy. • Myeloproliferative disorders.
   Pregnancy causes physiological neutrophilia.

Lymphocytosis (lymphocyte count $>3.5 \times 10^9$/L): Most commonly caused by viral infection. Lymphoproliferative disease, for example, CLL, lymphoma.

Eosinophilia (eosinophils $>0.5 \times 10^9$/L): Occurs in:
• Parasitic infections. • Allergy (asthma, drug reactions). • Inflammatory disease (e.g. polyarteritis nodosa). • Malignancy.

Lymphadenopathy

Enlarged lymph nodes may be an indicator of haematological disease, but can also occur in reaction to infection or inflammation (Box 14.2). Reactive nodes usually expand rapidly and are painful, whereas those caused by haematological disease are frequently painless and may be generalised. Initial investigations in lymphadenopathy should include:
• FBC: to detect neutrophilia in infection or evidence of haematological disease. • ESR. • CXR: to detect mediastinal lymphadenopathy.
   If the findings suggest malignancy, lymph node biopsy is required.

Splenomegaly

Causes of splenic enlargement are listed in Box 14.3. Massive splenomegaly occurs in CML, myelofibrosis, malaria and leishmaniasis. Hepatosplenomegaly is more suggestive of lympho- or myeloproliferative disease or liver disease. Coexisting lymphadenopathy makes a diagnosis of lymphoproliferative disease more likely.

   An enlarged spleen may cause abdominal discomfort; splenic infarction causes severe pain radiating to the shoulder tip. In rare cases, spontaneous or traumatic rupture may occur.

i	**14.3 Causes of splenomegaly**
Congestive	Portal hypertension, e.g. cirrhosis, portal vein thrombosis
	Cardiac, e.g. congestive cardiac failure
Infective	Bacterial, e.g. endocarditis, septicaemia, TB
	Viral, e.g. hepatitis, Epstein–Barr
	Protozoal, e.g. malaria, leishmaniasis (kala-azar)
	Fungal, e.g. histoplasmosis
Inflammatory/gran-ulomatous disorders	e.g. Felty's syndrome, SLE, sarcoidosis
Haematological	Red cell disorders, e.g. megaloblastic anaemia, haemoglobi-nopathies
	Autoimmune haemolytic anaemias
	Myeloproliferative disorders, e.g. chronic myeloid leukaemia, myelofibrosis, polycythaemia rubra vera, essential thrombo-cythaemia
	Neoplastic, e.g. leukaemias, lymphomas

Investigations should include • USS or CT: show splenic size and texture, and also the liver and abdominal lymph nodes. • FBC, blood film and CXR: required in all patients. • Further investigations: may include lymph node biopsy and bone marrow examination.

Bleeding

14

Normal haemostasis

Haemostasis depends upon interactions between the vessel wall, platelets and clotting factors. Initially, the damaged vessel constricts, and platelets aggregate to form a plug. This is followed by activation of the coagulation cascade, resulting in the formation of a cross-linked fibrin clot (Fig. 14.1). Clotting factors are synthesised by the liver, and several are dependent on vitamin K for their activation; activated factors are designated by the suffix 'a'. The extrinsic pathway is the main physiological mechanism in vivo.

Excessive coagulation is prevented by natural clotting inhibitors. Antithrombin is a serine protease inhibitor synthesised by the liver that destroys activated factors XIa and Xa and thrombin (IIa). Its activity against thrombin and Xa is enhanced by heparin and fondaparinux, explaining their anticoagulant effect. Protein C binds to its co-factor, protein S, and inactivates factors Va and VIIIa. Any reduction in these inhibitors results in a thrombotic tendency.

Clinical assessment

Abnormal bleeding may be caused by deficiency of coagulation factors, thrombocytopenia or occasionally excessive fibrinolysis following therapeutic fibrinolytic therapy.

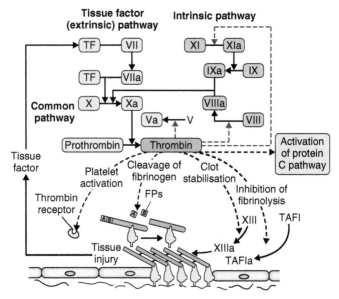

Fig. 14.1 Normal haemostasis. Injury breaches the endothelium, releasing TF; this activates the tissue factor (extrinsic) pathway, generating small amounts of thrombin. Platelets are activated by multiple mechanisms, including thrombin binding. Thrombin from the TF pathway then massively amplifies its own production; the 'intrinsic' pathway becomes activated, generating large amounts of thrombin (dotted red lines represent positive feedback). Thrombin forms clots by cleaving fibrinopeptides from fibrinogen to produce fibrin. Fibrin monomers are cross-linked by factor XIII (also activated by thrombin). Thrombin also regulates clot formation via: (a) activation of the protein C pathway, which opposes further coagulation; (b) activation of thrombin-activatable fibrinolysis inhibitor (TAFI).

Muscle and joint bleeds indicate a coagulation defect. Purpura, prolonged bleeding from cuts, epistaxis, GI haemorrhage, excessive postsurgical bleeding and menorrhagia suggest a platelet disorder, thrombocytopenia or von Willebrand's disease. Family history and duration of bleeding may indicate whether the disorder is congenital or acquired. Coexisting illness or drug therapy predisposing to bleeding should be sought.

On examination, check for:
• Bruising. • Purpura. • Telangiectasia on lips (indicates HHT). • Swollen joints/haemarthrosis. • Hepatomegaly. • Splenomegaly.

Investigations

Initial screening tests comprise:
• Platelet count. • Blood film. • Coagulation tests, including the prothrombin time (PT), activated partial thromboplastin time (APTT) and fibrinogen.

PT: Assesses the extrinsic system and is prolonged by deficiencies of factors II, V, VII and X, and by liver disease.

	14.4 Causes of thrombocytopenia
Marrow disorders	Hypoplasia
	Infiltration, e.g. leukaemia, myeloma, carcinoma, myelofibrosis
	Vitamin B_{12}/folate deficiency
Increased platelet consumption	Disseminated intravascular coagulation
	Idiopathic thrombocytopenic purpura
	Infections, e.g. Epstein–Barr virus, Gram-positive septicaemia
	Hypersplenism
	Thrombotic thrombocytopenic purpura
	Liver disease
	Drugs, e.g. vancomycin, heparin
	Haemolytic uraemic syndrome

APTT: Assesses the intrinsic system and is sensitive to deficiencies in factors II, V, VIII, IX, X, XI and XII.

INR: Used to assess the control of warfarin treatment, and is the ratio of the patient's PT to a normal control using an international reference thromboplastin. Concentrations of direct oral anticoagulants (DOACs) cannot be accurately assessed from the PT or the APTT, with which they correlate poorly.

Thrombocytopenia (low platelets)

Causes of thrombocytopenia are listed in Box 14.4. Purpura, bruising and spontaneous oral, nasal, GI or GU bleeding may occur, but not usually until the platelet count falls to less than 20×10^9/L. Blood film may be diagnostic (e.g. acute leukaemia). Bone marrow examination may reveal:
• Reduced megakaryocytes (platelet precursors) in cases of decreased platelet formation (e.g. hypoplastic anaemia). • Increased megakaryocytes, indicating excessive platelet destruction (e.g. ITP).

Platelet transfusion is rarely required and is usually confined to patients with bone marrow failure and platelet counts below 10×10^9/L, or to patients with actual or predicted serious haemorrhage.

Thrombocytosis (high platelets)

The platelet count may be raised as part of the inflammatory response (reactive thrombocytosis) or in patients with infection, connective tissue disease, malignancy or GI bleeding. Alternatively, it may be a feature of myeloproliferative disorders, such as primary thrombocythaemia, PRV and CML.

Blood products and transfusion

Blood transfusion from an unrelated donor inevitably carries some risk, including adverse immunological interactions between the host and infused blood and transmission of infections. Although there are many clinical indications for blood component transfusion, there are also many clinical circumstances in which the evidence for the effectiveness of transfusion is limited. In these settings, transfusion may be avoided by the use of low Hb thresholds for red cell transfusion, peri-operative blood salvage and anti-fibrinolytic drugs.

Blood products

Red cell concentrate (RCC): Used to increase red cell mass in patients with anaemia and in acute blood loss. Transfuse to maintain Hb at 70 g/L (90 g/L in cardiovascular disease).

Platelet concentrate: Used to treat and prevent bleeding caused by thrombocytopenia.

Fresh frozen plasma (FFP): Used to replace coagulation factors.

Cryoprecipitate: Obtained from plasma and used to replace fibrinogen, factor VIII and von Willebrand factor.

Coagulation factor concentrates: Used to treat haemophilia and von Willebrand's disease (factors VIII and IX).

For coagulation factor replacement, virus-inactivated or recombinant manufactured factors are now preferred where available to prevent the transmission of viral infection.

IV immunoglobulin: Used to prevent infection in patients with hypogammaglobulinaemia. It is also used in ITP and Guillain–Barré syndrome.

Every blood donation must be tested to exclude those containing transmissible agents. In the developed world, this includes:
• Hepatitis B. • Hepatitis C. • HIV. • HTLV.

Plasma donated in the UK is not used at present for producing pooled plasma derivatives, in view of concerns about transmission of variant CJD (p. 694).

Adverse effects of transfusion

Red cell incompatibility

There are four different ABO groups, determined by whether or not an individual's red cells express A or B antigens. Healthy individuals have antibodies directed against the A or B antigens that are not expressed on their own cells (Box 14.5). If red cells of an incompatible ABO group are transfused,

i 14.5 The ABO system		
Blood group	Red cell A or B antigens	Antibodies in plasma
0	None	Anti-A and anti-B
A	A	Anti-B
B	B	Anti-A
AB	A and B	None

the patient's antibodies bind to the transfused cells, causing red cell haemolysis. This is the main cause of an acute transfusion reaction, and can give rise to DIC, renal failure and death.

About 15% of Caucasians lack the Rhesus D (RhD) red cell antigen (meaning they are 'Rhesus-negative'). IgG antibodies to RhD-positive red cells are produced if such cells enter the circulation of an RhD-negative individual via fetomaternal haemorrhage during pregnancy. During a subsequent pregnancy with an RhD-positive fetus, these antibodies can cross the placenta and cause haemolytic disease of the newborn and severe neurological damage. Administration of anti-RhD immunoglobulin after delivery blocks the immune response to the RhD antigen and prevents the development of Rhesus antibodies in RhD-negative women.

Transfusion reactions

Temperature rise: A rise of less than 2°C to up to 38°C in an otherwise well patient indicates a febrile nonhaemolytic transfusion reaction. Paracetamol should be given, and the transfusion rate slowed.

Urticarial rash or itch: This is treated by giving an antihistamine (e.g. chlorphenamine 10 mg IV) and slowing the transfusion rate.

Severe allergic reactions: These patients present with bronchospasm, angioedema and hypotension. The transfusion should be stopped, and any unused units returned to the blood bank. The patient should be treated with oxygen, IV chlorphenamine, nebulised salbutamol and, if hypotensive, IM adrenaline (epinephrine; 0.5 mL of 1 in 1000).

ABO incompatibility: This causes red cell haemolysis, leading to fever, rigours, tachycardia, hypotension, chest and abdominal pain and shortness of breath. The transfusion is stopped, and an IV saline infusion given to maintain urine output more than 100 mL/hour. DIC should be treated with appropriate blood components.

Bacterial contamination: This should be considered if discoloration or damage of the pack is seen, or if the patient has a temperature greater than 39°C or hyper- or hypotension. The pack should be returned to the blood bank, blood cultures sent and broad-spectrum antibiotics given if infection seems likely. Transmission of malaria or Chagas's disease by transfusion occasionally occurs in endemic areas.

Breathlessness: This suggests fluid overload and is treated by stopping the transfusion and administering oxygen and IV furosemide.

Safe transfusion procedures

Red cells from the patient's blood sample are tested to determine the ABO and RhD type. The patient's plasma is tested to detect any red cell antibodies that could haemolyse transfused red cells. The transfusion laboratory then performs either a 'group and screen' or a 'cross-match'.
• Group and screen procedure: the sample is held in the laboratory, and compatible blood can be prepared rapidly if required. • Cross-matching: involves allocating specific red cell units to a particular patient.

It is essential to avoid all ABO-incompatible red cell transfusion. Most incompatible transfusions result from:
• Mistakes in taking and labelling the blood sample for pretransfusion testing. • Failure to perform standard checks before infusion to ensure the correct pack has been selected for the correct patient.

Transfusion in major haemorrhage

Frontline clinical staff must be trained to recognise significant blood loss early and to intervene before shock is established. Hospitals should have local major haemorrhage protocols, and all clinical staff must be familiar with them. FFP should be given as part of initial resuscitation in a 1:2 ratio with RCC until coagulation results are available. Platelets should be kept above 50×10^9/L.

Chemotherapy

Chemotherapy is the mainstay of treatment for most haematological cancers. Despite cancer cells being more sensitive, chemotherapy is non-specific and also kills some normal cells, leading to side effects such as transient bone marrow failure, mucositis and infertility. Supportive care is critical in overcoming these side effects.

Several cycles of a combination of drugs are given to achieve gradual reduction of tumour burden, to induce remission and, in some instances, to achieve a cure.

In recent years, chemotherapy has been improved by the addition of treatments such as targeted monoclonal antibodies and small molecules designed to exploit particular biochemical pathways in cancer cells.

Haematopoietic stem cell transplantation

HSCT offers the only hope of 'cure' for many blood diseases. The indications for HSCT are being refined and extended, and currently include:
• Leukaemias (AML, ALL, CML p. 574). • Myeloma. • Myelodysplastic syndrome. • Non-Hodgkin's lymphoma. • Severe aplastic anaemia.
• Myelofibrosis. • Severe immune deficiency syndromes.

The type of HSCT is defined according to the donor and source of stem cells.

Allogeneic HSCT

Stem cells from a donor—either related (usually an HLA-identical sibling) or a closely HLA-matched volunteer unrelated donor—are infused after planned ablation of the patient's own marrow. In addition to restoring marrow function, donor immune cells can attack recipient malignant cells ('graft versus disease effect').

There is considerable morbidity and mortality associated with HSCT. The best results are obtained in young patients with minimal residual disease. Reduced intensity (nonmyeloablative) conditioning using intense immunosuppression may help to reduce risk and allow less fit patients to achieve remission. Around 25% die from complications such as graft-versus-host disease (see later), and there remains a significant risk of disease relapse. The long-term survival for patients undergoing allogeneic HSCT in acute leukaemia is around 50%.

Graft-versus-host disease

GVHD is caused by the cytotoxic activity of donor T lymphocytes that become sensitised to their new host, regarding it as foreign.

Acute GVHD: Occurs in the first 100 days after transplant in around one-third of patients. It varies from mild to lethal, causing rashes, jaundice and diarrhoea. Prevention includes HLA-matching of the donor and immunosuppressant drugs.

Chronic GVHD: This may follow acute GVHD or arise independently. It often resembles a connective tissue disorder, and is usually treated with glucocorticoids and prolonged immunosuppression (e.g. ciclosporin).

Autologous HSCT

Stem cells are harvested from the patient's bone marrow or peripheral blood and frozen until required. After aggressive chemotherapy to treat disease (with associated myeloablation), stem cells are re-infused to restore marrow function. Autologous HSCT is used to allow aggressive chemotherapy for diseases that do not primarily involve the haematopoietic tissues, or for patients in whom very good remissions have been achieved. The most common indications are lymphomas and myeloma.

Anticoagulant and antithrombotic therapy

Antiplatelet agents (e.g. aspirin, clopidogrel) are more effective in preventing arterial thrombosis than VTE. They are therefore the drugs of choice in acute coronary and cerebrovascular disease, whereas warfarin and other anticoagulants are favoured in VTE and atrial fibrillation. Indications for anticoagulation are given in Box 14.6.

Heparin

14

Unfractionated heparin (UFH) produces its anticoagulant effect by potentiating the activity of antithrombin. This results in prolongation of the APTT. The low molecular weight heparins (LMWHs) augment antithrombin activity preferentially against factor Xa. LMWHs produce reliable dose-dependent anticoagulation when given as a daily subcutaneous injection in a weight-related dose. Blood monitoring is not required.

LMWHs are widely used for the treatment of VTE and have replaced UFH, except where rapid reversibility is important. The short half-life of UFH (~1 hour) makes it useful for those with a predisposition to bleeding (e.g. patients with a peptic ulcer). UFH is started with a loading dose of 80 U/kg IV, followed by a continuous infusion, initially of 18 U/kg/hour, adjusted to maintain the APTT at 1.5 to 2.5 times control. If a patient bleeds, it is usually sufficient just to discontinue the infusion; however, if bleeding is severe, it can be neutralised with IV protamine.

Heparin-induced thrombocytopenia

In a small proportion of patients treated with heparin, the platelet count falls after 5–14 days because of development of an antibody directed against

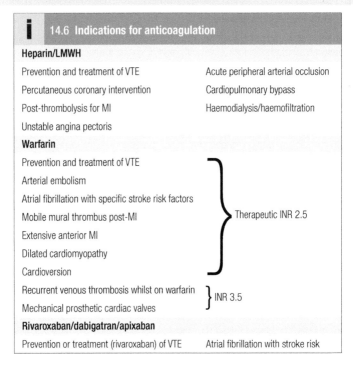

i **14.6 Indications for anticoagulation**

Heparin/LMWH

Prevention and treatment of VTE	Acute peripheral arterial occlusion
Percutaneous coronary intervention	Cardiopulmonary bypass
Post-thrombolysis for MI	Haemodialysis/haemofiltration
Unstable angina pectoris	

Warfarin

Prevention and treatment of VTE

Arterial embolism

Atrial fibrillation with specific stroke risk factors

Mobile mural thrombus post-MI   } Therapeutic INR 2.5

Extensive anterior MI

Dilated cardiomyopathy

Cardioversion

Recurrent venous thrombosis whilst on warfarin   } INR 3.5

Mechanical prosthetic cardiac valves

Rivaroxaban/dabigatran/apixaban

Prevention or treatment (rivaroxaban) of VTE	Atrial fibrillation with stroke risk

a factor on the platelet surface. Heparin should be discontinued immediately, and an alternative, such as the direct thrombin inhibitor argatroban, substituted.

Coumarins

Warfarin, the most commonly used coumarin, inhibits the vitamin K–dependent carboxylation of factors II, VII, IX and X in the liver. Indications for warfarin and appropriate target INRs are listed in Box 14.6. Warfarin must be initiated with a loading dose (e.g. 10 mg orally) on the first day; subsequent daily doses depend on the INR and can be predicted using an algorithm. The duration of warfarin therapy depends on the clinical indication. Preparation for cardioversion requires a limited duration, whereas anticoagulation to prevent cardioembolic stroke in atrial fibrillation is long-term.

Drug interactions are common through protein binding and metabolism by the cytochrome P450 system. Bleeding is the most common serious side effect of warfarin. If the INR is above the desired therapeutic level, the warfarin dose should be reduced or withheld. The anticoagulant effect of warfarin may be reversed by administering vitamin K, but this takes around 6 hours. In serious haemorrhage, reversal can be effected quickly by giving coagulation factor concentrate or FFP.

Direct oral anticoagulants

The DOACs are direct specific inhibitors of key proteases in the common pathway, and offer an alternative to coumarins in the management of VTE and the prevention of stroke in patients with atrial fibrillation. Dabigatran inhibits thrombin, whereas rivaroxaban, apixaban and edoxaban inhibit Xa. They are effective in fixed oral doses, have a short half-life (~10 hours), achieve peak plasma levels 2 to 4 hours after oral administration, have very few drug interactions and are all moderately dependent on renal function for excretion. The lack of specific reversal agents for these drugs was initially a problem, but new drugs to reverse each DOAC are becoming available.

DOACs are now licensed for the prevention of VTE following high-risk orthopaedic surgery (except edoxaban), the acute management and prevention of recurrence of VTE and the prevention of stroke and systemic embolism in patients with atrial fibrillation with risk factors.

Anaemias

Around 30% of the world population is anaemic; iron deficiency is the cause in half of these.

Iron deficiency anaemia

This occurs when iron losses exceed absorption:

Blood loss: The most common explanation in men and postmenopausal women is GI blood loss. This may result from gastric or colorectal malignancy, peptic ulceration, inflammatory bowel disease, diverticulitis or angiodysplasia. Worldwide, hookworm and schistosomiasis are common causes (p. 110). GI bleeding may be exacerbated by the use of aspirin or NSAIDs. In younger women, menstrual bleeding and pregnancy often contribute to iron deficiency.

Malabsorption: Gastric acid is required to release iron from food and helps keep it in the soluble ferrous state. Hypochlorhydria as a result of proton pump inhibitor treatment or previous gastric surgery may contribute to deficiency. Iron is absorbed actively in the upper small intestine, and absorption can be affected by coeliac disease.

Physiological demands: Increased demands for iron during puberty and pregnancy can cause deficiency.

Investigations

The blood film shows microcytic hypochromic red cells (low MCV, low mean cell Hb, MCH). Iron deficiency is confirmed by a low serum ferritin; however, ferritin may also be raised (up to 100 µg/L) by liver disease and in the acute phase response, even in the presence of iron deficiency. In these patients, measurement of transferrin saturation (<16%) and soluble transferrin receptor (raised) may be helpful.

The underlying cause of the iron deficiency should be established. Men older than 40 years of age and postmenopausal women should undergo investigation of the upper and lower GI tract by endoscopy or barium studies. Coeliac disease should be excluded by antibody testing at an early stage. In the tropics, stool and urine should be examined for parasites.

14

Management

Unless the patient has angina, heart failure or cerebral hypoxia, transfusion is not necessary, and oral iron supplementation (ferrous sulphate 200 mg three times daily for 3–6 months) is appropriate, together with treatment of the underlying cause. Patients with malabsorption or intolerance of oral preparations may need parenteral iron. The Hb should rise by 10 g/L every 7 to 10 days.

Anaemia of chronic disease

This common type of anaemia occurs with chronic infections, chronic inflammation and neoplasia. The anaemia is mild and usually associated with a normal MCV (normocytic, normochromic), although this may be reduced in long-standing inflammation. Hepcidin, a key regulatory protein, inhibits the export of iron from cells, resulting in anaemia despite high iron stores. Raised ferritin and reduced TIBC and soluble transferrin receptor help to distinguish ACD from iron deficiency. Measures that reduce the severity of the underlying disorder generally help to improve the anaemia.

Megaloblastic anaemia

This results from deficiency of vitamin B_{12} or folic acid, both of which are required for DNA synthesis. Deficiency leads to red cells with arrested nuclear maturation but normal cytoplasmic development within the bone marrow (megaloblasts). There is a macrocytic anaemia with an MCV often greater than 120 fl, and mature red cells are commonly oval in shape. Involvement of white cells and platelets can lead to neutrophils with hyper-segmented nuclei and, in severe cases, pancytopenia. Bone marrow examination reveals hypercellularity and megaloblastic changes.

▌Vitamin B_{12}

The average diet contains well over the 1 µg daily requirement of vitamin B_{12}, mainly in meat, eggs and milk. In the stomach, vitamin B_{12} is released from food by gastric enzymes and binds to a carrier protein (R protein). The gastric parietal cells produce intrinsic factor, a vitamin B_{12}-binding protein. As gastric emptying occurs, dietary vitamin B_{12} switches from the R protein to intrinsic factor. Vitamin B_{12} is absorbed in the terminal ileum and transported in plasma bound to transcobalamin II. The liver stores enough vitamin B_{12} for 3 years, so deficiency takes many years to appear, even if all dietary intake stops.

Vitamin B_{12} deficiency can cause neurological disease, including peripheral neuropathy (glove and stocking paraesthesiae) and subacute combined degeneration of the cord. The latter involves the posterior columns (causing diminished vibration sense and proprioception, leading to sensory ataxia) and corticospinal tracts (resulting in upper motor neuron signs). Dementia and optic atrophy can also occur.

Causes of vitamin B_{12} deficiency

Dietary deficiency: This occurs only in strict vegans.

Gastric factors: Gastric surgery (including gastrectomy) can cause vitamin B_{12} deficiency as a result of impaired secretion of gastric acid and intrinsic factor.

Pernicious anaemia: This is an autoimmune disorder characterised by loss of gastric parietal cells causing intrinsic factor deficiency, leading to vitamin B_{12} malabsorption. Pernicious anaemia has an average age of onset of 60 years and is associated with other autoimmune conditions including Hashimoto's thyroiditis, Graves' disease, vitiligo and Addison's disease. Antiparietal cell antibodies are present in 90% of cases, but also occur in 20% of normal females older than 60 years of age. The Schilling test (the absorption of oral radio-labelled vitamin B_{12}, before and after intrinsic factor replacement) is used less because of the development of autoantibody tests, greater caution in the use of radioactive tracers and limited availability of intrinsic factor.

Small bowel factors: Terminal ileal disease (e.g. Crohn's) and ileal resection result in vitamin B_{12} malabsorption. Motility disorders can cause bacterial overgrowth, and the resulting competition for free vitamin B_{12} leads to deficiency.

Folate

Leafy vegetables, fruits, liver and kidney provide rich sources of dietary folate. An average Western diet meets the daily requirement, but total body stores are small, and deficiency can develop rapidly. Causes of folate deficiency include:

• Diet, for example, poor intake of vegetables. • Malabsorption, for example, coeliac disease. • Increased demand, for example, pregnancy, haemolysis. • Drugs, for example, phenytoin, contraceptive pill, methotrexate.

Serum folate is very sensitive to dietary intake, and red cell folate is therefore a more accurate indicator of folate stores.

Management of megaloblastic anaemia

If a patient with severe megaloblastic anaemia requires treatment before vitamin B_{12} and red cell folate results are available, both folic acid and vitamin B_{12} are given. Folic acid therapy alone in vitamin B_{12} deficiency may cause worsening of neurological defects.

Vitamin B_{12} deficiency: Treated with IM hydroxycobalamin (1000 μg, six doses 2 or 3 days apart, followed by lifelong therapy of 1000 μg every 3 months). Hb should rise by 10 g/L per week, but neuropathy may take 6 to 12 months to correct.

Folate deficiency: Treated with oral folic acid 5 mg daily. Folic acid supplementation in pregnancy reduces the risk of neural tube defects. Prophylactic folic acid is also given in chronic haematological disease associated with reduced red cell lifespan (e.g. autoimmune haemolytic anaemia or haemoglobinopathies).

Haemolytic anaemia

Normal red cells have a lifespan of 120 days. Increased red cell destruction (haemolysis) leads to increased LDH, a modest increase in unconjugated bilirubin and mild jaundice. Compensatory bone marrow activity results in increased reticulocytes and immature granulocytes in peripheral blood. Blood films may also show the reason for haemolysis (e.g. spherocytosis). The erythroid hyperplasia may also cause folate deficiency, leading to megaloblastosis. When destruction exceeds production, haemolytic anaemia results.

The causes of haemolytic anaemia may be inherited (e.g. spherocytosis, haemoglobinopathies, G6PD deficiency) or acquired (e.g. autoantibody-mediated, infective, toxic or mechanical (as with metallic heart valves)).

Extravascular haemolysis: Occurs in the reticulo-endothelial cells of the liver and spleen, so avoiding free Hb in the plasma. In most haemolytic states, haemolysis is predominantly extravascular.

Intravascular haemolysis: Releases free Hb into the plasma, where it binds to haptoglobin (an α_2 globulin produced by the liver), resulting in a fall in haptoglobin levels. Once haptoglobins are saturated, free Hb is oxidised to form methaemoglobin. Excess free Hb may also be absorbed by renal tubular cells, where it is degraded, and the iron stored as haemosiderin. When the tubular cells are subsequently sloughed into the urine, they give rise to haemosiderinuria.

Red cell membrane defects

Hereditary spherocytosis

This is usually inherited as an autosomal dominant condition and has an incidence of 1:5000. The most common abnormalities are deficiencies of the red cell membrane proteins, beta spectrin or ankyrin. The cells lose their normal elasticity and undergo destruction when they pass through the spleen. The severity of spontaneous haemolysis varies. Most cases feature an asymptomatic compensated chronic haemolytic state with spherocytes on the blood film and a reticulocytosis. Pigment gallstones occur in up to 50% of patients and may cause cholecystitis.

The clinical course may be complicated by crises:
• Haemolytic crisis: occurs uncommonly, usually with infection. • Megaloblastic crisis: follows the development of folate deficiency. • Aplastic crisis: occurs in association with parvovirus (erythrovirus) infection; the virus directly invades red cell precursors and switches off red cell production.

Investigations:
• Hb levels: variable, depending on the degree of compensation. • Blood film: shows spherocytes and reticulocytes. • Direct Coombs test (see Fig. 14.2): negative, excluding immune haemolysis. • Bilirubin and LDH: raised. • Screening of family members.

Management: Folic acid prophylaxis (5 mg weekly) should be lifelong. Acute severe haemolytic crises require transfusion. Splenectomy should be considered in moderate to severe cases, but only after the age of 6 years because of the risk of sepsis. Before splenectomy, patients should receive vaccination against pneumococcus, *Haemophilus influenzae* type B, meningococcus group C and influenza. Thereafter they should undergo regular immunisation against pneumococcus and influenza, and receive lifelong penicillin V.

Hereditary elliptocytosis

This is less common and generally milder than hereditary spherocytosis. The blood film shows elliptocytic red cells with variable haemolysis. Most cases are asymptomatic and do not require specific treatment; more severe cases are managed like hereditary spherocytosis.

Direct antiglobulin test (DAT) (Coombs test)

Detects the presence of antibody bound to
the red cell surface, e.g.,
1. autoimmune haemolytic anaemia
2. haemolytic disease of newborn (HDN)
3. transfusion reactions

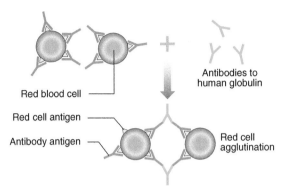

Indirect antiglobulin test (IAT) (indirect Coombs test)

Detects antibodies in the plasma, e.g., antibody screen
in pre-transfusion testing

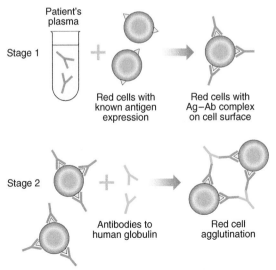

Fig. 14.2 Direct and indirect antiglobulin tests.

Red cell enzymopathies

Glucose-6-phosphate dehydrogenase deficiency (G6PD) is the commonest inherited enzymopathy, affecting 10% of the world's population. It is an X-linked condition principally affecting males. G6PD is pivotal in the hexose monophosphate shunt and helps to protect red cells against oxidative stress. Deficiency results in acute intravascular haemolysis secondary to infection, drugs (e.g. antimalarials, sulphonamides, nitrofurantoin) and ingestion of fava beans. It can also cause chronic haemolysis and neonatal jaundice. Management involves stopping any precipitant drugs or foods. Transfusion may be required in severe cases.

Autoimmune haemolytic anaemia

This results from increased red cell destruction caused by red cell autoantibodies. If an antibody avidly fixes complement, it will result in intravascular haemolysis, but if complement activation is weak, the haemolysis will be extravascular. Immune haemolysis is classified according to whether the antibodies bind best at 37°C (warm antibodies, 80% of cases) or 4°C (cold antibodies).

Warm autoimmune haemolysis

This occurs at all ages, but most commonly in middle age. Antibodies are usually IgG. No cause is identified in up to 50% of cases, but known causes include:

• Lymphoid neoplasms, for example, lymphoma. • Solid tumours, for example, lung, colon. • Connective tissue disease, for example, SLE, rheumatoid arthritis. • Drugs, for example, methyldopa. • HIV.

Investigations: There is evidence of haemolysis, spherocytes and polychromasia on the blood film. The diagnosis is confirmed by the direct Coombs or antiglobulin test (see Fig. 14.2), in which red cells are mixed with Coombs reagent containing antibodies against human IgG/IgM/complement. If the red cells have been coated by antibody *in vivo*, agglutination occurs. The test will miss IgA and IgE antibodies.

Management: Any underlying cause must be treated, and any implicated drugs stopped. Oral prednisolone (1 mg/kg) is the mainstay of treatment. It works by decreasing macrophage destruction of antibody-coated red cells and reducing antibody production. Transfusion may be required for severe anaemia. Second-line therapies include immunomodulation with rituximab, immunosuppression (e.g. azathioprine, cyclophosphamide) and splenectomy. All have risks: long-term immunosuppressants can cause malignancy, and splenectomy predisposes to overwhelming sepsis.

Cold agglutinin disease

This is as a result of antibodies ('cold agglutinins'), usually IgM, which bind to the red cells at 4°C, causing agglutination and intravascular haemolysis if complement fixation occurs. Causes include:

• Lymphoma. • Infections, for example, *Mycoplasma pneumoniae*, infectious mononucleosis. • Paroxysmal cold haemoglobinuria.

Cold antibodies optimally bind red cells at lower temperatures. Red cell agglutination therefore occurs in small vessels in exposed areas, causing cold, painful and blue fingers and toes (acrocyanosis).

Management: Any underlying cause must be treated. All patients should receive folate supplements. Patients must keep extremities warm, especially in winter. Glucocorticoid therapy and blood transfusion may be required.

Alloimmune haemolytic anaemia

This is caused by antibodies against nonself red cells. It occurs after unmatched blood transfusion or maternal sensitisation to paternal antigens on fetal cells (haemolytic disease of the newborn).

Nonimmune haemolytic anaemia

Disruption of the red cell membrane
This is characterised by red cell fragments on the blood film and positive tests for intravascular haemolysis. Causes include:

Mechanical heart valves: High flow through incompetent valves results in shear stress damage.

March haemoglobinuria: Prolonged marching or marathon running can cause red cell damage in the capillaries in the feet.

Thermal injury: Damage to red cells following burns.

Microangiopathic haemolytic anaemia: Fibrin deposition in capillaries can cause severe red cell disruption. Causes include malignant hypertension, haemolytic uraemic syndrome and DIC.

Infection
Plasmodium falciparum infection (malaria) may cause intravascular haemolysis with haemoglobinuria ('blackwater fever').

Clostridium perfringens sepsis in ascending cholangitis or necrotising fasciitis may cause intravascular haemolysis.

Haemoglobinopathies

14

Sickle-cell anaemia

The normal Hb molecule is composed of two α and two non-α globin polypeptide chains, each containing a Hb group. HbA (HbA-$\alpha_2\beta_2$) is the predominant form in adults. Sickle-cell disease results from a single glutamic acid to valine substitution at position 6 of the β-globin chain. It is inherited as an autosomal recessive trait.

Homozygotes produce only abnormal β chains that make hbS (HbS, termed SS), resulting in the clinical syndrome of sickle-cell disease. Heterozygotes produce a mixture of normal and abnormal β chains that make normal HbA and HbS (termed AS), causing sickle-cell trait, which was formerly thought to be asymptomatic but is now known to carry a risk of sudden cardiovascular death.

Individuals with sickle-cell trait are relatively resistant to falciparum malaria, which explains the high incidence of the sickle gene in equatorial Africa, where falciparum malaria is endemic.

Clinical features
When HbS is deoxygenated, the Hb molecules polymerise and the red cell membrane becomes distorted, producing characteristic sickle-shaped cells.

Sickling is precipitated by hypoxia, dehydration and infection. Sickled cells have a shortened survival and plug vessels in the microcirculation. This results in a number of acute syndromes termed 'crises' and chronic organ damage:

Vaso-occlusive crisis: Plugging of small vessels in the bone results in avascular necrosis, producing acute severe bone pain. Commonly affected sites include the femur, humerus, ribs, pelvis and vertebrae.

Stroke: Stroke or silent stroke occurs in 10% to 15% of children with sickle-cell disease.

Sickle chest syndrome: Bone marrow infarction results in fat emboli to the lungs, which cause sickling and infarction, leading to ventilatory failure.

Sequestration crisis: Thrombosis of the venous outflow from an organ causes loss of function and acute painful enlargement. Massive splenic enlargement may result in severe anaemia and circulatory collapse. Recurrent sickling in the spleen in childhood results in infarction, and adults may have no functional spleen. Sequestration in the liver leads to severe pain caused by capsular stretching.

Aplastic crisis: Infection with parvovirus results in severe red cell aplasia, causing severe anaemia.

Pregnancy: Pregnancy-related morbidity includes painful crisis, placental failure and thrombosis.

Investigations

Patients with sickle-cell disease have a compensated anaemia (usually 60–80 g/L) with a reticulocytosis and sickle cells on the blood film. Hb electrophoresis demonstrates a predominance of HbS with absent HbA.

Management and prognosis

Patients with sickle-cell disease should receive prophylaxis with folic acid. Pneumococcal infection may be lethal in the presence of hyposplenism; patients should therefore receive prophylaxis with daily penicillin V and vaccination against pneumococcus. They should also be vaccinated against *Haemophilus influenzae* B and hepatitis B.

Vaso-occlusive crises are managed by aggressive rehydration, oxygen and adequate analgesia (which often requires opiates) and antibiotics. Top-up transfusion may be used in sequestration or aplastic crises. Exchange transfusion, where a patient is simultaneously venesected and transfused to replace HbS with HbA, may be used in life-threatening crises. The oral cytotoxic agent hydroxycarbamide induces increased synthesis of fetal Hb (HbF-$\alpha_2\gamma_2$), which in turn inhibits polymerisation of HbS and reduces sickling; this may be helpful in individuals with recurrent severe crises. Allogeneic stem cell transplantation is rarely performed but may be potentially curative. Sickle-cell anaemia has mortality of 15% by the age of 20 years and 50% by the age of 40 years.

Thalassaemias

The thalassaemias are a group of inherited disorders of Hb production in which there is impaired synthesis of alpha or beta globin chains. The resultant imbalance in the ratio of alpha to beta chains leads to precipitation of the excess chains, causing membrane damage and reduced red cell survival.

Beta-thalassaemia

Failure to synthesise beta chains is the most common type of thalassaemia and occurs most frequently in the Mediterranean area.

Heterozygotes have beta-thalassaemia minor: they usually have mild microcytic anaemia, which may be detected only when iron therapy for microcytic anaemia fails. Homozygotes have beta-thalassaemia major and are either unable to synthesise HbA or produce very little. After the first 4 months of life, they develop profound transfusion-dependent hypochromic anaemia. Tests show red cell dysplasia and raised HbF.

Management: Cure is now a possibility for selected children, with allogeneic HSCT (p. 562). Prenatal diagnosis by chorionic villous sampling may be offered to parents with beta-thalassaemia minor, with the option of termination.

Alpha-thalassaemia

Reduced or absent alpha-chain synthesis is common in South-east Asia. There are two alpha gene loci on chromosome 16, and therefore four alpha genes, giving a range of features:
• One deletion: no clinical effect. • Two deletions: a mild microcytic hypochromic anaemia. • Three deletions: patient makes haemoglobin H, a beta tetramer that is functionally useless; treatment is similar to that of beta-thalassaemia of intermediate severity. • All four alpha genes deleted: the baby is stillborn (hydrops fetalis).

Haematological malignancies

Haematological malignancies arise when the proliferation or apoptosis of blood cells are corrupted because of acquired mutations in key regulatory genes. If mature differentiated cells are involved, indolent neoplasms arise, such as low-grade lymphomas and chronic leukaemias, where long survival is expected. Mutations in more primitive stem or progenitor cells produce rapidly progressive life-threatening illnesses, such as acute leukaemias and high-grade lymphomas.

Haematological neoplasms generally affect elderly patients, except for acute lymphoblastic leukaemia, which predominantly affects children, and Hodgkin lymphoma, which affects people aged 20 to 40 years.

Leukaemias

Leukaemias are malignant disorders of haematopoietic stem cells associated with increased numbers of white cells in the bone marrow and/or peripheral blood. The aetiology is unknown in most patients, but several factors are associated with the development of leukaemia:

Ionising radiation: Both wartime and iatrogenic exposure cause increased risk.

Cytotoxic drugs: Alkylating drugs can induce myeloid leukaemia after a latent period of several years. Industrial benzene exposure is associated with leukaemia.

Retroviruses: One rare form of T cell leukaemia is associated with retroviral infection.

Genetic: Increased incidence in identical twins of affected individuals. Incidence is increased in Down's syndrome. Ethnic variation also occurs; chronic lymphocytic leukaemia is rare in Chinese populations.

Immunological: Immunodeficiency states (e.g. hypogammaglobulinaemia).

Leukaemias are traditionally classified into four main groups:
• Acute lymphoblastic leukaemia (ALL). • Acute myeloid leukaemia (AML).
• Chronic lymphocytic leukaemia (CLL). • Chronic myeloid leukaemia (CML).

Lymphocytic and lymphoblastic cells are derived from the lymphoid stem cell (B cells and T cells). Myeloid refers to the other lineages: precursors of red cells, granulocytes, monocytes and platelets.

Acute leukaemia

In acute leukaemia there is proliferation of primitive stem cells leading to an accumulation of blast cells in the bone marrow, which causes bone marrow failure. Eventually, this proliferation spills into the blood. AML is about four times more common than ALL in adults. In children, the proportions are reversed, with ALL being more common. The presenting features are usually anaemia, bleeding and infection.

Investigations

FBC usually shows anaemia and thrombocytopenia. The leucocyte count varies from as low as 1×10^9/L to as high as 500×10^9/L or more. The appearance of blast cells on the blood film is usually diagnostic.

Bone marrow examination confirms the diagnosis. The marrow is usually hypercellular, with replacement of normal elements by leukaemic blast cells in varying proportions (but >20% of the cells). The presence of Auer rods in the cytoplasm of blast cells indicates myeloblastic leukaemia. Classification and prognosis are determined by immunophenotyping, chromosome and molecular analysis.

Management

Specific treatment for acute leukaemia is aggressive, has many side effects and may be inappropriate for very elderly patients or those with significant comorbidity. In these patients, supportive treatment only should be considered. Low-intensity chemotherapy may be offered to elderly frail patients but only induces remission in less than 20% of patients.

Specific therapy

Before specific therapy is started, any underlying infection should be treated. Anaemia and thrombocytopenia should be corrected with red cell and platelet transfusions. The aim of treatment is to destroy the leukaemic clone of cells without destroying the residual normal stem cell compartment. There are three phases:

Remission induction: A proportion of the tumour is destroyed by combination chemotherapy. This causes 3 to 4 weeks of severe bone marrow hypoplasia, requiring intensive inpatient support.

Remission consolidation: Residual disease is attacked by several courses of chemotherapy during the consolidation phase. This again results in periods of marrow hypoplasia. In poor-prognosis leukaemia, this phase may include allogeneic HSCT.

Remission maintenance: If the patient is still in remission after the consolidation phase for ALL, a period of outpatient maintenance therapy is given, consisting of repeating cycles of drugs. In ALL, prophylactic cranial irradiation and intrathecal methotrexate are used to ensure therapy penetrates the CNS.

Supportive therapy

Aggressive chemotherapy involves periods of bone marrow failure and requires adequate supportive care. The following problems are common:

Anaemia: This is treated with red cell transfusion.

Bleeding: Thrombocytopenic bleeding requires platelet transfusions. Prophylactic platelet transfusion should be given to maintain the platelet count greater than 10×10^9/L. Coagulation abnormalities should be treated appropriately (see earlier).

Infection: Fever (>38°C) lasting over 1 hour in a significantly neutropenic patient (neutrophil count $<1.0 \times 10^9$/L) indicates possible sepsis. IV broad-spectrum antibiotic therapy is essential. Empirical therapy is given with a combination of an aminoglycoside (e.g. gentamicin) and a broad-spectrum penicillin (e.g. piperacillin/tazobactam). This combination is synergistic and bactericidal. The organisms most commonly associated with severe neutropenia are skin-based Gram-positive bacteria such as *Staphylococcus aureus* and *S. epidermidis*, which gain entry via cannulae and central lines, and Gram-negative bacteria from the gut.

Patients with ALL are susceptible to infection with *Pneumocystis jirovecii*, which causes severe pneumonia with fever and hypoxia. Prophylactic oral co-trimoxazole helps to prevent this during chemotherapy. Diagnosis is by sputum induction, and treatment is with high-dose IV co-trimoxazole.

Oropharyngeal *Candida* is common and is treated with fluconazole. Patients receiving intensive chemotherapy receive prophylaxis against systemic fungal infections with itraconazole or posaconazole. Systemic fungal infection with *Candida* or *Aspergillus* is treated with IV liposomal amphotericin, caspofungin or voriconazole.

Herpes simplex infection frequently occurs around the lips and nose during chemotherapy, and is treated with aciclovir. Herpes zoster should be dealt with early using high-dose aciclovir, as it can be fatal in immunocompromised patients.

Metabolic problems: Continuous monitoring of renal and hepatic function is necessary. Renal toxicity occurs with some antibiotics (e.g. aminoglycosides) and antifungal agents (amphotericin). Cellular breakdown during induction therapy increases uric acid production, which may cause renal failure; allopurinol and IV hydration are given to prevent this.

Psychological support: Support from a trained multidisciplinary team is essential.

Haematopoietic stem cell transplantation

This is described on p. 562 and can increase 5-year survival from 20% to 50% in high-risk acute leukaemia. Reduced-intensity conditioning has allowed HSCT to be delivered to patients aged up to 65 years.

14

Prognosis

Without treatment, the median survival in acute leukaemia is around 5 weeks. Around 80% of adult patients aged younger than 60 years achieve remission with specific therapy; however, relapse rates remain high. Remission rates are lower for older patients. Better use of HSCT, novel drugs, monoclonal antibodies and receptor inhibitors have led to steady improvements in survival from leukaemia.

Chronic myeloid leukaemia

CML is a myeloproliferative stem cell disorder resulting in proliferation of all haematopoietic lineages, but predominantly the granulocytic series. Cell maturation proceeds fairly normally. The peak incidence is at the age of 55 years. The defining characteristic of CML is the chromosome abnormality (Philadelphia chromosome, Ph), a shortened chromosome 22 formed by reciprocal translocation with chromosome 9. A resulting chimeric gene (*BCR ABL*) codes for a protein with tyrosine kinase activity, which plays a causative role in the disease, influencing cellular proliferation and differentiation.

Clinical features

The disease has three phases:

Chronic phase: The disease is responsive to treatment and is easily controlled. Formerly, this stage lasted 3 to 5 years, but imatinib therapy has prolonged this to normal life expectancy in many patients.

Accelerated phase: Disease control becomes more difficult.

Blast crisis: The disease transforms into an acute leukaemia (AML in 70%, ALL in 30%), which is relatively refractory to treatment and often fatal. Imatinib therapy greatly reduces the number of patients per year who transform to blast crisis.

Common symptoms include lethargy, weight loss, abdominal discomfort, gout and sweating. About 25% of patients are asymptomatic at diagnosis. Splenomegaly is characteristic and may be massive; hepatomegaly occurs in 50% of cases.

Investigations

• FBC: usually shows a normocytic, normochromic anaemia. • Leucocyte count: varies from 10 to 600 × 10^9/L. • Platelet count: very high in around one-third of patients—up to 2000 × 10^9/L. • Blood film: neutrophils and myelocytes are the predominant cell type, although the full range of granulocyte precursors is seen. The number of circulating blasts increases dramatically in blast transformation. • Chromosome analysis of bone marrow reveals the Ph chromosome, and RNA analysis reveals the *BCR ABL* gene defect.

Management

Chronic phase: Tyrosine kinase inhibitors (TKIs) are the mainstay of treatment for CML. Imatinib, nilotinib and dasatinib normalise blood counts within a month and cause disappearance of the Ph chromosome in 3 to 6 months in 90% of patients. Monitoring is by 3-monthly quantitative PCR for BCR ABL mRNA in blood. Alternative TKIs are tried in nonresponders.

Allogeneic HSCT (p. 562) is reserved for patients who fail TKI therapy. Hydroxycarbamide is still useful in palliative situations, and interferon is used in women planning pregnancy.

Accelerated phase and blast crisis: For accelerated phase cases, the TKIs nilotinib or dasatinib are used. In blast crisis, acute leukaemia treatment is used. Response is better in lymphoblastic crisis than in myeloblastic crisis. In younger, fitter patients, allogeneic HSCT may achieve a return to chronic phase. Hydroxycarbamide or low-dose cytarabine can be used palliatively in older patients.

Chronic lymphocytic leukaemia

CLL is the most common variety of leukaemia, typically presenting between the ages of 65 and 70 years. There is uncontrolled proliferation of immuno-incompetent B lymphocytes, leading to impaired immunity and haematopoiesis.

Clinical features

The onset is very insidious. In around 70% of patients, the diagnosis is made incidentally on a routine FBC. Presenting problems include:
• Anaemia. • Infections. • Lymphadenopathy. • Systemic symptoms, such as night sweats and weight loss.

Investigations

Peripheral blood shows a mature lymphocytosis ($>5 \times 10^9$/L). Immunophenotyping confirms monoclonal B cells expressing CD19 and CD23. Serum immunoglobulins indicate the degree of hypogammaglobulinaemia. Direct Coombs test may show autoimmune haemolytic anaemia. Mutations in the *TP53* gene are a powerful prognostic marker in CLL. Bone marrow examination may be helpful in difficult cases, to monitor response and to judge prognosis.

The clinical stages of CLL are:
• A (60% of patients): no anaemia or thrombocytopenia; less than three areas of lymphadenopathy. • B (30%): as for A but three or more areas of lymphadenopathy. • C (10%): anaemia and/or thrombocytopenia.

Management and prognosis

Most stage A patients do not require treatment.

Treatment is indicated if there is bone marrow failure, massive lymphadenopathy or splenomegaly, systemic symptomology, rapidly increasing lymphocyte count, autoimmune anaemia or thrombocytopenia. Initial therapy for progressive stage A and stages B and C is based on age, fitness and *TP53* mutation status. For patients younger than 70 years of age who are fit and *TP53* mutation–negative, fludarabine, cyclophosphamide and rituximab (FCR) is standard care. For older, less fit patients, rituximab is combined with bendamustine or chlorambucil. Supportive care is required in progressive disease, for example, transfusions for symptomatic anaemia or thrombocytopenia and prompt treatment of infections.

The main prognostic factor is stage of disease. Most patients with stage A disease have a normal life expectancy. Patients with advanced CLL are more likely to die from their disease or infectious complications. In those treated with chemotherapy and rituximab, 90% are alive 4 years later.

14

Myelodysplastic syndromes

These predominantly affect elderly patients and are characterised by ineffective blood cell production and progression to AML. The underlying genetic abnormalities have been identified.

The blood film shows cytopenias and dysplastic blood cells with nuclear hypersegmentation. The bone marrow is hypercellular, with dysplastic changes.

Over time progressive dysplasia leads to bone marrow failure or progression to AML in 30% of cases. Supportive care with red cell and platelet transfusions is the main treatment. Erythropoietin and G–CSF may improve Hb and WCC. Allogeneic HSCT may allow a cure in patients with good performance status. In low-risk patients, median survival is 9 years, falling to 1 to 1.5 years in high-risk patients.

Lymphomas

These neoplasms arise from lymphoid tissues and are classified according to biopsy findings into Hodgkin's lymphoma and non-Hodgkin's lymphoma (NHL) further divided into high grade (aggressive) and low grade (indolent) tumours. Most are of B cell origin.

Hodgkin's lymphoma

Hodgkin's lymphoma typically affects adults aged 20 to 35 years, although there is a second peak at 50 to 70 years of age. The condition is more common in individuals with a previous history of infectious mononucleosis, although no causal link has been proved. Reed–Sternberg cells, large malignant lymphoid cells of B cell origin, are the histological hallmark of Hodgkin's lymphoma. Four histological patterns of classical Hodgkin's lymphoma are recognised, according to the WHO:
• Nodular sclerosing (common in young patients and women). • Mixed cellularity. • Lymphocyte-rich. • Lymphocyte-depleted (rare).

A nodular lymphocyte-predominant form of Hodgkin's lymphoma also occurs; it is slow-growing, localised and rarely fatal.

Clinical features

There is painless rubbery lymphadenopathy, usually in the neck or supraclavicular fossae. Some patients have no systemic 'B' symptoms; others have weight loss and drenching sweats. Hepatosplenomegaly may be present. Dry cough and breathlessness may occur in those with mediastinal adenopathy.

Investigations

• FBC: may be normal or show normocytic, normochromic anaemia. Lymphopenia or eosinophilia may be present. • ESR: may be raised. • Liver function: may be abnormal, with or without hepatic infiltration. • Raised LDH levels: indicate adverse prognosis. • CXR: may show a mediastinal mass. • CT and PET scanning of chest, abdomen and pelvis: permits staging (Box 14.7) and guides management. • Lymph node biopsy: required to confirm the diagnosis.

i	**14.7 Clinical stages of Hodgkin's lymphoma (Ann Arbor classification)**
Stage	Definition
I	Involvement of a single lymph node region or extralymphatic site
II	Involvement of two or more lymph node regions or an extralymphatic site and lymph node regions on the same side of the diaphragm
III	Involvement of lymph node regions on both sides of the diaphragm with or without localised extralymphatic involvement or involvement of the spleen or both
IV	Diffuse involvement of one or more extralymphatic tissues, e.g. liver or bone marrow
A	No systemic symptoms
B	Weight loss >10%, drenching sweats

Management and prognosis

Patients with early-stage disease (stages IA and IIA) should receive chemotherapy combined with radiotherapy. The ABVD regimen (doxorubicin, vinblastine, bleomycin and dacarbazine) is followed by radiotherapy to any involved lymph nodes. Radiotherapy can be omitted in most PET-negative patients to minimise damage to normal tissues. Treatment response is assessed clinically and by repeat CT/PET scanning.

Patients with advanced-stage disease are usually managed with chemotherapy alone. As with early disease, initial PET-negative remission predicts good treatment outcome. Cure rates are lower with advanced disease. Patients with relapsed or resistant disease may be considered for stem cell transplant (p. 572).

Over 90% of patients with early-stage HL achieve complete remission, and most are cured. Some 80% of those with advanced-stage HL can be cured with PET-guided treatment.

Non-Hodgkin lymphoma

NHL represents a monoclonal proliferation of lymphoid cells and may be of B cell (90%) or T cell (10%) origin. It has a peak incidence between 65 and 70 years of age. The most important factor influencing treatment and prognosis is grade.

High-grade NHL: Has high proliferation rates, rapidly produces symptoms and is fatal if untreated, but is potentially curable.

Low-grade NHL: Has low proliferation rates, may be asymptomatic for months to years and runs an indolent course, but is not curable by conventional therapy.

Clinical features

• Lymph node enlargement. • Systemic upset, for example, weight loss, sweats and fever. • Hepatosplenomegaly. • Extranodal disease: more common in NHL, with involvement of the bone marrow, gut, thyroid, lung and skin.

• Bone marrow involvement: more common in low-grade disease than in high-grade disease.

The same staging system (see Box 14.7) is used for both Hodgkin's lymphoma and NHL, but NHL is more likely to be stage III or IV at presentation.

Investigations

These are as for Hodgkin's lymphoma, but in addition patients should undergo: • Bone marrow aspiration and trephine. • Immunophenotyping to distinguish T cell and B cell tumours. • Cytogenetic analysis for translocations. • Urate levels—can cause renal failure during treatment. • HIV testing—a risk factor for lymphoma. • Hepatitis B and C testing—before rituximab therapy.

Management

Low-grade NHL: Asymptomatic patients may not require therapy. Indications for treatment include systemic symptoms, lymphadenopathy causing discomfort and bone marrow failure. Radiotherapy can be used for localised disease. Chemotherapy (cyclophosphamide, vincristine and prednisolone), in combination with rituximab, is first-line therapy. This increases survival but is not curative. High-dose chemotherapy with HSCT extends survival in relapsed disease.

High-grade NHL: The most common form, diffuse large B cell NHL, responds to cyclophosphamide, doxorubicin, vincristine, prednisolone and rituximab. Radiotherapy is used for residual localised disease after chemotherapy, cord compression or localised stage I disease. Autologous HSCT is used in relapsed disease.

Prognosis

Low-grade NHL runs an indolent remitting and relapsing course, with a median survival of 12 years. In high-grade NHL, 5-year survival ranges from 25% to 75% depending on stage and performance status.

Paraproteinaemias

Polyclonal gammopathies occur with infection, inflammation or malignancy. A monoclonal increase in a single immunoglobulin class may occur with normal or reduced levels of the other immunoglobulins. Such monoclonal proteins are called paraproteins or M-proteins.

Monoclonal gammopathy of uncertain significance

In this condition, a paraprotein is present in the blood, without any other features of myeloma. It predominantly affects asymptomatic elderly patients, and blood tests are otherwise normal. No specific treatment is required, but patients should receive annual monitoring to identify progression to myeloma (~1% per annum).

Waldenström's macroglobulinaemia

This rare, low-grade lymphoma occurs in the elderly and is associated with the production of an IgM paraprotein. Patients present with features of hyperviscosity, such as visual disturbance and confusion. Other features include anaemia, systemic symptoms, splenomegaly and lymphadenopathy. Plasma electrophoresis demonstrates an IgM paraprotein, and bone

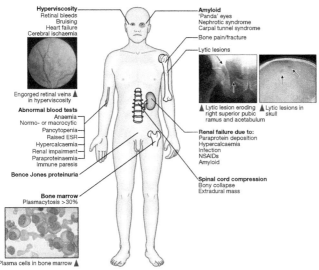

Fig. 14.3 Clinical and laboratory features of multiple myeloma.

marrow aspiration shows infiltration of lymphoid cells. Severe hyperviscosity may require plasmapheresis to remove IgM. Rituximab with chlorambucil or fludarabine is usual treatment.

Multiple myeloma

This is a malignant proliferation of plasma cells and has a peak incidence between the ages of 60 and 70 years. Normal plasma cells are derived from B cells and produce immunoglobulins containing heavy and light chains. In myeloma, plasma cells produce a monoclonal immunoglobulin (paraprotein). Light chains may appear in the urine as Bence Jones proteinuria. IgG is the most common paraprotein type in myeloma.

Clinical features and investigations

The clinical features are shown in Fig. 14.3. The diagnosis of myeloma requires two of the following:
• Increased malignant plasma cells on bone marrow aspiration. • Serum and/or urinary M-protein. • Lytic lesions on skeletal survey.

Other investigations include FBC, U&Es and serum calcium. ESR is usually elevated. Alkaline phosphatase and bone scans are normal in the absence of fractures.

Management

Asymptomatic patients without kidney, marrow or bone damage may not require treatment.

Supportive therapy:
• High fluid intake to treat renal impairment and hypercalcaemia.
• Analgesia for bone pain. • Allopurinol to prevent urate nephropathy.

• Bisphosphonates for hypercalcaemia and to prevent fractures. • Plasmapheresis for hyperviscosity.

Specific therapy: In older patients, thalidomide combined with melphalan and prednisolone has increased the median overall survival to more than 4 years. Thalidomide is both antiangiogenic and immunomodulatory but is highly teratogenic. In younger, fitter patients, chemotherapy is followed by autologous HSCT, which improves quality of life and prolongs survival but does not cure myeloma. Lenalidomide maintenance prolongs initial response. Bortezomib and lenalidomide are used for subsequent progression. Radiotherapy is used for bone pain and cord compression. Long-term bisphosphonates can reduce bone pain and protect bone.

Prognosis

The median survival of patients receiving standard treatment varies from 29 to 62 months, depending on disease stage.

Aplastic anaemias

Primary idiopathic acquired aplastic anaemia

This is a rare disorder in Europe and North America. It is characterised by autoimmune-mediated failure of pluripotent stem cells, resulting in hypoplasia of the bone marrow with pancytopenia. Usually no cause is found but known causes of secondary aplasia should be excluded.

Clinical features and investigations

Patients present with symptoms of bone marrow failure, including anaemia, bleeding and infection. FBC demonstrates pancytopenia with low reticulocytes. Bone marrow aspiration reveals hypocellularity.

Management

Patients require supportive treatment with red cell and platelet transfusions and aggressive management of infection. The curative treatment for patients younger than 35 years of age is allogeneic HSCT, which offers a 75% to 90% chance of long-term cure. Immunosuppressive therapy with antithymocyte globulin and ciclosporin is used in older patients.

Secondary aplastic anaemia

Causes of secondary aplastic anaemia are listed in Box 14.8. In some instances, the cytopenia is more selective and affects only one cell line, most often neutrophils. Clinical features and investigations are the same as for primary aplastic anaemia. Any underlying cause should be addressed.

Myeloproliferative neoplasms

These chronic conditions are characterised by clonal proliferation of marrow precursor cells, and include polycythaemia rubra vera (PRV), essential thrombocythaemia, myelofibrosis and CML (p. 576). Although most patients have one of these disorders, some have overlapping features or progress from one to another, for example, PRV to myelofibrosis. A mutation in the gene encoding the signal transduction molecule JAK-2 has been found in more than 90% of PRV cases and 50% of those with essential thrombocythaemia and myelofibrosis.

14.8 Causes of secondary aplastic anaemia

- Drugs:
    Cytotoxic drugs
    Antibiotics: chloramphenicol, sulphonamides
    Antirheumatic agents: penicillamine, gold
    Antithyroid drugs
    Anticonvulsants
    Immunosuppressives: azathioprine
- Chemicals:
    Benzene toluene solvent misuse: glue-sniffing
    Insecticides: organophosphates
- Radiation
- Viral hepatitis
- Pregnancy
- Paroxysmal nocturnal haemoglobinuria

Myelofibrosis

In myelofibrosis, the marrow is initially hypercellular, with an excess of abnormal megakaryocytes that release growth factors, resulting in fibroblast proliferation. As the disease progresses, the marrow becomes fibrosed.

Clinical features

Most patients present over the age of 50 years with fatigue, weight loss and night sweats. The spleen may be massively enlarged as a result of extramedullary haematopoiesis, and painful splenic infarcts may occur.

Investigations

There is anaemia with a leucoerythroblastic blood picture (circulating immature red cells and granulocyte precursors). The WCC and platelet count may be high, normal or low. Increased cell turnover commonly leads to high urate levels and folate deficiency. Bone marrow is often difficult to aspirate; trephine biopsy shows replacement by fibrous tissue. Finding the JAK-2 mutation supports the diagnosis.

Management

Supportive treatment includes transfusions for anaemia. Folic acid should be given to prevent deficiency. Hydroxycarbamide may help reduce the WCC and spleen size, but splenectomy may be required for massive splenomegaly. HSCT may be considered in younger patients. Ruxolitinib, a JAK-2 inhibitor, reduces systemic symptoms and splenomegaly. Survival is variable, with a median of 4 years.

Essential thrombocythaemia

Uncontrolled proliferation of megakaryocytes results in increased circulating platelets that are often dysfunctional. Reactive causes of increased platelets must be excluded before making the diagnosis. The JAK-2 mutation supports the diagnosis but is not universal. Patients present at a median

14

age of 60 years with vascular occlusion or bleeding events. A small percentage transform to acute leukaemia or myelofibrosis.

Aspirin should be considered for all patients to reduce the risk of thrombosis. Hydroxycarbamide may be used to control high platelet counts.

Polycythaemia rubra vera

PRV occurs mainly in patients over the age of 40 years. It is characterised by increased erythropoiesis caused by a primary increase in marrow activity.

Clinical features

Patients present with an incidental finding of a high Hb, or with symptoms of hyperviscosity such as lassitude, headaches, dizziness and pruritus. Some present with manifestations of peripheral arterial disease or a cerebrovascular accident. There is an increased risk of VTE. Peptic ulceration is common and is sometimes complicated by bleeding. Patients are often plethoric and have splenomegaly.

Investigations

The investigation of polycythaemia is covered on p. 554. High Hct plus the *JAK-2* mutation usually makes the diagnosis. In *JAK-2* mutation–negative cases, secondary polycythaemia (see Box 14.1) should be excluded. Neutrophil and platelet counts are often raised.

Management and prognosis

Aspirin reduces the risk of thrombosis. Venesection relieves hyperviscosity symptoms and should be repeated to maintain the Hct lower than 45%.

Hydroxycarbamide or interferon alfa can be used to suppress the underlying myeloproliferation. Radioactive phosphorus (^{32}P) is reserved for older patients, as it increases the risk of transformation to acute leukaemia six- to tenfold. Median survival exceeds 10 years. Conversion to myelofibrosis or acute leukaemia occurs in 15%.

Bleeding disorders

Disorders of primary haemostasis

Platelet functional disorders, thrombocytopenia, von Willebrand's disease and diseases affecting the vessel wall may all result in failure of platelet plug formation in primary haemostasis.

Vessel wall abnormalities

Hereditary haemorrhagic telangiectasia

This is a dominantly inherited condition characterised by abnormalities of vascular modelling.

Telangiectasia and small aneurysms occur on the fingertips, on the face, in the nasal passages, on the tongue, in the lung and in the GI tract. Many patients develop larger pulmonary arteriovenous malformations that cause arterial hypoxaemia and are associated with stroke and cerebral abscess as a result of paradoxical embolism; these should be treated by percutaneous embolisation. Patients present with recurrent bleeds (particularly epistaxis) or with iron deficiency as a result of occult GI bleeding.

Treatment includes iron therapy and local cautery or laser therapy to prevent lesions from bleeding.

Thrombocytopenia

Causes of thrombocytopenia are listed in Box 14.4, and treatment is discussed on p. 559.

Idiopathic thrombocytopenic purpura

The presence of autoantibodies directed against platelets results in platelet destruction. Spontaneous bleeding occurs mainly with platelet counts lower than 20×10^9/L. At higher counts, the patient may complain of easy bruising, epistaxis or menorrhagia. Many cases with counts higher than 50×10^9/L are discovered by chance.

In adults, ITP more commonly affects females and may have an insidious onset. Unlike ITP in children, there is usually no history of a preceding viral infection. Patients aged older than 65 years should have a bone marrow examination to exclude an accompanying B cell malignancy and autoantibody testing if connective tissue disease is likely. HIV testing should be considered. There is a greatly reduced platelet count, and the bone marrow reveals increased megakaryocytes.

Management

Most cases of childhood ITP are self-limiting and resolve within a few weeks. Indications for oral prednisolone include severe purpura, bruising or epistaxis, and a platelet count less than 10×10^9/L. Adults are also treated with prednisolone, although this is often less effective than in children. IV IgG raises the platelet count and is indicated if the bleeding is immediately life-threatening. Persistent or potentially life-threatening bleeding should be treated with platelet transfusion. Splenectomy should be considered for relapsing disease.

14

Coagulation disorders

Coagulation factor disorders can arise from deficiency of a single factor (usually congenital, e.g. haemophilia A) or of multiple factors (often acquired, e.g. liver disease).

Congenital bleeding disorders

Haemophilia A

Factor VIII deficiency (haemophilia A) is the most common congenital coagulation disorder. It affects 1:10 000 individuals. Factor VIII is manufactured by liver and endothelial cells; the gene is located on the X chromosome. Haemophilia A is inherited as an X-linked recessive disorder, and patients are therefore male. All daughters of haemophiliacs are carriers. If a carrier has a son, he will have a 50% chance of having haemophilia, and a daughter will have a 50% chance of being a carrier. Antenatal screening is possible in affected families.

i 14.9 Severity of haemophilia		
Degree of severity	Factor VIII or IX level	Clinical presentation
Severe	<0.01 U/mL	Spontaneous haemarthroses and muscle haematomas
Moderate	0.01–0.05 U/mL	Mild trauma or surgery causes haematomas
Mild	>0.05–0.4 U/mL	Major injury or surgery results in excess bleeding

Clinical features and investigations

The diagnosis is normally made after the age of 6 months, when babies become more mobile and first experience bruising or haemarthrosis. The features of haemophilia A are related to the plasma factor VIII level (Box 14.9). Individuals with severe haemophilia experience recurrent haemarthroses in large joints, which over time lead to chronic haemophilic arthropathy. Although joints and muscles are the most common sites for haemorrhage, bleeding can occur at almost any site. Intracranial haemorrhage is often fatal.

Management

In affluent countries, treatment is based on prophylactic coagulation factor replacement with recombinant factor concentrates, which reduces bleeding episodes in men with severe haemophilia, preventing joint damage, the major long-term morbidity.

In less affluent countries, bleeding episodes are treated with factor VIII concentrate. Freeze-dried factor VIII concentrates can be stored at 4°C in domestic refrigerators, and many patients are therefore able to treat themselves at home. The concentrates are prepared from blood donor plasma that has been screened for hepatitis B, hepatitis C and HIV, and has undergone a viral inactivation process during manufacture. Recombinant factor VIII concentrates are also widely available now and, although more expensive, carry less infection risk than those derived from plasma. In individuals with mild haemophilia A, IV or intranasal desmopressin can be used to increase factor VIII levels. This is often sufficient to treat a mild bleed or cover minor surgery such as dental extraction.

Complications of therapy

Before 1986, concentrates were not virally inactivated, and many patients became infected with hepatitis B, hepatitis C or HIV. All potential recipients of pooled blood products should therefore be offered hepatitis A and B immunisation. There is now concern that variant CJD may be transmissible via pooled plasma products, so these are now prepared from plasma from countries with a low incidence of bovine spongiform encephalopathy.

The other serious consequence of factor VIII infusion is the development of antifactor VIII antibodies, which arise in around 20% to 30% of severe haemophiliacs. Such antibodies rapidly neutralise therapeutic infusions, making treatment relatively ineffective. Infusion of factor VIIa may stop bleeding.

Haemophilia B (Christmas disease)

This is caused by deficiency of factor IX and is also an X-linked condition. The disorder is clinically indistinguishable from haemophilia A but is less common. Treatment is with factor IX concentrate.

Von Willebrand's disease

Von Willebrand's disease is a common but usually mild bleeding disorder with autosomal dominant inheritance. Von Willebrand factor (vWF) is a protein that performs two principal functions:
• It acts as a carrier protein for factor VIII; deficiency of vWF therefore results in a secondary reduction in the plasma factor VIII level. • It facilitates platelet binding to subendothelial collagen; deficiency therefore also leads to impaired platelet plug formation.

Clinical features

Patients present with haemorrhagic manifestations similar to those in individuals with reduced platelet function. Superficial bruising, epistaxis, menorrhagia and GI haemorrhage are common. Bleeding episodes are usually far less common and severe than in severe haemophilia.

Investigations

There is a reduced level of vWF, with secondary reduction in factor VIII. Mutation analysis is informative in most cases.

Management

• Mild haemorrhage: desmopressin, which raises the vWF level. • Mucosal bleeding: tranexamic acid. • Severe bleeding: factor VIII/vWF concentrates.

Acquired bleeding disorders

Disseminated intravascular coagulation

DIC may cause bleeding but begins with intravascular coagulation and is covered on (p. 590)

Liver disease

In severe parenchymal liver disease, bleeding may arise from many different causes. These include reduced synthesis of coagulation factors, DIC and thrombocytopenia secondary to hypersplenism. Cholestatic jaundice reduces vitamin K absorption and leads to deficiency of factors II, VII, IX and X. This deficiency can be treated with parenteral vitamin K.

Renal disease

Advanced renal failure is associated with platelet dysfunction and bleeding, especially GI bleeding.

Thrombotic disorders

Venous thromboembolism

Predisposing conditions for VTE are listed in Box 14.10. Although the most common presentations are deep vein thrombosis (DVT, p. 70)

14.10 Factors predisposing to venous thrombosis

Patient factors

- Increasing age
- Obesity
- Varicose veins
- Family history of unprovoked VTE when young
- Previous DVT
- Pregnancy/puerperium
- Oestrogens: oral contraceptives, HRT
- Immobility
- IV drug use (femoral vein)

Surgical conditions

- Major surgery, especially >30 minutes' duration
- Abdominal or pelvic surgery, especially for cancer
- Major lower limb orthopaedic surgery, e.g. joint replacement and hip fracture surgery

Medical conditions

- MI
- Heart failure
- Inflammatory bowel disease
- Malignancy
- Nephrotic syndrome
- Pneumonia
- Neurological conditions causing immobility, e.g. stroke, paraplegia

Haematological disorders

- Polycythaemia rubra vera
- Essential thrombocythaemia
- Deficiency of antithrombin, proteins C and S
- Paroxysmal nocturnal haemoglobinuria
- Prothrombotic mutations: factor V Leiden, prothrombin gene *G20210A*
- Myelofibrosis
- Lupus anticoagulant
- Anticardiolipin antibody

and/or pulmonary embolism (p. 84), similar principles apply to jugular vein thrombosis, upper limb DVT, cerebral sinus thrombosis (p. 666) and intra-abdominal venous thrombosis.

VTE has an annual incidence of approximately 1:1000 in Western populations. All forms of VTE are increasingly common with age, and many of the deaths are related to coexisting medical conditions, such as cancer or inflammatory disease, that predispose the patient to thrombosis in the first place.

Management of VTE

The mainstay of treatment is anticoagulation. Conventionally, LMWH is followed by a coumarin such as warfarin. Treatment of acute VTE with LMWH

14.11 Antithrombotic prophylaxis

Patients in the following categories should be considered for specific antithrombotic prophylaxis:

Moderate risk of DVT

- Major surgery in patients >40 years of age or with other risk factor
- Major medical illness, e.g. heart failure, sepsis, malignancy, inflammatory bowel disease, stroke or other reason for immobility

High risk of DVT

- Major abdominal or pelvic surgery for malignancy or with history of DVT or known thrombophilia
- Specific surgical risk: major hip or knee surgery, neurosurgery

should continue for a minimum of 5 days. Patients treated with warfarin should achieve a target INR of 2.5 (range 2–3) with LMWH continuing until the INR is greater than 2. Alternatively, patients may be treated with a DOAC (p. 565). Rivaroxaban and apixaban may be used immediately from diagnosis, without the need for LMWH. In patients with cancer underlying VTE, maintenance anticoagulation with LMWH reduces recurrence.

Patients with VTE provoked by a temporary risk factor that is then removed can be treated for short periods (e.g. 3 months); anticoagulation for more than 6 months does not alter recurrence rate following discontinuation. If there are unchangeable ongoing risk factors, for example, active cancer, long-term anticoagulation is usually recommended, provided bleeding risk is not excessive.

In unprovoked VTE, the optimum duration of anticoagulation can be difficult to establish. Recurrence of VTE is about 2% to 3% per annum in patients with a temporary risk factor and 7% to 10% per annum in those with apparently unprovoked VTE. This plateaus at around 30% to 40% at 5 years. Therefore many patients with unprovoked episodes of VTE will benefit from long-term anticoagulation. The strongest predictors of recurrence after unprovoked VTE are male sex and a positive D-dimer measured 1 month after stopping anticoagulants.

Prevention of venous thrombosis

All patients admitted to hospital should be assessed for their risk of developing VTE (Box 14.11). Early mobilisation of all patients is important to prevent DVTs. Patients at medium or high risk may require additional antithrombotic measures such as graduated compression stockings and LMWH; those at high risk may need prolonged prophylaxis.

Several inherited conditions predispose to VTE; none of them is strongly associated with arterial thrombosis, however. All carry a slightly increased risk in pregnancy. Apart from antithrombin deficiency and homozygous factor V Leiden, most carriers will never have an episode of VTE. Detection of these abnormalities does not predict recurrence of VTE. None of these conditions per se requires treatment with anticoagulants, unless thrombosis occurs or particular risk factors are also present.

14.12 Antiphospholipid syndrome

Clinical manifestations

- Adverse pregnancy outcome
  - Recurrent first trimester abortion (≥3)
  - Unexplained death of morphologically normal fetus after 10 weeks' gestation
  - Severe early preeclampsia
- Venous thromboembolism
- Arterial thromboembolism
- Livedo reticularis, catastrophic antiphospholipid syndrome, transverse myelitis, skin necrosis, chorea

Conditions associated with secondary antiphospholipid syndrome

- Systemic lupus erythematosus
- Rheumatoid arthritis
- Systemic sclerosis
- Behçet's disease
- Temporal arteritis
- Sjögren's syndrome

Targets for antiphospholipid antibodies

- β_2-glycoprotein 1
- Protein C
- Annexin V
- Prothrombin (may result in haemorrhagic presentation)

Antithrombin deficiency: Antithrombin is a protein that inactivates factors IIa (thrombin), IXa, Xa and XIa. Its activity is greatly potentiated by heparin. Familial deficiency of antithrombin is an autosomal dominant disorder that is associated with a marked predisposition to VTE.

Protein C and S deficiencies: Protein C and S are natural anticoagulants involved in switching off coagulation factor activation (factors Va and VIIIa) and thrombin generation. Inherited deficiency of either protein C or S therefore results in a prothrombotic state.

Factor V Leiden: Factor V Leiden results from a mutation that prevents the cleavage and hence inactivation of activated factor V. This causes a relative risk of venous thrombosis of 5 in heterozygotes and >50 in rare homozygotes.

Antiphospholipid syndrome: In this syndrome, antiphospholipid antibodies (which include lupus anticoagulant and anticardiolipin antibodies) interact with the coagulation cascade, causing arterial and venous thromboembolism. The syndrome sometimes occurs alone (primary antiphospholipid syndrome) or as a complication of rheumatic disease, for example, systemic lupus erythematosus (secondary antiphospholipid syndrome). Clinical features and associations are summarised in Box 14.12.

Disseminated intravascular coagulation

DIC can be initiated by many conditions, including infections, malignancy, drug toxicity, burns and obstetric problems (e.g. placental abruption, amniotic fluid embolism). Systemic activation of the pathways involved in coagulation and its regulation, either via cytokine pathways or by tissue factor, causes the generation of intravascular fibrin clots leading to multi-organ failure, with simultaneous coagulation factor and platelet consumption causing bleeding. This may be exacerbated by activation of the fibrinolytic system secondary to the deposition of fibrin.

Investigations

• Thrombocytopenia. • Prolonged PT and APTT caused by coagulation factor deficiency. • Low fibrinogen. • Increased levels of D-dimer (a fibrin degradation product).

Management

Therapy should be aimed at treating the underlying condition causing DIC (e.g. IV antibiotics for septicaemia). Blood products such as platelets and/ or FFP should be given to control active bleeding.

Thrombotic thrombocytopenic purpura

This is a rare autoimmune disorder in which thrombosis is accompanied by paradoxical thrombocytopenia. It is characterised by five features:
• Thrombocytopenia. • Microangiopathic haemolytic anaemia. • Neurological sequelae. • Fever. • Renal impairment.

Microvascular occlusion by platelet thrombi affects the brain, kidneys and other organs. It may occur alone or in association with drugs (ticlopidine, ciclosporin), HIV, Shiga toxins and malignancy. Treatment is by emergency plasma exchange; glucocorticoids, aspirin and rituximab also have a role. Untreated, mortality rates are 90% in the first 10 days.

14

Rheumatology and bone disease

Disorders of the musculoskeletal system affect all ages and ethnic groups, accounting for around 25% of general practice consultations in the UK. Musculoskeletal diseases affect bones, joints, muscles or connective tissues such as skin and tendon, causing pain and impairment of locomotor function. They are the most common cause of physical disability in older people.

Presenting problems in musculoskeletal disease

Acute monoarthritis

The most important causes of acute arthritis in a single joint are crystal arthritis, sepsis, spondyloarthritis (SpA) and oligoarticular juvenile idiopathic arthritis (JIA; p. 616). Other potential causes are shown in Box 15.1. Gout classically affects the first MTP joint, whereas the hand/wrist ankle, knee or hip are typical sites for pseudogout. Rapid onset (6–12 hours) favours crystal arthritis; joint sepsis develops slowly and progresses until treated. Haemarthrosis typically causes a large effusion in an injured joint. Recent diarrhoeal illness or genital infection suggests reactive arthritis, whereas intercurrent illness, dehydration or surgery may trigger crystal-induced arthritis.

Joint aspiration with or without washout is normally required to exclude sepsis and to look for crystals. Serum uric acid is usually raised in gout but may be normal. Ruling out primary hyperparathyroidism is essential if there is pseudogout.

Polyarthritis

Polyarthritis is inflammation affecting five or more joints. Inflammatory arthritis causes early morning stiffness and worsening of symptoms with inactivity, along with synovial swelling and tenderness on examination. The pattern of joint involvement and associated features help to determine the underlying

Clinical examination of the musculoskeletal system

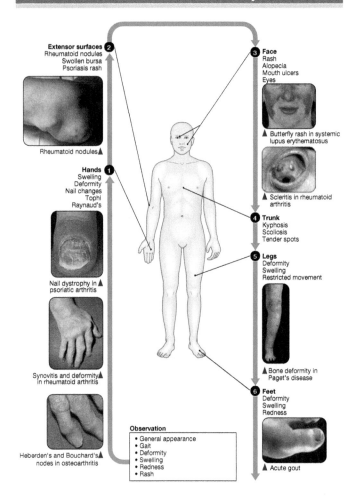

Extensor surfaces 2
Rheumatoid nodules
Swollen bursa
Psoriasis rash

Rheumatoid nodules ▲

Hands 1
Swelling
Deformity
Nail changes
Tophi
Raynaud's

Nail dystrophy in ▲
psoriatic arthritis

Synovitis and deformity ▲
in rheumatoid arthritis

Heberden's and Bouchard's ▲
nodes in osteoarthritis

Face 3
Rash
Alopecia
Mouth ulcers
Eyes

▲ Butterfly rash in systemic
lupus erythematosus

▲ Scleritis in rheumatoid
arthritis

Trunk 4
Kyphosis
Scoliosis
Tender spots

Legs 5
Deformity
Swelling
Restricted movement

▲ Bone deformity in
Paget's disease

Feet 6
Deformity
Swelling
Redness

▲ Acute gout

Observation
• General appearance
• Gait
• Deformity
• Swelling
• Redness
• Rash

15.1 Causes of acute monoarthritis

Common

- Septic arthritis
- Gout
- Pseudogout
- Trauma
- Haemarthrosis
- Spondyloarthritis
- Psoriatic arthritis
- Reactive arthritis
- Enteropathic arthritis

Less common

- Rheumatoid arthritis
- Juvenile idiopathic arthritis
- Pigmented villonodular synovitis
- Foreign body reaction
- Gonococcal infection
- Tuberculosis
- Leukaemia
- Osteomyelitis

cause (Box 15.2). RA is characterised by symmetrical involvement of the small joints of the hands and feet, wrists, ankles and knees. PsA is strongly associated with enthesitis and nail pitting. Asymmetry, lower limb predominance and greater involvement of large joints are characteristic of spondyloarthritis.

Blood should be checked for inflammatory markers and viral serology. USS or MRI is used to detect synovitis. Treatment is that of the underlying condition.

Fracture

Fractures are a common presenting symptom of osteoporosis but also occur with metastases, osteopenia and in normal bone.

Clinical Assessment

There is localised bone pain, worsened by movement, usually with a history of trauma; however, spontaneous fractures can occur in severe osteoporosis. Fractures are distinguished from soft tissue injury by marked pain and swelling, abnormal movement, crepitus or deformity. Femoral neck fractures produce a shortened, painful, externally rotated leg.

Investigations

X-rays in two planes should be examined for discontinuity of the cortical outline. They may also reveal underlying osteoporosis, Paget's disease or osteomalacia.

Management

This involves adequate pain relief, reduction of the fracture and immobilisation, using a cast or splint, or by internal fixation. Femoral neck fractures often require joint replacement surgery.

| **i** | **15.2 Causes of polyarthritis** |

Cause	Characteristics
Rheumatoid arthritis	Symmetrical, any joint, upper and lower limbs
Viral arthritis	Symmetrical, small joints; with rash and prodromal illness
Osteoarthritis	Symmetrical, targets DIP joints in hands, knees, hips, back and neck; Heberden's and Bouchard's nodes
Psoriatic arthritis	Asymmetrical, targets PIP and DIP joints of hands and feet, nail pitting, large joints also affected
Axial spondylarthritis and enteropathic arthritis	Large joints, lower > upper limbs, possible history of back pain
Systemic lupus erythematosus	Symmetrical, small joints, synovitis unusual
Juvenile idiopathic arthritis	Symmetrical, any joint, upper and lower limbs
Chronic gout	Distal > proximal joints, acute attacks
Chronic sarcoidosis	Symmetrical, any joint
Calcium pyrophosphate arthritis	Chronic polyarthritis of hands, wrists, ankles, knees

Generalised musculoskeletal pain

The differential diagnosis includes:
• Malignant disease with bone metastases: relentlessly progressive pain with weight loss. • Paget's disease: usually more focal and localised to the site of involvement. • osteoarthritis (OA): localised to affected sites, for example, lumbar spine, hips, knees and hands. • Osteomalacia: generalised bone pain and tenderness with limb girdle weakness. • Fibromyalgia: generalised pain particularly affecting the trunk, back and neck.

Regional musculoskeletal pain

Back pain

Back pain is extremely common. In the UK, 7% of the adult population consult their GP each year with back pain.

Clinical assessment

The aim of history and examination is to distinguish the few patients with serious spinal pathology from the majority who have self-limiting mechanical pain.

Mechanical pain: This accounts for more than 90% of back pain episodes, usually affecting patients aged 20 to 55 years. It is more common in heavy manual workers, and often starts suddenly while lifting or bending. Symptoms are worsened by activity and relieved by rest. Pain is typically asymmetrical and confined to the lumbosacral region, buttock or thigh, with no clear-cut nerve root distribution (unlike radicular pain). Examination may reveal paraspinal muscle spasm with painful restriction of movement. Prognosis is good, with 90% recovery at 6 weeks. Psychological factors (e.g. job dissatisfaction, depression) increase the risk of progression to chronic disability.

Pain because of serious pathology: Causes include bony destruction because of malignancy, fracture or infection. 'Red flag' features suggesting serious spinal pathology include: • Age younger than 20 or older than 50 years. • Constant, progressive pain unrelieved by rest. • Thoracic pain. • History or symptoms of malignancy or TB. • Systemic glucocorticoid use. • Constitutional symptoms: sweats, malaise, weight loss.

Examination: Examination may reveal painful spinal deformity with signs at multiple nerve root levels. In all cases it is important to exclude signs of cauda equina syndrome (see later).

Degenerative disc disease: This causes nerve root pain (Box 15.3) in young adults, most commonly at L4 or L5. Around 70% of patients improve by 4 weeks. Compression of multiple nerve roots in the cauda equina occurs in Paget's disease and spinal OA and requires urgent treatment.

Inflammatory pain: Pain attributed to spondylitis is gradual in onset and often occurs before the age of 40 years. It is associated with morning stiffness and improves with movement. Spondylolisthesis may cause back pain that is typically aggravated by standing and walking.

Investigations

Investigations are not required for mechanical back pain. Those with persistent pain (>6 weeks) or 'red flags' should undergo MRI, which can demonstrate spinal stenosis, cord or nerve root compression, inflammatory axial spondyloarthritis, malignancy or sepsis. Plain X-rays can be of value if vertebral compression fractures, OA and degenerative disc disease are suspected. If metastatic disease is suspected, bone scintigraphy is useful. Additional investigations include:

15

15.3 Features of radicular pain

Nerve root pain

- Unilateral leg pain worse than low back pain
- Radiates beyond knee
- Paraesthesia in same distribution
- Nerve irritation signs (reduced straight leg raising, reproduces pain)
- Motor, sensory or reflex signs (limited to one nerve root)

Cauda equina syndrome

- Difficulty with micturition
- Loss of anal sphincter tone or faecal incontinence
- Saddle anaesthesia
- Gait disturbance
- Pain, numbness or weakness affecting one or both legs

i 15.4	Causes of neck pain
Mechanical	Postural, 'whiplash', disc prolapse, cervical spondylosis
Inflammatory	Infection, spondylarthritis, rheumatoid arthritis, polymyalgia rheumatica
Neoplasia	Metastases, myeloma, lymphoma, intrathecal tumours
Other	Fibromyalgia, torticollis
Referred pain	Pharynx, teeth, angina, Pancoast's tumour, cervical lymph nodes

• Biochemistry and haematology, including ESR and CRP (for sepsis and inflammatory disease). • Protein and urinary electrophoresis (for myeloma). • Prostate-specific antigen (for prostate carcinoma).

Management

Treatment of mechanical back pain involves reassurance, education, simple analgesia and early mobilisation. Bed rest is not helpful and increases the risk of chronic disability. Physiotherapy may be required in individuals not settling with the above measures. Surgery is required for less than 1% of patients. The management of serious spinal pathology is dictated by the cause.

Neck pain

Neck pain is a common symptom that can occur following injury, after falling asleep in an awkward position, as a result of stress or in association with OA of the spine. Causes are shown in Box 15.4. Most cases resolve spontaneously or with a short course of NSAID or analgesics, or some exercise therapy. Patients with persistent pain in a nerve root distribution and those with neurological signs and symptoms should be referred for an MRI scan and, if necessary, a neurosurgical opinion.

Shoulder pain

Rotator cuff syndrome: In this common condition, tendinitis or bursitis around the glenohumeral joint causes pain that is reproduced by resisted movement. Treatment is by physiotherapy, analgesia and glucocorticoid injections.

Adhesive capsulitis ('frozen shoulder'): This presents with pain associated with marked restriction of elevation and external rotation. Adhesive capsulitis is commonly associated with diabetes mellitus and neck/radicular lesions. Treatment comprises analgesia, local glucocorticoid injection and regular 'pendulum' exercises of the arm. Complete recovery sometimes takes up to 2 years. For severe or persistent symptoms, joint distension and manipulation under anaesthesia may help.

Elbow pain

Common causes are shown in Box 15.5. Olecranon bursitis may also complicate infection, gout and RA. Management is by rest, analgesics and topical or systemic NSAIDs. Local glucocorticoid injection is used in resistant cases.

i	**15.5 Local causes of elbow pain**	
Lesion	Pain	Examination findings, tests
Lateral humeral epicon-dylitis 'Tennis elbow'	Lateral epicondyle Radiation to extensor forearm	Tenderness over epicondyle- Pain reproduced by resisted active wrist extension
Medial humeral epicon-dylitis 'Golfer's elbow'	Medial epicondyle Radiation to flexor forearm	Tenderness over epicondyle- Pain reproduced by resisted active wrist flexion
Olecranon bursitis	Olecranon	Tender swelling

Hand and wrist pain

Pain from hand or wrist joints is localised to the affected joint, except for pain from the first carpometacarpal joint, which often radiates down the thumb and to the radial aspect of the wrist. Nonarticular causes of hand pain include:

• Tenosynovitis: affects flexor or extensor tendons; pain and tenderness over lesions, 'claw-like' morning stiffness. De Quervain's tenosynovitis involves the tendon sheaths of abductor pollicis longus and extensor pollicis brevis. It produces pain and tenderness maximal over the radial aspect of the distal forearm and wrist and marked pain on forced ulnar deviation of the wrist with the thumb held across the patient's palm. • Raynaud's phenomenon (digital vasospasm triggered mostly by cold). • C6, 7 or 8 radiculopathy. • Carpal tunnel syndrome: hand position-dependent and/or nocturnal pain, numbness and paraesthesia of thumb and second to fourth digits.

Lower limb pain

Common causes of lower limb pain are shown in Box 15.6.

15

Muscle pain and weakness

It is important to distinguish between a subjective feeling of generalised weakness or fatigue, and 'true' weakness with objective loss of muscle power. The former is a non-specific manifestation of many systemic conditions. Proximal muscle weakness causes difficulty in standing from a seated position, walking up steps, squatting and lifting overhead. Causes of proximal myopathy are listed in Box 15.7. Weakness should be graded on the MRC 6-point scale (0 = no power, 5 = full power).

Investigations include biochemistry and haematology, ESR, CRP and CK. Serum 25(OH) vitamin D, parathyroid hormone, serology for parvovirus, hepatitis B/C and HIV, serum and urine electrophoresis and autoantibodies including ANA and anti-Jo-1 should also be checked. Muscle biopsy (guided by MRI detection of abnormal muscle) and EMG are usually required to make the diagnosis. If underlying malignancy is suspected, CT chest/abdo/pelvis and upper and lower GI endoscopy are often required.

i	**15.6 Common causes of lower limb pain**	
Lesion	**Pain**	**Examination findings**
Trochanteric bursitis	Upper lateral thigh, worse on lying on that side at night	Tender over greater trochanter
Adductor tendinitis	Upper inner thigh Usually clearly sports-related	Tender over adductor origin/tendon/muscle Pain reproduced by resisted active hip adduction
Prepatellar bursitis	Anterior patella	Tender fluctuant swelling in front of patella
Popliteal cyst (Baker's cyst)	Popliteal fossa	Tender swelling of popliteal fossa, usually reducible by massage with knee in mid-flexion
Plantar fasciitis	Under heel, worse on standing and walking	Tender under distal calcaneus/plantar fascia insertion site
Osteochondritis (Osgood–Schlatter disease)	Anterior upper tibia	Affects adolescents Pain on resisted active knee extension
Achilles tendinitis	Localised to tendon	Tender on squeezing tendon Pain reproduced by standing on toes or resisted plantar flexion

i	**15.7 Causes of proximal muscle pain and weakness**
Inflammatory	Polymyositis, dermatomyositis, polymyalgia rheumatica
Endocrine	Hypothyroidism, hyperthyroidism, Cushing's syndrome, Addison's disease
Metabolic	Myophosphorylase/phosophofructokinase deficiency, hypokalaemia, osteomalacia
Drugs/toxins	Alcohol, glucocorticoids, fibrates, statins, cocaine, penicillamine, zidovudine
Infections	HIV, cytomegalovirus, Epstein–Barr virus, staphylococci, TB, schistosomiasis

Principles of management of rheumatological disorders

Key aims of management of rheumatological conditions are:
• Patient education. • Pain control. • Optimisation of function. • Beneficial modification of the disease process.

These therapeutic objectives are achieved most effectively via a multidisciplinary team approach.

Non-pharmacological interventions

Patient education: This has been shown to reduce pain and disability. Local strengthening exercise should be combined with aerobic and local strengthening exercises to maximise benefit. Adverse mechanical factors should be addressed; examples include shock-absorbing footwear, walking aids and weight loss in obese patients. Tuition in coping strategies (e.g. yoga, relaxation, avoidance of maladaptive pain behaviour) can assist patients with incurable disease.

Physical and occupational therapy: Local heat, ice packs, hydrotherapy, wax baths and local external applications can induce muscle relaxation with temporary relief of symptoms in many rheumatic diseases. Manipulative techniques may help improve restricted movement. Splints can give temporary rest and support for painful joints and periarticular tissues. Orthoses are more permanent appliances used to reduce instability and abnormal movement. They are particularly suited to severely disabled patients in whom surgery is inappropriate, and often need to be custom-made. An assessment by an occupational therapist can identify aids to help patients with activities of daily living. Examples include a raised toilet seat or chair, extended tap handles, thick-handled cutlery, and devices to pull on tights and socks.

Surgery: Soft tissue release and tenosynovectomy may reduce inflammatory symptoms and improve function. Synovectomy does not prevent disease progression but may provide pain relief when other measures have failed. Surgery may involve osteotomy (cutting bone to alter joint mechanics), excision arthroplasty (removing part or all of the joint), joint replacement or arthrodesis (joint fusion).

Pharmacological treatment

Analgesia

Paracetamol is effective for the treatment of mild to moderate pain. It acts by inhibiting central prostaglandin synthesis but has little effect on peripheral prostaglandin production. It is safe, has few contraindications and drug interactions, and is low in cost. It is therefore an appropriate first-line analgesic in most patients. If paracetamol fails to control pain, it can be combined with codeine (in co-codamol) or dihydrocodeine (in co-dydramol). The centrally acting analgesics tramadol and meptazinol are used for temporary control of unresponsive severe pain. Although these drugs are more effective than paracetamol, side effects include constipation, headache, confusion, dizziness and somnolence, especially in the elderly. Withdrawal symptoms may occur after chronic use. The nonopioid nefopam (30–90 mg three times daily) can help moderate pain, although side effects (nausea, anxiety, dry mouth) limit its use. Patients with severe pain may require oxycodone and morphine, but risk of dependency should be considered.

Non-steroidal anti-inflammatory drugs

NSAIDs (e.g. ibuprofen, diclofenac) are effective in combating pain and stiffness associated with inflammatory disease. They also help reduce bone pain because of metastatic deposits. They act by inhibiting COX

15

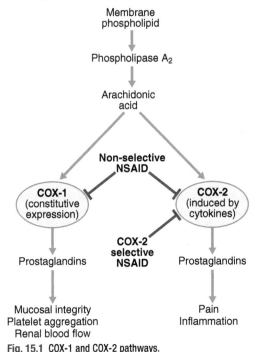

Fig. 15.1 COX-1 and COX-2 pathways.

and thereby reducing prostaglandin synthesis (Fig. 15.1). There are two isoforms of COX, encoded by distinct genes. The main side effects of NSAIDs are GI ulceration, bleeding and perforation and renal impairment. Dosage and toxicity of commonly used NSAIDs are summarised in Box 15.8.

Disease-modifying antirheumatic drugs

DMARDs are small-molecule inhibitors of the immune response used to treat many rheumatic diseases. The most common drugs and indications are summarised in Box 15.9. Most can cause bone marrow suppression or liver dysfunction, so they require regular blood monitoring.

Glucocorticoids

Glucocorticoids have powerful antiinflammatory and immunosuppressive effects. They are used orally, intravenously, intramuscularly and by intra-articular injection in the treatment of many rheumatic diseases. High dose systemic therapy is used to induce remission and to treat disease flares in RA, JIA, AxSpA, PsA, polymyalgia rheumatica, vasculitis and SLE.

i	15.8 Commonly used NSAIDs and their GI risk profile		
Drug	**Daily adult dose**	**Doses/ day**	**Idiosyncratic side-effects, comments**
Low risk			
Celecoxib	100–200 mg	1-2	Selective COX-2 inhibitor
Etoricoxib	60–120 mg	1	Selective COX-2 inhibitor
Medium risk			
Ibuprofen	1600–2400 mg	3 – 4	Gastrointestinal adverse effects more likely than with COX-2 inhibitors, even with PPI therapy
Naproxen	500–1000 mg	1 – 2	
Diclofenac	75–150 mg	2 – 3	
High risk			
Indometacin	50–200 mg	3 – 4	High incidence of dyspepsia and CNS side-effects
Ketoprofen	100–200 mg	2 – 4	
Piroxicam	20–30 mg	1-2	Restricted use in those >60 years

i	15.9 Commonly used disease-modifying antirheumatic drugs		
Drug	**Disease indications**	**Side effects (N.B. All can cause rash and GI upset.)**	**Monitoring requirement[a]**
Methotrexate	RA, PsA, AxSpA, JIA	Mouth ulcers, alopecia, hepatotoxicity, pneumonitis	FBC, LFTs
Sulfasalazine	RA, PsA, AxSpA, JIA	Hepatitis, neutropenia	FBC, LFTs
Hydroxychloro-quine	RA, SLE	Diarrhoea, headache, corneal deposits, retinopathy	Visual function pretreatment and 12-monthly
Leflunomide	RA, PsA, AxSpA	Alopecia, hepatitis, hypertension	FBC, LFTs, BP
Penicillamine	RA	Stomatitis, metallic taste, proteinuria, thrombocytopenia	FBC, urine (protein)
Azathioprine	SLE, SV	Marrow suppression	FBC, LFTs
Cyclophospha-mide	SLE, SV	Marrow suppression, haem-orrhagic cystitis	FBC, LFTs, eGFR
Mycophenylate mofetil	SLE, SV	Marrow suppression	FBC, LFTs
Gold	RA	Stomatitis, alopecia, pro-teinuria, thrombocytopenia	FBC, urine (protein)
Ciclosporin A	RA, PsA	Renal impairment, hypertension	BP, eGFR

[a]Monitoring–initially every 2 weeks for 6 weeks, then monthly for 3 months, then 3 monthly.

15

Intra-articular methylprednisolone is primarily used for problem joints with persistent synovitis despite good general disease control.

Biologics

This group of medications includes monoclonal antibodies, fusion proteins and decoy receptors, used in the treatment of inflammatory rheumatic diseases. The commonly used drugs and their side effects are summarised in Box 15.10. Their main adverse effect is an increased risk of infections. They are more expensive than DMARDs, and use is restricted in many countries.

Anti-TNF therapy

Most inhibitors of TNF are monoclonal antibodies that bind to and neutralise TNF, but etanercept is a decoy receptor that prevents TNF binding to its receptor. Anti-TNF therapy has traditionally been co-prescribed with MTX as the first-line biologic in RA when DMARD therapy has been ineffective. It has also traditionally been the first-line biologic in PsA and AxSpA, but anti IL-17A therapy is an equally effective alternative. Anti-TNF therapy is contraindicated in patients with active infections or indwelling catheters, because of the risk of infection.

Rituximab

Rituximab is an antibody against the CD20 receptor, which is expressed on B lymphocytes and immature plasma cells. It causes B-cell lymphopenia for several months because of complement-mediated lysis of CD20+ cells. Rituximab is typically employed as a third-line treatment in patients with RA who have not responded to first-line therapy and in whom TNF inhibitors have been ineffective. It is also used in place of cyclophosphamide to induce remission in patients with ANCA-positive vasculitis.

 15.10 Causes of hyperuricaemia and gout

Diminished renal excretion (>90% of cases)

- Inherited reduction in renal tubular excretion of urate
- Renal failure
- Drug therapy (e.g. thiazide and loop diuretics, low-dose aspirin, ciclosporin)
- Lead toxicity (e.g. in 'moonshine' drinkers)
- Lactic acidosis (alcohol)

Increased intake

- Game, red meat, seafood, offal

Increased production

- Myeloproliferative or lymphoproliferative disorders, chemotherapy for leukaemias, psoriasis
- High fructose intake
- Rarely: glycogen storage disease, inherited disorders

Topical agents

NSAID and capsaicin (chilli extract) creams provide safe and effective pain relief from arthritis (especially OA) and periarticular lesions. They may be used as monotherapy or as an adjunct to oral analgesics. Topical capsaicin causes pain fibres to discharge substance P. Initial application results in a burning sensation, but continued use reduces substance P activity with consequent pain reduction.

Osteoarthritis

OA is by far the most common form of arthritis and is a major cause of pain and disability in older people. Up to 45% of all people develop knee OA, and 25% hip OA, at some point during life. It is characterised by focal loss of articular cartilage with new bone proliferation and remodelling of the joint contour with enlargement of affected joints.

Genetic and environmental factors contribute to OA. Family studies show that the heritability (usually polygenic) of OA ranges from 43% at the knee to 60% to 65% at the hip and hand. Repetitive adverse loading of joints during occupation or sports is a predisposing factor in farmers, miners and athletes. For most people, however, sport does not increase the risk of OA. Congenital joint abnormalities (e.g. slipped femoral epiphysis), Paget's disease and obesity are also associated with OA, presumably caused by abnormal load distribution within the joint. In obesity, cytokines released from adipose tissue may also play a role. Oestrogen appears to play a role; women who use hormone replacement therapy have lower rates of OA.

Degeneration of articular cartilage is the defining feature of OA, with fissuring and thinning of the cartilage surface (Fig. 15.2). Cysts develop within the subchondral bone, possibly caused by osteonecrosis resulting from increased pressure on the bone as the cartilage fails. At the joint margins, new fibrocartilage grows and then ossifies, forming osteophytes. Bone remodelling and cartilage thinning gradually alter the shape of the OA joint. This is accompanied by wasting of the surrounding muscles, synovial hyperplasia and thickening of the joint capsule.

Clinical features

OA has a characteristic distribution, mainly targeting the hips, knees, PIP and DIP joints of the hands, neck and lumbar spine (Fig. 15.3).

Symptoms:
• Pain and functional restriction. • Insidious onset over months or years. • Pain worsened by movement and relieved by rest. • Only brief (<15 minutes) morning stiffness and brief 'gelling' after rest (in contrast to inflammatory arthritis). • Usually only one or a few painful joints.

Examination:
• Restricted range of movement. • Palpable coarse crepitus. • Bony swelling and deformity around joint margins. • Joint-line or periarticular tenderness. • Muscle wasting. • Synovitis mild or absent.

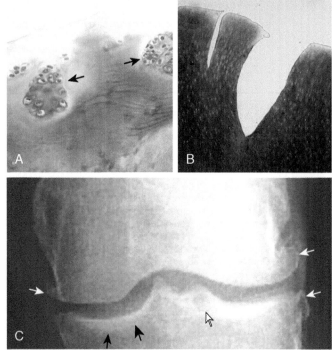

Fig. 15.2 Pathological changes in OA. (A) Abnormal nests of proliferating chondro-cytes (arrows) interspersed with matrix devoid of normal chondrocytes. **(B)** Fibrillation of cartilage. **(C)** X-ray changes of OA in a knee joint: osteophytes at the joint margin (white arrows), subchondral sclerosis (black arrows) and subchondral cyst (open arrow).

Generalised nodal OA

This common form of OA has a strong genetic predisposition and is more common in middle-aged women. Patients develop pain, stiffness and swelling affecting the interphalangeal joints (distal and proximal). Associ-ated joint swellings develop that harden to become Heberden's (DIP) and Bouchard's (PIP) nodes (Fig. 15.4). Involvement of the first carpometacarpal joint is also common. The condition is associated with a good functional prognosis. There is, however, an increased risk of OA at other sites ('gener-alised OA'), especially the knee.

Knee OA

OA of the knee may be primary, or secondary to trauma; the latter is more common in men and is typically unilateral. Pain is usually localised to the anterior and medial aspects of the knee. Functional difficulties include those involved in prolonged walking, rising from a chair and bending to put on shoes. Examination reveals:

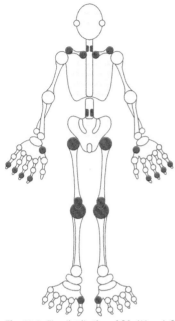

Fig. 15.3 The distribution of OA. Although OA can affect any synovial joint, those shown in red are the most commonly targeted.

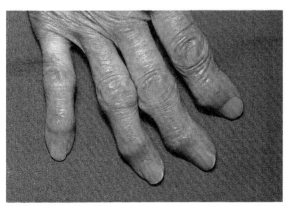

Fig. 15.4 Nodal OA. Heberden's nodes and lateral deviation of the distal interphalangeal joints, with mild Bouchard's nodes at the proximal interphalangeal joints.

• A jerky, asymmetric, 'antalgic' gait (less time weight-bearing on the painful side). • Deformity: varus, less commonly valgus, fixed flexion. • Bony swelling around the joint line. • Wasting of the quadriceps. • Joint line and/or periarticular tenderness. • Restricted flexion/extension with coarse crepitus.

Hip OA

Pain because of hip OA is usually maximal deep in the anterior groin, with variable radiation to the buttock, thigh or knee. Lateral hip pain, worse on lying on that side with tenderness over the greater trochanter, suggests secondary trochanteric bursitis. Functional difficulties are similar to those in knee OA. Examination shows:
• An antalgic gait. • Wasting of quadriceps and gluteal muscles. • Pain and restriction of internal rotation with the hip flexed (the earliest sign of hip OA); other movements may subsequently be affected. • Anterior groin tenderness. • Fixed flexion, external rotation deformity of the hip.

Spine OA

This affects the cervical and lumbar spine (cervical and lumbar spondylosis, respectively), presenting with neck or lower back pain. Radiation of pain to the arms, buttocks and legs also occurs because of nerve root compression. On examination, the range of movement is limited, loss of lumbar lordosis is typical, and neurological signs may confirm nerve root compression.

Investigations

Plain X-rays may reveal joint space narrowing, subchondral sclerosis, osteophytes and bone cysts. However, correlation between radiographic changes, symptoms and disability is variable. MRI is indicated if nerve root compression is suspected. Routine blood tests are normal in OA.

Management

Treatment follows the same principles as set out on pp. 600–604 and includes:
• Full education on the nature of OA. • Local strengthening and aerobic exercises. • Reduction of adverse mechanical factors (e.g. weight loss if obese, shock-absorbing footwear, walking aids). • Local physical therapies such as heat or cold. • Analgesia (initially paracetamol, then consider topical NSAID or capsaicin, then paracetamol plus oral NSAIDs; opioids may occasionally be required for severe pain). • Intra-articular glucocorticoid injection: may temporarily relieve knee pain. • Chondroitin sulphate and glucosamine sulphate slightly improve knee pain. • Surgery: osteotomy and joint replacement should be considered for patients with uncontrolled pain and progressive functional impairment despite medical treatment.

Crystal-induced arthritis

Crystal deposition in and around joints can result in acute and chronic inflammatory arthritis.

Gout

Gout is caused by the deposition of monosodium urate monohydrate (MSUM) crystals at synovial joints. It has a prevalence of 1% to 2%, and is more common in men, in certain ethnic groups and with increasing age. Uric acid mainly comes from the metabolism of purines within the body, but some is ingested with food. Gout is becoming more common with increased longevity and prevalence of metabolic syndrome (p. 425), of which hyperuricaemia is a component. Causes of hyperuricaemia are shown in Box 15.11.

Clinical Features

Acute gout: This presents with rapid onset of severe pain in a single distal joint, commonly the first metatarsophalangeal joint (Fig. 15.5A). Other common sites include the ankle, midfoot, knee, hand, wrist and elbow. Examination reveals marked synovitis with swelling, red shiny skin and extreme tenderness. Fever may also be present. Symptoms are usually self-limiting over 5 to 14 days. The differential diagnosis includes septic arthritis, cellulitis and reactive arthritis.

Recurrent and chronic gout: Following an acute attack, many patients go on to experience a second attack within a year. The frequency of attacks increases with time. Involvement of several joints with continued MSUM deposition eventually leads to joint damage and chronic pain.

Chronic tophaceous gout: MSUM crystal deposits produce irregular firm nodules ('tophi') around extensor surfaces of fingers (Fig. 15.5B), forearms, elbows, Achilles tendons and ears. Tophi are usually a late feature of gout.

Renal and urinary tract manifestations: Chronic hyperuricaemia may be complicated by renal stone formation (p. 241) and sometimes renal impairment because of interstitial nephritis caused by urate deposition in

15

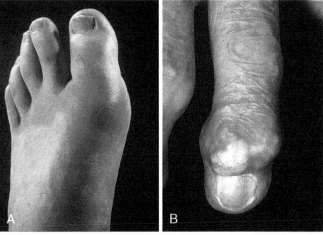

Fig. 15.5 Gout. (A) Acute gout causing inflammation of the first metatarsophalangeal joint (podagra). **(B)** Tophus.

i 15.11 Criteria for diagnosis of rheumatoid arthritis	
Criterion	Score
Joints affected	
1 large joint	0
2–10 large joints	1
1–3 small joints	2
4–10 small joints	3
>10 joints (at least 1 small joint)	5
Serology	
Negative RF and ACPA	0
Low positive RF or ACPA	2
High positive RF or ACPA	3
Duration of symptoms	
<6 weeks	0
>6 weeks	1
Acute phase reactants	
Normal CRP and ESR	0
Abnormal CRP or ESR	1
Patients with a score ≥6 are considered to have definite RA.	
European League Against Rheumatism/American College of Rheumatology 2010 Criteria.	

the kidney. This particularly affects patients with chronic tophaceous gout who are on diuretics.

Investigations

Joint aspiration reveals long, needle-shaped MSUM crystals, which are negatively birefringent under polarised light. Synovial fluid in acute gout appears turbid because of the high neutrophil count (>90%). Serum uric acid is usually elevated, but levels may be normal during an attack. Serum creatinine should be checked to exclude renal impairment. There is neutrophilia with a raised CRP and ESR in acute gout. Tophaceous gout may be accompanied by modest chronic elevation in ESR and CRP. Joint X-rays are usually normal in early gout. Changes of secondary OA and gouty erosions may develop with chronic disease.

Management

Acute attacks: Oral colchicine (0.5 mg two to three times daily) is the treatment of choice, but common adverse effects include nausea, vomiting and diarrhoea. NSAIDs are also effective, but may exacerbate coexisting cardiovascular, cerebrovascular or kidney disease. Joint aspiration and intra-articular glucocorticoid injections are effective in more severe cases.

Long-term management: Allopurinol lowers serum uric acid levels by inhibiting xanthine oxidase, which reduces conversion of hypoxanthine and xanthine to uric acid. It is indicated in patients with recurrent attacks of acute gout, tophi, joint damage or renal impairment. Allopurinol initiation can trigger an acute attack; it should therefore be started after the acute attack has settled and should be co-prescribed with colchicine or an NSAID when introduced.

Predisposing factors should be addressed:
• Weight loss: advised in obese patients. • Excess beer: avoid. • Thiazides and ACE inhibitors: stop if possible. • High-purine diet (seafood and offal): avoid.

Calcium pyrophosphate dihydrate crystal deposition

CPPD crystal deposition within articular cartilage causes chondrocalcinosis. Risk factors include age, OA and primary hyperparathyroidism. Rarely, it is associated with metabolic disease (e.g. haemochromatosis, hypophosphataemia, hypomagnesaemia and Wilson's disease). It is often clinically silent but can cause episodes of acute synovitis ('pseudogout') or occur as a chronic arthritis that is associated with OA.

Clinical features

Acute synovitis ('pseudogout'): This is the most common cause of acute monoarthritis in the elderly. The knee is the most common site, followed by the wrist, shoulder and ankle. The typical attack resembles acute gout with rapid onset of pain, stiffness and swelling. Examination reveals erythema, marked joint tenderness and signs of synovitis (large effusion, warmth and restricted movement). Fever may be present. Septic arthritis and gout are the main differential diagnoses.

Chronic CPPD arthritis: Chronic symptoms usually occur in elderly women. The distribution is similar to that of pseudogout. Symptoms are chronic pain with variable early morning stiffness. Affected joints show features of OA (bony swelling, crepitus, restriction) with varying degrees of synovitis.

Investigations

Joint fluid aspiration in acute pseudogout reveals small, rhomboid-shaped CPPD crystals that are positively birefringent under polarised light. Gram stain and culture of the fluid will exclude sepsis. X-rays may show chondrocalcinosis within the articular cartilage. Blood tests should be performed to exclude metabolic causes of CPPD crystal deposition in younger patients and in individuals with polyarticular disease.

Management

• Joint aspiration with intra-articular glucocorticoid injection: provides rapid pain relief. • Oral NSAIDs and colchicine: effective for acute pseudogout.

15

Fibromyalgia

This is a common cause of generalised pain and disability and is frequently associated with medically unexplained symptoms in other systems. The prevalence in the UK is around 2% to 3%. It increases in prevalence with age, to reach a peak of 7% in women aged over 70 years. There is a female predominance of around 10:1. Risk factors include stressful life events, such as marital disharmony, previous abuse, alcoholism in the family, injury or assault and low income.

No structural, inflammatory or metabolic abnormality has been identified, although abnormalities of non-REM sleep and of central pain processing have been postulated as potential aetiological factors.

Clinical features and investigations

The main presenting feature is widespread pain, affecting the neck, back, both arms and both legs, which is unresponsive to analgesics and NSAIDs. Patients commonly report fatigability, particularly in the morning, and reported disability is often marked. Although people can usually dress and groom themselves, they may struggle with daily tasks such as shopping and housework and may have given up work because of pain and fatigue.

Examination usually reveals hyperalgesia on moderate digital pressure (enough just to whiten the nail) over multiple sites. Although there are no abnormal investigations associated with fibromyalgia, it is important to screen for alternative musculoskeletal conditions.

Management

The patient should be reassured that their widespread pain does not reflect inflammation, tissue damage or disease. Low-dose amitriptyline with or without fluoxetine may be useful. Graded exercise may improve well-being. Coping strategies such as relaxation and cognitive behavioural therapy should be encouraged, and unresolved psychological issues addressed. Patient organisations can provide valuable support.

Bone and joint infections

Septic arthritis

Septic arthritis is a medical emergency. It usually arises from haematogenous spread of bacterial infection from another site, commonly the skin or upper respiratory tract. Infection from direct puncture wounds or that secondary to joint aspiration is uncommon. Risk factors include increasing age, preexisting joint disease (especially RA), diabetes mellitus, immunosuppression and IV drug misuse.

Clinical features

The usual presentation is with acute or subacute monoarthritis. The joint is usually swollen, hot and red, with pain at rest and on movement. The knee and hip are the most common sites. The usual culprit organism is *Staphylococcus aureus*. Disseminated gonococcal infection is another cause in young, sexually active adults. This presents with migratory arthralgia and low-grade fever, followed by the development of oligo- or monoarthritis.

Painful pustular skin lesions may also be present. Gram-negative bacilli or group B, C and G streptococci are important causes among the elderly and intravenous drug users.

Investigations

Joint fluid aspiration for Gram stain and culture is essential, under image guidance if deep. Aspirated fluid often looks turbid or blood-stained. Culture yield is high, except in gonococcal infection where concurrent cultures from the genital tract are indicated. Blood tests may reveal leucocytosis with raised ESR and CRP, although these may be absent in elderly or immunocompromised patients.

Management

• Pain relief. • Flucloxacillin (2 g IV four times daily): the antibiotic of choice pending culture results. IV treatment is usually continued for 2 weeks, followed by oral treatment for a further 4 weeks. • Daily joint aspiration in the initial stages to minimise the effusion. If this is unsuccessful, surgical drainage may be required. • Early mobilisation.

Viral arthritis

The usual presentation is with acute polyarthritis, fever and rash. Parvovirus B19 is the most common cause of viral arthritis; other causes include hepatitis B and C, rubella and HIV. Symptoms are usually self-limiting. Diagnosis is confirmed by viral serology.

Osteomyelitis

Infection of bone usually arises in children from haematogenous spread, although directly introduced infection from a compound fracture, penetrating injury or surgery is more important in adults. Organisms most frequently implicated are *S. aureus*, *S. epidermidis* and streptococci. Risk factors include diabetes, immunodeficiency and sickle-cell disease. Infection results in a florid inflammatory response complicated by localised osteonecrosis.

Clinical features and investigations

Presentation is with localised bone pain and tenderness, fever and night sweats. A discharging sinus may form in advanced cases. X-rays may show osteolysis or osteonecrosis, but MRI is the imaging method of choice because it is much more sensitive. Confirmation of the diagnosis should be obtained by blood culture and culture of a bone aspirate or biopsy.

Management

• Pain relief. • 2 weeks of IV antibiotics, followed by 4 weeks of oral antibiotics. • Surgical decompression and removal of any dead bone. • Rehabilitation.

Discitis

This is an unusual infection of the intervertebral disc (usually by *S. aureus*), often extending into the epidural space or paravertebral soft tissues. Risk factors include diabetes, immunodeficiency and intravenous drug use. It presents with back pain, fever, high ESR and CRP and neutrophilia. MRI, blood cultures and image-guided biopsy are required. Management is as for osteomyelitis.

15

Tuberculosis

Musculoskeletal TB usually targets the spine (Pott's disease), hip, knee or ankle. The presentation is with pain, swelling and fever. X-rays are non-specific, and mycobacteria are seldom identified in synovial fluid, so tissue biopsy is required for diagnosis. Antibiotic treatment is described on p. 339. Occasionally, surgical debridement of joints or stabilisation and decompression of the spine is required.

Rheumatoid arthritis

RA is the most common persistent inflammatory arthritis, and occurs worldwide and in all ethnic groups. The prevalence is around 0.8% to 1.0% in Europe and the Indian subcontinent, with a female:male ratio of 3:1. The prevalence is lower in South-East Asia (0.4%). The clinical course is chronic, with exacerbations and remissions.

RA has genetic and environmental components. Concordance is higher in monozygotic twins (12%–15%) than in dizygotic twins (3%). Nearly 100 genetic loci (particularly *HLA* and other immune regulatory genes) are associated with risk of RA. It is believed that RA occurs when an environmental stimulus (possibly infection) triggers autoimmunity in a genetically susceptible host by modifying host proteins through processes like citrullination. Smoking is an important environmental risk factor.

The earliest change is swelling and congestion of the synovial membrane and the underlying connective tissues, with infiltration by lymphocytes, plasma cells and macrophages. TNF plays a central role in triggering local inflammation and regulating cytokines responsible for the systemic effects of RA. Hypertrophy of the synovial membrane occurs, and inflammatory granulation tissue (pannus) directly invades bone and cartilage to cause joint erosions. Muscles adjacent to inflamed joints atrophy and may be infiltrated with lymphocytes. Subcutaneous rheumatoid nodules are granulomatous lesions consisting of a central area of fibrinoid material surrounded by proliferating mononuclear cells. Granulomatous lesions may occur in the pleura, lung and pericardium.

Clinical features

The most common presentation is with a gradual onset of symmetrical arthralgia and synovitis of small joints of the hands, feet and wrists. Large joint involvement, systemic symptoms and extra-articular features may also occur. Clinical criteria for the diagnosis of RA are shown in Box 15.11.

Sometimes RA has a very acute onset, with florid morning stiffness, polyarthritis and pitting oedema. This occurs more commonly in old age. Another presentation is with proximal muscle stiffness mimicking polymyalgia rheumatica (p. 600). Occasionally, the onset is palindromic, with relapsing and remitting episodes of pain, stiffness and swelling that last for only a few hours or days.

Examination typically reveals swelling and tenderness of the affected joints. Erythema is unusual and suggests coexistent sepsis. In the absence of modern aggressive treatment, characteristic deformities develop over time including 'swan neck' deformity, the boutonnière ('button hole') deformity and Z deformity of the thumb (Fig. 15.6). Dorsal subluxation of the ulna at the distal radio-ulnar joint may occur and contribute to rupture of the fourth and fifth extensor tendons. Trigger fingers may occur because of nodules in the flexor tendon sheaths.

Subluxation of the MTP joints in the feet may result in pain on weight-bearing on the exposed metatarsal heads. Popliteal (Baker's) cysts usually complicate knee synovitis. Cyst rupture, often induced by knee flexion with a large effusion, leads to calf pain and swelling that may mimic DVT.

Systemic features

Anorexia, weight loss and fatigue are common, and may occur throughout the disease course. Extra-articular features (Box 15.12) are more common in patients with long-standing seropositive erosive disease, but may occur at presentation, especially in men.

Rheumatoid nodules occur in seropositive patients, usually at pressure sites such as the extensor surfaces of the forearm, Achilles tendon and toes. Rheumatoid vasculitis occurs in older seropositive patients, ranging from benign nail-fold infarcts to widespread cutaneous ulceration.

Ocular complications are covered on p. 717 (Box 17.5).

Cardiac involvement occurs in up to 30% of seropositive patients but is usually asymptomatic. The risk of cardiovascular disease is, however, increased in RA. Pulmonary fibrosis can occur in RA and may cause dyspnoea (p. 626).

Median nerve compression in the carpal tunnel is common, and bilateral compression can occur as an early presenting feature of RA.

Investigations

Diagnosis is based on clinical criteria (see Box 15.11). ESR and CRP are usually elevated in patients with active disease. Anti-citrullinated peptide antibodies (ACPA) are positive in around 70% of cases and are highly specific for RA, often occurring before clinical onset of disease. RF is positive in around 70%, many of whom also have positive ACPA. RF, however, is less specific and is found in other diseases.

Ultrasound examination and MRI are mainly used in uncertain cases to detect synovitis. Plain X-rays are of limited value in early RA, but periarticular osteoporosis and marginal joint erosions are characteristic in advanced disease. Patients who are suspected of having atlanto-axial disease should have MRI. In patients with suspected Baker's cyst, ultrasound may be required to establish the diagnosis and exclude DVT.

Management

DMARDs: DMARDs should be offered to all patients because they improve outcome. Glucocorticoids are used for induction of remission. An algorithm for the escalation of therapy in RA is shown in Fig. 15.7. Regular monitoring of DMARD therapy is essential, because of the risk of liver and haematological toxicity. Some DMARDs are contraindicated in pregnancy, especially during the first trimester. Further details of individual DMARDs are given in Box 15.9. Partial or nonresponse to DMARDs necessitates dose escalation, use of an additional DMARD, or progression to biological drugs (Box 15.13) if necessary.

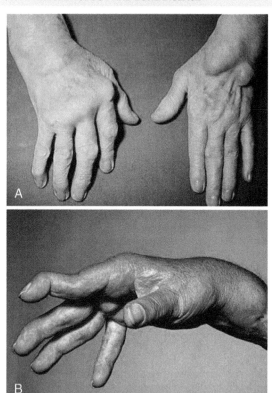

Fig. 15.6 The hand in rheumatoid arthritis. (A) Ulnar deviation of the fingers with wasting of the small muscles of the hands and synovial swelling at the wrists, the extensor tendon sheaths, the metacarpophalangeal and proximal interphalangeal joints. **(B)** 'Swan neck' deformity of the fingers.

Non-pharmacological interventions: These important aspects of treatment are covered on p. 601.

Surgery: Synovectomy of wrist or finger tendon sheaths may provide pain relief when medical interventions have failed. Osteotomy, arthrodesis or arthroplasties may be beneficial in later stages of disease.

Juvenile idiopathic arthritis

JIA includes several forms of arthritis affecting children. The most common is oligoarthritis, which is characterised by asymmetrical large joint arthritis, uveitis and positive ANA. Polyarthritis affects over five joints, and systemic JIA (formerly Still's disease) features fever, rash, arthralgia and hepatosplenomegaly without autoantibodies.

i	**15.12 Extra-articular manifestations of rheumatoid disease**
Systemic	Fever, fatigue, weight loss, susceptibility to infection
Musculoskeletal	Muscle-wasting, tenosynovitis, bursitis, osteoporosis
Haematological	Anaemia, eosinophilia, thrombocytosis
Lymphatic	Splenomegaly, Felty's syndrome (RA, splenomegaly and neutropenia)
Nodules	Sinuses, fistulae
Ocular	Episcleritis, scleritis, scleromalacia, keratoconjunctivitis sicca
Vasculitis	Digital arteritis, ulcers, pyoderma gangrenosum, mononeuritis multiplex, visceral arteritis
Cardiac	Pericarditis, myocarditis, endocarditis, conduction defects, coronary vasculitis, granulomatous aortitis
Pulmonary	Nodules, pleural effusions, pulmonary fibrosis, Caplan's syndrome (RA plus pneumoconiosis), bronchiolitis, bronchiectasis
Neurological	Cervical cord compression, compression neuropathies, peripheral neuropathy, mononeuritis multiplex
Amyloidosis	Nephrotic syndrome, cardiomyopathy, peripheral neuropathy

i	**15.13 Biological drugs for inflammatory rheumatic disease**		
Drug	**Maintenance dose**	**Mechanism of action**	**Indications**
Etanercept	50 mg weekly SC	Decoy receptor for TNFα	RA, PsA, AxSpA, JIA
Infliximab	3–5 mg/kg 8-weekly IV	Antibody to TNFα	RA, PsA, AxSpA, JIA
Adalimumab	40 mg 2-weekly SC		
Rituximab	2 × 1 g 2 weeks apart IV	Antibody to CD20	RA, vasculitis
Belimumab	10 mg/kg 4-weekly IV	Antibody to BAFF	SLE
Abatacept	125 mg weekly SC	Inhibits T-cell activation	RA
Tocilizumab	162 mg weekly SC	Blocks IL-6 receptor	RA, JIA
Ustenkinumab	45 mg 12-weekly SC	Antibody to IL-12 and IL-23	PsA
Secukinumab	150 mg 4-weekly SC	Antibody to IL-17A	PsA, AxSpA

15

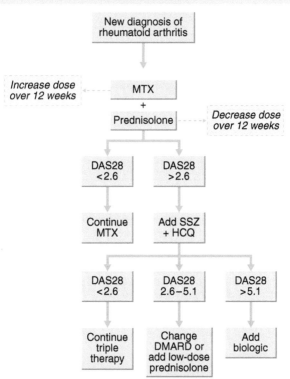

Fig. 15.7 Algorithm for the management of rheumatoid arthritis. DAS28 = Disease Activity Score 28 (see www.4s-dawn.com/das28); DMARD = disease-modifying antirheumatic drug; HCQ = hydroxychloroquine; MTX = methotrexate; SSZ = sulfasalazine)

The key goal is rapid control of inflammation, usually starting with methotrexate. Leflunomide is an alternative, and azathioprine and ciclosporin are used in uveitis. TNF blockers and other biological agents are used for resistant cases.

Oligoarthritis frequently resolves at puberty, but those with polyarticular or systemic manifestations have a poorer prognosis; around 50% of cases persist into adulthood, requiring transition to adult rheumatology services.

Spondyloarthropathies

This term refers to a group of inflammatory musculoskeletal diseases with overlapping clinical features (Box 15.14), which share an association with HLA-B27:

• Axial spondyloarthritis. • Ankylosing spondylitis. • Reactive arthritis, including Reiter's disease. • Psoriatic arthropathy. • Arthritis associated with inflammatory bowel disease (enteropathic arthritis).

---

i 15.14 Features common to spondyloarthropathies

- Asymmetrical inflammatory oligoarthritis (lower > upper limb)
- History of inflammatory back pain
- Sacroiliitis and spinal osteitis
- Enthesitis (e.g. gluteus medius insertion, plantar fascia origin)
- Tendency for familial aggregation
- HLA-B27 association
- Psoriasis (of skin and/or nails)
- Uveitis
- Sterile urethritis and/or prostatitis
- Inflammatory bowel disease
- Aortic root lesions (aortic incompetence, conduction defects)

(HLA = human leucocyte antigen)

Unlike RA, the SpAs frequently cause nonsynovial musculoskeletal inflammation affecting ligaments, tendons, periosteum and bones. Enthesitis (inflammation at the bony insertion of a ligament or tendon) is typical, and dactylitis (inflammation of a whole digit) also occurs.

The association with HLA-B27 is particularly strong for ankylosing spondylitis (>95%). The suggested pathogenesis is an aberrant response to infection in genetically predisposed individuals. In some situations, a triggering organism can be identified, as in Reiter's disease following bacterial dysentery or chlamydial urethritis, but in others the environmental trigger remains obscure.

Axial spondyloarthropathy

Axial spondyloarthropathy includes classical ankylosing spondylitis (AS) as well as axial spondyloarthritis (axSpA). Inflammatory changes in the entire axial skeleton (visible on MRI) are characteristic of AxSpA; bony changes with syndesmophytes and ankylosis develop later. Not all patients with AxSpA will go on to develop AS.

Clinical features

The cardinal feature of AxSpA is low back pain radiating to the buttocks or posterior thighs, and early morning stiffness. Symptoms are exacerbated by inactivity and relieved by movement. Musculoskeletal symptoms may be prominent at entheses. If persistent, these can cause widespread pain mistaken for fibromyalgia. Fatigue is common. If there is progression to AS, sacroiliitis and structural spinal changes are seen on X-ray, which may eventually progress to bony fusion of the spine. Examination reveals a reduced range of lumbar spine movements and pain on sacroiliac stressing. Secondary vertebral osteoporosis frequently occurs, causing an increased fracture risk.

Spinal fusion is usually mild, but a few patients develop incapacitating thoracic and cervical kyphosis with fixed flexion contractures of hips or knees. Pleuritic chest pain is common, and results from costovertebral joint involvement. Plantar fasciitis, Achilles tendinitis and tenderness over bony prominences such as the iliac crest and greater trochanter may occur, reflecting inflammation at tendon insertions (enthesitis).

15

Up to 40% of patients also have asymmetrical peripheral musculoskeletal symptoms, affecting entheses of large joints such as the hips, knees, ankles and shoulders.

Fatigue is common and reflects both chronic sleep disturbance by pain and systemic inflammation with direct effects of inflammatory cytokines on the brain. Anterior uveitis is the most common extra-articular feature, which occasionally precedes joint disease.

Investigations

The diagnosis is aided by ultrasound or MRI of entheses, or by MRI of the sacroiliac joints and spine. In established ankylosing spondylitis, X-rays show sacroiliitis with irregularity, sclerosis, joint space narrowing and fusion. Lateral thoracolumbar spine X-rays may show bridging syndesmophytes, ossification of the anterior longitudinal ligament and facet joint fusion ('bamboo' spine).

The ESR and CRP are usually raised in active disease but may be normal. HLA-B27 is usually present. Faecal calprotectin is a useful screening test for associated inflammatory bowel disease.

Management and prognosis

Patient education, NSAID use (once daily or slow release taken at bedtime) and physical therapy with mobilising exercises are the key interventions. For severe and/or persistent peripheral musculoskeletal features of SpA, both sulfasalazine and methotrexate are reasonable therapy choices. These medications have no impact on spinal symptoms or disease progression. For patients who fail to respond or cannot tolerate NSAIDs, biologic therapy with either TNF inhibitors or secukinumab should be considered.

Local glucocorticoid injections may help persistent plantar fasciitis, other enthesitis and peripheral arthritis. Severe hip, knee, ankle or shoulder symptoms may require arthroplasty.

Reactive arthritis

Reactive (spondylo)arthritis classically affects young men. It follows an episode of bacterial dysentery (because of *Salmonella*, *Shigella*, *Campylobacter* or *Yersinia*) or nonspecific urethritis (attributed to *Chlamydia*). The syndrome of chlamydial urethritis, conjunctivitis and reactive arthritis was formerly known as Reiter's disease.

Clinical features

Patients present with acute-onset, inflammatory enthesitis, spinal inflammation and/or oligoarthritis affecting the lower limbs 1 to 3 weeks following sexual exposure or an attack of dysentery. Symptoms of urethritis and conjunctivitis may be present. It occasionally presents with insidious onset of single joint involvement, minimal features of urethritis and conjunctivitis, and no clear history of 'trigger' illness. Achilles tendinitis or plantar fasciitis may occur.

Additional extra-articular features include:
• Circinate balanitis: causes vesicles (often painless) on the prepuce and glans. • Buccal erosions. • Keratoderma blennorrhagica: waxy yellow–brown skin lesions, particularly affecting the palms and soles. • Nail dystrophy identical to psoriatic nail dystrophy.

The first attack of reactive arthritis is usually self-limiting, with spontaneous remission within 2 to 4 months. Recurrent arthritis develops in more than 60% of patients. Uveitis is rare with the first attack but occurs in 30% of patients with recurring arthritis.

Investigations

The diagnosis is clinical:

• Raised ESR and CRP. • Aspirated synovial fluid: leucocyte-rich with multinucleated macrophages. • High vaginal swab: may reveal *Chlamydia*. • Stool cultures: usually negative by the time the arthritis presents. • Serum RF, ACPA and ANA: negative. • X-ray changes: usually absent during the acute attack, other than soft tissue swelling. Joint space narrowing and marginal erosions may develop with recurrent disease.

Management

Rest and NSAIDs provide symptomatic relief during the acute phase. Intra-articular corticosteroid injections may help severe synovitis. Nonspecific chlamydial urethritis is treated with a short course of doxycycline. DMARDs are occasionally used for severe progressive arthritis and keratoderma blennorrhagica. Anterior uveitis is a medical emergency requiring topical or systemic glucocorticoids.

Psoriatic arthropathy

Psoriatic arthritis affects up to 40% of patients with psoriasis. It typically presents between the ages of 25 and 40 years. The seronegative arthritis usually occurs in individuals with preexisting cutaneous psoriasis but can predate the skin disease.

Clinical features

Five major presentations of joint disease are recognised:

Asymmetrical inflammatory oligoarthritis (40%): May affect lower and upper limb joints. Involvement of a finger or toe by synovitis, together with enthesitis and inflammation of intervening tissue, can give rise to a 'sausage digit' or dactylitis. Usually only one or two large joints are involved, mainly knees.

Symmetrical polyarthritis (25%): May strongly resemble RA, with symmetrical involvement of small and large joints in both upper and lower limbs. However, nodules and other extra-articular features of RA are absent.

Distal interphalangeal joint arthritis (15%): Predominantly affects men, almost invariably with accompanying nail disease.

Psoriatic spondylitis (15%): Presents with inflammatory back or neck pain and prominent stiffness.

Arthritis mutilans (5%): This deforming erosive arthritis targets fingers and toes. Marked cartilage and bone attrition results in loss of the joint and instability.

Enthesitis-predominant: This presents with pain and stiffness at the insertion sites of tendons and ligaments into bone. Symptoms can be extensive or localized.

Extra-articular features include:

• Skin lesions. • Nail changes: pitting, onycholysis (separation of the nail from the nail bed) and subungual hyperkeratosis. • Uveitis (in HLA-B27–positive cases with spondylitis).

Investigations

• ESR and CRP: may be raised but are often normal. • Serum RF and ANA: negative. • X-rays: may be normal or show erosive change with joint space narrowing. MRI reveals enthesitis.

Management and prognosis

Simple analgesics and NSAIDs provide symptomatic relief. Intra-articular glucocorticoids may help control isolated synovitis or enthesitis. Regular exercise is important in preventing ankylosis. DMARDs may be required for persistent unresponsive synovitis. Methotrexate is the treatment of choice, as it may also help severe skin psoriasis. Anti-TNF therapy should be considered in those unresponsive to DMARDs. Ustekinumab and secukinumab are monoclonal antibodies used for resistant cases.

Enteropathic (spondylo)arthritis

This inflammatory arthritis is associated with ulcerative colitis and Crohn's disease, predominantly affecting large lower limb joints. The arthritis coincides with exacerbations of the underlying bowel disease and improves with effective treatment of the bowel disease. Sacroiliitis and ankylosing spondylitis indistinguishable from classic ankylosing spondylitis also occur with bowel disease but are not correlated with the activity of the bowel disease.

Autoimmune connective tissue disease

These diseases share overlapping clinical features, characterised by dysregulation of immune responses, autoantibody production often directed at components of the cell nucleus and widespread tissue damage.

Systemic lupus erythematosus

SLE is a rare multisystem connective tissue disease, mainly occurring in women (90%), with a peak age at onset between 20 and 30 years. Prevalence is 0.2% in Afro-Caribbeans and 0.03% in Caucasians.

Several autoantibodies are associated with SLE. Many of the target autoantigens are intracellular and intranuclear components. It is likely that the wide spectrum of autoantibody production results from polyclonal B- and T-cell activation. Although the triggers that lead to autoantibody production in SLE are unknown, one mechanism may be exposure of intracellular antigens on the cell surface during apoptosis.

Clinical features

Fever, weight loss and mild lymphadenopathy occur during flares of disease activity; fatigue, malaise and low-grade joint pains are not particularly associated with active disease.

Arthritis: This is a common symptom, occurring in 90% of patients and often associated with early morning stiffness. Tenosynovitis may also be a feature, but clinically apparent synovitis with joint swelling is rare.

Raynaud's phenomenon: Arthralgia or arthritis in combination with Raynaud's phenomenon (digital vasospasm) is a common presentation of SLE. Raynaud's phenomenon in a teenage girl with no other associated symptoms is likely to be idiopathic 'primary' Raynaud's. By contrast, onset in a male, or in a woman over the age of 30 years suggests underlying connective tissue disease.

Skin: Skin involvement is common and takes several forms:
• The classic butterfly (malar) facial rash: raised and painful or pruritic, and spares the nasolabial folds (Fig. 15.8). • The discoid lupus rash: characterised by hyperkeratosis and follicular plugging, with scarring alopecia if it occurs on the scalp. • Urticarial eruptions. • Livedo reticularis, which is also a feature of the antiphospholipid syndrome, and can become vasculitic if severe.

Kidney: The typical renal lesion is a proliferative glomerulonephritis, characterised by haematuria, proteinuria and casts on urine microscopy.

Cardiovascular: Pericarditis is the most common feature. Myocarditis and Libman–Sacks endocarditis (sterile fibrin containing vegetations) also occur. Atherosclerosis, stroke and myocardial infarction are increased because of the adverse effects of inflammation on the endothelium, chronic glucocorticoid therapy and the procoagulant effects of antiphospholipid antibodies.

Lung: Pleurisy can cause pleuritic chest pain, a rub or a pleural effusion. Alveolitis, lung fibrosis and diaphragmatic paralysis can also occur.

Neurological: Fatigue, headache and poor concentration are common. Cerebral lupus causes visual hallucinations, chorea, organic psychosis, transverse myelitis and lymphocytic meningitis.

Haematological: Neutropenia, lymphopenia, thrombocytopenia and haemolytic anaemia occur.

GI: Mouth ulcers are common. Mesenteric vasculitis can cause bowel infarction.

15

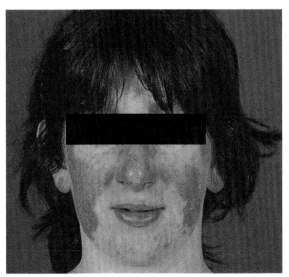

Fig 15.8 Butterfly (malar) rash of systemic lupus erythematosus.

Investigations

The criteria for diagnosis of SLE are given in Box 15.15. Blood should be sent for haematology, biochemistry, ANAs, ENAs and complement levels. Urinalysis is mandatory. Patients with active SLE test positive for ANA. Rarely, some authorities diagnose ANA-negative SLE with antibodies to the Ro antigen. Anti-dsDNA antibodies are positive in many, but not all, patients. Patients with active disease tend to have low C3 because of complement consumption, but this may reflect inherited complement deficiency that predisposes to SLE. A raised ESR, leucopenia and lymphopenia are typical of active SLE, as are anaemia, haemolytic anaemia and thrombocytopenia. CRP is often normal in active SLE, except in the presence of serositis; elevated CRP suggests coexisting infection.

Management

The goals are education, symptom control and the prevention of organ damage. Patients should avoid sun exposure and use high-factor sun blocks.

Mild disease: Disease restricted to skin and joints may require only analgesics, NSAIDs, hydroxychloroquine and sometimes also glucocorticoids with methotrexate or azathioprine. Increased oral glucocorticoids may be needed for disease flares (e.g. synovitis, pleuro-pericarditis).

i	**15.15 American Rheumatism Association criteria for SLE**	
Features	**Characteristics**
Malar rash	Fixed erythema, flat or raised, sparing nasolabial folds
Discoid rash	Erythematous raised patches, keratotic scarring, follicular plugging
Photosensitivity	Rash on sunlight exposure
Oral ulcers	Oral or nasopharyngeal; may be painless
Arthritis	Nonerosive, ≥2 peripheral joints
Serositis	Pleuritis *or* pericarditis
Renal disorder	Persistent proteinuria > 0.5 g/day *or* cellular casts
Neurological	Seizures or psychosis, without provoking drugs/metabolic derangement
Haematological disorder	Haemolytic anaemia *or* leucopenia[a] ($<4 \times 10^9$/L) *or* lymphopenia[a] ($<1 \times 10^9$/L) *or* thrombocytopenia[a] ($<100 \times 10^9$/L) not because of drugs
Immunological	Raised anti-DNA antibodies *or* antibody to Sm antigen *or* positive antiphospholipid antibodies
ANA disorder	Abnormal ANA titre by immunofluorescence

SLE is diagnosed if any four of these 11 features are present serially or simultaneously.
[a]On two separate occasions.

Life-threatening disease (e.g. renal, cerebral, cardiac): This requires high-dose glucocorticoids (IV methylprednisolone) in combination with IV cyclophosphamide, repeated at intervals of 2 to 3 weeks. Haemorrhagic cystitis is an important complication of cyclophosphamide treatment. Mycophenolate is a less toxic alternative to cyclophosphamide.

Maintenance therapy: Azathioprine, methotrexate and MMF are used for maintenance. Patients with thrombosis and the antiphospholipid syndrome require lifelong anticoagulation.

Systemic sclerosis

SScl is an autoimmune disorder of connective tissue that causes fibrosis affecting the skin, internal organs and vasculature. The peak age of onset is in the fourth and fifth decades, and it has a 4:1 female:male ratio. It is subdivided into diffuse cutaneous systemic sclerosis (dcSScl) and limited cutaneous systemic sclerosis (lcSScl). Some patients with lcSScl have calcinosis and telangiectasia. Poor prognostic factors in SScl include older age, diffuse skin disease, proteinuria, high ESR, TLCO and pulmonary hypertension.

The aetiology of systemic sclerosis is unknown. Early in the disease, there is skin infiltration by T lymphocytes and abnormal fibroblast activation, leading to increased production of collagen in the dermis. This results in symmetrical thickening, tightening and induration of the skin, and then sclerodactyly in the fingers. In addition to skin changes, there is arterial and arteriolar narrowing because of intimal proliferation and vessel wall inflammation. Endothelial injury causes release of vasoconstrictors and platelet activation, resulting in further ischaemia.

Clinical features

Skin: The skin of the fingers becomes tight, shiny and thickened (sclerodactyly, Fig. 15.9). Raynaud's phenomenon occurs early in the disease. In the distal extremities, the combination of intimal fibrosis and vasculitis may cause tissue ischaemia, skin ulceration and localised infarcts. Involvement

15

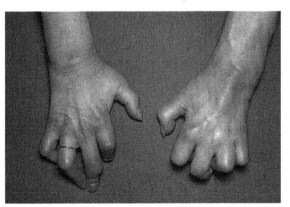

Fig. 15.9 Systemic sclerosis. Hands showing tight shiny skin, sclerodactyly and flexion contractures of the fingers.

of the face causes thinning and radial furrowing of the lips. Telangiectasia may be present. Skin involvement restricted to sites distal to the elbow or knee (apart from the face) is classified as lcSScl; more proximal involvement is classified as dcSScl.

Musculoskeletal features: Arthralgia and flexor tenosynovitis are common. Restricted hand function is usually because of skin rather than joint disease.

GI features: Smooth muscle atrophy and fibrosis in the lower oesophagus lead to acid reflux with erosive oesophagitis; this may in turn progress to further fibrosis. Dysphagia may also occur. Involvement of the stomach causes early satiety and occasionally outlet obstruction. Small intestine involvement may lead to malabsorption because of bacterial overgrowth and intermittent bloating or pain. Dilatation of the bowel because of autonomic neuropathy may cause pseudo-obstruction.

Pulmonary involvement: Pulmonary fibrosis mainly affects patients with diffuse disease. Pulmonary hypertension is a complication of long-standing limited disease, particularly lcSScl, characterised by progressive exertional dyspnoea and right heart failure.

Renal features: One of the main causes of death is hypertensive renal crisis characterised by rapidly developing accelerated phase hypertension and renal failure. It is much more common in patients with dcSScl.

Investigations

The diagnosis is primarily a clinical one. Renal and liver function should be checked. ANA is positive in 70%. Antitopoisomerase I (anti-Scl-70) antibodies occur in 30% of those with dcSScl, and anticentromere antibodies occur in 60% of those with lcSScl. Echocardiography and respiratory function should be checked to assess cardiopulmonary involvement.

Management and prognosis

Raynaud's and digital ulcers: Patients should avoid cold exposure; conventional or heated mittens can be effective. Calcium channel blockers, losartan, fluoxetine and sildenafil have efficacy, and prostacyclin infusions may be helpful for severe disease. Bosentan is licensed for treating ischaemic digital ulcers.

Oesophageal reflux: This should be treated with PPI and prokinetic agents such as metoclopramide.

Hypertension: This should be treated aggressively with ACE inhibitors.

Pulmonary hypertension: This is managed with the oral endothelin 1 antagonist bosentan, but if severe may require heart–lung transplantation.

Mixed connective tissue disease

This is an overlap connective tissue disease with features of SLE, SScl and myositis. Most patients have anti-RNP antibodies, although these can also occur in SLE without overlap features.

Primary Sjögren's syndrome

This disorder is characterised by lymphocytic infiltration of salivary and lacrimal glands, leading to glandular fibrosis and exocrine failure. It predominantly affects women, and has a peak onset between the ages of 40 and

50 years. There is an association with HLA-B8 and DR3. The disease may be primary or secondary in association with other autoimmune diseases (secondary Sjögrens syndrome).

Clinical features

• Dry eyes (keratoconjunctivitis sicca) because of a lack of tears. • Dry mouth (xerostomia). • Vaginal dryness. • Other features: fatigue, nonerosive arthritis and Raynaud's phenomenon. • There is a fortyfold increase in lifetime risk of lymphoma.

Investigations

The diagnosis can be established by the Schirmer test, which measures the flow of tears using an absorbent paper strip placed in the lower eyelid; a normal result is more than 6 mm of wetting over 5 minutes. If the diagnosis is in doubt, lip biopsy may identify lymphocytic infiltration of the minor salivary glands.

• ESR: usually elevated. • Autoantibodies: RF, ANA, anti-Ro (SS-A) and anti-La (SS-B).

Management

Treatment is largely symptomatic:

• Artificial tears and lubricants for dry eyes. • Artificial saliva for xerostomia. • Lubricants for vaginal dryness. • Hydroxychloroquine is often used for skin and musculoskeletal features and may help fatigue.

Polymyositis and dermatomyositis

These rare connective tissue disorders are characterised by muscle weakness and inflammation. The onset is usually between 40 and 60 years of age. Both conditions are associated with underlying malignancy.

Clinical features

The typical presentation is with symmetrical proximal muscle weakness over a few weeks, usually affecting the lower limbs more than the upper, in adults between 40 and 60 years of age. Patients report difficulty rising from a chair, climbing stairs and lifting, often with muscle pain. Systemic features include fever, weight loss and fatigue. Respiratory or pharyngeal muscle involvement can lead to ventilatory failure or aspiration. Interstitial lung disease occurs in up to 30% of patients and is strongly associated with antisynthetase (Jo-1) antibodies.

In DM, the skin lesions include Gottron's papules, which are scaly, erythematous or violaceous, plaques occurring over the extensor surfaces of PIP and DIP joints (Fig. 18.14) and a violaceous discoloration of the eyelid with periorbital oedema ('heliotrope rash'). Similar rashes occur on the upper back, chest and shoulders. Nail-fold capillaries are often enlarged and tortuous.

Investigations

Muscle biopsy shows typical features of fibre necrosis and inflammatory cell infiltration. MRI can help identify areas of abnormal muscle. CK is usually raised and tracks disease activity. ANA and anti-Jo1 antibodies may be positive. EMG may confirm the presence of myopathy. Occult malignancy should be excluded (CT chest/abdo, mammography and PSA).

15

Management

Oral glucocorticoids are the mainstay of initial treatment. Patients with severe weakness or respiratory or pharyngeal involvement may require IV methylprednisolone. Additional immunosuppressive therapy (e.g. azathioprine or methotrexate) is often required.

Vasculitis

Vasculitis is characterised by inflammation and necrosis of blood vessel walls with associated damage to skin, kidney, lung, heart, brain and gastrointestinal tract. Clinical features (Box 15.16) result from both local tissue ischaemia and the systemic effects of widespread inflammation. Systemic vasculitis should be considered in any patient with fever, weight loss, fatigue, multiorgan involvement, rashes, raised inflammatory markers and abnormal urinalysis.

Antineutrophil cytoplasmic antibody-associated vasculitis

ANCA antibodies (perinuclear or p-ANCA and cytoplasmic or c-ANCA) are associated with two types of small-vessel vasculitis:

Microscopic polyangiitis (MPA) A necrotising small-vessel vasculitis associated with rapidly progressive glomerulonephritis, alveolar haemorrhage, neuropathy and pleural effusions. Patients are usually p-ANCA–positive.

Granulomatosis with polyangiitis (formerly Wegener's granulomatosis): Characterised by granuloma formation in the nasopharynx, airways and kidney (glomerulonephritis). It presents with epistaxis, nasal crusting and sinusitis, but haemoptysis, mucosal ulceration and deafness are also seen. Proptosis occurs because of retro-orbital inflammation, causing diplopia or visual loss. Untreated nasal disease may erode bone and cartilage. Pulmonary infiltrates and cavitating nodules occur in 50% of patients. Patients are usually c-ANCA–positive, with elevated CRP and ESR. MRI is useful in localising abnormalities, but the diagnosis should be confirmed by biopsy of the kidney or upper airway lesions.

Initial treatment is to give high-dose glucocorticoids with cyclophosphamide or rituximab; maintenance treatment is with lower-dose glucocorticoids and azathioprine, methotrexate or mycophenolate. A chronic relapsing course is usual.

i	**15.16 Clinical features of systemic vasculitis**
Systemic	Malaise, fever, night sweats, weight loss, arthralgia, myalgia
Rashes	Palpable purpura, pulp infarcts, ulceration, livedo reticularis
ENT	Epistaxis, sinusitis, deafness
Respiratory	Haemoptysis, cough, poorly controlled asthma
GI	Abdominal pain (mucosal inflammation or enteric ischaemia), mouth ulcers, diarrhoea
Neurological	Sensory or motor neuropathy

Takayasu arteritis

This is a granulomatous vasculitis affecting the aorta and its major branches, and occasionally the pulmonary arteries. The typical age at onset is 25 to 30 years, with an 8:1 female:male ratio. The usual presentation is with claudication, fever, arthralgia and weight loss. Examination may reveal loss of pulses, bruits and aortic incompetence. Diagnosis is by angiography, which shows coarctation, occlusion and aneurysmal dilatation. Treatment is as for ANCA-associated vasculitis.

Kawasaki's disease

This rare vasculitis causes coronary arteritis in children aged under 5 years. It presents with fever, rash and pericarditis, myocarditis or infarction.

Polyarteritis nodosa

PAN is a necrotising vasculitis of medium and small arteries, presenting age 20 to 40 years, with a 2:1 male preponderance. Hepatitis B is a risk factor for PAN.

Presentation is with myalgia, arthralgia, fever and weight loss, together with manifestations of multisystem disease. Skin involvement can cause a palpable purpuric rash, ulceration, infarction and livedo reticularis. Arteritis of the vasa nervorum leads to a symmetrical sensory and motor neuropathy. Severe hypertension and renal impairment may occur because of multiple renal infarctions. Diagnosis is confirmed by finding multiple aneurysms and narrowing of the mesenteric, hepatic or renal vessels on angiography. Muscle or sural nerve biopsy may also be diagnostic. Treatment is as for ANCA-associated vasculitis.

Giant cell arteritis and polymyalgia rheumatica

GCA is a granulomatous arteritis affecting large and medium-sized arteries. It is commonly associated with PMR, which causes pain and stiffness in the shoulders and hips. Because many patients with GCA have symptoms of PMR, and many patients with PMR go on to develop GCA if untreated, they may be different manifestations of one underlying disorder. Both are rare under the age of 60 years. The average age at onset is 70 years, with a female preponderance of around 3:1. The overall prevalence is around 20/100 000 in those aged over 50 years.

Clinical features

The cardinal symptom of GCA is temporal or occipital headache, which may be accompanied by scalp tenderness. Jaw pain develops in some patients, brought on by chewing or talking. Visual disturbance (e.g. amaurosis) can occur, and GCA may present with blindness in one eye because of occlusion of the posterior ciliary artery. On fundoscopy, the optic disc may appear pale and swollen with haemorrhages, but these changes take 24 to 36 hours to develop, and the fundi may initially appear normal. Rarely, transient ischaemic attacks, brainstem infarcts and hemiparesis may occur. Constitutional symptoms, such as weight loss, fatigue, malaise and night sweats, are common.

PMR presents with symmetrical muscle pain and stiffness affecting the shoulder and pelvic girdles. Symptoms usually appear over a few days, but onset may be more insidious. Examination reveals stiffness and painful restriction of active shoulder movement, but passive movements are preserved. Muscles may be tender to palpation, but weakness and muscle-wasting are absent.

Investigations

• Raised ESR and CRP. • Normochromic, normocytic anaemia. • Abnormal liver function. Confirmation of GCA is important, this can be by temporal artery biopsy, ultrasound of the temporal arteries and [19]FDG PET scan. Multiple biopsies are needed because the lesions are focal, and false negatives may occur with 'skip' lesions. A positive PET scan is specific, but sensitivity is low.

Management

Prednisolone should be commenced urgently in suspected GCA to prevent visual loss. Symptoms will completely resolve within 48 to 72 hours of starting glucocorticoids in virtually all patients. The prednisolone dose should be reduced progressively, guided by symptoms and ESR, until an acceptable dose is achieved (5–7.5 mg daily). If symptoms recur, the dose should be temporarily increased again. Most patients need glucocorticoids for an average of 12 to 24 months. Prophylaxis against osteoporosis should be given in patients with low bone mineral density.

Eosinophilic granulomatosis with polyangiitis (Churg–Strauss syndrome)

This is a small-vessel vasculitis presenting with skin lesions (purpura or nodules), mononeuritis multiplex and eosinophilia on a background of resistant asthma. Pulmonary infiltrates may be present. Mesenteric vasculitis can cause abdominal symptoms. Either c-ANCA or p-ANCA is present in around 60% of cases. Diagnosis is by biopsy of an affected site, and treatment is as for ANCA-associated vasculitis.

Henoch–Schönlein purpura

This small-vessel vasculitis is caused by immune complex deposition, and usually affects children and young adults. Typical presentation is with purpura over the buttocks and lower legs, abdominal symptoms (pain and bleeding) and arthritis (knee or ankle) following an upper respiratory tract infection. Nephritis may result in renal impairment. The diagnosis is confirmed by demonstrating IgA within blood vessel walls. Henoch–Schönlein purpura is usually self-limiting, but glucocorticoids and immunosuppressants are used for severe disease, for example, nephritis.

Cryoglobulinaemic vasculitis

This is a small-vessel vasculitis that occurs when immunoglobulins precipitate in the cold. The typical presentation is with a vasculitic rash over the legs, arthralgia, Raynaud's phenomenon and neuropathy. Some cases are secondary to hepatitis B or C or to autoimmune disease. Glucocorticoids and immunosuppressive therapy are often used, but their efficacy is uncertain.

Behçet's disease

This rare vasculitis characteristically targets venules. The diagnosis is clinical, and is based on the presence of recurrent oral ulceration together with two of the following:

• Recurrent genital ulceration. • Eye lesions: anterior or posterior uveitis, retinal vasculitis. • Skin lesions: erythema nodosum, papulopustular lesions, acneiform nodules. • Positive pathergy test: skin pricking with a needle results in pustule development within 48 hours.

Other features include meningitis, encephalitis and recurrent thromboses. Oral ulceration is treated with topical glucocorticoids. Thalidomide is effective for resistant oral and genital ulceration but is highly teratogenic. Glucocorticoids and immunosuppressants are indicated for uveitis and neurological disease.

Diseases of bone

Osteoporosis

Osteoporosis is the most common bone disease. It is characterised by reduced BMD with an increased risk of fracture and increases markedly with age. Lifetime fracture risk is about 33% in women and 20% in men aged 50 years and over. In normal individuals, bone mass increases to reach a peak between the ages of 20 and 45 years but falls thereafter. Bone turnover throughout life depends on the balance between bone formation by osteoblasts and bone resorption by osteoclasts. There is an accelerated phase of bone loss in women after the menopause as a result of oestrogen deficiency, which alters this balance in favour of increased bone resorption. This leads to an increased risk of osteoporosis and fractures, particularly in women with a low peak bone mass. Conditions increasing the risk of osteoporosis are shown in Box 15.17.

Glucocorticoids are an important cause of osteoporosis. Although there is no 'safe' dose of glucocorticoid, the risk increases when the dose of prednisolone exceeds 7.5 mg daily for more than 3 months. Glucocorticoids mainly cause osteoporosis by inhibiting bone formation and causing apoptosis of osteoblasts and osteocytes. They also inhibit intestinal calcium absorption and increase renal calcium excretion, leading to secondary hyperparathyroidism with increased osteoclastic bone resorption.

15

i	**15.17 Risk factors for osteoporosis**	
Genetics	Polygenic inheritance, rarely single gene disorders
Endocrine disease	Early menopause, hypogonadism, hyperthyroidism, hyperparathyroidism, Cushing's syndrome
Inflammatory disease	Inflammatory bowel disease, RA, ankylosing spondylitis
Drugs	Corticosteroids, anticonvulsants, heparin, alcohol excess
GI disease	Malabsorption, chronic liver disease
Respiratory disease	COPD, cystic fibrosis
Miscellaneous	Myeloma, anorexia nervosa, lack of exercise, immobilisation, poor diet/low body weight, smoking, HIV

Clinical features

Osteoporosis is asymptomatic until a fracture occurs. The most common sites are the forearm (Colles fracture), spine (vertebral fractures causing back pain, height loss and kyphosis) and femur (hip fracture).

Investigations

Bone mineral density is measured using dual energy X-ray absorptiometry (DEXA) of the lumbar spine and hip. DEXA should be performed in patients sustaining low trauma fractures or other features of osteoporosis, and individuals with a 10-year fracture risk greater than 10% as judged by a risk-assessment tool (e.g. www.shef.ac.uk/FRAX/).

DEXA yields a T-score that measures by how many standard deviations the patient's BMD value differs from that of a young, healthy control. Osteoporosis is diagnosed when the T-score value falls to −2.5 or below. T-scores between −1.0 and −2.5 indicate osteopenia, and values above −1.0 are regarded as normal. If osteoporosis is confirmed by bone densitometry, any predisposing factors should be sought (see Box 15.17). Relevant blood tests include:
• U&Es, calcium, phosphate. • TFTs. • Immunoglobulins. • ESR. • Anti-tissue transglutaminase (for coeliac disease). • 25(OH) vitamin D. • PTH. • Sex hormone and gonadotrophin levels.

Management

Nonpharmacological interventions:

• Cessation of smoking. • Limitation of alcohol intake. • Adequate dietary calcium intake (1500 mg daily). • Regular exercise. • Refer to a multidisciplinary falls prevention team if unsteady on a 'get up and go' test.

Osteopenic patients should be offered a repeat BMD measurement in 2 to 3 years.

Pharmacological interventions:

Bisphosphonates: These are first-line drugs for treatment of osteoporosis. They reduce bone resorption by osteoclasts and reduce fracture risk. Oral bisphosphonates (e.g. alendronic acid) should be taken on an empty stomach, with no food for 30 to 45 minutes after administration. Intravenous zolendronic acid is given to those unable to tolerate or unresponsive to oral bisphoshonates. Osteonecrosis of the jaw is a rare but important side effect.

Denosumab: A monoclonal antibody which inhibits bone resorption, denosumab is given SC six monthly.

Teriparitide: A fragment of PTH, teriparitide is given by daily SC injection, and stimulates new bone formation.

Calcium and vitamin D supplements: Calcium (1 g daily) and vitamin D supplements (800 IU daily) are used as an adjunct to other treatments. As monotherapy, they do not reduce fracture risk in osteoporosis.

Hormone replacement therapy: HRT with oestrogen and progestogens prevents postmenopausal bone loss and reduces vertebral and nonvertebral osteoporotic fractures. It is mainly used to prevent osteoporosis in women with an early menopause and those with osteoporosis and troublesome menopausal symptoms. HRT should be avoided in women over 60 years of age because it increases the risk of breast cancer and cardiovascular disease.

Osteomalacia, rickets and vitamin D deficiency

Osteomalacia and rickets result from defective bone mineralisation most commonly because of vitamin D deficiency. In adults, osteomalacia describes a syndrome of bone pain, bone fragility and fractures. Rickets is the equivalent in children and features enlargement of the growth plate and bone deformity. The disease remains prevalent in frail older people with a poor diet and limited sunlight exposure, and in some Muslim women.

Vitamin D deficiency can result from lack of sunlight exposure, dietary deficiency or malabsorption in patients with GI disease. In normal individuals, around 70% is made in the skin from 7-dehydrocholesterol under the influence of ultraviolet light, whereas the remaining 30% is derived from the diet. Lack of vitamin D is accompanied by a reduction in $25(OH)D_3$ synthesis in the liver. This causes reduced production of the active metabolite $1,25(OH)_2D_3$ in the kidneys, reduced intestinal calcium absorption and low serum calcium. Low serum calcium stimulates PTH secretion, resulting in secondary hyperparathyroidism and subsequent increased osteoclastic bone resorption, reduced renal calcium excretion and increased renal phosphate excretion. This sequence represents an attempt by the parathyroid glands to restore serum calcium levels to normal; however, this cannot be achieved with continuing vitamin D deficiency, so there is progressive loss of both calcium and phosphate from bone and defective mineralisation.

Osteomalacia also occurs in association with defects of vitamin D metabolism and function:

Chronic renal failure: Renal synthesis of the active metabolite of vitamin D $(1,25(OH)_2D_3)$ fails.

Mutations in the renal 1α-hydroxylase enzyme: These mutations render the enzyme unable to convert $25(OH)D_3$ to $1,25(OH)_2D_3$ and cause vitamin D-resistant rickets type I.

Mutations in the vitamin D receptor: These mutations render the receptor resistant to activation by $1,25(OH)_2D_3$ and cause vitamin D-resistant rickets type II.

Clinical features

In children, rickets causes enlargement of epiphyses at the lower end of the radius and swelling of the costochondral junctions ('rickety rosary').

Osteomalacia in adults presents more insidiously and may be asymptomatic. When symptomatic, it causes bone pain, pathological fractures and proximal muscle weakness, causing a waddling gait and difficulty climbing stairs or rising from a chair.

Investigations

Serum $25(OH)D_3$, PTH, calcium, phosphate and alkaline phosphatase levels should be measured. Vitamin D-deficient osteomalacia is suggested by low or low–normal calcium and phosphate, raised alkaline phosphatase, low $25(OH)D_3$ and raised PTH. X-rays are of limited value in diagnosis but may show focal radiolucent areas (Looser's zones) in advanced cases. Osteopenia is a common finding. Bone biopsy can be used to confirm the diagnosis.

15

Management

Rickets and osteomalacia caused by vitamin D deficiency respond rapidly to oral vitamin D and calcium supplementation. Higher doses may be required in patients with malabsorption. Osteomalacia caused by renal failure and vitamin D-resistant rickets type I requires treatment with active vitamin D metabolites ($1\text{-}\alpha\text{-}(OH)D_3$ or $1,25(OH)_2D_3$) because these bypass the defect in $1\text{-}\alpha$-hydroxylation of $25(OH)D_3$. Serum calcium and alkaline phosphatase should be monitored to assess response to treatment.

Paget's disease of bone

PDB is characterised by focal areas of increased and disorganised bone remodelling. It increases in frequency with age, affecting 8% of the UK population by the age of 85 years. Genetic factors are implicated in the aetiology of PDB; mutations in the *SQSTM1* gene are a common cause of classical PDB. The presence of inclusion bodies within osteoclasts has led to speculation that a slow virus infection may also play a role. The primary abnormality in PDB is increased osteoclastic bone resorption accompanied by increased osteoblast activity. The resultant bone is architecturally abnormal and has reduced mechanical strength. Other features of PDB are marrow fibrosis and increased bone vascularity.

Clinical features

PDB most commonly affects the pelvis, femur, tibia, lumbar spine and skull. Patients classically present with bone pain, deformity and pathological fractures, although many cases are asymptomatic. Clinical signs include bone deformity and expansion with increased warmth over affected bones. Bone deformity is most evident in the femur, tibia and skull. Neurological complications include deafness and spinal cord compression. The deafness is often conductive in nature because of osteosclerosis of the temporal bone. Other rare complications include high-output cardiac failure (because of increased bone vascularity) and osteosarcoma.

Investigations

Alkaline phosphatase is raised with normal calcium and phosphate levels. X-rays show areas of osteosclerosis alternating with areas of radiolucency, together with bone expansion and deformity. Radionuclide bone scanning is useful in confirming PDB and documenting its extent. Bone biopsy is not usually required to make the diagnosis but can occasionally be helpful in differentiating PDB from sclerotic bony metastases.

Management

Inhibitors of bone resorption are used to control of bone pain which results from increased metabolic activity. If paracetamol and NSAIDs are ineffective, then bisphosphonates (e.g. oral risedronate, IV pamidronate, IV zoledronic acid) are helpful in suppressing bone turnover and controlling pain. Currently, there is no evidence to show that bisphosphonates are effective in preventing complications such as deafness, bone deformity and fracture.

Scheuermann's osteochondritis

This predominantly affects adolescent boys, who develop a dorsal kyphosis with irregular radiographic ossification of the vertebral end plates. It has a strong genetic component and may be inherited as an autosomal dominant trait. Most patients are asymptomatic, but back pain, aggravated by exercise and relieved by rest, may occur. Management consists of avoidance of excessive activity and provision of protective postural exercises. Rarely, corrective surgery may be required for severe deformity.

Osteogenesis imperfecta

This rare disease is characterised by bone fragility presenting with multiple fractures in infancy and childhood. It is caused by genetic defects of collagen production. Other common features include blue sclerae and abnormal dentition. Treatment is multidisciplinary, involving orthopaedic surgery for the management of fractures and limb deformities, physiotherapy and occupational therapy.

Primary bone tumours

Primary bone tumours are less common than secondary bone metastases. They have a peak incidence in childhood and adolescence, although osteosarcoma secondary to PDB affects adults over 40 years of age.

Primary bone tumours present with local pain and swelling. Plain X-rays show expansion of the bone, CT and MRI are used for staging, and diagnosis is confirmed by biopsy. Treatment usually involves surgical removal followed by chemotherapy and radiotherapy. The prognosis is generally good in cases presenting in childhood and adolescence, but poor in elderly patients with osteosarcoma related to PDB.

15

Neurology

The complexity of the brain differentiates us from other species, and its interactions with the spinal cord and peripheral nerves combine to allow us to perceive and react to the external world while maintaining a stable internal environment.

In the UK, some 10% of the population consult their GP each year with a neurological symptom, and neurological disorders account for 20% of acute medical admissions and a large proportion of chronic physical disability.

Presenting problems in neurological disease

Headache and facial pain

Most headaches are chronic disorders, but acute headache is an important symptom in emergency medical care (dealt with on p. 68). Headache may be divided into:
• Primary (benign): for example, migraine, tension headache, cluster headache, thunderclap headache (p. 70). • Secondary: for example, medication overuse, intracerebral bleed, infection, temporal arteritis, referred pain.

Most patients have primary syndromes.

Ocular pain

Assuming ocular disease (see p. 715) has been excluded, ocular pain may be caused by TACs or, rarely, inflammatory or infiltrative lesions at the apex of the orbit or the cavernous sinus, when 3rd, 4th, 5th or 6th cranial nerve involvement is usually evident.

Facial pain

Pain in the face can be caused by dental, temporomandibular joint or sinus problems, but this is usually apparent from other features. Facial pain is common in migraine, but some syndromes can present solely with facial pain. The most common neurological causes are trigeminal neuralgia, herpes zoster (shingles) and postherpetic neuralgia; all cause severe pain. In trigeminal neuralgia, the patient describes brief bouts of lancinating pain ('electric shocks'), most frequently in the second and third divisions of the nerve, triggered by talking or chewing. Facial shingles most commonly affects the ophthalmic division of the trigeminal nerve, and pain usually precedes the rash. Postherpetic neuralgia may follow, typically a continuous burning pain throughout the affected territory, with marked sensitivity to light touch (allodynia) and resistance to treatment. Destructive lesions of the trigeminal nerve usually cause numbness rather than pain.

Clinical examination of the nervous system

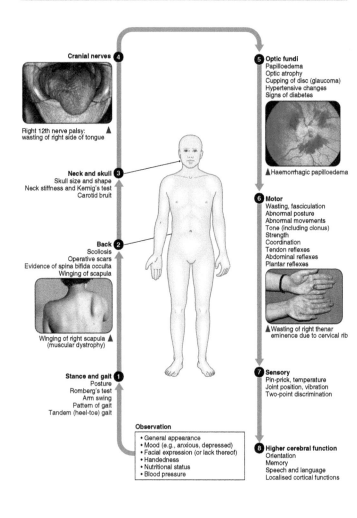

Cranial nerves 4

Right 12th nerve palsy: wasting of right side of tongue ▲

Neck and skull 3
Skull size and shape
Neck stiffness and Kernig's test
Carotid bruit

Back 2
Scoliosis
Operative scars
Evidence of spina bifida occulta
Winging of scapula

Winging of right scapula ▲
(muscular dystrophy)

Stance and gait 1
Posture
Romberg's test
Arm swing
Pattern of gait
Tandem (heel-toe) gait

Observation
• General appearance
• Mood (e.g., anxious, depressed)
• Facial expression (or lack thereof)
• Handedness
• Nutritional status
• Blood pressure

Optic fundi 5
Papilloedema
Optic atrophy
Cupping of disc (glaucoma)
Hypertensive changes
Signs of diabetes

▲ Haemorrhagic papilloedema

Motor 6
Wasting, fasciculation
Abnormal posture
Abnormal movements
Tone (including clonus)
Strength
Coordination
Tendon reflexes
Abdominal reflexes
Plantar reflexes

▲ Wasting of right thenar
eminence due to cervical rib

Sensory 7
Pin-prick, temperature
Joint position, vibration
Two-point discrimination

Higher cerebral function 8
Orientation
Memory
Speech and language
Localised cortical functions

Dizziness, blackouts and 'funny turns'

Acute onset of dizziness or blackouts will present to the acute medical department. In neurological practice, it is common to deal with patients presenting with a history of multiple events. Although detailed questioning will be dealt with in the relevant section (p. 63), the neurologist will have to tease out the pattern of each of the different attack types experienced by the patient to be able to form a treatment and investigation plan, one of the challenges of clinical neurology.

Status epilepticus

Status epilepticus is seizure activity not resolving spontaneously, or recurrent seizure without recovery of consciousness in between. It is an emergency with a recognised mortality.

Diagnosis is clinical, based on the description of prolonged rigidity and/or clonic movements with loss of awareness. Cyanosis, pyrexia, acidosis and sweating may occur, and complications include aspiration, hypotension, arrhythmias and renal or hepatic failure.

In patients with preexisting epilepsy, the most common cause is a subtherapeutic antiepileptic drug level. In de novo status epilepticus, precipitants such as infection (meningitis, encephalitis), neoplasia and metabolic derangement (hypoglycaemia, hyponatraemia, hypocalcaemia) should be excluded. Management is outlined in Box 16.1.

16.1 Management of status epilepticus

Initial

- Check airway, pulse, BP, blood glucose stick, respiratory rate
- Secure IV access
- Send blood for glucose, U&Es, calcium, magnesium, LFTs, drug levels
- If seizures continue >5 minutes, give midazolam 10 mg buccaly or nasally *or* lorazepam 4 mg IV *or* diazepam 10 mg IV (or rectally); repeat *once only* after 15 minutes
- Correct any metabolic trigger, e.g. hypoglycaemia

Ongoing

If seizures continue >30 minutes

- IV infusion (with cardiac monitoring) with one of:
  Phenytoin: 15 mg/kg at 50 mg/min
  Sodium valproate: 20–30 mg/kg at 40 mg/min
  Phenobarbital: 10 mg/kg at 100 mg/min

If seizures still continue after 30–60 minutes

- Transfer to ICU for intubation and ventilation, and general anaesthesia using propofol or thiopental, EEG monitor

Once status controlled

- Commence longer-term anticonvulsant medication with one of:
  Sodium valproate 10 mg/kg IV over 3–5 minutes, then 800–2000 mg/day
  Phenytoin: give loading dose (if not already used) of 15 mg/kg, infuse at <50 mg/min, then 300 mg/day
  Carbamazepine 400 mg by nasogastric tube, then 400–1200 mg/day
- Investigate cause

16

Coma

Coma and loss of consciousness usually present to the acute medical admissions department (p. 78). Clarification of cause and prognosis may require specialist neurological input.

Delirium

Delirium describes cortical dysfunction and replaces the older term 'acute confusional state'. It has a range of primary causes, and given its role in precipitating acute admission, is covered on p. 66.

Amnesia

Memory disturbance is common. In the absence of significant functional impairment, many patients prove to have benign memory dysfunction related to age, mood or psychiatric disorders. Publicity about dementia has led to more patients presenting with memory loss; however, many have benign symptoms. Diagnosis and treatment of dementia is discussed later (p. 680). Temporary memory loss may be as a result of delirium secondary to infection, a postictal state or transient global amnesia. These are distinguished from the history.

Transient global amnesia

This predominantly affects middle-aged people with an abrupt, discrete loss of anterograde memory function, leading to repetitive questioning. Consciousness is preserved, and after 4 to 6 hours, memory and behaviour return to normal. There are none of the phenomena associated with seizures, and transient global amnesia recurs in only 10% to 20%. There are no physical signs and, provided there is a typical history (which requires a witness), no investigation is necessary.

Persistent amnesia

This more commonly signifies serious disease. When short-term memory is affected, Korsakoff's syndrome (often secondary to alcohol) is likely. Progressive loss should lead to testing for dementia. Depression may present as a 'pseudo-dementia', with concentration and memory impairment that may respond to antidepressants. However patients with dementia (particularly Alzheimer's) may develop depression in the early stages.

Weakness

Lesions in various parts of the motor system produce distinctive patterns of motor deficit.

The motor system

A programme of movement formulated by the premotor cortex is converted into a series of muscle movements in the motor cortex and then transmitted to the spinal cord in the pyramidal tract (Fig. 16.1). The effect of lesions at different levels in this motor pathway is summarised in Fig. 16.2.

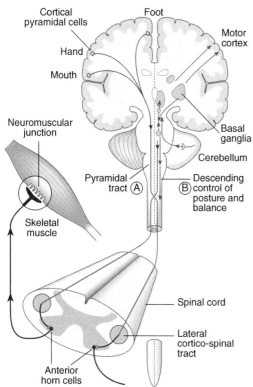

Fig. 16.1 The motor system. Neurons from the motor cortex descend as the pyramidal tract in the internal capsule and cerebral peduncle to the ventral brainstem, where most cross low in the medulla (A). In the spinal cord, the upper motor neurons form the cortico-spinal tract in the lateral column before synapsing with the lower motor neurons in the anterior horns. The activity in the motor cortex is modulated by influences from the basal ganglia and cerebellum. Pathways descending from these structures control posture and balance (B).

16

Lower motor neuron lesions: These cause loss of contraction in their units' muscle fibres, and the muscle will be weak and flaccid. Denervated muscle fibres atrophy, causing wasting. Re-innervation from neighbouring motor neurons occurs, but the neuromuscular junctions are unstable, causing fasciculations (visible to the naked eye because the motor units are larger than normal).

Upper motor neuron (pyramidal) lesions: Upper motor neurons have both excitatory and inhibitory influences on anterior horn cells. Upper motor neuron lesions cause increased tone, most evident in the strongest muscle groups (i.e., leg extensors and arm flexors); weakness is conversely more pronounced in the opposing muscle groups. Loss of inhibition leads to

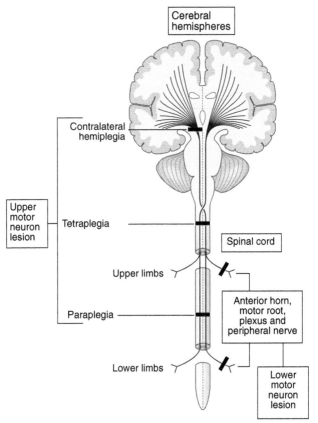

Fig. 16.2 Patterns of motor loss according to the anatomical site of the lesion.

brisk reflexes, an extensor plantar response and enhanced reflex patterns of movement, such as flexion withdrawal to noxious stimuli and spasms of extension.

Extrapyramidal lesions: These affect circuits connecting the basal ganglia with the cortex. There is an increase in tone, which is continuous throughout the range of movement at any speed of stretch ('lead-pipe' rigidity). Involuntary movements are present, and a tremor combined with rigidity produces typical 'cogwheel' rigidity. Rapid movements are slowed (bradykinesia). Extrapyramidal lesions also cause postural instability, precipitating falls.

Cerebellar lesions: These cause lack of coordination on the same side of the body. The initial movement is normal, but accuracy deteriorates as the target is approached, producing an 'intention tremor'.

16.2 How to assess weakness

Clinical finding	Likely level of lesion/diagnosis
Pattern and distribution	
Isolated muscles	Radiculopathy or mononeuropathy
Both limbs on one side (hemiparesis)	Cerebral hemisphere, less likely cord or brainstem
One limb	Neuronopathy, plexopathy, cord/brain
Both lower limbs (paraparesis)	Spinal cord; look for a sensory level
Fatigability	Myasthenia gravis
Bizarre, fluctuating, not following anatomical rules	Functional
Signs	
Upper motor neuron	Brain/spinal cord
Lower motor neuron	Peripheral nervous system
Evolution of the weakness	
Sudden and improving	Stroke/mononeuropathy
Evolving over months or years	Meningioma, cervical spondylotic my-elopathy
Gradually worsening over days or weeks	Cerebral mass, demyelination
Associated symptoms	
Absence of sensory involvement	Motor neuron disease, myopathy, myasthenia

The distances of targets are misjudged (dysmetria), resulting in 'past-pointing'. The ability to produce rapid, regularly alternating movements is impaired (dysdiadochokinesis). Disorders of the central vermis of the cerebellum produce a characteristic ataxic gait.

Clinical assessment of weakness

The pattern of symptoms and signs usually indicates the nature of the lesion (Box 16.2, Fig. 16.2). It is important to establish whether the patient has loss of power, altered sensation or generalised fatigue. Pain may restrict movement, mimicking weakness, whereas sensory neglect (p. 646) may leave patients unaware of severe weakness.

Patients with parkinsonism may complain of weakness; examination reveals rigidity (cogwheel or lead pipe), bradykinesia should be evident, and there is a resting tremor, usually asymmetrical (p. 681). Inspection of gait may be diagnostic. Movement restricted by pain should be apparent to observation, as should contractures, wasting, fasciculations and abnormal movements/postures.

16

Functional weakness is common. Clinical examination findings are often variable (e.g. the patient can walk but appears to have no leg movement when assessed on the couch), and strength may appear to 'give way', with the patient able to achieve full power for brief bursts, which does not occur in disease. In functional weakness, one may see hip extension weakness (rarely organic), which then returns to full strength on testing contralateral hip flexion. This sign may be demonstrated to the patient in a nonconfrontational manner, to show that the potential limb power is intact.

Facial nerve palsy (Bell's palsy)

One of the most common causes of facial weakness is Bell's palsy, a lower motor neuron lesion of the 7th (facial) nerve within the facial canal, affecting all ages and both sexes. It is more common following upper respiratory tract infections, during pregnancy, and in patients with diabetes, immunosuppression and hypertension.

Symptoms develop subacutely over a few hours, with pain around the ear preceding unilateral lower motor neurone facial weakness. Patients often describe numbness, but there is no objective sensory loss (except to taste, if the chorda tympani is involved). Hyperacusis indicates if the nerve to stapedius is involved, and there may also be diminished salivation and tear secretion. Vesicles in the ear or on the palate may indicate primary herpes zoster infection (p. 637).

Glucocorticoids speed recovery if started within 72 hours but antiviral drugs are ineffective. Artificial tears and taping the eye shut overnight helps prevent exposure keratitis and corneal abrasion. About 80% of patients recover spontaneously within 12 weeks. Unlike Bell's palsy, lesions with an upper motor neuron origin partly spare the upper face.

Sensory disturbance

Sensory symptoms are common and frequently benign, but sensory examination is difficult for both doctor and patient. Although neurological disease can cause sensory symptoms, systemic disorders can also be responsible. Perioral and digital tingling occurs with hyperventilation or hypocalcaemia (p. 397). When there is dysfunction of the relevant cerebral cortex, the patient's perception of the relevant part of the body may be distorted.

Numbness and paraesthesia

In the history, the most useful features are:
• Anatomical distribution. • Mode of onset of numbness. • Paraesthesia or pain.

Certain patterns can be recognised (Fig. 16.3). For example, in migraine the aura may consist of a front of paraesthesia followed by numbness that takes 20 to 30 minutes to spread over one half of the body. Sensory loss as a result of a vascular lesion, on the other hand, will occur more or less instantaneously. The numbness and paraesthesia of spinal cord lesions often ascend one or both lower limbs to a level on the trunk over hours or days. In psychogenic sensory change, the distribution usually neither conforms to a known anatomical pattern nor fits with any organic disease.

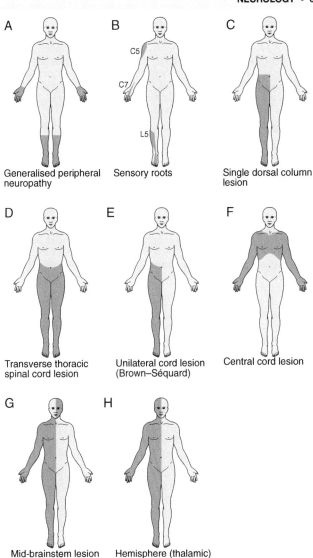

Fig. 16.3 Patterns of sensory loss. (A) Generalised peripheral neuropathy. **(B)** Sensory roots. **C** Single dorsal column lesion (proprioception and some touch loss). **(D)** Transverse thoracic spinal cord lesion. **(E)** Unilateral cord lesion (Brown–Séquard): ipsilateral dorsal column (and motor) deficit and contralateral spinothalamic deficit. **(F)** Central cord lesion: 'cape' distribution of spinothalamic loss. **(G)** Mid-brainstem lesion: ipsilateral facial sensory loss and contralateral loss on body. **(H)** Hemisphere (thalamic) lesion: contralateral loss on one side of face and body.

16

Sensory loss in peripheral nerve lesions

In peripheral nerve lesions, the symptoms are usually of sensory loss and paraesthesia. Single peripheral nerve lesions will cause disturbance in the sensory distribution of that nerve. In diffuse neuropathies the longest neurons are affected first, giving the characteristic 'glove and stocking' distribution. Diabetes typically affects small fibres, preferentially impairing temperature and pinprick, whereas demyelination may particularly affect large fibres subserving vibration and proprioception.

Sensory loss in nerve root lesions

Pain is a prominent feature of lesions of nerve roots within the spine or in the limb plexuses. It is often felt in the muscles innervated by a root. The site of nerve root lesions may be deduced from the dermatomal pattern of sensory loss.

Sensory loss in spinal cord lesions

Sensory information ascends the nervous system in two anatomically discrete systems, differential involvement of which is often of diagnostic assistance (Fig. 16.4).

Transverse spinal cord lesions: There is loss of all modalities below that segmental level. Often a band of paraesthesia or hyperaesthesia is found at the top of the area of loss. If vascular in origin (e.g. because of anterior spinal artery thrombosis), the posterior one-third of the spinal cord (dorsal column modalities) may be spared.

Unilateral spinal cord lesions: There is loss for spinothalamic modalities (pain and temperature) on the opposite side of the lesion. There is also loss for dorsal column modalities (joint position and vibration) on the same side as the lesion (e.g. Brown–Séquard syndrome).

Central spinal cord lesions (e.g. syringomyelia): These spare the dorsal columns but affect spinothalamic fibres crossing the cord from both sides over the length of the lesion. The sensory loss is therefore dissociated (in terms of the modalities affected) and suspended (segments above and below the lesion are spared).

Isolated dorsal column lesion (e.g. MS): The patient experiences an unpleasant tight feeling over the limb involved. There is loss of proprioception without any loss of pinprick or temperature sensation.

Sensory loss in brainstem lesions

Brainstem lesions produce complex patterns of sensory disturbance, including facial pain and numbness, depending on the anatomy of the lesion and its influence on the trigeminal nuclei.

Sensory loss in hemispheric lesions

These may affect all modalities of sensation. In the thalamus, discrete lesions (e.g. small lacunar strokes) can cause loss of sensation over the whole contralateral half of the body. Cortical lesions often produce mixed sensory and motor loss. Large lesions of the parietal cortex (e.g. large strokes) may cause severe loss of proprioception and even loss of conscious awareness of the existence of the affected limb (neglect).

Neuropathic pain

Pain is of two main types:
• Nociceptive pain, arising from a pathological process in a body part. • Neuropathic pain, caused by dysfunction of the pain perception apparatus itself.

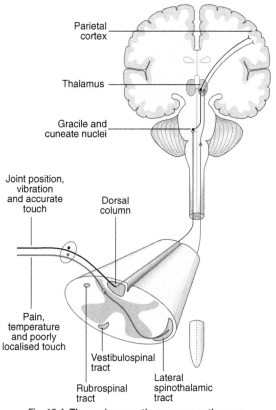

Fig. 16.4 The main somatic sensory pathways.

16

Neuropathic pain is a very unpleasant persistent burning sensation, often with increased sensitivity such that light touch causes pain (allodynia). The most common syndromes include partial damage to peripheral nerves ('causalgia'), the trigeminal nerve (postherpetic neuralgia) or the thalamus. Drugs (gabapentin, carbamazepine or tricyclics) may help, but usually only partially. Neurosurgical attempts to interrupt pain pathways sometimes succeed. Implantation of electrical stimulators has occasionally proved successful.

Abnormal movements

Abnormal movements usually imply a disorder in the basal ganglia, in which there is disinhibition of intrinsic rhythm generators or a disorder of postural control. They can be hypokinetic or hyperkinetic, and diagnosis requires observation and pattern recognition.

Tremor

The many causes of tremor have different characteristics:

Parkinsonian: 'Pill-rolling', asymmetrical and present at rest.

Physiological: Fine, enhanced by anxiety, emotion, drugs and toxins.

Essential: Slower than physiological tremor; often familial and responsive to propranolol.

Dystonic: Affects head, arms and legs; jerky, associated with dystonias.

Functional: Variable pattern; disappears on distraction.

Other hyperkinetic syndromes

Chorea: Jerky, brief, purposeless involuntary movements, appearing as fidgety; they suggest disease in the caudate nucleus. Causes include:
• Hereditary (Huntington's disease, Wilson's disease). • Drugs (levodopa, antipsychotics, anticonvulsants, oral contraceptives). • Autoimmune disease (e.g. Sydenham's chorea, antiphospholipid syndrome, systemic lupus erythematosus). • Endocrine factors (pregnancy, thyrotoxicosis, hypoparathyroidism, hypoglycaemia). • Other: vascular causes, demyelination, brain tumour, cerebral trauma or birth injury.

Athetosis: Slower writhing movements of the limbs—are often combined with chorea and share similar causes.

Ballism: This dramatic form of chorea causes flinging movements of the limbs (usually unilateral, hemiballism) in vascular lesions of the subthalamic nucleus.

Dystonia: Sustained involuntary muscle contraction causes abnormal postures or movement. It may be generalised (usually in genetic syndromes) or, more commonly, focal/segmental (such as torticollis, when the head twists repeatedly to one side). Some dystonias occur with specific tasks, such as writer's cramp or other occupational 'cramps'. The associated dystonic tremor is asymmetrical and of large amplitude.

Myoclonus: Brief, isolated, random, jerks of muscle groups. They occur normally at the onset of sleep (hypnic jerks). Myoclonus can occur in epilepsy, from subcortical structures or from segments of the spinal cord.

Tics: Repetitive stereotyped movements, such as blinking, winking, grinning or screwing up of the eyes. Unlike with other involuntary movements, patients can suppress tics, at least for a short time.

Abnormal perception

The parietal lobes are involved in the higher processing and integration of sensory information. This takes place in areas of 'association' cortex, damage to which causes sensory (including visual) inattention, disorders of spatial perception, and disruption of spatially orientated behaviour, leading to apraxia. Apraxia is the inability to perform complex, organised activity in the presence of normal basic motor, sensory and cerebellar function (after weakness, numbness and ataxia have been excluded). Examples of complex motor activities include dressing, using cutlery and geographical orientation. Other abnormalities that can result from damage to the association cortex involve difficulty reading (dyslexia) or writing (dysgraphia), or the inability to recognise familiar objects (agnosia).

Altered balance and vertigo

Disorders of balance can arise from abnormalities affecting:
• Input: loss of vision, vestibular disorders or lack of joint position sense.
• Processing: damage to vestibular nuclei or cerebellum. • Motor function: spinal cord lesions, leg weakness of any cause.

Disturbance of cerebellar function may also cause nystagmus, dysarthria or ataxia.

Disordered balance because of failure of proprioception or cerebellar function causes unsteadiness, whereas failure of the vestibular and labyrinthine apparatus causes vertigo, an illusory sensation of movement of the environment or self.

Vertigo occurs as a result of a mismatch between the information about a person's position reaching the brain from the eyes, limb proprioception and the vestibular system. Vertigo arising from inappropriate labyrinthine input is usually short-lived, although it may recur, whereas vertigo arising from central (brainstem) disorders is often persistent and accompanied by other signs of brainstem dysfunction.

Abnormal gait

Patterns of weakness, loss of coordination and proprioceptive sensory loss produce a range of abnormal gaits. Neurogenic disorders need to be distinguished from skeletal abnormalities, usually characterised by pain producing an antalgic gait, or limp.

Pyramidal gait: Upper motor neuron lesions cause extension of the leg. The tendency for the toes to strike the ground on walking requires the leg to swing outwards at the hip (circumduction). In hemiplegia, there is asymmetry between affected and normal sides, whereas in paraparesis, both legs move slowly, swung from the hips and dragged on the ground in extension.

Foot drop: Weakness of ankle dorsiflexion disrupts normal gait. Descent of the foot is less controlled, making a slapping noise, and the foot may be lifted higher, producing a high-stepping gait.

Myopathic gait: In proximal muscle weakness, usually caused by muscle disease, weak hip abductors allow pelvic tilt, causing exaggerated trunk movements, with a rolling or waddling gait.

Ataxic gait: Patients with lesions of the central parts of the cerebellum (the vermis) walk with a characteristic broad-based gait, 'as if drunk'. Patients with acute vestibular disturbances walk similarly but also experience vertigo.

Proprioceptive defects also impair walking, especially in poor light. The feet are placed with greater emphasis (to enhance proprioceptive input), causing a 'stamping' gait.

Apraxic gait: There is normal power, cerebellar function and proprioception, yet the patient cannot formulate the motor act of walking. This higher cerebral dysfunction occurs in bilateral hemisphere disease, such as normal pressure hydrocephalus and diffuse frontal lobe disease.

16

Marche à petits pas: This gait is characterised by small, slow steps and marked instability. The usual cause is small-vessel cerebrovascular disease, and there are accompanying bilateral upper motor neuron signs.

Extrapyramidal gait: Patients have difficulty initiating walking and controlling the pace of their gait. This produces the festinant gait: initial stuttering steps that quickly increase in frequency while decreasing in length.

Abnormal speech and language

Speech disturbance may be isolated to disruption of sound output (dysarthria) or may involve language disturbance (dysphasia). Dysphonia (reduction in the sound/volume) is usually caused by mechanical laryngeal disruption, whereas dysarthria is more typically neurological in origin. Dysphasia is always neurological and localises to the dominant cerebral hemisphere (usually left, regardless of handedness).

Dysphonia

Dysphonia describes hoarse or whispered speech. The commonest cause is laryngitis, but lesions of the vagus nerve or disease of the vocal cords also cause dysphonia. Parkinsonism may cause hypophonia with reduced speech volume, often with dysarthria, making speech hard to understand.

Dysarthria

Dysarthria means poorly articulated or slurred speech and can occur in association with lesions of the cerebellum, brainstem and lower cranial nerves, as well as in myasthenia or myopathic disease. Language function is not affected.

Dysphasia

Dysphasia (or aphasia) is a disorder of the language content of speech that causes an inability to produce the correct word. It can occur with lesions over a wide area of the dominant hemisphere. It is categorised as fluent or nonfluent. Fluent (or receptive) aphasias are impairments to the input or reception of language. Speech is easy and fluent, but output of language may also be affected, with paraphasia (substitution of similar-sounding nonwords, or incorrect words) and neologisms (nonexistent words). In nonfluent (expressive) aphasias, such as Broca's aphasia, verbal comprehension may be preserved. Patients with large lesions over much of the speech area have no language production and have 'global aphasia'.

Disturbance of smell

Symptomatic olfactory loss is most commonly attributed to local causes (nasal obstruction), but may follow head injury. Hyposmia may predate motor symptoms in Parkinson's disease. Frontal lobe lesions are a rare cause. Positive olfactory symptoms may arise in Alzheimer's disease or epilepsy.

Visual disturbance and ocular abnormalities

Visual disturbance

Visual loss as a result of ocular disease is covered in Chapter 17.

The visual pathway from the retina to the occipital cortex is topographically organised, so the pattern of visual field loss allows localisation of the site of the lesion (Fig. 16.5, Box 16.3). Patients often present with transient visual loss. Visual loss lasting less than 15 minutes is likely to have a vascular cause. This can affect one eye (amaurosis fugax) or one visual

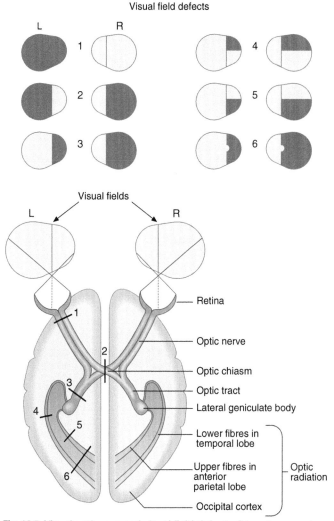

Fig. 16.5 Visual pathways and visual field defects. Schematic representation of eyes and brain in transverse section.

16.3 Clinical manifestations of visual field loss

Site	Common causes	Complaint	Visual field loss	Associated physical signs
Retina/ optic disc	Vascular disease (including vasculitis) Glaucoma Inflammation	Partial/complete visual loss depending on site	Altitudinal field defect Arcuate scotoma	Reduced acuity Visual distortion (macula) Abnormal retinal appearance
Optic nerve	Optic neuritis Sarcoidosis Tumour Leber's hereditary optic neuropathy	Partial/complete loss of vision in one eye Often painful Central vision particularly affected	Central scotoma Paracentral scotoma Monocular blindness	Reduced acuity Reduced colour vision Relative afferent pupillary defect
Optic chiasm	Pituitary tumours Craniopharyngioma Sarcoidosis	May be none Rarely diplopia ('hemifield slide')	Bitemporal hemianopia	Pituitary function abnormalities
Optic tract	Tumour Inflammatory disease	Disturbed vision to one side of midline	Incongruous contralateral homonymous hemianopia	
Temporal lobe	Stroke Tumour Inflammatory disease	Disturbed vision to one side of midline	Contralateral homonymous upper quadrantanopia	Memory/ language disorders
Parietal lobe	Stroke Tumour Inflammatory disease	Disturbed vision to one side of midline Bumping into things	Contralateral homonymous lower quadrantanopia	Contralateral sensory disturbance Asymmetry of optokinetic nystagmus
Occipital lobe	Stroke Tumour Inflammatory disease	Disturbed vision to one side of midline Difficulty reading Bumping into things	Homonymous hemianopia (may be macula-sparing)	Damage to other structures supplied by posterior cerebral circulation

field. The field loss may be monocular (carotid circulation) or a homonymous hemianopia (vertebro-basilar circulation). Transient visual disturbance lasting 10 to 60 minutes suggests migraine, especially if accompanied by headache and/or positive visual phenomena (e.g. zigzag lines, flashing coloured lights).

Visual hallucinations may be caused by drugs or epilepsy.

Eye movement disorders

The control of eye movements begins in the cerebral hemispheres, and the pathway descends to the brainstem with input from the visual cortex and cerebellum. Horizontal and vertical gaze centres in the pons and midbrain coordinate output to the ocular motor nerve nuclei (3, 4 and 6). These are connected to each other by the medial longitudinal fasciculus. The extraocular muscles are innervated by the trochlear (4th, supplying superior oblique), abducens (6th, supplying lateral rectus) and oculomotor (3rd, supplying the remaining extraocular muscles) nerves.

Double vision

The pattern of double vision and associated features allow localisation of the lesion, whilst the mode of onset and subsequent behaviour suggest the aetiology (e.g. fatigability in myasthenia). Monocular diplopia suggests ocular disease, whereas binocular diplopia (cancelled by closing one eye) suggests a neurological cause. Causes of ocular motor nerve palsies are given in Box 16.4.

Nystagmus

Nystagmus describes a repetitive to-and-fro movement of the eyes, with slow drifts followed by rapid correction movements. The direction of the fast phase is designated as the direction of the nystagmus because it is easier to see, although the abnormality is the slower drift of the eyes off target.

Brainstem/cerebellar lesions: Lesions allow the eyes to drift back in towards primary position, producing nystagmus with fast component that beats in the direction of gaze. They are bidirectional and not accompanied by vertigo. Brainstem disease may also cause vertical nystagmus. Unilateral cerebellar lesions may cause nystagmus in the direction of the lesion (fast phases are directed towards the side of the lesion).

Vestibular lesions: Damage to the horizontal canal allows output from the healthy, contralateral side to cause the eyes to drift towards the side of the lesion. Recurrent compensatory fast movements away from the lesion cause unidirectional horizontal nystagmus to the opposite side. Nystagmus of peripheral labyrinthine lesions fatigues quickly and is always accompanied by vertigo and/or nausea and vomiting. Central vestibular nystagmus is more persistent.

Other causes: These include physiological (in response to vestibular stimulation), toxicity (especially drugs), nutritional (thiamin) deficiency and congenital ('pendular' rather than 'jerking') causes.

16

Ptosis

Ptosis may result from a 3rd nerve palsy (Box 16.4), sympathetic nerve damage (Horner's syndrome) or muscle disorders (e.g. myasthenia gravis or myotonic dystrophy).

Abnormal pupillary responses

These may arise from lesions at several points between the retina and brainstem. Lesions of the 3rd nerve, ciliary ganglion and sympathetic supply produce characteristic pupillary disorders:

16.4 Common causes of damage to cranial nerves 3, 4 and 6			
Site	Common pathology	Nerve(s) involved	Associated features
Brainstem	Infarction Haemorrhage Demyelination Intrinsic tumour	3 (mid-brain) 6 (ponto-medullary junction)	Contralateral pyramidal signs Ipsilateral lower motor neuron 7 palsy Other brainstem/cerebellar signs
Intrameningeal	Meningitis Raised intracranial pressure	3, 4 and/or 6 6	Meningism Papilloedema Features of space-occupying lesion
		3 (uncal herniation)	
	Aneurysms	3 (posterior communicating artery)	Pain
		6 (basilar artery)	Features of subarachnoid haemorrhage
	Cerebello-pontine angle tumour	6	8, 7, 5 lesions Ipsilateral cerebellar signs
	Trauma	3, 4 and/or 6	Other features of trauma
Cavernous sinus	Infection/thrombosis Carotid artery aneurysm Carotico-cavernous fistula	3, 4 and/or 6	May be 5th nerve involvement also Pupil may be fixed, mid-position
Superior orbital fissure	Tumour (e.g. sphenoid wing meningioma) Granuloma	3, 4 and/or 6	May be proptosis, chemosis
Orbit	Vascular, infections, tumour, granuloma, trauma	3, 4 and/or 6	Pain Pupil often spared in vascular 3 palsy

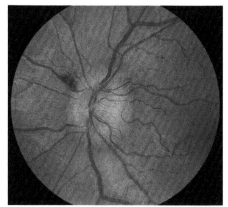

Fig. 16.6 Optic disc oedema (papilloedema). Fundus photograph of the left eye showing optic disc oedema with a small haemorrhage on the nasal side of the disc.

• Third nerve lesions: pupillary dilatation, complete ptosis and extraocular muscle palsy. • Sympathetic lesions (e.g. Horner's syndrome): partial ptosis and pupillary constriction. • Holmes–Adie pupils: dilation and constriction to accommodation but not to light. • Afferent pupillary disorders (in optic nerve damage): impairment of the direct light reflex–consensual response from stimulation of the normal eye remains intact.

Optic disc swelling

This occurs with:
• Raised intracranial pressure ('papilloedema'). • Venous obstruction (cavernous sinus or retinal). • Systemic disorders affecting retinal vessels (hypertension, hypercapnia, vasculitis). • Optic nerve damage (e.g. demyelination, ischaemia, sarcoid, glioma).

There is the cessation of normal venous pulsation at the disc, and the disc margins then become red and indistinct; the whole disc is raised up, often with haemorrhages in the retina (Fig. 16.6).

Optic atrophy

Optic nerve damage makes the optic disc appear pale (Fig. 16.7). Causes include:
• Previous optic neuritis. • Ischaemic damage. • Chronic papilloedema.
• Optic nerve compression. • Trauma. • Degenerative conditions.

Hearing disturbance

Each cochlear organ has bilateral cortical representation, so unilateral hearing loss indicates peripheral organ damage. Bilateral hearing dysfunction is usual and is usually caused by age-related degeneration or noise damage, although infection and drugs (particularly diuretics and aminoglycoside antibiotics) can cause deafness.

16

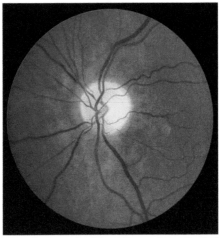

Fig. 16.7 Fundus photograph of the left eye of a patient with familial optic atrophy. Note marked pallor of optic disc.

Bulbar symptoms–dysphagia and dysarthria

Swallowing is a complex activity involving the lips, tongue, soft palate, pharynx, larynx and cranial nerves 7, 9, 10, 11 and 12. Structural causes of dysphagia are considered on p. 449. Neurological mechanisms usually cause dysphagia accompanied by dysarthria. Acute onset suggests a brainstem stroke or a rapidly developing neuropathy, such as Guillain–Barré syndrome or diphtheria. Intermittent fatigable muscle weakness (including dysphagia) suggests myasthenia gravis. Dysphagia developing over weeks or months occurs in motor neuron disease, basal meningitis and inflammatory brainstem disease. More slowly developing dysphagia suggests a myopathy or possibly a brainstem or skull-base tumour.

Pathologies affecting lower cranial nerves (9–12) frequently manifest bilaterally, producing dysphagia and dysarthria. 'Bulbar palsy' is the term for lower motor neuron lesions either within or outside the brainstem. The tongue may be wasted and fasciculating, and palatal movement reduced.

Upper motor neuron innervation of swallowing is bilateral, so persistent dysphagia is unusual with a unilateral upper motor lesion (except in the acute stages of a hemispheric stroke). Widespread lesions above the medulla will cause upper motor neuron bulbar paralysis, known as 'pseudobulbar palsy'. Here the tongue is small and contracted and moves slowly; the jaw jerk is brisk.

Bladder, bowel and sexual disturbance

Bladder

The bladder is analogous to skeletal muscle in that neural control can be divided into upper and lower motor neuron components.

Atonic (lower motor neuron) bladder: Distended with overflow, and loss of perineal sensation. It occurs in disease affecting the sacral cord or roots.

Hypertonic (upper motor neuron) bladder: Damage to the pons or spinal cord results in parasympathetic over-activity with frequency, urgency and urge incontinence. More severe spinal cord lesions can cause painless retention as bladder sensation is disrupted.

Damage to the frontal lobes causes loss of awareness of bladder fullness and consequent incontinence. Coexisting cognitive impairment may result in inappropriate micturition.

Rectum

The rectum has an excitatory cholinergic input from the parasympathetic sacral outflow, and inhibitory sympathetic supply similar to that of the bladder. Continence depends on skeletal muscle contraction in the pelvic floor muscles supplied by the pudendal nerves, as well as the internal and external anal sphincters.

Damage to the autonomic components usually causes constipation. Lesions affecting the conus medullaris, the somatic S2–4 roots and the pudendal nerves cause faecal incontinence.

Erectile failure and ejaculation failure

These related functions are under autonomic control via the pelvic (parasympathetic, S2–4) and hypogastric nerves (sympathetic, L1–2). Erection is largely parasympathetic and is impaired by several anticholinergic, antihypertensive and antidepressant drugs. Sympathetic activity is important for ejaculation and may be inhibited by α-adrenoceptor antagonists.

Personality change

Although this is often because of psychiatric illness, neurological conditions that alter the function of the frontal lobes can cause personality change and mood disorder. These include structural damage as a result of stroke, trauma, tumour or hydrocephalus. Three main patterns are seen:

Mesial frontal lesions: Cause patients to become withdrawn, unresponsive and mute, often with urinary incontinence, gait apraxia and increased tone.

Dorsolateral prefrontal cortical lesions: Cause difficulties with speech, motor planning and organisation.

Orbitofrontal lesions: Cause disinhibited or irresponsible behaviour. Memory is substantially intact, and there may be focal physical signs such as a grasp reflex, palmo-mental response or pout.

Functional symptoms

Many patients presenting with neurological symptoms do not have a defined neurological disease and are described as having functional symptoms. Such patients often have symptoms in multiple systems and a long list of consultations and negative tests from other specialties. Diagnosing functional symptoms may save the patient further unnecessary anxiety and investigation.

Weakness and sensory change predominate in functional neurological disorders, but pain or loss of consciousness can also occur. Associated tiredness, lethargy, poor concentration, bowel or and gynaecological complaints are common. The clinician must approach the patient's symptoms in a sensitive and nonjudgemental manner. Assessment for an underlying or exacerbating mood disorder is vital, ensuring that depression and anxiety are managed to minimise their secondary effects on symptoms.

Stroke

Stroke is a common medical emergency with an annual incidence of between 180 and 300 per 100 000. The incidence rises with age. About 20% of stroke patients die within a month of the event, and at least half of those who survive will be left with physical disability.

Acute stroke

Pathophysiology

Cerebral infarction

Cerebral infarction (85%) is mostly caused by thromboembolic disease secondary to atherosclerosis in the major extracranial arteries (carotid artery and aortic arch). About 20% are as a result of embolism from the heart, and 20% are as a result of intrinsic disease of small perforating vessels, producing so-called 'lacunar' infarctions. Perhaps 5% have rare causes, including vasculitis, endocarditis and cerebral venous disease. Risk factors for ischaemic stroke are similar to those for coronary artery disease (p. 276).

In the affected territory, as blood flow falls below the threshold for the maintenance of electrical activity, neurological deficit develops. At this point, the neurons are still viable; if the blood flow increases again, function returns, and the patient will have had a transient ischaemic attack (TIA). If the blood flow falls further, however, a level is reached at which irreversible cell death (infarction) occurs.

Intracerebral haemorrhage

Intracerebral haemorrhage (10%) usually results from rupture of a blood vessel within the brain parenchyma: a primary intracerebral haemorrhage. It may also occur with subarachnoid haemorrhage (5%) if the artery ruptures into the brain substance, as well as the subarachnoid space. Haemorrhage frequently occurs into an area of brain infarction; if large, it may be difficult to distinguish from primary intracerebral haemorrhage. Risk factors for intracerebral haemorrhage include:
• Age. • Hypertension. • Impaired clotting. • Intracranial vascular malformations. • Substance misuse.

> # ℹ️ 16.5 Differential diagnosis of stroke and TIA
>
> **'Structural' stroke mimics**
>
> - Primary cerebral tumours
> - Metastatic cerebral tumours
> - Subdural haematoma
> - Cerebral abscess
> - Peripheral nerve lesions (vascular or compressive)
> - Demyelination
>
> **'Functional' stroke mimics**
>
> - Todd's paresis (after epileptic seizure)
> - Hypoglycaemia
> - Migrainous aura (with or without headache)
> - Focal seizures
> - Ménière's disease or other vestibular disorder
> - Conversion disorder
> - Encephalitis

Clinical features

Both acute stroke and TIA are characterised by a rapid-onset (in minutes) loss of function affecting an identifiable brain area. With this history, there is a 95% chance of a vascular cause. Nonvascular 'stroke mimics' are listed in Box 16.5. If symptoms progress over hours or days, other diagnoses must be excluded. Delirium and memory or balance disturbance are more often caused by stroke mimics. Transient syncope or dizziness are often mistakenly attributed to TIA. Public stroke awareness campaigns stress that face or arm weakness, or speech disturbance are the most common presentations.

The common clinical stroke syndromes depend on which vascular territories are affected and the size of the lesion (Fig. 16.8). This may affect management, for example, suitability for carotid endarterectomy. The neurological deficit can be identified from the history and (if persistent) the neurological examination. A unilateral motor deficit, aphasia, neglect or a visual field defect usually indicate a cerebral hemisphere lesion. Ataxia, diplopia, vertigo and/or bilateral weakness usually indicate a brainstem or cerebellar lesion.

Reduced conscious level usually indicates a large cerebral hemisphere lesion but may result from a brainstem lesion or complications such as obstructive hydrocephalus, hypoxia or systemic infection. Severe headache and vomiting at the onset suggests intracerebral haemorrhage.

Stroke can also be classified by the time course of the deficit:

TIA: Symptoms resolve completely within 24 hours. This includes amaurosis fugax (retinal vascular occlusion).

16

Clinical syndrome	Common symptoms
Total anterior circulation syndrome (TACS) 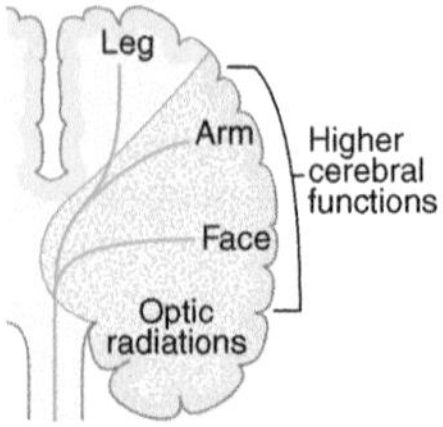 Leg Arm — Higher cerebral functions Face Optic radiations	Combination of: Hemiparesis Higher cerebral dysfunction (e.g., aphasia) Hemisensory loss Homonymous hemianopia (damage to optic radiations)
Partial anterior circulation syndrome (PACS) 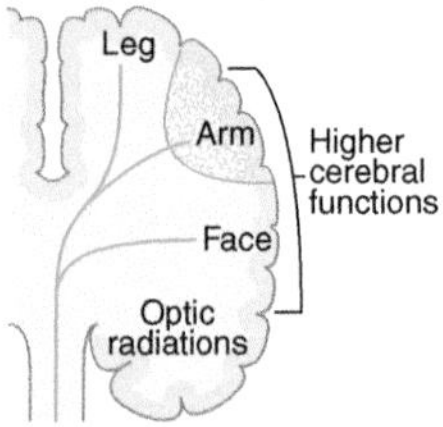 Leg Arm — Higher cerebral functions Face Optic radiations	Isolated motor loss (e.g., leg only, arm only, face) Isolated higher cerebral dysfunction (e.g., aphasia, neglect) Mixture of higher cerebral dysfunction and motor loss (e.g., aphasia with right hemiparesis)
Lacunar syndrome (LACS) 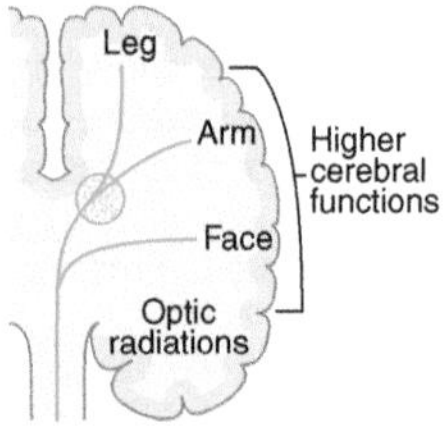 Leg Arm — Higher cerebral functions Face Optic radiations	Pure motor stroke – affects two limbs Pure sensory stroke Sensory-motor stroke No higher cerebral dysfunction or hemianopia
Posterior circulation stroke (POCS) (lateral view) 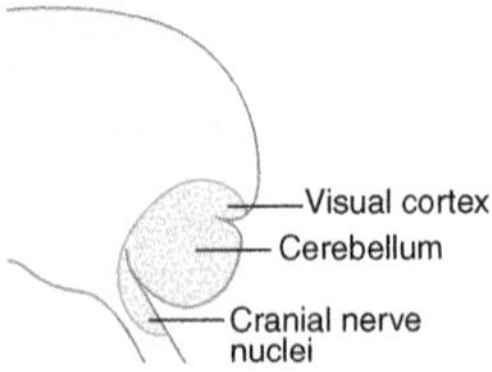 Visual cortex Cerebellum Cranial nerve nuclei	Homonymous hemianopia (damage to visual cortex) Cerebellar syndrome Cranial nerve syndromes

Fig. 16.8 Clinical and radiological features of the stroke syndromes.
The top three diagrams show coronal brain sections, the bottom one a sagittal section. Infarcted areas (shown in red) can cause damage to the relevant cortex (PACS), nerve tracts (LACS) or both (TACS). In corresponding CT scans, the lesion is highlighted by arrows.

Common cause	CT scan features
Middle cerebral artery occlusion (Embolism from heart or major vessels)	
Occlusion of a branch of the middle cerebral artery or anterior cerebral artery (Embolism from heart or major vessels)	
Thrombotic occlusion of small perforating arteries (Thrombosis in situ)	
Occlusion in vertebral, basilar or posterior cerebral artery territory (Cardiac embolism or thrombosis in situ)	

16

Fig. 16.8 cont'd

Stroke: Symptoms last more than 24 hours. The term 'minor stroke' is sometimes used to refer to symptoms lasting over 24 hours but not causing significant disability.

Progressing stroke ('stroke in evolution'): Focal neurological deficit worsens after the patient first presents. It may be caused by increasing volume of infarction, haemorrhagic transformation or cerebral oedema.

Completed stroke: Focal deficit persists but is not progressing.

Investigations

Investigation aims to:
• Confirm the vascular nature of the lesion. • Distinguish cerebral infarction from haemorrhage. • Identify the underlying vascular disease and risk factors (Box 16.6).

Further investigations are indicated if the nature of the stroke is uncertain, especially for younger patients who are less likely to have atherosclerotic disease.

Neuroimaging

CT or MRI should be performed in all patients. CT (Figs. 16.8 and 16.9) can exclude nonstroke lesions (e.g. subdural haematomas, tumours) and demonstrate intracerebral haemorrhage. CT changes in cerebral infarction may be absent in the first few hours after symptom onset. Usually, CT scan within the first day or so is adequate. However, an immediate CT scan is essential if the patient has abnormal coagulation, a progressing deficit or suspected cerebellar haematoma, or if thrombolysis is planned. More recently, CT angiography is being used to show vessel occlusion suitable for clot retrieval. MRI detects infarction earlier than CT and is more sensitive for strokes affecting the brainstem and cerebellum.

Vascular imaging

Detection of extracranial vascular disease can reveal the cause of an ischaemic stroke, and may lead to specific treatments, including carotid

i 16.6 Investigation of a patient with an acute stroke	
Is it a vascular lesion?	CT/MRI
Is it ischaemic or haemorrhagic?	CT/MRI
Is it a subarachnoid haemorrhage?	CT, LP
Is there any cardiac source of embolism?	ECG, 24-hr ECG, echocardiogram
What is the underlying vascular disease?	Duplex USS of carotids MRA CTA Contrast angiography
What are the risk factors?	FBC, cholesterol, glucose
Is there an unusual cause?	ESR, protein electrophoresis, clotting and thrombophilia screen

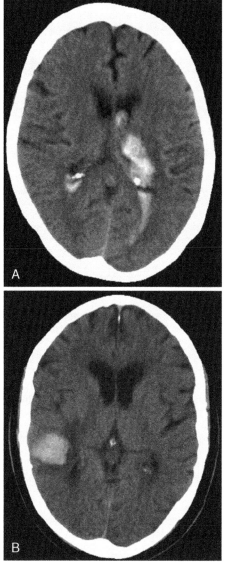

Fig. 16.9 CT scans showing intracerebral haemorrhage. (A) Basal ganglia haemorrhage with intraventricular extension. **(B)** Small cortical haemorrhage.

16

endarterectomy, to reduce further stroke risk. A carotid bruit is not a reliable measure of carotid stenosis. Extracranial arterial disease can be noninvasively identified with duplex USS, MR angiography or CT angiography.

Cardiac investigations

The most common causes of cardiac embolism are atrial fibrillation, prosthetic heart valves, other valvular abnormalities and recent myocardial infarction. A transthoracic or transoesophageal echocardiogram can identify an unsuspected source such as endocarditis, atrial myxoma, intracardiac thrombus or patent foramen ovale.

Management

Management is aimed at:
• Identifying the cause • Minimising the volume of brain that is irreversibly damaged. • Preventing complications. • Reducing disability and handicap through rehabilitation. • Reducing the risk of recurrent episodes.

Rapid admission to a specialised stroke unit facilitates coordinated care from a multidisciplinary team and reduces mortality and residual disability amongst survivors. In the acute phase it may be useful to refer to a checklist (Box 16.7) to ensure that all the factors that might influence outcome have been addressed.

Neurological deficits may worsen during the hours or days after their onset. This may be caused by extension of the area of infarction, haemorrhagic transformation of an infarction or the development of oedema with mass effect. It is important to distinguish this from deterioration caused by complications (hypoxia, sepsis, seizures, metabolic abnormalities), which may be more easily reversed. Patients with cerebellar haematomas or infarcts with mass effect may develop obstructive hydrocephalus and may benefit from insertion of a ventricular drain and/or decompressive surgery. Patients with massive cerebral oedema may benefit from antioedema agents (mannitol), artificial ventilation and/or surgical decompression to reduce intracranial pressure.

Reperfusion (thrombolysis and thrombectomy)

Rapid reperfusion in ischaemic stroke can reduce the extent of brain damage. IV thrombolysis with recombinant tissue plasminogen activator (rt-PA) increases the risk of haemorrhagic transformation of the cerebral infarct, with potentially fatal results. However, if given within 4.5 hours of symptom onset to carefully selected patients, the haemorrhagic risk is offset by an improved overall outcome. Mechanical clot retrieval (thrombectomy) in patients with a large-vessel occlusion can also reduce subsequent disability.

Aspirin and heparin

Aspirin (300 mg daily) should be started immediately after an ischaemic stroke unless rt-PA has been given, in which case it should be withheld for at least 24 hours. Aspirin reduces the risk of early recurrence and improves long-term outcome. Heparin does not improve outcomes and should not be used in acute stroke.

Coagulation abnormalities

In intracerebral haemorrhage, coagulation abnormalities (most commonly caused by oral anticoagulants) should be reversed immediately to reduce the likelihood of the haematoma enlarging.

Management of risk factors

The average risk of a further stroke is 5% to 10% within the first week of a stroke or TIA, 15% in the first year and 5% per year thereafter. The benefits of secondary prevention are expressed as the number needed to treat (NNT) to avoid a recurrent stroke. Patients with ischaemic events should receive long-term antiplatelet drugs (NNT 100) and statins (NNT 60). For patients in atrial fibrillation, warfarin anticoagulation reduces risk substantially (NNT 15). Direct oral anticoagulants (e.g. rivaroxaban, apixaban) now offer improved safety and effectiveness at increased cost. The risk of recurrent ischaemic and haemorrhagic strokes is reduced by blood pressure reduction (NNT 50).

Carotid endarterectomy and angioplasty

Patients with a carotid territory ischaemic event and more than 50% carotid artery stenosis on the side of the brain lesion have a higher risk of stroke recurrence. For those without major residual disability, removal of the stenosis reduces the overall risk of recurrence (NNT 15), although the operation itself carries a 5% risk of stroke. Carotid angioplasty and stenting are technically feasible, but the long-term effects are unclear.

i	**16.7 Acute stroke management: admission checklist**
Airway	Perform a swallow screen and keep patient nil by mouth if swallowing unsafe
Breathing	Check respiratory rate, O_2 saturation; give oxygen if SaO_2 <95%
Circulation	Check peripheral perfusion, pulse and BP are adequate
Hydration	If dehydrated, give IV or NG fluids if swallow is unsafe
Nutrition	Consider nutritional supplements; if persistent dysphagia, feed via NG tube
Medication	If dysphagic, consider alternative routes for essential medications
BP	Unless there is heart failure/renal failure/hypertensive encephalopathy/aortic dissection, do not lower BP in first week, as it compromises cerebral perfusion. BP usually normalises within a few days
Blood glucose	If blood glucose ≥11.1 mmol/L, use insulin (via infusion or GKI) to normalise levels. Check for and correct any hypoglycaemia.
Temperature	If pyrexial, investigate and treat cause, but give antipyretics early
Pressure areas	Anticipate and manage risk: treat infection, maintain nutrition, provide a pressure-relieving mattress and turn immobile patients regularly
Incontinence	Ensure patient is not constipated or in urinary retention; avoid catheterisation unless retention or incontinence is threatening pressure areas
Mobilisation	Avoid bed rest

16

Subarachnoid haemorrhage

About 85% of cases of subarachnoid haemorrhage are caused by rupture of saccular ('berry') aneurysms at bifurcations of the cerebral arteries; 10% are nonaneurysmal haemorrhages (usually benign prognosis); and 5% are caused by rarities (arteriovenous malformations, vertebral artery dissection). Subarachnoid haemorrhage is rare (affecting about 6/100000); women are more frequently affected, and most present younger than 65 years of age. The immediate mortality is around 30%. Survivors have a rebleed rate of 40% in the first 4 weeks and 3% annually thereafter.

Clinical features

There is typically a sudden, severe 'thunderclap' headache (often occipital), which lasts for hours or even days, often accompanied by vomiting. Physical exertion, straining and sexual excitement are common antecedents. Usually the patient is distressed and irritable, with photophobia, but there may be loss of consciousness. Neck stiffness, focal hemisphere signs and subhyaloid haemorrhage on fundoscopy may be found.

Investigations

About 1 patient in 8 with a sudden severe headache has subarachnoid haemorrhage; therefore, all should be investigated to exclude it, starting with a CT scan. If the CT scan is negative (small amounts of blood may not be visible), then CSF should be obtained by LP at least 12 hours after symptom onset, to detect blood and xanthochromia. If either is positive, cerebral angiography is indicated.

Management

Nimodipine (30–60 mg IV) is given to prevent delayed ischaemia in the acute phase. Endovascular insertion of coils into an aneurysm or surgical clipping of the aneurysm neck reduces recurrence.

Cerebral venous disease

Thrombosis of cerebral veins and venous sinuses is relatively uncommon.
Predisposing systemic causes include:
• Dehydration. • Pregnancy. • Thrombophilia. • Oral contraceptives. • Hypotension. • Behçet's disease.
Local causes include:
• Paranasal sinusitis. • Meningitis. • Facial skin infection. • Otitis media, mastoiditis. • Penetrating head/eye wounds. • Skull fracture.
Anticoagulation is usually given, and management of underlying causes and complications is important.

Cortical vein thrombosis

This may present with focal cortical deficits (aphasia, hemiparesis) or epilepsy, according to the area involved.

Cerebral venous sinus thrombosis

Cavernous sinus thrombosis causes proptosis, ptosis, headache, ophthalmoplegias, papilloedema and numbness in the trigeminal first division dermatome. Superior sagittal sinus thrombosis causes headache, papilloedema and seizures. Transverse sinus thrombosis causes hemiparesis, seizures and papilloedema.

About 10% of cases are associated with infection and require antibiotics; otherwise, treatment is by anticoagulation.

Headache syndromes

The general approach to headache is described on p. 68. The primary headache syndromes are described here.

Tension-type headache

This is the most common type of headache.

Clinical features

The pain is constant and generalised, but often radiates forward from the occipital region. It is described as 'dull', 'tight' or like a 'pressure'. It may be episodic or persistent, although the severity may vary. There is no vomiting or photophobia. The pain often progresses throughout the day, but it is rarely disabling, and the patient appears well. Tenderness may be present over the skull.

Management

Discussion of likely precipitants and explanation that the symptoms are not caused by sinister pathology are more likely to help than analgesics. Excessive use of analgesics, particularly codeine, may worsen the headache (analgesic headache). Physiotherapy (with muscle relaxation and stress management) may be useful, as may low-dose amitriptyline. Patients benefit most from reassurance and rigorous assessment. Imaging is unhelpful and may raise anxiety.

Migraine

Migraine affects 20% of women and 6% of men at some point. The aetiology is largely unknown. The headache phase is associated with vasodilatation of extracranial vessels. There is often a family history, suggesting a genetic predisposition. The female preponderance hints at hormonal influences. The contraceptive pill appears to exacerbate migraine in many patients. Doctors and patients often over-estimate the role of dietary precipitants such as cheese, chocolate or red wine. When psychological stress is involved, the migraine attack often occurs after the period of stress.

Clinical features

A prodrome of malaise, irritability or behavioural change may occur. In around 20% of patients, migraine starts with aura (previously called 'classical' migraine). Shimmering, silvery zigzag lines (fortification spectra) spread across the visual fields for up to 40 minutes, sometimes leaving a trail of temporary field loss (scotoma). Patients may feel tingling followed by numbness, spreading over 20 to 30 minutes, from one part of the body to another. Transient speech or motor disturbance occurs less commonly. Aura without headache is also seen. Some 80% of patients have migraine without aura (previously 'common' migraine).

16

Migraine headache is usually severe and throbbing, with photophobia, phonophobia and vomiting lasting 4 to 72 hours. Movement exacerbates pain, and patients seek a quiet, dark room.

Rarely, the aura may persist, leaving permanent neurological disturbance. This persistent migrainous aura may occur with or without evidence of brain infarction.

Management

Prevention: Avoidance of identified triggers or exacerbating factors. Women with aura should avoid oestrogen treatment for contraception or HRT, although the risk of ischaemic stroke is minimal. For frequent attacks (>2 per month), prophylaxis with propranolol, amitriptyline or antiepileptic drugs (e.g. sodium valproate) should be considered.

Acute attack: Simple analgesia with aspirin or paracetamol, often with an antiemetic. Severe attacks can be treated with one of the 'triptans' (e.g. sumatriptan), 5-HT agonists.

Medication overuse headache

Headache syndromes perpetuated by analgesia intake (particularly codeine and other opiate-containing preparations) are becoming more common. Medication overuse headache is usually associated with use on more than 10 to 15 days per month.

Management is by withdrawal of the responsible analgesics; patients should be warned that the initial effect will be to exacerbate the headache.

Cluster headache (migrainous neuralgia)

Clinical features

This is much less common than migraine. Males predominate, and onset is usually in the third decade. The syndrome comprises repeated identical episodes of severe, unilateral periorbital pain accompanied by unilateral lacrimation, nasal congestion and conjunctival injection, lasting 30 to 90 minutes. The cluster extends for a number of weeks, followed by months of respite before another cluster occurs.

Management

Acute attacks are usually halted by SC injections of sumatriptan or inhalation of 100% oxygen. Attacks can sometimes be prevented by verapamil, sodium valproate or short courses of glucocorticoids. Severe, debilitating clusters can be helped with lithium therapy.

Trigeminal neuralgia

Clinical features

Trigeminal neuralgia causes unilateral lancinating facial pains in the second and third divisions of the trigeminal nerve territory. The pain is severe and very brief but repetitive, causing the patient to flinch as if with a motor tic. It may be precipitated by touching trigger zones within the trigeminal territory or by eating. There is a tendency for the condition to remit and relapse over years.

Management

The pain often responds to carbamazepine. If patients cannot tolerate carbamazepine, oxcarbazine, gabapentin, pregabalin, amitriptyline or glucocorticoids may help.

Surgical treatment should be considered, especially where response is incomplete in younger patients. Decompression of the vascular loop encroaching on the trigeminal root is said to have a 90% success rate. Otherwise, localised injection of alcohol or phenol into a peripheral branch of the nerve may be effective.

Epilepsy

A seizure is defined as signs and/or symptoms caused by abnormal, excessive or synchronous neuronal activity in the brain. The lifetime risk of an isolated seizure is about 5%. Epilepsy is the tendency to have unprovoked seizures, but it can also be diagnosed after a single seizure with a high probability of recurrence. The prevalence of epilepsy is around 0.5% in European countries.

Modern classification (Box 16.8) distinguishes focal seizures, in which abnormal activity is limited to part of the cortex, from generalised seizures in which the electrophysiological abnormality involves both hemispheres simultaneously.

Focal seizures can result from any cortical disturbance including infection, tumour or scarring. The symptoms depend on the cortical area affected. For temporal areas, awareness of the environment becomes impaired. When both hemispheres become involved, the seizure becomes generalised.

Seizures that are generalised at onset (~30% of all epilepsy) arise in the central mechanisms controlling cortical activation and spread rapidly. Generalised seizures almost always present before the age of 35.

Clinical features

To classify seizure type, establish first whether there is a focal onset, and second whether the seizures conform to one of the recognised patterns (Box 16.8). Where activity remains focal, signs may indicate the site. Even when generalised tonic–clonic seizures occur, seizures beginning in one cortical area will cause neurological symptoms and signs corresponding to the function of that area.

• Occipital onset: causes visual changes (lights/blobs of colour). • Temporal lobe onset: false recognition (déjà vu). • Sensory strip involvement: sensory alteration (burning, tingling). • Motor strip involvement: jerking.

Focal seizures

These may be idiopathic or may reflect focal structural lesions. The latter may be:

• Genetic (e.g. tuberous sclerosis). • Developmental. • Cerebrovascular (e.g. arteriovenous malformation). • Neoplastic. • Traumatic. • Infective. • Inflammatory (e.g. vasculitis).

Focal neurological signs may localise the source but spread to the temporal or frontal lobes may cause impairment of awareness or bizarre behaviour. Patients may stop and stare blankly, sometimes displaying stereotyped actions. After a few minutes, consciousness returns, but the patient may be muddled and drowsy for up to an hour.

16

16.8 Classification of seizures (2010 International League Against Epilepsy classification)

Generalised seizures

- Tonic–clonic (in any combination)
- Absence:
    - Typical
    - Atypical
    - Absence with special features
- Myoclonic absence
- Eyelid myoclonia
- Myoclonic:
    - Myoclonic
    - Myoclonic atonic
    - Myoclonic tonic
- Clonic
- Tonic
- Atonic

Focal seizures

- Without impairment of consciousness or awareness (was 'simple partial'):
    - Focal motor
    - Focal sensory
- With impairment of consciousness or awareness (was 'complex partial')
- Evolving to a bilateral, convulsive seizure (was 'secondarily generalised seizure'):
    - Tonic
    - Clonic
    - Tonic–clonic

Unknown

- Epileptic spasms

Generalised seizures

Tonic–clonic seizures: May be preceded by an initial 'aura'. The patient then becomes rigid and unconscious and may fall heavily. Breathing stops and they become cyanosed. After a few moments, clonic jerks appear for up to 2 minutes. Urinary incontinence or tongue-biting may occur. After a period of flaccid coma, the patient then regains consciousness, but is drowsy or delirious for some hours.

Absence seizures: Generalised seizures, which always start in child-hood. The child goes blank and stares for a few seconds only. The attacks are brief but frequent and are not associated with postictal confusion. They may be mistaken for daydreaming.

Myoclonic seizures: Brief, jerking movements, predominating in the arms. They occur in the morning or on waking, or may be provoked by fatigue, alcohol or sleep deprivation.

Atonic seizures: Seizures involving brief loss of muscle tone, usually resulting in heavy falls with or without loss of consciousness.

Tonic seizures: Associated with a generalised increase in tone and an associated loss of awareness. Atonic and tonic seizures are usually seen as part of an epilepsy syndrome.

Clonic seizures: Similar to tonic–clonic seizures, but without a preceding tonic phase.

Many patients with epilepsy follow specific patterns of seizure type(s), age of onset and treatment responsiveness: the so-called electroclinical syndromes. Genetic testing may ultimately demonstrate similarities in molecular pathophysiology.

Investigations

These are summarised in Box 16.9.

Single seizure

All patients with transient loss of consciousness should have a 12-lead ECG. After a possible seizure, MRI or CT imaging is indicated, although without focal signs the yield is low.

Recurrence occurs in around 40% of patients, usually within 1 to 2 months.

Epilepsy

Inter-ictal EEG is only abnormal in around 50% of patients with recurrent seizures, so it cannot exclude epilepsy. Prolonged recordings, including sleep, increase sensitivity, but do not replace a detailed history. Imaging for a structural cause is indicated for:

---

i 16.9 Investigation of epilepsy

From where is the epilepsy arising?

- Standard EEG
- Sleep EEG
- EEG with special electrodes (foramen ovale, subdural)

What is the cause of the epilepsy?

Structural lesion?

- CT
- MRI

Metabolic disorder?

- Urea and electrolytes
- Liver function tests
- Blood glucose
- Serum calcium, magnesium

Inflammatory or infective disorder?

- Full blood count, erythrocyte sedimentation rate, C-reactive protein
- Chest x-ray
- Serology for syphilis, HIV, collagen disease
- CSF examination

Are the attacks truly epileptic?

- Ambulatory EEG
- Videotelemetry

16

• Onset age younger than 16 years of age. • Focal features. • EEG suggesting focal source. • Difficult-to-control seizures.

Management

Explain the nature and cause of seizures to patients and their relatives. Instruct relatives in the first aid management of major seizures. Emphasise that epilepsy is common, and that full control can be expected in around 70% of patients.

The recognised mortality of epilepsy should be discussed sensitively with patients to encourage a serious approach to lifestyle modification and adherence to medication.

Immediate care: Little can or need be done for a person whilst a convulsive seizure is occurring, except for first aid and common-sense manoeuvres (Box 16.10).

Lifestyle advice: Patients should be advised to avoid activities where they might place themselves or others at risk if they have a seizure. This includes work or recreational activities involving exposure to heights, dangerous machinery, open fires or water. Prolonged cycle journeys should be discouraged until good control has been achieved. In the UK and many other countries, legal restrictions regarding vehicle driving apply to patients with epilepsy.

Antiepileptic drugs: Drug treatment should be considered where risk of seizure recurrence is high (usually two or more prior seizures). Drug regimens should be discussed with the patient and kept simple to promote adherence. In most patients, full control is achieved with a single drug. Guidelines are listed in Box 16.11. For focal epilepsies, lamotrigine is the best-tolerated monotherapy, and has few side effects. Unclassified generalised epilepsies respond best to valproate, although teratogenicity precludes valproate use in women of reproductive age unless the benefits outweigh the risks. The initial choice should be an established first-line drug, with more recently introduced drugs as second choice. Newer drugs have predictable pharmacokinetics, so drug levels are used mainly to monitor adherence. Gradual medication withdrawal may be considered after 2

 16.10 Immediate care of seizures

First aid (by relatives and witnesses)

- Move person away from danger (fire, water, machinery, furniture)
- After convulsions cease, turn into 'recovery' position (semi-prone)
- Ensure airway is clear, but do **not** insert anything in mouth (tongue-biting occurs at onset and cannot be prevented)
- If convulsions continue for >5 minutes or recur without person regaining consciousness, summon urgent medical attention
- Person may be drowsy/delirious for 30–60 minutes, and should not be left alone until recovered

Immediate medical attention

- See Box 16.1

16.11 Guidelines for choice of antiepileptic drugs

Epilepsy type	First-line	Second-line
Focal onset and/or secondary GTCS	Lamotrigine	Carbamazepine Levetiracetam Sodium valproate Topiramate Zonisamide
GTCS	Sodium valproate Levetiracetam	Lamotrigine Topiramate Zonisamide
Absence	Ethosuximide	Sodium valproate
Myoclonic	Sodium valproate	Levetiracetam Clonazepam

Use as few drugs as possible. GTCS = generalised tonic-clonic seizure

seizure-free years. Childhood-onset epilepsy carries the best prognosis for successful drug withdrawal. Overall recurrence rate after drug withdrawal is around 40%.

Surgery: Some patients with drug-resistant epilepsy respond to resection of epileptogenic foci or nerve stimulation.

Prognosis

Generalised seizures are more readily controlled than partial seizures. A structural lesion makes complete control less likely. After 20 years:
• 50% have been seizure-free for the last 5 years without medication. • 20% are seizure-free with medication. • 30% continue to have seizures despite medication.

Nonepileptic attack disorder ('dissociative attacks')

Patients may present with attacks resembling seizures but caused by psychological phenomena, with a normal EEG. The distinction from frontal lobe epilepsy may be especially difficult, requiring videotelemetry with prolonged EEG recording. Prevention requires psychotherapy rather than medication.

Vestibular disorders

Vertigo is the typical symptom of vestibular dysfunction, and most patients with vertigo have acute vestibular failure, benign paroxysmal positional vertigo or Ménière's disease. Central (brain) causes of vertigo are rare by comparison, with the exception of migraine.

Acute vestibular failure (labyrinthitis, vestibular neuronitis): Usually presents as severe vertigo, with vomiting and unsteadiness. The vertigo is most severe at onset and settles down over the next few days but may be provoked by head movement for longer. Nystagmus is present for a few days during the attack. Symptomatic relief can be achieved with short-term use of vestibular sedatives (e.g. cinnarizine, prochlorperazine, betahistine). A few patients have persisting symptoms requiring vestibular rehabilitation by a physiotherapist.

Benign paroxysmal positional vertigo: Paroxysms of vertigo occurring with certain head movements may be caused by otolithic debris affecting endolymph flow in the labyrinth. Each attack lasts seconds, but patients may become reluctant to move their head, producing a muscle tension-type headache. The diagnosis can be confirmed by using the 'Hallpike manœuvre', in which the head is swung briskly back to demonstrate positional nystagmus. The vertigo fatigues with repetitive positioning of the head and can be treated with vestibular exercises.

Ménière's disease: Patients usually present with tinnitus and deafness, and then develop episodic vertigo accompanied by a sense of fullness in the ear. Examination shows sensorineural hearing loss on the affected side. Vestibular sedatives may be helpful for acute attacks.

Sleep disorders

Sleep disturbances include too much sleep (hypersomnolence or excessive daytime sleepiness), insufficient or poor-quality sleep (insomnia) and abnormal behaviour during sleep (parasomnias). Insomnia is usually caused by psychological or psychiatric disorders, shift work, pain or other environmental causes.

Hypersomnolence

The most common cause of excessive daytime sleepiness is obstructive sleep apnoea (p. 361).

Narcolepsy

This is easily distinguished from hypersomnolence by the history. Sudden, irresistible sleep 'attacks' occur, interrupting normal activities. Patients also report at least one of the classical symptoms:
• Cataplexy (sudden loss of muscle tone, triggered by surprise, laughter or emotion). • Frightening ('hypnagogic') hallucinations at sleep onset. • Sleep paralysis.

Narcolepsy can be treated with modafinil or sodium oxybate. Cataplexy responds to sodium oxybate, clomipramine or venlafaxine.

Parasomnias

Parasomnias are abnormal motor behaviours occurring in either REM or non-REM sleep.

Non-REM parasomnias: These manifest as night terrors, sleep walking and confusional arousals. Patients have little or no recollection of episodes, even though they appear 'awake'. Treatment is usually not required, but clonazepam can be used.

REM sleep behaviour disorder: Patients 'act out' their dreams during REM sleep because of failure of the usual muscle atonia. Sleep partners describe patients 'fighting' or 'struggling' in their sleep, sometimes injuring themselves or their partner. Polysomnography confirms the diagnosis, and clonazepam is the most successful treatment.

Restless leg syndrome: This is common, with a prevalence of around 10%. Unpleasant sensations in the legs that are eased by moving the legs occur when the patient is tired and at sleep onset. Restless legs can also be symptomatic of a peripheral neuropathy, iron deficiency, Parkinson's disease or uraemia. Treatment, if required, is with dopaminergic drugs or benzodiazepines.

Neuro-inflammatory diseases

Multiple sclerosis

MS is an important cause of chronic disability in adults. In the UK the prevalence is around 120/100000, with an annual incidence of 7/100000. Although the exact cause is uncertain, an interplay of genetic and environmental factors is probably responsible. The incidence is higher at temperate than equatorial latitudes, and the disease is twice as common in women as men. The risk of familial occurrence is 15%. Pathogenesis involves recurrent cell-mediated autoimmune attack on the myelin-producing oligodendrocytes of the CNS. Histologically, the characteristic lesion is a plaque of demyelination in the periventricular regions of the brain, the optic nerves or the subpial regions of the spinal cord.

Clinical features

The diagnosis of MS requires the demonstration of otherwise unexplained CNS lesions separated in time and space. There are several recognisable clinical courses:
• Relapsing and remitting clinical course (80%) with variable recovery.
• Primary progressive clinical course (10%–20%). • Secondary progressive disease (supersedes relapse and remission phase). • Fulminant disease (<10%), leading to early death.

There are a number of clinical syndromes suggestive of MS (Box 16.12). Demyelinating lesions cause symptoms and signs that come on over days or weeks and resolve over weeks or months. Frequent relapses with incomplete recovery indicate a poor prognosis. In a minority, there is an interval of years between attacks, and in some there is no recurrence. The physical signs depend on the anatomical site of demyelination. Combinations of spinal cord and brainstem signs are common, maybe with evidence of previous optic neuritis. Significant intellectual impairment is unusual until late in the disease.

Prognosis is difficult to predict, especially early. Those with relapsing and remitting symptoms have on average 1 to 2 relapses every 2 years. About 5% of patients die within 5 years of onset, but slightly more have very good long-term outcome with minimal disability. After 10 years, around one-third of patients are sufficiently disabled to need help with walking.

Investigations

There is no specific test for MS, and the clinical diagnosis should be supported by investigations to:

• Exclude other conditions. • Provide evidence of an inflammatory disorder.
• Identify multiple sites of neurological involvement.

MRI: The most sensitive test for demyelinating lesions in the brain and spinal cord (Fig. 16.10), which excludes other causes of the neurological deficit. However, appearances may be confused with small-vessel disease or cerebral vasculitis.

Visual evoked potentials: Detect clinically silent lesions in up to 70% of patients.

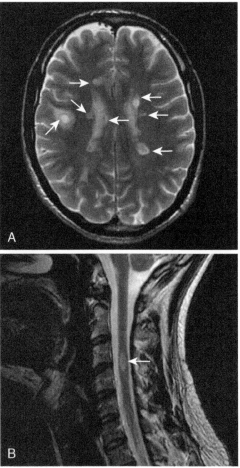

Fig. 16.10 Multiple sclerosis. (A) Brain MRI in MS: multiple high-signal lesions (arrows) are seen particularly in the paraventricular region on T2 image. **(B)** Demyelinating lesion in cervical spinal cord: high-signal T2 image (sagittal plane).

16.12 Clinical features of MS

Common presentations of MS

- Optic neuritis
- Relapsing and remitting sensory symptoms
- Subacute painless spinal cord lesion
- Acute brainstem syndrome
- Subacute loss of function of upper limb (dorsal column deficit)
- 6th cranial nerve palsy

Other symptoms and syndromes suggestive of CNS demyelination

- Afferent pupillary defect and optic atrophy (previous optic neuritis)
- Lhermitte's symptom (tingling in spine or limbs on neck flexion)
- Progressive noncompressive paraparesis
- Partial Brown–Séquard syndrome
- Internuclear ophthalmoplegia with ataxia
- Postural ('rubral', 'Holmes') tremor
- Trigeminal neuralgia <50 years of age
- Recurrent facial palsy

CSF: Lymphocytic pleocytosis in the acute phase and oligoclonal bands of IgG in 70% to 90% of patients between attacks. Oligoclonal bands (which are absent in the serum) denote intrathecal inflammation and occur in a range of other disorders.

Management

This involves treatment of the acute relapse, prevention of future relapses, treatment of complications and management of disability.

Acute relapse: Pulses of high-dose glucocorticoids, either IV or orally, shorten the duration of relapse, but do not affect long-term outcome. Pulsed glucocorticoids can be given up to three times per year, but should be restricted to significant function-threatening deficits. Prophylaxis against osteoporosis should be considered.

Disease-modifying treatments: These reduce annual relapse rates and the number and size of lesions on MRI, and some may reduce disability. Given orally, subcutaneously or intravenously, they are not indicated for early MS. Interferon beta, glatiramer acetate, dimethyl furoate and fingolimod are used in less severe cases, and reduce relapse rates by 30% to 50%. Alemtuzumab and natalizumab, given IV in severe cases, reduce relapse rates by more than 50%. A range of adverse effects is seen, so careful patient selection, counselling and expert supervision are necessary.

Complications: Treatment of complications is summarised in Box 16.13. Specialist nurses are of great value in managing the chronic phase of the disease. Physiotherapy and occupational therapy may improve functional capacity in patients who become disabled. Bladder care is particularly important. Urgency and frequency may be treated pharmacologically, but this may lead to retention and infection. Retention can be managed initially by intermittent self-catheterisation, but an in-dwelling catheter may become necessary.

16

i	**16.13 Treatment of complications of MS**	
Spasticity	Physiotherapy Baclofen, dantrolene, gabapentin, sativex, tizanidine Local IM botulinum toxin, chemical neuronectomy
Dysaesthesia	Carbamazepine, gabapentin, phenytoin, amitriptyline
Bladder symptoms	Anticholinergics for hypertonic bladder, intermittent catheterisation
Fatigue	Amantadine, modafinil, amitriptyline
Erectile dysfunction	Sildenafil, tadalafil

Acute disseminated encephalomyelitis

This is an acute monophasic condition with areas of perivenous demyelination throughout the brain and spinal cord. The illness often occurs a week or so after a viral infection (e.g. measles, chickenpox, recent vaccination), suggesting that it is immunologically mediated.

Clinical features
• Headache, vomiting, pyrexia, delirium and meningism, often with focal brain and spinal cord signs. • Occasionally, seizures or coma.

Investigations
MRI shows multiple high-signal areas in a pattern similar to that of MS. CSF may be normal or show an increase in protein and lymphocytes; oligoclonal bands may be found acutely, but do not persist on recovery (unlike in MS).

Management
The prognosis is generally good, although occasionally it may be fatal (<10%). Treatment is with high-dose IV methylprednisolone.

Transverse myelitis

Transverse myelitis is an acute, monophasic, inflammatory demyelinating disorder affecting the spinal cord. Patients present with a subacute paraparesis with a sensory level, often with severe neck or back pain at onset. MRI is needed to distinguish this from a compressive spinal cord lesion. CSF examination shows cellular pleocytosis, and oligoclonal bands are usually absent. Treatment is with high-dose IV methylprednisolone. The outcome is variable; in some cases, near-complete recovery occurs despite a severe initial deficit. Some patients go on to develop MS.

Paraneoplastic neurological disease

Neurological disease may occur with systemic malignant tumours in the absence of metastases. In most cases, tumour antigens lead to the development of autoantibodies to parts of the CNS.

Clinical features

These are summarised in Box 16.14. The neurological disease often precedes clinical presentation of the primary neoplasm.

Investigations

Characteristic autoantibodies are present in many cases (e.g. anti Jo-1 in dermatomyositis). CT of the chest or abdomen or PET scanning is often necessary to find the causative tumour. CSF often shows increased protein and lymphocytes with oligoclonal bands.

Management

This is directed at the primary tumour. Some improvement may occur following administration of IV immunoglobulin.

16.14 Paraneoplastic syndromes		
Syndrome	Clinical features	Associated tumours
CNS		
Limbic encephalitis	Memory loss, progressive dementia, seizures	SCLC, testicular, breast, thymoma, ovarian/testicular teratoma
Myelopathy	Progressive spinal cord lesion (usually cervical)	SCLC, thymoma
Cerebellar degeneration	Progressive ataxia, nystagmus, vertigo	SCLC, breast, ovarian, lymphoma
Motor neuron disease	Sub-acute, patchy progressive, usually lower limb, weakness and wasting	SCLC, others
Peripheral		
Sensory neuropathy	Limb pain, paraesthesia, distal numbness	Lymphoma, SCLC, others
Sensorimotor polyneuropathy	Mild, non disabling peripheral limb numbness and paraesthesia	Lymphoma, SCLC, others
Lambert–Eaton syndrome	Weakness of proximal limb muscles, fatigue with exertion after initial improvement, areflexia	SCLC
Dermatomyositis/ polymyositis	Proximal limb weakness and pain, heliotrope skin rash, Gottron's papules on knuckles	Lung, breast
Myasthenia gravis	Muscle fatigue reversible with anticholinesterase	Thymoma

16

Neurodegenerative diseases

Although MS is the most common cause of disability in young people in the UK, vascular and neurodegenerative diseases are increasingly important in later life. These diseases lead to specific neuronal death, causing relentlessly progressive symptoms that increase with age. Degeneration of the cerebral cortex causes dementia. Degeneration of the basal ganglia results in movement disorder. Cerebellar degeneration usually causes ataxia. Degeneration can also occur in the spinal cord or peripheral nerves, giving rise to motor, sensory or autonomic disturbance.

Degenerative causes of dementia

Dementia is characterised by a loss of previously acquired intellectual function in the absence of impairment of arousal and affects 5% of those aged over 65 years and 20% of those aged over 85 years. It is defined as a global impairment of cognitive function and is typically progressive and nonreversible. Although memory is most affected initially, deficits in visuo-spatial function, language ability, concentration and attention gradually become apparent. Alzheimer's disease and diffuse vascular disease are the most common causes, but rarer causes, which should be sought actively in younger patients and those with short histories, include:
• MS. • Chronic head trauma. • Prion disease. • Alcohol. • HIV. • Syphilis.
• Thiamin or vitamin B_{12} deficiency. • Hydrocephalus.

Alzheimer's disease

This is the most common cause of dementia. About 15% of cases are familial. The brain is atrophic, with senile plaques and neurofibrillary tangles in the cerebral cortex. Many different neurotransmitter abnormalities have been described, in particular impairment of cholinergic transmission.

Clinical features

The key feature is impairment of the ability to remember new information. Memory impairment is gradual and usually associated with disorders of other cortical functions. Both short-term memory and long-term memory are affected. Later in the disease, patients commonly deny their disabilities, and additional features are apraxia, visuo-spatial impairment, depression and aphasia.

Investigations and management

Investigation is aimed at excluding the less common treatable causes of dementia (see earlier). Anticholinesterases (donepezil, rivastigmine, galantamine) and the NMDA receptor antagonist memantine have been shown to be of some benefit. Depression should be treated with antidepressants. Support for carers is crucial.

Fronto-temporal dementia

This term encompasses a number of different syndromes, including Pick's diseases and primary progressive aphasia; all are much rarer than Alzheimer's disease. Patients may present with personality change because of frontal lobe involvement or with language disturbance as a result of temporal lobe involvement. Memory is relatively preserved in the early stages. There is no specific treatment.

Lewy body dementia

This is a neurodegenerative disorder clinically characterised by dementia and signs of Parkinson's disease. The cognitive state often fluctuates, and there is a high incidence of visual hallucinations. Affected individuals are particularly sensitive to the side effects of antiparkinsonian medication and also to antipsychotic drugs. There is no curative treatment, but anticholinesterase agents may slow progression.

Wernicke–Korsakoff syndrome

This is a rare but important effect of chronic alcohol misuse. It is an organic brain disorder resulting from damage to the mamillary bodies, dorsomedial nuclei of the thalamus and adjacent areas of periventricular grey matter. It is caused by a deficiency of thiamin (vitamin B_1), most commonly from long-standing heavy drinking and an inadequate diet. It can also arise from malabsorption or even protracted vomiting. Without prompt treatment, the acute presentation of Wernicke's encephalopathy (nystagmus, ophthalmoplegia, ataxia and delirium) can progress to the irreversible deficits of Korsakoff's syndrome (severe short-term memory deficits and confabulation).

This syndrome must be considered in any confused patient; if in doubt, treat anyway. Prevention of the Wernicke–Korsakoff syndrome requires the immediate use of high doses of thiamin, which is initially given parenterally in the form of Pabrinex (two vials three times daily for 48 hours) and then orally (100 mg three times daily). There is no treatment for Korsakoff's syndrome once it has arisen.

Movement disorders

Movement disorders present with a wide range of symptoms. They may be genetic or acquired, and the most important is Parkinson's disease. Most movement disorders are categorised clinically, with few confirmatory investigations available other than for those with a known gene abnormality.

Idiopathic Parkinson's disease

Parkinsonism is a clinical syndrome characterised by bradykinesia, increased tone (rigidity), tremor and loss of postural reflexes. Although it may be caused by drugs, degenerative disease (e.g. Alzheimer's), anoxic or other injury or genetic conditions (e.g. Huntington's disease), more than 80% of cases are because of PD. PD has an annual incidence of 18/100 000 in the UK and a prevalence of 180/100 000. Average age of onset is around 60 years; less than 5% present under 40 years of age.

Single-gene mutations have been identified in a few cases, but most cases are idiopathic. Having a first-degree relative with PD confers a 2 to 3 times increased risk of developing PD. It is progressive and incurable, with a variable prognosis. Although motor symptoms are the usual presenting features, cognitive impairment, depression and anxiety become increasingly prominent as the disease progresses, and significantly reduce quality of life.

Clinical features

The presentation is usually asymmetrical, for example, a resting tremor in an upper limb. Typical features of an established case include:

Bradykinesia: Slowness in initiating or repeating movements, impaired fine movements (causing small handwriting) and expressionless face. The patient is slow to start walking, with reduced arm swing, rapid small steps and a tendency to run (festination).

Tremor: Present at rest (3–4 Hz), diminished on action; it starts in the fingers/thumb and may affect arms, legs, feet, jaw and tongue.

Rigidity: 'Cogwheel' type (tremor plus rigidity) mostly affects upper limbs; 'lead-pipe' rigidity also occurs.

Nonmotor symptoms may precede typical motor symptoms by years and include:
• Depression. • Anxiety. • Cognitive impairment: develops in one-third of patients as the disease progresses.

Investigations

Diagnosis is clinical. CT may be needed if any features suggest pyramidal, cerebellar or autonomic involvement, or if the diagnosis is in doubt, but is usually normal for age. Younger patients should be investigated for Huntington's and Wilson's diseases.

Management: drug therapy

Levodopa: This remains the most effective treatment, together with a peripheral-acting dopa-decarboxylase inhibitor. Therapy should be started when symptoms are impacting on daily life. Decarboxylase inhibitors (carbidopa and benserazide) reduce peripheral side effects and are available as combination preparations with levodopa (Sinemet and Madopar). Levodopa is particularly effective at improving bradykinesia and rigidity. Side effects are:
• Postural hypotension. • Nausea and vomiting. • Involuntary movements (orofacial dyskinesias, limb and axial dystonias). • Occasionally, depression, hallucinations and delusions.

Late deterioration despite levodopa occurs after 3 to 5 years in up to 50% of patients. The simplest form is end-of-dose deterioration; this may be improved by using smaller, more frequent doses or a slow-release preparation. More complex fluctuations present as periods of severe parkinsonism alternating with dyskinesia and agitation (the 'on–off' phenomenon).

Dopamine receptor agonists: Oral ergot-derived agonists (e.g. bromocriptine) are no longer recommended because of fibrotic adverse reactions. Alternative agonists include subcutaneous apomorphine and oral pramipexole. Apart from apomorphine, all are considerably less effective than LD in relieving parkinsonism and have more adverse effects (nausea, vomiting, disorientation and hallucinations, impulse control disorders).

MAOI-B inhibitors: Monoamine oxidase B facilitates breakdown of dopamine in the synapse. Two inhibitors are used in PD: selegiline and rasagiline. The effects of both are modest, although usually well tolerated. Neither is neuroprotective.

COMT inhibitors: When used with levodopa, entacapone prolongs the effects of each dose and is most useful for early wearing-off.

Amantadine: This has a mild, short-lived effect on bradykinesia, but may be useful early in the disease. It can help control the dyskinesias produced by dopaminergic treatment later on. Side effects include: • Livedo reticularis. • Peripheral oedema. • Delirium and seizures.

Anticholinergic drugs: These were the main treatment for PD before the introduction of levodopa. Their role is now limited by lack of efficacy (except sometimes against tremor) and adverse effects, including dry mouth, blurred vision, constipation, urinary retention, delirium, hallucinosis and possibly cognitive impairment.

Management: nonpharmacological

Surgery: Stereotactic surgery most commonly involves deep brain stimulation (DBS), rather than the destructive approach of previous eras. Various targets have been identified, including the thalamus (only effective for tremor), globus pallidus and subthalamic nucleus. DBS is usually reserved for patients with medically refractory tremor or motor fluctuations.

Physiotherapy and speech therapy: Physiotherapy reduces rigidity and corrects abnormal posture. Speech therapy may help dysarthria and dysphonia.

Other parkinsonian syndromes

Cerebrovascular disease and drug-induced parkinsonism are the most common alternative causes of parkinsonism. There are several degenerative conditions that cause parkinsonism, including multiple systems atrophy, progressive supranuclear palsy and corticobasal degeneration. They typically have a more rapid progression than PD and tend to be resistant to levodopa.

Multiple systems atrophy

Features of parkinsonism are combined with degrees of autonomic failure, cerebellar involvement and pyramidal tract dysfunction. Diagnosis is assisted by autonomic function tests. Falls are more common than in idiopathic Parkinson's disease, and life expectancy is reduced.

Progressive supranuclear palsy

Presents with symmetrical parkinsonism, cognitive impairment, falls and bulbar symptoms. A characteristic impairment of up- and down-gaze develops as a late feature. There is no treatment.

Wilson's disease

An autosomal recessive disorder of copper metabolism. It is a treatable cause of tremor, dystonia, parkinsonism and ataxia. Psychiatric symptoms may also occur.

16

Huntington's disease

This is an autosomal dominant inherited disorder, usually presenting in adults. It is caused by expansion of a trinucleotide repeat on chromosome 4, and frequently demonstrates anticipation (younger onset in successive generations).

Clinical features: Gradually progressive chorea and behavioural disturbance are the earliest symptoms. There is cognitive impairment, progressing to frank dementia. Seizures may occur late in the disease.

Investigations: The diagnosis is confirmed by genetic testing; presymptomatic testing for family members is available but must be preceded by counselling. Brain imaging may show caudate atrophy but is not reliable.

Management: Chorea may respond to risperidone or tetrabenazine. Depression is common and may be helped by medication.

Ataxias

This is a group of inherited disorders in which degenerative changes occur to varying extents in the cerebellum, brainstem, pyramidal tracts, spino-cerebellar tracts and optic and peripheral nerves. They usually present in childhood with ataxia, and sometimes with other neurological deficits, for example, spasticity and impaired cognitive function. Genetic testing facilitates diagnosis and counselling in some.

Motor neuron disease

In this disease there is progressive degeneration of upper and lower motor neurons in the spinal cord, cranial nerve nuclei and motor cortex. Annual incidence is 2/100000, and prevalence is 7/100000. Most cases are sporadic but 10% are familial. Average age at onset is 65 years, with 10% presenting before the age of 45 years.

Clinical features

These are summarised in Box 16.15. Most patients present ALS, a combination of lower and upper motor neuron signs without sensory involvement. Up to 50% have some cognitive impairment on formal testing, and around 10% develop frontotemporal dementia.

Investigations

The diagnosis is clinical. Exclude potentially treatable disorders (e.g. cervical myeloradiculopathy, immune-mediated multifocal motor neuropathy).

16.15 Clinical features of MND

Onset

- Usually >50 years of age
- Very uncommon <30 years of age
- Affects males more commonly than females

Symptoms

- Limb weakness, cramps, twitching
- Disturbance of speech/swallowing (dysarthria/dysphagia)
- Cognitive and behavioural features similar to frontotemporal dementia

Signs

- Muscle wasting and fasciculation
- Weakness of muscles of limbs, tongue, face and palate
- Pyramidal tract involvement: spasticity, exaggerated tendon reflexes, extensor plantar responses
- External ocular muscles and sphincters usually spared
- No objective sensory deficit
- Evidence of cognitive impairment with frontotemporal dominance

Course

- Symptoms often begin focally, spreading gradually but relentlessly to become widespread

EMG confirms widespread denervation. Nerve conduction studies may show low-amplitude motor action potentials. Genetic testing is useful in familial MND.

Management and prognosis

Multidisciplinary team management is required, including physiotherapists, occupational therapists, speech therapists, dietitians and palliative care specialists. Riluzole has a modest effect in ALS. Percutaneous gastrostomy feeding may be necessary in advanced disease. Noninvasive ventilatory support significantly prolongs survival and improves or maintains quality of life in ALS.

Infections of the nervous system

Meningitis

Acute infection of the meninges presents with pyrexia, headache, photophobia and meningism (neck stiffness). Meningism can also occur with subarachnoid haemorrhage. Causes are listed in Box 16.16. Abnormalities in the CSF (Box 16.17) are helpful in distinguishing the cause of meningitis.

Viral meningitis

This is the most common cause of meningitis and is benign unless there is associated encephalitis.

i 16.16 **Causes of meningitis**	
Infective	
Bacteria	Adults: *Neisseria meningitidis, S. pneumoniae, Listeria, Mycobacterium tuberculosis, S. aureus, Haemophilus influenzae* Young children: *H. influenzae, N. meningitidis, S. pneumoniae, M. tuberculosis* Neonates: Gram-negative bacilli, group B streptococci, *Listeria*
Viruses	Enteroviruses (echo, Coxsackie, polio), mumps, influenza, Herpes simplex, varicella zoster, EBV, HIV
Protozoa and parasites	*Cysticerci, Amoeba*
Fungi	*Cryptococcus, Candida, Histoplasma, Coccidioides, Blastomyces*
Noninfective ('sterile')	
Malignant disease	Breast cancer, bronchial cancer, leukaemia, lymphoma
Inflammatory disease (may be recurrent)	Sarcoidosis, systemic lupus erythematosus, Behçet's disease

16

Clinical features

The condition occurs mainly in children or young adults, with acute headache, pyrexia, irritability and meningism. Headache is usually the most severe feature.

Investigations

CSF contains an excess of lymphocytes, but glucose and protein are commonly normal or the protein may be raised. This picture can also be found in partially treated bacterial meningitis.

Management

There is no specific treatment. Disease is usually benign and self-limiting. Treat the patient symptomatically in a quiet environment. Recovery usually occurs within days.

Meningitis may also occur as a complication of viral infection in other organs (e.g. mumps, measles, infectious mononucleosis, herpes zoster and hepatitis). Complete recovery without specific therapy is the rule.

Bacterial meningitis

Many bacteria can cause meningitis and certain organisms are particularly common at different ages (see Box 16.16). Bacterial meningitis is usually secondary to a bacteraemic illness. Several of the organisms are normal upper respiratory tract commensals, and infection may complicate otitis media, skull fracture or sinusitis. *Streptococcus pneumoniae* and *Neisseria meningitidis* (meningococcus) are the most frequent causes in Western Europe, whereas *Haemophilus influenzae* and *S. pneumoniae* are most common in India. Epidemics of meningococcal meningitis occur, particularly in cramped conditions or hot, dry climates. In sub-Saharan Africa, drought and dust storms are often associated with meningococcal outbreaks.

Clinical features

Headache, drowsiness, fever and neck stiffness are the usual presenting features. Around 90% of patients with meningococcal meningitis have two of the following:

• Fever. • Neck stiffness. • Altered consciousness. • Purpuric rash.

When accompanied by sepsis, signs may evolve rapidly, with abrupt obtundation caused by cerebral oedema and circulatory collapse. Pneumococcal meningitis may be associated with pneumonia, and occurs especially in older patients, alcoholics and patients with hyposplenism. *Listeria monocytogenes* is seen increasingly as a cause of meningitis and brainstem encephalitis in the immunosuppressed, people with diabetes, alcoholics and pregnant women.

Investigations

LP: CSF is cloudy because of neutrophils. Protein is significantly elevated, and glucose is reduced. A Gram film and culture may identify the organism.

CT head: If there is drowsiness, focal neurological signs or seizures, CT is required before LP because of the risk of coning.

Other: Blood cultures may be positive. PCR of blood and CSF can identify bacterial DNA.

	16.17 CSF findings in meningitis and subarachnoid haemorrhage

	Normal	Subarachnoid haemorrhage	Acute bacterial meningitis	Viral meningitis	Tuberculous meningitis
Pressure	50–250 mmH$_2$O	Increased	Normal/ increased	Normal	Normal/ increased
Colour	Clear	Blood-stained Xanthochromic	Cloudy	Clear	Clear/cloudy
Red cell count × 10^6/L	0–4	Raised	Normal	Normal	Normal
White cell count × 10^6/L	0–4	Normal/slightly raised	1000–5000 polymorphs	10–2000 lympho-cytes	50–5000 lymphocytes
Glucose	>50%–60% of blood level	Normal	Decreased	Normal	Decreased
Protein	<0.45 g/L	Increased	Increased	Normal/ increased	Increased
Microbiology	Sterile	Sterile	Organisms on Gram stain and/ or culture	Sterile/virus detected	Ziehl–Niels-en/auramine stain or TB culture positive
Oligo-clonal bands	Negative	Negative	Can be positive	Can be positive	Can be positive

16

Management

If bacterial meningitis is suspected, the patient should be given parenteral antibiotics immediately and admitted to hospital. Before the cause of meningitis is known, patients should receive cefotaxime (2 g IV four times daily) or ceftriaxone (2 g IV twice daily). The antibiotic regimen may be modified after CSF examination, depending on the infecting organism (Box 16.18). Adjunctive glucocorticoid therapy reduces complications in both children and adults.

Prevention of meningococcal infection: Close contacts of patients with meningococcal infections should be given 2 days of oral rifampicin. In adults, a single dose of ciprofloxacin is an alternative. If not treated with ceftriaxone, meningitis patients should be given similar treatment to clear nasopharyngeal carriage. Vaccines against meningococcus are available, but not for the most common subgroup (B).

i	16.18 Chemotherapy of bacterial meningitis when cause is known		
Pathogen	**Regimen of choice**	**Alternative agent(s)**	
N. meningitidis	Benzylpenicillin 2.4 g IV six times daily for 5–7 days	Cefuroxime, ampicillin Chloramphenicol[a]	
S. pneumoniae or S. suis (sensitive to β-lactams)	Cefotaxime 2 g IV four times daily or ceftriaxone 2 g IV twice daily for 10–14 days	Chloramphenicol[a]	
S. pneumoniae (resistant to β-lactams)	As above plus vancomycin 1 g IV twice daily or rifampicin 600 mg IV twice daily	Vancomycin + rifampicin[a]	
H. influenzae	Cefotaxime 2 g IV four times daily or ceftriaxone 2 g IV twice daily for 10–14 days	Chloramphenicol[a]	
L. monocytogenes	Ampicillin 2 g IV six times daily plus gentamicin 5 mg/kg IV daily	Ampicillin 2 g six times daily + co-trimoxazole 50 mg/kg daily in two doses	

[a]For patients with a history of anaphylaxis to β-lactam antibiotics.

Tuberculous meningitis

Tuberculous meningitis is uncommon in developed countries except in immunocompromised individuals, but remains common in developing countries, where it is seen more frequently as a secondary infection in AIDS. It may occur as part of a primary infection in childhood or as part of miliary TB. The usual source is a caseous focus in the meninges or brain.

Clinical features

There is a slow onset of headache, low-grade fever, vomiting, lassitude, depression, delirium and behavioural changes. Signs include meningism, oculomotor palsies, papilloedema, reduced conscious level and focal hemisphere signs. Untreated tuberculous meningitis is fatal. Complete recovery is the rule if treatment is started before focal signs or stupor. When treatment is started later, the risk of death or serious neurological deficit is 30%.

Investigations

CSF is clear and under increased pressure and contains up to 500×10^6 cells/L, predominantly lymphocytes. There is elevated protein and markedly reduced glucose. CSF culture takes up to 6 weeks, and so treatment must be started empirically. Brain imaging may show hydrocephalus, brisk meningeal enhancement on enhanced CT and/or an intracranial tuberculoma.

Management and prognosis

Chemotherapy should be started with a regimen including pyrazinamide (p. 339). Glucocorticoids may improve mortality, but not focal neurological damage. Surgical ventricular drainage may be needed if obstructive hydrocephalus develops.

Parenchymal viral infections

Viral encephalitis

Infection of nervous tissues will produce both focal dysfunction (deficits and/or seizures) and general signs of infection. Only a minority report recent systemic viral infection. In Europe, the most serious cause is herpes simplex. In some countries, viruses transmitted by mosquitoes and ticks (arboviruses) are an important cause. Zika virus has mutated recently to become a more significant global health problem. Acute or subacute encephalitis may occur in HIV infection.

Clinical features

Viral encephalitis presents with acute onset of headache, fever, focal neurological signs (aphasia and/or hemiplegia) and seizures. Disturbance of consciousness, ranging from drowsiness to deep coma, supervenes early. Meningism is common.

Investigations

CT (which should precede LP) may show low-density lesions in the temporal lobes, but MRI is more sensitive to early abnormalities. CSF usually contains excess lymphocytes, but polymorphs may predominate early. Protein may be elevated, but glucose is normal. The EEG is usually abnormal in the early stages, especially in herpes simplex encephalitis. Virological investigations of the CSF, including PCR, may reveal the cause, but treatment should not await this.

Management

In herpes simplex encephalitis, aciclovir (10 mg/kg IV three times daily for 2–3 weeks) reduces mortality from 70% to 10%. This should be given early to all patients with suspected viral encephalitis. Raised intracranial pressure is treated with dexamethasone, and seizures with antiepileptic treatment.

Brainstem encephalitis

This presents with ataxia, dysarthria, diplopia or other cranial nerve palsies. The CSF is lymphocytic, with a normal glucose. The causative agent is presumed to be viral. However, *L. monocytogenes* may cause a similar syndrome and requires specific treatment with ampicillin (500 mg four times daily).

Rabies

Rabies is caused by a rhabdovirus, which infects the central nervous tissue and salivary glands of mammals. It is usually conveyed by saliva through bites. Humans are most frequently infected from dogs. The incubation period varies but is usually between 4 and 8 weeks.

Clinical features

A prodromal period of 1 to 10 days leads to 'hydrophobia'; although the patient is thirsty, drinking provokes violent contractions of the diaphragm and inspiratory muscles. Delusions and hallucinations may develop, with lucid intervals. Cranial nerve lesions and terminal hyperpyrexia are common. Death ensues, usually within a week of symptoms.

Investigations

The diagnosis is made on clinical grounds. Rapid immunofluorescent techniques can detect antigen in corneal smears or skin biopsies.

Management

A few patients have survived; all received postexposure prophylaxis and needed ICU facilities. Only palliative treatment is possible once symptoms have appeared. The patient should be heavily sedated with diazepam, supplemented by chlorpromazine if necessary.

Prevention

Preexposure prophylaxis: This is required by those who professionally handle potentially infected animals, work with rabies virus in laboratories or live at special risk in rabies-endemic areas. Protection is afforded by two injections of human diploid cell strain vaccine given 4 weeks apart, followed by yearly boosters.

Postexposure prophylaxis: The wounds should be cleaned, damaged tissues excised and the wound left unsutured. Rabies can usually be prevented if treatment is started within a day or two of biting. For maximum protection, hyperimmune serum (human rabies immunoglobulin) and vaccine (human diploid cell strain vaccine) are required.

Poliomyelitis

The disease is caused by one of three polioviruses. It is much less common in developed countries following the use of oral vaccines. Infection occurs through the nasopharynx, causing a lymphocytic meningitis and infecting the grey matter of the nervous system. There is a propensity to damage anterior horn cells.

Clinical features

The incubation period is 7 to 14 days. Many patients recover fully after a few days of mild fever and headache. In others, there is recurrence of pyrexia, headache and meningism. Weakness may start later and can progress to widespread paresis. Respiratory failure may supervene if intercostal muscles or the medullary motor nuclei are involved. Death occurs from respiratory paralysis. Gradual recovery may take place over several months. Muscles showing no signs of recovery after 1 month will probably not regain function.

Investigations

CSF shows a lymphocytic pleocytosis, raised protein and normal glucose. Poliomyelitis virus may be cultured from CSF and stool.

Management

Bed rest is imperative, as exercise appears to worsen or precipitate the paralysis. A tracheostomy and ventilation are required for respiratory difficulties. Subsequent treatment is by physiotherapy and orthopaedic measures.

Prevention is by immunisation with live (Sabin) vaccine. Killed vaccine is used increasingly in countries where polio is rare.

Subacute sclerosing panencephalitis

This is a rare, chronic, progressive and eventually fatal complication of measles. It occurs in children and adolescents, usually many years after the primary virus infection. The onset is insidious, with intellectual deterioration, apathy and clumsiness, followed by myoclonic jerks, rigidity and dementia. The EEG is distinctive, with periodic bursts of triphasic waves. Antiviral therapy is ineffective, and death ensues within years.

Progressive multifocal leucoencephalopathy

This is an infection of oligodendrocytes by human polyomavirus JC, which causes widespread demyelination of the white matter of the cerebral hemispheres. It is found most frequently as a feature of AIDS or complicating therapeutic immunosuppression, but also occurs in lymphoma and leukaemia. Clinical signs include dementia, hemiparesis and aphasia, which progress rapidly, leading to death within weeks or months. MRI reveals diffuse high signal in the cerebral white matter. Restoring the immune system may be beneficial.

Parenchymal bacterial infections

Cerebral abscess

Bacteria can enter the cerebi through injury, spread from sinuses or via the circulation in congenital heart disease. The site of abscess formation and the causative organism are both related to the source of infection (Box 16.19).

Clinical features

A cerebral abscess may present acutely with fever, headache, meningism and drowsiness, but more commonly presents over days or weeks as a cerebral mass lesion with little or no evidence of infection, making distinction from tumour difficult. Seizures, raised ICP and focal hemisphere signs occur alone or in combination.

Investigations

LP is potentially hazardous in the presence of raised intracranial pressure, and CT should always precede it. CT reveals single or multiple low-density areas, which show ring enhancement and surrounding cerebral oedema. There may be an elevated WBC and ESR with active infection. Cerebral toxoplasmosis or tuberculous disease secondary to HIV infection should always be considered.

Management and prognosis

Antimicrobial therapy is indicated once the diagnosis is made (see Box 16.19). Surgical treatment by burr-hole aspiration or excision may be necessary. Epilepsy frequently develops and is often resistant to treatment. The mortality rate remains high at 10% to 20%.

Spinal epidural abscess

The characteristic clinical features are pain in a root distribution and progressive transverse spinal cord syndrome with paraparesis, sensory impairment and sphincter dysfunction. Infection is usually

16

	16.19 Aetiology and treatment of bacterial cerebral abscess		
Site of abscess	**Source of infection**	**Likely organisms**	**Recommended treatment**
Frontal lobe	Paranasal sinuses Teeth	Streptococci Anaerobes	Cefotaxime 2–3 g IV four times daily *plus* metronidazole 500 mg IV three times daily
Temporal lobe	Middle ear	Streptococci Enterobacteriaceae	Ampicillin 2–3 g IV three times daily *plus* metronidazole 500 mg IV three times daily *plus either* ceftazidime 2 g IV three times daily *or* gentamicin[a] 5 mg/kg IV daily
Cerebellum	Sphenoid sinus Mastoid/middle ear	*Pseudomonas* spp. Anaerobes	As for temporal lobe
Any site	Penetrating trauma	Staphylococci	Flucloxacillin 2–3 g IV four times daily *or* cefuroxime 1.5 g IV three times daily
Multiple	Metastatic and cryptogenic	Streptococci Anaerobes	Benzylpenicillin 1.8–2.4 g IV four times daily if endocarditis or cyanotic heart disease Otherwise cefotaxime 2–3 g IV four times daily *plus* metronidazole 500 mg IV three times daily
[a]Monitor gentamicin levels.			

haematogenous. Staphylococcal infection, often linked to IV drug misuse, has contributed to a marked rise in incidence. MRI or myelography should precede urgent neurosurgical intervention. Decompressive laminectomy with abscess drainage relieves the pressure on the dura. This, together with appropriate antibiotics, may prevent complete and irreversible paraplegia.

Neurosyphilis

Neurosyphilis may involve the meninges, blood vessels and/or the brain and spinal cord. The incidence of syphilis increased recently, because of misguided relaxation of safe sex precautions after development of effective treatments for AIDS. Early diagnosis and treatment remain essential.

Clinical features

The three most common presentations are summarised in Box 16.20. The 'Argyll Robertson' pupil (pupil small, reacts to convergence but not to light) may accompany any neurosyphilitic syndrome.

	16.20 Clinical and pathological features of neurosyphilis

Type (interval from primary)	Pathology	Clinical features
Meningovascular (5 years)	Endarteritis obliterans Meningeal exudates Granuloma (gumma)	Stroke Cranial nerve palsies Seizures/mass lesion
General paralysis of the insane (5–15 years)	Degeneration in cerebral cortex/cerebral atrophy Thickened meninges	Dementia Tremor Bilateral upper motor signs
Tabes dorsalis (5–20 years)	Degeneration of sensory neurons Wasting of dorsal columns Optic atrophy	Lightning pains Sensory ataxia Visual failure Abdominal crises Incontinence Trophic changes
Any of the above		Argyll Robertson pupils

Investigations

Routine screening is warranted in many neurological patients. Treponemal antibodies are positive in most patients but CSF examination is essential; active disease is suggested by a lymphocytosis, and protein may be elevated.

Management

Procaine benzylpenicillin and probenecid are given for 17 days. Further courses must be given if symptoms persist/recur or if the CSF continues to show signs of active disease.

Diseases caused by bacterial toxins

Tetanus

This results from infection with *Clostridium tetani*, a commensal in the gut of humans and domestic animals, which is found in soil. Infection enters the body through wounds. It is rare in the UK (affecting gardeners, farmers and IV drug misusers) but is common in many developing countries. Spores germinate and bacilli multiply in areas of tissue necrosis. The bacilli remain localised but produce an exotoxin with an affinity for motor nerve endings and cells. The anterior horn cells are affected, resulting in rigidity and convulsions. Symptoms appear from 2 days to several weeks after injury—the shorter the incubation period, the worse the prognosis.

Clinical features

The most important early symptom is trismus—painless spasm of the masseter muscles ('lockjaw'). The tonic rigidity spreads to the muscles of the face, neck and trunk. Contraction of facial muscles leads to the so-called 'risus sardonicus'. The back is usually slightly arched ('opisthotonus'), and there is a board-like abdominal wall. In more severe cases, painful violent

16

spasms or convulsions can occur, which may lead to exhaustion, asphyxia or aspiration pneumonia. Autonomic involvement may cause cardiovascular complications such as hypertension.

Investigations and management

The diagnosis is made on clinical grounds. Treatment of an established case involves:
• Human tetanus antitoxin (3000 U IV) to neutralise absorbed toxin. • Debridement of wounds. • IV benzylpenicillin (or metronidazole if allergic). • Nursing in a quiet room and avoidance of unnecessary stimuli. • Diazepam IV to control spasms; if ineffective, paralyse and ventilate. • Fluid and nutritional support.

Prevention

• Debridement of contaminated injuries. • Penicillin (1.2 g injection followed by a 7-day oral course). • IM injection of 250 U of human tetanus antitoxin, along with toxoid (repeated at 1 and 6 months). • If already immunised: only a booster of toxoid is required.

Botulism

Botulism means paralysis and neurological dysfunction produced by the neurotoxins of *Clostridium botulinum*. Common contaminated sources include sealed and preserved foods, and honey. Wound botulism is a growing problem in injection drug-users. Ingestion of even picogram amounts of this potent neurotoxin causes bulbar and ocular palsies (dysphagia, blurred or double vision, ptosis), progressing to limb weakness and respiratory paralysis. Management includes ventilation and supportive measures until the toxin dissociates from nerve endings at 6 to 8 weeks following ingestion. Antitoxin is available against some toxin types.

Prion diseases

Prions are unique amongst infectious agents in that they are devoid of nucleic acid and are not inactivated by cooking or conventional sterilization. Transmission may occur by consumption of infected CNS tissue or by inoculation, but prion diseases also occur spontaneously or as an inherited disorder. Histopathology shows cortical spongiform change, neuronal cell loss, gliosis and deposition of abnormal prion protein.

Creutzfeldt–Jakob disease

CJD is the best-characterised human prion disease. Some 10% of cases arise from a mutation in the gene coding for the prion protein. The sporadic form is the most common, presenting in middle-aged to elderly patients with rapidly progressive dementia, myoclonus and a characteristic EEG pattern (repetitive slow wave complexes). Death occurs after a mean of 4 to 6 months. There is no known treatment.

Variant CJD

This type of CJD affected a small number of UK patients in the 1990s. The source was cows with bovine spongiform encephalopathy, and the incidence fell sharply with changes in public health and farming practice.

Intracranial mass lesions and raised intracranial pressure

Intracranial mass lesions may be:
• Traumatic: subdural or extradural haematoma. • Vascular: intracranial haemorrhage. • Infective: for example, abscess, tuberculoma, cysticercosis. • Neoplastic: benign or malignant.

Symptoms and signs are produced by direct effects on adjacent tissue, raised intracranial pressure and false localising signs.

Raised intracranial pressure

Raised ICP may be caused by mass lesions, cerebral oedema, obstruction to CSF circulation causing hydrocephalus, impaired CSF absorption and cerebral venous obstruction.

Clinical features

In adults, intracranial pressure is less than 10 to 15 mmHg. If pressure increases slowly, compensatory alteration in the volume of fluid in CSF spaces and venous sinuses may minimise symptoms. Rapid pressure increase overwhelms this compensation, causing early symptoms, including sudden death. Papilloedema may be absent.

False localising signs (i.e., signs distant from the primary pathology) occur in raised ICP. Cerebral swelling may stretch or compress the 6th cranial nerve against the petrous temporal bone ridge. Transtentorial herniation of the uncus may compress the ipsilateral 3rd nerve, causing a dilated pupil; however, a contralateral 3rd nerve palsy may also occur because of compression by the tentorial margin. Vomiting, coma, bradycardia and arterial hypertension are later features of raised ICP.

Downward displacement of the medial temporal lobe (uncus) through the tentorium because of a cortical mass may cause 'temporal coning'. This may stretch the 3rd and/or 6th cranial nerves, or compress the contralateral cerebral peduncle (causing ipsilateral upper motor neuron signs), usually with progressive coma. Downward movement of the cerebellar tonsils through the foramen magnum may compress the medulla—'tonsillar coning', causing brainstem haemorrhage and/or acute obstruction of the CSF pathways. Unless the condition is treated rapidly, coma and death occur.

Management is that of the causative lesion.

Brain tumours

Primary and secondary brain tumours

Common sources of metastases from extracranial primary tumours are bronchus, breast and GI tract. Primary intracerebral tumours are classified by their cell of origin and degree of malignancy (Box 16.21). Even when malignant, they do not metastasise outside the nervous system.

Clinical features

Rapidly growing tumours present with a short history of mass effects (headache, nausea), whereas indolent tumours present with slowly progressive focal deficits, reflecting their location; generalised or focal seizures are common. Headache, if present, is accompanied by focal deficits or seizures; isolated stable headache is almost never caused by intracranial tumour.

i 16.21 Primary intracranial tumours

Histological type	Common site	Age
Malignant		
Glioma (astrocytoma)	Cerebral hemisphere	Adulthood
	Cerebellum	Childhood/adulthood
	Brainstem	Childhood/young adulthood
Oligodendroglioma	Cerebral hemisphere	Adulthood
Medulloblastoma	Posterior fossa	Childhood
Ependymoma	Posterior fossa	Childhood/adolescence
Cerebral lymphoma	Cerebral hemisphere	Adulthood
Benign		
Meningioma	Cortical dura, parasagittal, sphenoid ridge, suprasellar, olfactory groove	Adulthood
Neurofibroma	Acoustic neuroma	Adulthood
Craniopharyngioma	Suprasellar	Childhood/adolescence
Pituitary adenoma	Pituitary fossa	Adulthood
Colloid cyst	Third ventricle	Any age
Pineal tumours	Quadrigeminal cistern	Childhood (teratomas) Young adult (germ cell)

The size of a brain tumour is of far less prognostic significance than its location. Brainstem tumours cause early neurological deficits, whereas frontal tumours may be large before symptoms occur.

Investigations

Diagnosis is by neuroimaging and pathological grading following biopsy, or resection where possible. The more malignant tumours are more likely to demonstrate contrast enhancement on imaging. If the tumour appears metastatic, further investigation to find the primary is required.

Management

Medical: Dexamethasone (orally or IV in acute raised ICP) lowers intracranial pressure by resolving the reactive oedema. Seizures should be treated with anticonvulsants. Prolactin or growth hormone-secreting pituitary tumours may respond to dopamine agonists.

Surgical: Surgery is the mainstay of treatment. Only partial excision may be possible if tumour is inaccessible or if removal will cause unacceptable brain damage. Biopsy should be considered even if tumour cannot be removed (histology has implications for management). Meningiomas and acoustic neuromas offer the best prospects for complete removal. Pituitary adenomas may be removed by a trans-sphenoidal route, avoiding craniotomy.

Radiotherapy and chemotherapy: These have only a marginal effect on cerebral metastases and malignant gliomas in adults, although temozolomide may slightly extend survival in grade IV glioblastomas. Radiotherapy reduces recurrence of pituitary adenoma after surgery. Radiotherapy may be an adjunct to surgery for meningiomas that cannot be completely excised or whose histology suggests an increased tendency to recurrence.

Prognosis

Histological grade is a powerful predictor of prognosis in primary CNS tumours, although it does not yet take account of individual biomarkers. For each tumour type and grade, advancing age and deteriorating functional status are the next most important negative prognostic features. The overall 5-year survival rate of about 14% in adults masks a wide variation that depends on tumour type.

Acoustic neuroma

This is a benign tumour of Schwann cells of the 8th cranial nerve, which may arise in isolation or as part of neurofibromatosis (see later). As an isolated finding, it occurs after the third decade and is more frequent in females.

Clinical features

There is unilateral hearing loss, often with tinnitus. Vertigo is an unusual symptom, as slow growth allows compensatory brainstem mechanisms to develop. Distortion of the brainstem or cerebellum may cause ataxia and/ or cerebellar signs. Distortion of the fourth ventricle and cerebral aqueduct may cause hydrocephalus.

Investigations and management

MRI is the investigation of choice. Management involves surgical removal. If this is complete, the prognosis is excellent. Deafness and facial weakness may result from the operation.

Neurofibromatosis

Neurofibromatosis encompasses two clinically and genetically separate conditions, with an autosomal dominant pattern of inheritance. Multiple fibromatous tumours develop from the neurilemmal sheaths of peripheral and cranial nerves.

16

Type 1 (NF1): Caused by a mutation on chromosome 17. Clinical features include multiple cutaneous neurofibromas, café au lait spots in the skin, plexiform and spinal neurofibroma, scoliosis and endocrine tumours. Investigation and treatment are only indicated if there are new symptoms or if malignant change is suspected.

Type 2 (NF2): Caused by a mutation on chromosome 22. Characterised by schwannomas (benign nerve sheath Schwann cell tumours), with little skin involvement. Clinical manifestations include acoustic and/or spinal schwannomas, meningiomas, ependymomas and ocular hamartomas or meningiomas.

Von Hippel–Lindau disease

This rare dominantly inherited disease is characterised by the combination of retinal and intracranial (typically cerebellar) haemangiomas and haemangioblastomas. There may be associated extracranial hamartomatous lesions.

Hydrocephalus

Hydrocephalus (dilatation of the ventricular system) may be caused by increased CSF production, reduced absorption or obstruction of CSF circulation. Causes are given in Box 16.22. In obstructive hydrocephalus, diversion of the CSF by a shunt placed between the ventricular system and peritoneal cavity or right atrium may relieve symptoms.

Normal pressure hydrocephalus

Dilatation of the ventricular system is caused by intermittent rises in CSF pressure. It occurs in old age and is suggested by gait apraxia and dementia, often with urinary incontinence. The result of shunting procedures is unpredictable.

Idiopathic intracranial hypertension

This usually occurs in obese young women. Raised ICP develops without a structural lesion, hydrocephalus or other identifiable cause. The aetiology is uncertain, but there is an association with obesity in females. It can be precipitated by drugs (tetracycline, vitamin A, retinoids).

Clinical features

Headache is present, sometimes with diplopia and visual disturbance. There are usually no signs other than papilloedema.

Investigations

Brain imaging is required to exclude a structural or other cause (e.g. cerebral venous sinus thrombosis). LP (after CT) confirms normal CSF constituents at pressure greater than 30 cm H_2O.

 16.22 Causes of hydrocephalus

Congenital malformations

- Aqueduct stenosis
- Chiari malformations
- Dandy–Walker syndrome
- Benign intracranial cysts
- Vein of Galen aneurysms
- Congenital CNS infections
- Craniofacial anomalies

Acquired causes

- Mass lesions (esp. posterior fossa):
    - Tumour
    - Colloid cyst of third ventricle
    - Abscess
    - Haematoma
- Absorption blockages:
    - Inflammation (e.g. meningitis, sarcoidosis)
    - Intracranial haemorrhage

Management

Avoid precipitants; reduce weight if obese. Acetazolamide or topiramate may lower intracranial pressure. Repeated LP helps headache but is often poorly tolerated. Patients failing to respond, in whom chronic papilloedema threatens vision, may require optic nerve sheath fenestration or a lumbo-peritoneal shunt.

Disorders of the spine and spinal cord

Cervical spondylosis

Degeneration of the intervertebral discs and osteoarthritis of the cervical vertebrae is often asymptomatic but may cause neurological dysfunction. The C5/6, C6/7 and C4/5 vertebral levels affecting C6, C7 and C5 roots, respectively, are most commonly affected.

Cervical radiculopathy

Compression of a nerve root occurs when a disc prolapses laterally, which may develop acutely or more gradually because of osteophytic encroachment of the intervertebral foramina.

Clinical features

Neck pain may radiate in the distribution of the affected nerve root. Neck movements may exacerbate pain. Paraesthesia and sensory loss may be found in the affected segment, and there may be lower motor neuron signs (Box 16.23).

Investigations

X-rays are unhelpful, except for trauma or destructive lesions. MRI is the investigation of choice for radicular symptoms. Electrophysiological studies rarely add to clinical examination.

Management

Analgesia and physiotherapy usually suffice. A minority require surgery (discectomy or radicular decompression).

Cervical myelopathy

Dorsomedial herniation of a disc or dorsal osteophytes may compress the spinal cord or the anterior spinal artery (which supplies the anterior two-thirds of the cord).

16

i	16.23 Physical signs in cervical root compression		
Root	Muscle weakness	Sensory loss	Reflex loss
C5	Biceps, deltoid, spinati	Upper lateral arm	Biceps
C6	Brachioradialis	Lower lateral arm, thumb, index finger	Supinator
C7	Triceps, finger and wrist extensors	Middle finger	Triceps

Clinical features

The onset is usually insidious and painless, but acute deterioration may occur after trauma. Spasticity in the legs, together with numbness, tingling and proprioceptive loss in the hands, is a common pattern. Disturbance of micturition is a very late feature.

Investigations

MRI or rarely myelography will direct surgical intervention.

Management and prognosis

Surgery, including laminectomy and anterior discectomy, may arrest progression, but neurological improvement is not the rule. The decision whether to operate may be difficult. Manual manipulation of the cervical spine is of no benefit and may cause acute deterioration.

Lumbar spondylosis

This term covers degenerative disc disease and osteoarthritic change in the lumbar spine. Pain in the distribution of the lumbar or sacral roots ('sciatica') is usually caused by disc protrusion, but can rarely be a feature of spinal tumour, pelvic malignancy or vertebral TB.

Lumbar disc herniation

Acute lumbar disc herniation is often precipitated by lifting heavy weights while the spine is flexed.

Clinical features

The onset may be sudden or gradual. Constant aching pain in the lumbar region may radiate to the buttock, thigh, calf and foot. Pain is exacerbated by straining but may be relieved by lying flat. Root pressure is suggested by limited hip flexion on the affected side if the straight leg is raised (Lasègue's sign). If the L3 or L4 is involved, back pain may be induced by hyperextension of the hip (femoral nerve stretch test). The roots most frequently affected are L4, L5 and S1 (Box 16.24).

Investigations

MRI is the investigation of choice; plain x-rays of the lumbar spine are of little value.

i	**16.24 Physical signs in lumbar root compression**			
Disc level	Root	Sensory loss	Weakness	Reflex loss
L3/L4	L4	Inner calf	Inversion of foot	Knee
L4/L5	L5	Outer calf and dorsum of foot	Dorsiflexion of hallux/toes	Hamstring
L5/S1	S1	Sole and lateral foot	Plantar flexion	Ankle

Management

Some 90% of patients recover with analgesia and early mobilisation. Physical manœuvres likely to strain the lumbar spine should be avoided. Local anaesthetic or glucocorticoid injections may help in ligamentous injury or joint dysfunction. Consider surgery if there is no response to conservative treatment or if there is a progressive neurological deficit. Central disc prolapse with bilateral symptoms and sphincter dysfunction requires urgent surgical decompression.

Lumbar canal stenosis

This is congenital narrowing of the lumbar spinal canal, exacerbated by age-related degenerative change. Patients are usually elderly. There is exercise-induced weakness and paraesthesia in the legs, which is quickly relieved by rest ('spinal claudication'). Peripheral pulses are preserved, and ankle reflexes are absent. MRI will demonstrate narrowing of the lumbar canal. Lumbar laminectomy often results in complete relief of symptoms.

Spinal cord compression

Acute spinal cord compression is a common neurological emergency and is most commonly caused by trauma or metastatic tumours. Rarer causes include intervertebral disc prolapse, epidural abscess, tuberculoma and tumours of the meninges or spinal cord. The early stages of damage are reversible, but severely damaged neurons do not recover; patients with a short history should therefore be investigated urgently.

Clinical features

The onset is usually slow but may be acute with trauma or metastases.
• Pain: localised over the spine or in a root distribution, which may be aggravated by coughing, sneezing or straining. • Sensory: paraesthesia, numbness or cold sensations, especially in the lower limbs, which spread proximally, often to a level on the trunk. • Motor: weakness, heaviness or stiffness of the limbs, most commonly the legs. • Sphincters: urgency or hesitancy of micturition, leading eventually to urinary retention.

i	**16.25 Signs of spinal cord compression**
Cervical, above C5	Upper motor neuron signs and sensory loss in all four limbs Diaphragm weakness (phrenic nerve)
Cervical, C5–T1	Lower motor neuron signs and segmental sensory loss in the arms; upper motor neuron signs in the legs Respiratory (intercostal) muscle weakness
Thoracic cord	Spastic paraplegia with a sensory level on the trunk. Sacral loss of sensation and extensor plantar responses
Cauda equina	Spinal cord ends at approximately the T12/L1 spinal level; lesions below this can only cause lower motor neuron signs by affecting the cauda equina

16

The Brown–Séquard syndrome (see Fig. 16.3) results if damage is confined to one side of the cord.

Box 16.25 lists the expected signs, according to the level of cord damage.

Investigations

• Urgent MRI of the spine: the investigation of choice. • Plain X-rays: may show bony destruction and soft-tissue abnormalities. • Routine investigations, including CXR: may reveal systemic disease. • Needle biopsy: required before radiotherapy to establish tumour histology.

Management

Benign tumours: These should be surgically excised. Recovery is good unless there is a marked neurological deficit before diagnosis.

Extradural compression because of malignancy: Prognosis is poor; useful function may be regained if treatment is initiated within 24 hours of severe weakness or sphincter dysfunction. Surgical decompression may be appropriate in some; outcome is similar to that of radiotherapy.

Spinal cord compression because of TB: Surgical treatment is performed if the patient is seen early. Appropriate antituberculous chemotherapy should be given.

Traumatic lesions of the vertebral column: These require specialised neurosurgical treatment.

Intrinsic diseases of the spinal cord

There are many disorders that interfere with spinal cord function due to noncompressive involvement of the spinal cord itself (Box 16.26). The symptoms and signs are similar to those of extrinsic compression, although a suspended sensory loss can occur only with intrinsic disease such as syringomyelia. Investigation starts with imaging, which is important for excluding a compressive lesion. MRI provides the most information about structural lesions (e.g. diastematomyelia, intrinsic tumour or syringomyelia; Fig. 16.11). Nonspecific signal change may be seen in inflammatory, infective or metabolic conditions. LP or blood tests may be required to make a specific diagnosis.

Diseases of peripheral nerves

Pathological processes may affect the nerve roots (radiculopathy), the nerve plexuses (plexopathy) and/or the individual nerves (neuropathy). Nerve fibres of different types (motor, sensory or autonomic) may be involved. Disorders may be primarily directed at the axon, the myelin sheath (Schwann cells) or both. An acute or chronic peripheral nerve disorder may be focal (affecting a single nerve: mononeuropathy), multifocal (several nerves: mononeuritis multiplex) or generalised (polyneuropathy). Neurophysiological tests, and sometimes nerve biopsy, will help determine whether the pathology is primarily affecting the nerve axon (axonal neuropathy) or the myelin sheath (demyelinating neuropathy).

Causes of polyneuropathy include:
• Genetic: for example, CMT disease. • Toxins: alcohol, lead, thallium, many drugs. • Metabolic disease: diabetes, chronic kidney disease. • Inflammatory: for example, Guillain–Barré syndrome, polyarteritis nodosa, systemic lupus erythematosus, rheumatoid arthritis. • Infections: for example, HIV,

i	16.26 Intrinsic diseases of the spinal cord	
Type of disorder	**Condition**	**Clinical features**
Congenital	Diastematomyelia (spina bifida)	LMN features, deformity and sensory loss of legs, sphincter dysfunction Hairy patch or pit over low back Incidence ↓ by maternal intake of folic acid during pregnancy
	Hereditary spastic paraplegia	Autosomal dominant; onset usually in adult life. Slowly progressive UMN features (legs >arms), little sensory loss
Infective/ inflamma- tory	Transverse myelitis (viruses, e.g. HZV, HIV), schistosomia- sis, MS, sarcoidosis	Weakness, sensory loss pain, developing over hours to days UMN features below lesion, impaired sphincter function
Vascular	Anterior spinal artery infarct (atherosclero- sis, aortic dissection, embolus)	Abrupt onset LMN signs at level of lesion, UMN features below it Spinothalamic sensory loss below lesion (spared dorsal column sensation)
	Spinal AVM/dural fistula	Onset variable (acute to slowly progressive) Variable LMN, UMN, sensory and sphincter disturbance
Neoplastic	Glioma, ependy- moma	Weakness, sensory loss, pain, developing over months/years UMN features below lesion; LMN features in conus; sphincter dysfunction
Metabolic	Vitamin B$_{12}$ deficiency (sub-acute combined degeneration)	Progressive spastic paraparesis with propriocep- tion loss, absent reflexes because of peripheral neuropathy, optic nerve and cerebral involvement
Degenera- tive	Motor neuron disease Syringomyelia	Progressive LMN and UMN features, bulbar weakness, no sensory loss Gradual onset over months or years, pain in cervical segments LMN signs at level of lesion, UMN features below it Suspended spinothalamic sensory loss at lesion, dorsal columns preserved

16

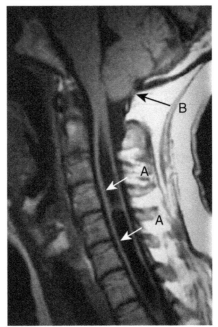

Fig. 16.11 MRI scan showing syrinx (arrows A), with herniation of cerebellar tonsils (arrow B).

brucella, leprosy. • Neoplasms: lymphoma, carcinoma, myeloma. • Vitamin deficiencies: especially B_{12}, thiamin, pyridoxine, E.

Investigations required in peripheral neuropathy reflect the spectrum of causes (Box 16.27).

Entrapment neuropathy

Focal compression is the usual cause of a mononeuropathy Box 16.28. Certain conditions predispose to entrapment neuropathies, including diabetes, excess alcohol or toxins and some genetic syndromes. Unless axonal loss has occurred, entrapment neuropathies will recover, provided the pressure on the nerve is relieved, either by avoidance of precipitating activities or by surgical decompression.

Multifocal neuropathy (mononeuritis multiplex)

When multiple nerve root, peripheral nerve or cranial nerve lesions occur serially or concurrently, the pathology is due either to involvement of the vasa nervorum or to malignant infiltration of the nerves. Vasculitis is a common cause, or it may complicate a polyneuropathy (e.g. diabetes).

16.27 Investigation of peripheral neuropathy

Initial tests

- Glucose (fasting)
- ESR, C-reactive protein
- Full blood count
- Urea and electrolytes
- Liver function tests
- Serum protein electrophoresis
- Vitamin B12, folate
- ANA, ANCA
- Chest x-ray
- HIV testing

If initial tests are negative

- Nerve conduction studies
- Vitamins E and A
- Genetic testing
- Lyme serology (p. 131)
- Angiotensin-converting enzyme
- Serum amyloid

Polyneuropathy

The clinical effects of a generalised pathological process occur in the longest peripheral nerves first, affecting the distal lower limbs before the upper limbs, with sensory symptoms and signs of an ascending 'glove and stocking' distribution. In inflammatory demyelinating neuropathies, the pathology may be patchier and variations from this ascending pattern occur.

Guillain–Barré syndrome

Guillain–Barré syndrome is a heterogeneous group of immune-mediated conditions with an incidence of 1 to 2 per 100 000 per year. In Europe and North America, the most common variant is acute inflammatory demyelinating polyneuropathy (AIDP). Axonal or sensorimotor variants are more common in China and Japan (often associated with *Campylobacter jejuni*). The hallmark is an acute paralysis evolving over days or weeks, with loss of reflexes. About two-thirds of those with AIDP have a prior history of infection, and an autoimmune response triggered by the preceding infection causes demyelination.

Clinical features

Distal paraesthesia and pain precede weakness that ascends rapidly from lower to upper limbs and is more marked proximally than distally. Facial and bulbar weakness is common, and respiratory weakness requiring ventilation occurs in 20% of cases. Weakness progresses for up to 4 weeks. Rapid deterioration to respiratory failure can develop within hours. Examination shows diffuse weakness with loss of reflexes. A rare variant, Miller Fisher syndrome, presents with internal and external ophthalmoplegia, ataxia and areflexia.

Investigations

CSF protein is elevated (or may initially be normal), but there is usually no rise in CSF cell number. Electrophysiology shows conduction block and

16

	16.28 Symptoms and signs in common entrapment neuropathies		

Nerve	Symptoms	Muscle weakness/ muscle-wasting	Area of sensory loss
Median (at wrist; carpal tunnel syndrome)	Pain and paraesthesia on palmar aspect of hands. Pain may extend to arm and shoulder	Abductor pollicis brevis	Lateral palm and thumb, index, middle and lateral half 4th finger
Ulnar (at elbow)	Paraesthesia on medial border of hand, wasting and weakness of hand muscles	All small hand muscles, excluding abductor pollicis brevis	Medial palm and little finger, and medial half 4th finger
Radial	Weakness of extension of wrist and fingers, often precipitated by sleeping in abnormal posture, e.g. arm over back of chair	Wrist and finger extensors, supinator	Dorsum of thumb
Common peroneal	Foot drop, trauma to head of fibula	Dorsiflexion and eversion of foot	Nil or dorsum of foot
Lateral cutaneous nerve of the thigh	Tingling and dysaesthesia on lateral border of the thigh	Nil	Lateral border of thigh

motor slowing after a week. Other causes of neuromuscular paralysis should be excluded (e.g. poliomyelitis, botulism, diphtheria, spinal cord syndromes or myasthenia).

Management and prognosis

• Plasma exchange or IV immunoglobulin therapy: shorten the illness and improve prognosis if started within 14 days. • Regular monitoring of vital capacity to detect respiratory failure. • Supportive measures to protect the airway and prevent pressure sores and venous thrombosis.

Overall, 80% of patients recover completely within 3 to 6 months, 4% die and the remainder suffer residual neurological disability. Adverse prognostic features include older age, rapid deterioration to ventilation and evidence of axonal loss on EMG.

Chronic polyneuropathy

A chronic symmetrical axonal polyneuropathy, evolving over months or years, is the most common form of chronic neuropathy. Diabetes mellitus is the most common cause, but in around 25% to 50%, no cause can be found.

Hereditary neuropathy

Charcot–Marie–Tooth disease (CMT) is an umbrella term for the inherited neuropathies. This group of syndromes has varied clinical and genetic features. The most common CMT is the autosomal dominantly inherited CMT type 1, which causes distal wasting ('inverted champagne bottle' legs), often with pes cavus, and predominantly motor involvement. X-linked and recessive forms of CMT also occur.

Chronic demyelinating polyneuropathy

The acquired chronic demyelinating neuropathies include chronic inflammatory demyelinating peripheral neuropathy (which responds to glucocorticoids, plasma exchange or IV immunoglobulin), multifocal motor neuropathy and paraprotein-associated demyelinating neuropathy (sometimes associated with a lymphoproliferative malignancy). They may also demonstrate positive antibodies to myelin-associated glycoprotein.

Brachial plexopathy

Trauma usually damages either the upper or the lower parts of the brachial plexus, according to the mechanics of the injury. The clinical features depend upon the site of damage (Box 16.29). The lower brachial plexus is vulnerable to breast or apical lung tumours, therapeutic irradiation, birth trauma or compression by thoracic outlet anomalies such as a cervical rib.

Lumbosacral plexopathy

This may be caused by neoplastic infiltration or compression by retroperitoneal haematomas. A small-vessel vasculopathy can produce a lumbar plexopathy, especially in association with diabetes mellitus ('diabetic amyotrophy') or a vasculitis. This presents with painful wasting of the quadriceps and an absent knee reflex.

Spinal root lesions

These are caused by compression at or near spinal exit foramina by prolapsed intervertebral discs or degenerative spinal disease. Clinical features include muscle weakness and wasting and dermatomal sensory loss with reflex changes reflecting the roots involved. Pain in the muscles innervated by the affected roots is common.

16

i 16.29 Physical signs in brachial plexus lesions			
Site	Root	Affected muscles	Sensory loss
Upper plexus (Erb–Duchenne)	C5/6	Biceps, deltoid, spinati, rhomboids, brachioradialis	Patch over deltoid
Lower plexus (Déjerine–Klumpke)	C8/T1	Small hand muscles, lumbricals (claw hand), ulnar wrist flexors	Ulnar border hand/forearm
Thoracic outlet syndrome	C8/T1	Small hand muscles, lumbricals (claw hand), long finger flexors	Ulnar border hand/forearm/ medial surface of upper arm

Disorders of the neuromuscular junction

Myasthenia gravis

This is characterised by progressive fatigable weakness, particularly of the ocular, neck, facial and bulbar muscles. In 80% of cases it is caused by autoantibodies to acetylcholine receptors in the neuromuscular junction. About 15% of patients have a thymoma, and a majority of the remainder have thymic follicular hyperplasia. Penicillamine can trigger an antibody-mediated myasthenic syndrome, and some drugs (e.g. aminoglycosides and quinolones) may exacerbate the neuromuscular blockade.

Clinical features

The disease usually presents between 15 and 50 years of age, with women affected more often than men in the younger age groups and the reverse at older ages. The cardinal symptom is abnormal fatigable weakness of the muscles; movement is initially strong, but rapidly weakens. Worsening towards the end of the day or following exercise is characteristic. Intermittent ptosis or diplopia is common, but weakness of chewing, swallowing, speaking or limb movement also occurs. Respiratory muscle weakness is an avoidable cause of death. Aspiration may occur, and cough may be ineffectual. Ventilatory support is required where weakness is severe or of abrupt onset.

Investigations

Tensilon test: IV injection of an anticholinesterase, edrophonium, causes improved muscle power within 30 seconds, which persists for 2 to 3 minutes.

Nerve conduction studies: Repetitive stimulation may show a characteristic decremental response.

Autoantibodies: Antiacetylcholine receptor antibody is found in more than 80% of cases, and antimuscle-specific kinase antibodies in others. Screen for associated autoimmune disorders.

Thoracic CT: Required to exclude thymoma (may not be visible on plain X-ray).

Management

Anticholinesterases: These maximise activity of acetylcholine at receptors in the neuromuscular junction using anticholinesterases, for example, pyridostigmine. Muscarinic side effects may be controlled by propantheline. Anticholinesterase over-dosage may cause a cholinergic crisis (muscle fasciculation, paralysis, pallor, sweating, salivation and small pupils); this may be distinguished from a myasthenic crisis clinically and, if necessary, by a dose of edrophonium.

Immunological treatment: Acutely, plasma exchange or IV immunoglobulin reduces antibody levels and causes marked, although brief, improvement. This is mainly used for severe myasthenia or preoperative preparation. For long-term treatment, glucocorticoids (which may initially exacerbate symptoms) may be used, with azathioprine to minimise dose and side effects. Thymectomy should be considered in young female patients with generalised disease but is less likely to cause remission in older patients. Rapid progression of the disease more than 5 years after onset is uncommon.

Lambert–Eaton myasthenic syndrome

In this condition, transmitter release is impaired often with antibodies to prejunctional calcium channels. The cardinal sign is absent tendon reflexes, which return after sustained contraction of the relevant muscle. LEMS is frequently associated with underlying malignancy. It is diagnosed electro-physiologically, and treatment is with 3,4-diaminopyridine, or pyridostig-mine with immunosuppression.

Diseases of muscle

Disease of voluntary muscle most commonly presents as proximal sym-metrical weakness (proximal myopathy). Other presenting symptoms include myotonia (an abnormality of muscle relaxation) and muscle pain. Diagnosis depends on the clinical picture, along with EMG studies, muscle biopsy and sometimes genetic studies.

Muscular dystrophies

These inherited disorders are characterised by progressive degeneration of muscle groups, sometimes with cardiac or respiratory involvement or nonmyopathic features (Box 16.30).

Clinical features

Onset is often in childhood, with symmetrical wasting and weakness. There is no fasciculation and no sensory loss. Tendon reflexes are preserved until a late stage, except in myotonic dystrophy.

Investigations

• Specific genetic testing, with EMG and muscle biopsy if necessary.
• Creatine kinase: markedly elevated in Duchenne and Becker muscu-lar dystrophies but normal or moderately elevated in other dystrophies.
• Screening for cardiomyopathy or dysrhythmia: important.

Management

There is no specific therapy, but physiotherapy and occupational therapy help with managing disability. Glucocorticoids can be used in Duchenne muscular dystrophy, but side effects limit their use. Treat-ment of associated cardiac failure or arrhythmia (by pacemaker) may be required; similarly, management of respiratory complications (including nocturnal hypoventilation) can improve quality of life. Improvements in noninvasive ventilation have led to significant improvements in survival for patients with Duchenne muscular dystrophy. Genetic counselling is important.

	16.30 The muscular dystrophies			
Type	Genetics	Age of onset (years)	Muscles affected	Other features
Myotonic dystrophy	AD; expanded triplet repeat chromosome 19q	Any	Face (including ptosis), sternomastoids, distal limb, generalised later	Myotonia, cognitive impairment, cardiac conduction abnormalities, lens opacities, frontal balding, hypogonadism
Proximal myotonic myopathy	AD; quadruplet repeat in chromosome 3q	8–50	Proximal, especially thigh, muscle hypertrophy	As earlier, but cognition not affected Muscle pain
Duchenne	X-linked; deletions in *dystrophin* gene	<5	Proximal and limb girdle	Cardiomyopathy and respiratory failure
Becker	X-linked; deletions in *dystrophin* gene	Childhood/ early adult	Proximal and limb girdle	Cardiomyopathy; respiratory failure uncommon
Limb girdle	Many mutations on different chromosomes	Childhood/ early adult	Limb girdle	Variable with mutation. Some have cardiorespiratory involvement
Facioscapulohumeral	AD; repeat deletion chromosome 4q	7–30	Face and upper limb girdle; distal leg	Pain in shoulder girdle common, deafness
Oculopharyngeal	AD or AR	30–60	Ptosis, ophthalmoplegia, dysphagia, tongue	Mild leg weakness
AD = autosomal dominant, AR = autosomal recessive				

Inherited metabolic myopathies

There are many rare inherited disorders that affect muscle function and present with weakness, pain or myotonia:

- Disordered biochemical pathways affecting ATP synthesis, for example, myophosphorylase deficiency (McArdle's disease)
- Mitochondrial disorders—inherited in the maternal line
- Channelopathies—disordered sodium, potassium or calcium channel function; autosomal inheritance

i	**16.31 Causes of acquired proximal myopathy**	
Inflammatory	Polymyositis, dermatomyositis
Endocrine and metabolic	Hypothyroidism, hyperthyroidism, acromegaly, Cushing's syndrome, Addison's disease, Conn's syndrome, osteomalacia, hypokalaemia (liquorice, diuretic and purgative abuse), hypercalcaemia (disseminated bony metastases)
Toxic	Alcohol, amphetamines, cocaine, heroin, vitamin E, organophosphates, snake venoms
Drugs	Glucocorticoids, chloroquine, amiodarone, β-blockers, statins, clofibrate, ciclosporin, vincristine, zidovudine, opiates
Paraneoplastic	Carcinomatous neuromyopathy, dermatomyositis

Acquired myopathies

Muscle weakness may be caused by a range of acquire metabolic, endocrine, toxic or inflammatory disorders (Box 16.31).

Medical ophthalmology

Visual impairment has significant socioeconomic impact, and although progress has occurred in prevention and treatment of ocular infections, cataract and glaucoma, age-related conditions such as macular degeneration, diabetic retinopathy and retinal vein occlusion are increasing in frequency. Medical ophthalmology requires a good grounding in dermatology, diabetes and endocrinology, infectious diseases, medical genetics, neurology, rheumatology and stroke medicine. Neuro-ophthalmology is covered in Chapter 16. This chapter concentrates mainly on intraocular inflammation and conditions that require intravitreal injection therapy.

Investigation of visual disorders

History is the key to diagnosing visual disorders, with examination and investigations used to confirm or refute the provisional diagnosis.

Perimetry

Mainly used for monitoring glaucoma, perimetry also has a role in assessing neuro-ophthalmic disorders. All methods of perimetry rely on patient cooperation and mental agility.

Amsler chart: The simplest perimetry method, best for following up the scotomata in macular disorders.

Tangent/Goldmann kinetic perimetry: The operator introduces moving targets into the patient's visual field. Used to distinguish functional peripheral field loss (tunnel vision) from pathological field loss (funnel vision).

Automated threshold perimetry: Tests the threshold of the eye's ability to see at various points within the visual field.

Imaging

See Fig. 17.1.

Photography: For the retina, red-free imaging is superior for discriminating red haemorrhages or abnormal new vessels from the red background of the retina.

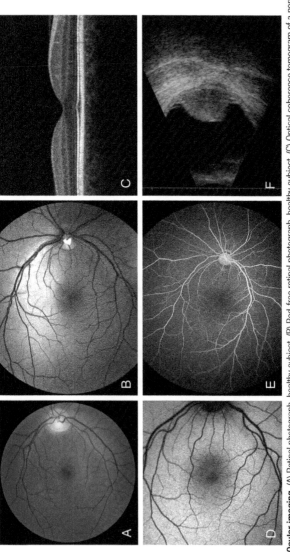

Fig. 17.1 Ocular imaging. (A) Retinal photograph, healthy subject. (B) Red-free retinal photograph, healthy subject. (C) Optical coherence tomogram of a normal eye, showing the layers of the retina and normal foveal indentation. (D) Fundus autofluorescence, normal subject, showing typical reduced signal at the optic disc. (absence of autofluorescent material) and retinal vessels (absorption). Intensity decreased over the fovea due to absorption of light by yellow macular pigment. (E) Fundal fluorescein angiogram, normal retina. (F) Ocular ultrasound showing typical biconvex appearance of a choroidal melanoma. (A, B, C and F, Courtesy of Aberdeen Royal Infirmary; D, From Schmitz-Valckenberg S, Fleckenstein M, Hendrik PN, et al. Fundus autofluorescence and progression of age-related macular degeneration. Survey Ophthalmol 2009; 54(1):96–117; E, From Witmer MT, Szilárd K. Wide-field imaging of the retina. Survey Ophthalmol 2013; 58(2):143–154)

Optical coherence tomography: The optical equivalent of ultrasound, used for assessing the integrity of the layers of the retina and detecting macular oedema.

Autofluorescence: Images autofluorescent lipofuscin pigment in the retina. Increased in certain inherited retinal dystrophies, at the edge of atrophic macular degeneration or with drug deposition, (e.g. hydroxychloroquine).

Fluorescein angiography: An invasive technique used in the diagnosis of retinal vasculitis, retinal and choroidal neovascularisation and capillary occlusion.

Ocular ultrasound: Useful when the retina is obscured, for example, by cataract or vitreous haemorrhage, and for diagnosing choroidal melanoma, using its distinctive internal reflectivity.

Visual electrophysiology

Used to localise disorders to the photoreceptors (electroretinogram), the retinal ganglion cells (pattern electroretinogram) or the optic pathways (visual evoked potential).

Presenting problems in ophthalmic disease

Presenting problems of predominantly neurological disease (e.g. ptosis, diplopia, oscillopsia, nystagmus and pupillary abnormalities) are discussed in Chapter 16. Opthalmic features of non-opthalmological conditions are listed in Boxes 17.1 - 17.7.

Watery/dry eye

The most common cause of a watery eye is a dry eye triggering reflex lacrimation. Patients may complain of a foreign body or gritty sensation or intermittent visual blurring triggered by reduced blinking, as occurs when reading or when concentrating on a distant object.

Pruritus

The most common causes are an acute allergic response to airborne or contact allergens. Some people are allergic to topical chloramphenicol, which is used for many minor ocular ailments.

Pain/headache

The key sign when assessing ocular pain and/or headache is whether there is a ciliary flush (red eye) or not (white eye).

Red eye

The presence of a ciliary flush at the limbus (the corneal margin of the sclerae) is a key finding in intraocular causes of pain. Watery discharge is not a discriminatory feature, and over-reliance on this symptom often results in anterior uveitis being misdiagnosed as viral conjunctivitis.

17.1 Ophthalmic features of haematological disease

Condition	Ophthalmic findings
Severe anaemia	Flame & preretinal haemorrhages, cotton wool spots, Roth spots
Megaloblastic anaemia	Optic neuropathy
Sickle-cell anaemia	Conjunctival vasculopathy, peripheral retinal neovascularisation
Leukaemia	Flame haemorrhages, Roth spots, retinal oedema, retinal vein occlusion, pseudohypopyon
Lymphoma	Lacrimal gland infiltrates, posterior uveitis
Hyperviscosity	Retinal vein occlusion
Cerebral venous thrombosis	Papilloedema

 17.2 Ophthalmic features of endocrine disease

Condition	Ophthalmic findings
Diabetes	Proliferative retinopathy, macular oedema, cataract
Thyrotoxicosis	Lid retraction
Graves' disease	Exposure keratopathy, periorbital oedema, proptosis, optic neuropathy
Thyroid cancer	Horner's syndrome
Parathyroid disease	Band keratopathy, corneal calcium deposition
Phaeochromocytoma	Hypertensive retinopathy
Cushing's syndrome	Cataract, diabetic retinopathy, central serous retinopathy

 17.3 Ophthalmic features of cardiovascular disease

Condition	Ophthalmic findings
Arteriosclerosis	Arteriovenous nipping, retinal vein occlusion, retinal artery macroaneurysm, ischaemic optic neuropathy, III/VI nerve palsy
Hypertension	Cotton wool spots, flame haemorrhages, papilloedema ± macular oedema
Infective endocarditis	Flame haemorrhages, Roth spots, endophthalmitis
Drugs	Amiodarone: vortex keratopathy, bilateral optic neuropathy
Thromboembolism	Retinal artery occlusion, hemianopia in stroke

White eye

In the absence of a ciliary flush, ocular or periorbital pain is most commonly caused by migraine.

Pain on eye movement is a cardinal feature of optic neuritis (eye is white) and scleritis (eye is red, except in posterior scleritis). Posterior scleritis, in which

17.4 Ophthalmic features of respiratory disease

Condition	Ophthalmic findings
COPD	Papilloedema (type 2 respiratory failure)
CF	Diabetic retinopathy
TB	Anterior uveitis, choroidal granuloma, serpiginous choroiditis, peripheral retinal arteritis, optic neuropathy (from ethambutol)
Sarcoidosis	Panuveitis, choroidal granuloma, iris nodules, keratitic precipitates
Lung cancer	Horner's syndrome, retinopathy

17.5 Ophthalmic features of rheumatological/ musculoskeletal disease

Condition	Ophthalmic findings
Rheumatoid arthritis	Keratoconjuncitivitis sicca, scleritis, scleromalacia, peripheral ulcerative keratitis, painless episcleritis
Seronegative spondyloarthritides	Anterior uveitis, conjunctivitis (in reactive arthritis)
Dermatomyositis	Periorbital oedema with violaceous eyelid rash
Sjögren's syndrome	Dry eyes
Giant cell arteritis	Central/branch retinal artery occlusion, ischaemic optic neuropathy
Behçet's disease	Occlusive retinal vasculitis, anterior uveitis with hypopyon
Granulomatosis with polyangiitis	Sclerokeratitis, retro-orbital inflammation
Polyarteritis nodosa	Peripheral ulcerative keratitis, scleritis, retinal arteritis

17.6 Ophthalmic features of gastrointestinal disease

Condition	Ophthalmic findings
Malabsorption	Corneal and conjunctival keratinisation, rod photoreceptor loss
Chronic pancreatitis	Diabetic retinopathy
Inflammatory bowel disease	Episcleritis, nonnecrotising scleritis, anterior uveitis
Large bowel tumour	Atypical congenital retinal pigment epithelium hypertrophy
Wilson's disease	Kayser-Fleischer corneal rings, sunflower cataracts
Haemochromatosis	Diabetic retinopathy

17

the visible sclera is white, should be diagnosed only with positive signs such as disc swelling and exudative retinal detachment, or with confirmation by ocular ultrasound. A more common cause of severe ocular/periocular pain, with photophobia and lacrimation, is cluster headache (p. 668), often misdiagnosed as scleritis. Both respond to glucocorticoids, adding to diagnostic confusion.

| **i** | **17.7 Ophthalmic features of skin disease** |

Condition	Ophthalmic findings
Rosacea	Posterior blepharitis, keratitis
Acne vulgaris	Dry eye (from isotretinoin), papilloedema (from tetracycline)
Psoriasis	Anterior uveitis
Eczema	Atopic keratoconjunctivitis
Urticaria	Angioedema
Bullous disease	Ocular cicatricial pemphigoid, Stevens–Johnson syndrome
Skin melanoma	Melanoma-associated retinopathy
Tumours	Basal cell carcinoma, squamous carcinoma of eyelid
Infections	Stye (folliculitis), chronic conjunctivitis (molluscum contageosum), acute blepharoconjunctivitis (herpes simplex)

Intermittent subacute angle closure glaucoma can cause headache, but usually accompanying corneal oedema causes visual blurring or haloes (glare with rainbow colours when looking at lights).

Giant cell arteritis is an uncommon, but usually striking, cause of headache, seen mainly in the elderly. Rarely, it presents with sudden, painless visual loss in the absence of raised inflammatory markers. Diagnosis can be made by fluorescein angiography.

Photophobia/glare

Excessive sensitivity to light, rather than fear of light, usually indicates ciliary muscle spasm caused by inflammation in the iris. Common causes are corneal abrasion, acute anterior uveitis and contact lens-related keratitis.

Occasionally, photophobia can be a symptom of congenital retinal dystrophies, especially cone photoreceptor deficiency. Photophobia may also be a feature of meningitis, usually with accompanying neck stiffness and headache (meningism, p. 685).

Glare is a common early feature of cataract, particularly triggered by oncoming headlights during night driving. It is a relatively common indication for surgery. It may also be an issue where there is insufficient melanin in the retinal pigment epithelium, for example, in atrophic age-related macular degeneration, in ocular albinism or following extensive laser therapy. If surgery is not an option, or pending surgery, glare may be reduced by wearing a broad-brimmed hat.

Photopsia

A flickering light sensation is indicative of photoreceptor activity, either through traction (e.g. posterior vitreous detachment), or inflammation, (e.g. autoimmune or paraneoplastic retinopathy). Rarely, photopsia occurs in occipital lobe epilepsy, usually with an accompanying homonymous hemianopia.

17.8 Red flag symptoms in visual loss

Symptom	Possible causes
Sudden onset	Retinal artery occlusion, ischaemic optic neuropathy
Headache	Giant cell arteritis (age >55 years)
Eye pain	Angle closure glaucoma, keratitis, scleritis, anterior uveitis
Pain on eye movement	Optic neuritis, scleritis

Distortion	Choroidal neovascular membrane:
	  Age-related macular degeneration, pathological
	    myopia, posterior uveitis, idiopathic
	Macular hole
	Epiretinal membrane

Worse in the morning	Macular oedema:
	  Diabetic macular oedema, retinal vein occlusion,
	    uveitis

Any of these symptoms in a patient with visual loss requires emergency ophthalmology referral.

Blurred vision

With this, patients can see what they are looking at, but it is out of focus. The most common intermittent cause is dry eye; the most common cause of permanent blurred vision is cataract. If vision is worse in the morning and eases later, this suggests macular oedema.

Loss of vision

In visual loss, patients are no longer able to see all or part of what they are looking at. Some symptoms associated with visual loss require urgent ophthalmological assessment (Box 17.8).

The most common cause of transient visual loss is migraine, usually a positive phenomenon with the object of regard seemingly hidden by something in the way, rather than a negative phenomenon in which part or all of what is being looked at is missing. With positive visual phenomena, the obstruction is often white or coloured, expanding across the visual field, or stationary but shimmering.

Negative visual phenomena, with absence of vision (blackness) occupying part or all the visual field, are typical of ocular, usually retinal, ischaemia. Transient ocular ischaemia is usually embolic, but occasionally occurs in giant cell arteritis, suggesting critical optic nerve ischaemia. Permanent monocular negative visual phenomena usually indicate previous optic nerve or retinal infarction. Tiny negative visual phenomena may also be seen in diabetic retinopathy, where patchy macular capillary occlusion may cause letters to be missing from words on reading.

17

Distortion of vision

Distortion is a cardinal symptom of disruption of foveal photoreceptor alignment, usually caused by choroidal neovascularisation. Less commonly, posterior hyaloid surface scarring causes foveal traction.

Objects appear not only misshapen but also smaller (micropsia), as a result of the photoreceptors being pulled apart. Macropsia, where objects look bigger than normal, is uncommon. It is sometimes seen in 'Alice in Wonderland' syndrome, a paediatric variant of migraine.

Eyelid retraction

Eyelid retraction is usually caused by inflammatory thyroid eye disease or thyrotoxicosis (see p. 372). In thyroid eye disease, enlargement of the inferior rectus tethers the eye, restricting upgaze. Compensatory overactivity of the superior rectus and levator palpebrae superioris causes eyelid retraction.

In thyrotoxicosis, increased sympathetic activity causes bilateral eyelid retraction that resolves with β-blockade and treatment of thyrotoxicosis.

Optic disc swelling

Optic disc swelling can be caused by a congenital variant (pseudopapilloedema), optic nerve pathology or widespread nerve fibre oedema, as with retinal vein occlusion. Neurological causes of optic disc swelling are discussed on p. 655.

Proptosis

Proptosis with eyelid retraction is most commonly caused by thyroid eye disease, when it is termed exophthalmos. Proptosis is a sign of retro-orbital tissue expansion. When expansion is within the cone of extraocular muscles, then forward eye displacement will be in line with the visual axis. When outside, the eye is additionally displaced to the side.

The primary clinical concerns are optic nerve compression, corneal exposure and diplopia. In thyroid eye disease, diplopia may be absent in symmetrical disease. Instead, restricted ocular movements make patients move their head to track moving objects. To the patient, however, the overarching concern is often appearance.

Specialist ophthalmological conditions

Ocular inflammation

In exposed structures, particularly the cornea and conjunctiva, inflammation is most commonly caused by infection. In other structures, such as the uveal tract and sclera, inflammation is more commonly caused by autoimmunity, although infection or malignancy also occur. Although the latter conditions may be obvious, they are sometimes discovered only after failure to respond to immunosuppression.

Most noninfective forms of ocular inflammation are idiopathic; all occur more commonly with other autoimmune conditions. Some occur asynchronously with other disease manifestations, for example, anterior uveitis in ankylosing spondylitis (p. 618). Others are direct manifestations of an underlying inflammatory condition, for example, keratoscleritis in granulomatosis with polyangiitis (formerly Wegener's granulomatosis).

Sjögren's syndrome

Sjögren's syndrome is either primary or secondary to other autoimmune conditions e.g. SLE, systemic sclerosis or primary biliary cholangitis (see p. 626). Inflammation of the lacrimal gland, its conjunctival accessory glands and the parotid gland leads to hyposecretion of tears and saliva. Lacrimal gland inflammation is one cause of keratoconjunctivitis sicca (dry, irritated eyes).

Treatment of the eyes in Sjögren's syndrome is symptomatic, involving artificial tears (e.g. hypromellose) and reducing tear loss by humidification. If symptoms persist, tear drainage may be reduced using surgical punctal plugs and punctal occlusion.

Peripheral ulcerative keratitis

Peripheral ulcerative keratitis ('corneal melting') is an autoimmune disorder affecting the limbus, sometimes with adjacent scleritis. It may be associated with disorders forming immune complexes, for rheumatoid arthritis, SLE and granulomatosis with polyangiitis. Pain and redness are usual, but are not always present. Systemic immunosuppression is always required, but topical glucocorticoids should be used cautiously to avoid keratolysis (corneal thinning). Secondary infection should be prevented with topical antibiotics, and corneal hydration should be maintained using artificial tears.

More common causes of peripheral corneal ulceration are blepharitis and acne rosacea, causing ocular irritation rather than pain. Hypersensitivity to staphylococcal exotoxin leads to stromal infiltrate adjacent to, but sparing, the limbus (marginal keratitis). This is self-limiting, but resolution can be assisted using topical chloramphenicol with or without topical glucocorticoids.

Scleritis

Scleritis usually causes severe pain that is worse on eye movement and often wakes the patient at night. Anterior scleritis is usually visible, with diffuse or nodular erythema (although it may be under the eyelids). Posterior uveitis is often accompanied by reduced vision and oedema of the retina, choroid and extraocular muscles.

White patches of necrosis within the erythema are indicative of systemic vasculitis. Nonnecrotising scleritis is commonly idiopathic, but may occur with autoimmune conditions, for example, rheumatoid arthritis and inflammatory bowel disease. It is also common with herpes zoster ophthalmicus, intraocular involvement being indicated by the involvement of the lateral external nose (Hutchison's sign).

Necrotising scleritis requires aggressive immunosuppression; nonnecrotising scleritis can occasionally be managed by topical glucocorticoids or NSAIDs but usually requires oral glucocorticoids.

Some patients with gradual, prolonged or recurrent scleritis develop scleral thinning (scleromalacia), revealing the underlying blue choroid.

17

17.9 Aetiology of uveitis

Idiopathic

- Anterior uveitis often associated with HLA-B27, even without other manifestations

Primary ophthalmic conditions

- Trauma, including penetrating injury and ophthalmic surgery
- Fuchs' heterochromic cyclitis
- Posner-Schlossman syndrome

Rheumatological

- HLA-B27-associated (seronegative) spondyloarthropathies: ankylosing spondylitis, psoriatic arthritis, reactive arthritis
- Juvenile idiopathic arthritis

Systemic vasculitides

- Behçet's disease
- Polyarteritis nodosa
- Granulomatosis with polyangiitis (formerly Wegener's)

Systemic infections

- Brucellosis
- Herpes virus infections (cytomegalovirus, herpes simplex virus, varicella zoster virus)
- Leptospirosis
- Lyme borreliosis
- Syphilis
- Toxoplasmosis
- Tuberculosis
- Whipple's disease

Gastrointestinal conditions

- Inflammatory bowel disease

Malignancy

- Primary CNS lymphoma (rare)

Systemic conditions of unknown cause

- Multiple sclerosis
- Sarcoidosis

Episcleritis

Episcleritis is a benign, self-limiting, idiopathic condition, occasionally associated with other inflammatory disorders. Sectoral redness of the episclera is usual, although nodules can form. Often confused with scleritis, topical phenylephrine blanches inflamed episclera, but has no effect on the redness in scleritis. Treatment is with cold artificial tears; occasionally topical NSAIDs or glucocorticoids are required.

Uveitis

Uveitis denotes inflammation anywhere in the uveal tract, retina or vitreous. It may be classified by speed of onset, location, specific features or aetiology (Box 17.9). Syphilis can cause all forms of uveitis. Active tuberculosis may present with an occlusive vasculitis or serpiginous (snake-like) choroiditis emanating from the optic disc. In latent tuberculosis, treatment of uveitis with biologics may induce active systemic infection. Furthermore, the most commonly used biologic for uveitis—antitumour necrosis factor therapy (e.g. adalimumab, infliximab)—may trigger demyelination.

The most common uveitis is anterior uveitis, which is usually idiopathic but may be associated with autoimmune conditions, particularly HLA-B27–related spondyloarthropathies (p. 618); it is rarely caused directly by infection. Acutely, dilating drops are used to prevent the inflamed iris from sticking to the lens (posterior synechiae), obstructing the outflow of aqueous fluid, whereas a tapering dose of topical glucocorticoids (4–6 weeks) mitigates the local self-resolving inflammation. Inadequate treatment can lead to pupil block glaucoma and cataract. Macular oedema can also develop, the main cause of visual impairment in uveitis.

Intermediate uveitis is associated with demyelination, sarcoidosis and inflammatory bowel disease. The predominant symptom is floaters, caused by inflammation of the vitreous base. Unlike anterior uveitis, pure intermediate uveitis spares the iris; instead, leucocytes appear predominantly in the anterior vitreous, with a few in the anterior chamber. Treatment is challenging. Topical therapy is ineffective beyond the anterior chamber, but symptoms of floaters rarely justify systemic immunosuppression. Vitritis (vitreous inflammation) or macular oedema may cause visual impairment. Occasionally, retinal neovascular proliferation may occur, either as an inflammatory response or secondary to capillary occlusion.

Posterior uveitis usually presents with visual impairment caused by macular oedema, vitritis or choroiditis. More chronic forms also exist, and these present with photopsia, visual field defects or distortion inducing choroidal neovascular membranes.

Infectious conditions

Conjunctivitis

Conjunctivitis is predominantly caused by bacteria or viruses and is usually self-limiting in 7 to 10 days. Bacterial conjunctivitis is associated with a purulent discharge, and viral conjunctivitis with a watery discharge, the latter often being confused with the photophobia and reflex lacrimation of anterior uveitis. Chlamydial infection should always be considered with persistent thick, mucopurulent discharge (p. 175).

Allergic conjunctivitis is also common, either in hay fever (with allergic rhinitis, p. 361) or as an allergy to chloramphenicol, used to treat conjunctivitis.

Rare causes of conjunctivitis include pemphigoid and Stevens–Johnson syndrome (p. 773). Secondary damage to the cornea can be devastating. Other causes of conjunctival scarring include trachoma (p. 148), chemical burns and orbital radiotherapy.

Infectious keratitis/corneal ulceration

Infections are an important cause of corneal inflammation (Box 17.10). Central ulceration is more serious than peripheral ulceration, as it affects vision. Cultures from corneal scraping or biopsy may be required, although much infectious keratitis is treated empirically on clinical features.

17

i 17.10 Common causes of infectious keratitis

Organism	Features/comments	Treatment
Viruses		
Herpes simplex	'Dendritic' ulcer is the commonest form, often recurrent	Topical/systemic aciclovir (with topical glucocorticoid once the epithelium is healed)
Varicella zoster	Herpes zoster ophthalmicus	Systemic aciclovir
Bacteria		
Pseudomonas aeruginosa *Staphylococcus aureus* Coagulase-positive staphylococci *Propionibacterium* spp.	Coagulase-negative staphylococci and *Propionibacterium* spp. are skin flora, and must not be dismissed as contaminants	Topical fluoroquinolone (e.g. ofloxacin)–subsequent treatment depends on sensitivity testing
Fungi		
Fusarium sp. *Aspergillus* sp. *Candida* sp.	*Fusarium* and *Aspergillus* keratitis often associated with soil +/– corneal trauma or contact lens-related *Candida* causes postkeratoplasty keratitis	Options include topical natamycin (if available), amphotericin B, voriconazole and other azoles (e.g. econazole) and systemic fluconazole or voriconazole
Parasites		
Acanthamoeba castellanii (free-living amoeba)	Associated with poor contact lens hygiene	Topical polyhexamethylene biguanide
Onchocerca volvulus (nematode)	See p. 165	

In the West, the most common cause of infectious keratitis is herpes simplex virus, usually type 1 (Fig. 17.2). All corneal layers may be involved: the epithelium shows dendritic ulceration; the stroma a white infiltrate and occasionally necrosis; and the endothelium localised oedema and keratitic precipitates. Loss of sensation is common following herpes simplex keratitis, and neurotrophic keratopathy may result. Epithelial disease is self-limiting, but topical or oral antivirals reduces the risk of stromal involvement and scarring. Stromal and endothelial disease require additional topical glucocorticoids once any epithelial defect has healed. Like herpes labialis, herpes keratitis commonly recurs. Frequent recurrences may warrant long-term antivirals. Corneal grafting may be required, but the risk of recurrence remains.

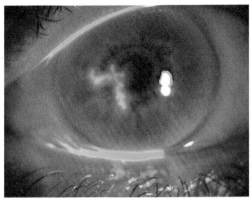

Fig. 17.2 Herpes simplex dendritic ulcer stained with fluorescein.

Bacteria also cause keratitis, especially following corneal trauma or contact lens misuse. Other risk factors for microbial keratitis include topical glucocorticoids and preexisting ocular surface disease. Some causes of bacterial keratitis are resistant to chloramphenicol, so topical quinolones are first-line agents. Rarely, the free-living amoeba *Acanthamoeba castellanii* may cause contact lens-associated keratitis, presenting subacutely and leading to corneal nerve infiltration, keratitis and scleritis.

In developing countries, infectious keratitis is most commonly caused by *Fusarium* fungi, particularly when associated with corneal trauma and contact with soil or plant matter. Fungal keratitis has no particular distinguishing features, and delayed diagnosis is common. If suspected, cultures should be undertaken and antifungal treatment started promptly. Corneal transplantation is often required.

Endophthalmitis

Endophthalmitis is infection of the anterior and posterior chambers of the eye. It may be exogenous (e.g. penetrating trauma or surgery) or, less commonly, endogenous, caused by bacteraemia and fungaemia. Microorganisms enter the eye via the choroid and the ciliary body. Gram-positive bacteria are most common, followed by Gram-negative bacteria and then fungi.

Presentation is usually with unilateral visual blurring and/or visual loss. Ocular findings range from a few deposits in the retina/choroid (chorioretinitis) to panendophthalmitis, with severe inflammation in both anterior and posterior chambers. A specific retinal appearance is described for *Candida* endophthalmitis, with creamy-white retinal or chorioretinal lesions (Fig. 17.3). It is vitally important to sample the vitreous, as this may provide the only opportunity to determine the most appropriate therapy. Treatment is with systemic and/or intravitreal antibiotics or antifungal agents, depending on the cause and severity. Vitrectomy may also be required.

17

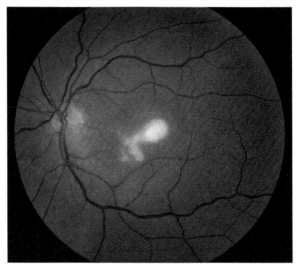

Fig. 17.3 Focal chorioretinitis in endogenous *Candida* endophthalmitis. Patient was an intravenous drug user and improved with oral fluconazole. (From Ryan SJ (ed). Retina, 5th edn. Saunders, Elsevier Inc.; 2013. (Case courtesy of Jeffrey K. Moore, MD).)

Cataract

Cataract is permanent lens opacity. Globally, untreated cataract is the most common cause of visual impairment, although where surgery is available, age-related macular degeneration is more common.

The normal lens thickens and opacifies with age, and cataract can be detected in more than half the population over the age of 65 years (senile cataract). Many diseases can predispose to cataract, the most common being uveitis and diabetes mellitus. Wilson's disease (p. 543) causes a characteristic 'sunflower' cataract. Excessive exposure to ultraviolet light, radiation and glucocorticoids are also predisposing factors.

The characteristic symptoms are progressive loss of vision and glare. If these become serious enough to require treatment, surgical intervention will be required, usually in the form of ultrasonic phacoemulsification with intraocular lens implantation.

Diabetic eye disease

Diabetic retinopathy

Diabetic retinopathy is the most common cause of visual impairment in people of working age in developed countries. The prevalence increases with the duration of diabetes. Almost all individuals with type 1 diabetes, and most with type 2 diabetes, will have some degree of retinopathy after 20 years.

Pathogenesis

Hyperglycaemia-induced capillary occlusion stimulates production of retinal vascular endothelial growth factor, which increases capillary permeability, leading to retinal oedema, and stimulates angiogenesis, leading to new vessel formation.

Clinical features

Capillary occlusion is visible only on retinal angiography. Adjacent capillaries form discrete swellings (microaneurysms), which leak fluid and blood, causing oedema and retinal haemorrhages (Fig. 17.4).

Clinically, microaneurysms appear as isolated red dots, the capillaries being too small to see. Lipids precipitate out of the fluid, forming exudates. When capillaries occlude, their microaneurysms turn white before disappearing. Capillary occlusion causes patches of retinal ischaemia, inducing secretion of vascular endothelial growth factor and the growth of new vessels.

Within ischaemic patches, diseased capillaries form intraretinal microvascular abnormalities, and retinal veins develop beading; signs best seen on fluorescein angiography.

New vessels and their glial tissue grow into the vitreous, triggering local inflammation and scarring. The vitreous pulls back on the new vessels, triggering further bleeding, inflammation and scarring. Ultimately, tractional retinal detachment and blindness may occur.

Other retinal lesions in the nerve-fibre layer in diabetic retinopathy include flame haemorrhages and cotton wool spots (soft exudates). Cotton wool spots occur mainly nasal to the optic disc. When combined with an enclosing flame haemorrhage, this is termed a Roth spot.

Management of proliferative diabetic retinopathy

Untreated proliferative retinopathy causes visual impairment through vitreous haemorrhage and retinal detachment. Pan-retinal laser photocoagulation is extremely effective at preserving vision if applied before complications develop.

Historically, laser therapy was used empirically to ablate the retina extensively, but this resulted in optic atrophy and night blindness (nyctalopia), interfering with driving. Modern laser treatment is tailored to the sites of ischaemia, and is relatively free of side effects, only occasionally preventing driving. In the UK it is obligatory to inform the driver licensing authority if there is bilateral retinopathy, irrespective of treatment.

Intravitreal injections of anti-VEGF (e.g. ranibizumab) cause temporary regression of proliferative retinopathy, whereas pan-retinal laser therapy causes permanent regression. After bilateral laser treatment, patients can be safely discharged to a retinal screening programme.

Management of diabetic macular oedema

Traditionally, oedema was categorised (using slit-lamp fluorescein angiography) into three patterns of leakage:

- Focal leakage from microaneurysms
- Diffuse leakage from diseased capillaries
- Ischaemia (no leakage) from thrombosis of the perifoveal capillaries

Previously, preventative laser was used to reduce leakage before the fovea was affected. However, screening programmes show that extrafoveal macular oedema often resolves spontaneously, so treatment has changed

17

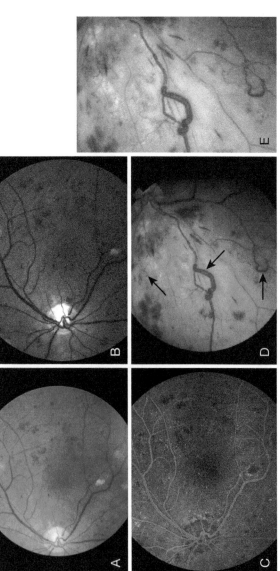

Fig. 17.4 Diabetic retinopathy. (A) Colour photograph of severe background diabetic retinopathy: multiple blot haemorrhages, microaneurysms, microaneurysmal bleeds and cotton wool spots. (B) Red-free image shows extensive haemorrhages more clearly. (C) Fluorescein angiogram reveals entrapment of fluorescein within multiple microaneurysms. (D) Colour photograph showing three consequences of capillary occlusion: intra-retinal microvascular anomalies (top arrow); venous reduplication with venous beading, occurring where capillaries are occluded either side of the vein (middle arrow); and new vessel formation at the border between diseased and healthy retina (bottom arrow). (E) Red-free image shows these features clearly. Note the relative pallor compared with the right side of the image, which indicates widespread capillary occlusion. Absolute pallor never occurs, as it is 'masked' by the underlying highly vascularised choroid. (A–E, Courtesy of Aberdeen Royal Infirmary.)

to treating those who are already symptomatic from centre-involving foveal oedema using intravitreal anti-VEGF injections, which rescue vision in 50% of those treated, regardless of the mechanism. Although this treatment is more effective, monthly injections may be required indefinitely.

Prevention

There is a clear relationship between glycaemic control and diabetic retinopathy. Good control of both glycaemia and blood pressure also slows the progression of retinopathy.

When blood glucose is rapidly lowered in type 1 diabetes, however, there can be a transient deterioration of retinopathy as a result of the development of cotton wool spots and, occasionally, new vessel formation. This can accompany reinstitution of insulin in nonadherent patients, for example, during hospitalisation for other reasons or when the patient suddenly decides to adhere to treatment, leading to dramatic improvement in glycaemic control.

Screening

Systematic screening for asymptomatic proliferative retinopathy is cost effective, and occurs routinely in many countries. There is little evidence that screening asymptomatic patients for macular oedema is cost-effective, although it may be detected during retinopathy screening.

Although ophthalmoscopy has poor sensitivity compared with slit-lamp examination or retinal photography, any screening is better than none. Currently, optical coherence tomography is being added to the screening pathway to reduce false-negative referrals for macular oedema.

Annual screening is usual, but patients with type 2 diabetes and repeated normal screens can safely be screened every 2 years.

In pregnancy, the placenta generates angiogenic growth factors, so although the risk of developing retinopathy during pregnancy remains low, pregnant women should be screened every trimester.

Other causes of visual loss in people with diabetes

Around 50% of visual loss in type 2 diabetes results from causes other than retinopathy. These include cataract, age-related macular degeneration, retinal vein occlusion, retinal arterial occlusion, nonarteritic ischaemic optic neuropathy and glaucoma. Some of these conditions relate to cardiovascular risk factors (e.g. hypertension, hyperlipidaemia and smoking), which are prevalent in type 2 diabetes.

Metabolic changes in the lens cause premature cataract, including the rare 'snowflake' cataract in young patients with poorly controlled diabetes. This does not usually affect vision but tends to make fundal examination difficult. Indications for cataract surgery in diabetes are as for the non-diabetic population, plus the need to operate if assessment of the fundus and/or retinal laser therapy becomes impossible.

Retinal vascular occlusion

Retinal vein occlusion (thrombosis)

This is an important vascular cause of visual impairment, the visual loss resulting from macular oedema or occasionally neovascularisation, both managed as in diabetes.

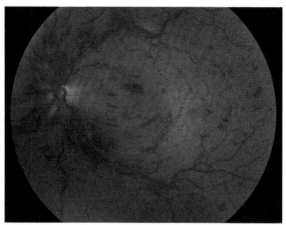

Fig. 17.5 Central retinal vein occlusion (thrombosis) showing flame haemorrhages, cotton wool spots, macular oedema and a swollen optic disc. (Courtesy of Aberdeen Royal Infirmary.)

The most common mechanism is probably compression of a vein by an adjacent arteriosclerotic artery. Where retinal arteries and veins cross, they share a common tunica adventitia, so that arteriosclerotic thickening of an artery directly compresses the adjacent vein (arteriovenous nipping).

A less common cause of retinal vein occlusion is inflammation (periphlebitis), also called retinal vasculitis (unlike in systemic vasculitis, the arterial system is spared). Periphlebitis should be suspected in younger patients and those with no obvious risk factors for arteriosclerosis. Diagnosis is by fluorescein angiography, and treatment is with systemic immunosuppression with or without adjunctive intravitreal therapy.

Retinal vein occlusion is associated with hypertension, and occasionally with hyperviscosity caused by multiple myeloma, Waldenström's macroglobulinaemia or leukaemia. Glaucoma is another associated disease, but whether this is a causal link or a comorbidity is unknown.

Presentation is with unilateral painless loss of central vision (central retinal vein thrombosis) or an area of peripheral vision (branch retinal vein thrombosis). Fundoscopic features include flame haemorrhages, cotton wool spots, macular oedema and a swollen optic disc (Fig. 17.5).

Management is twofold: management of the cause and management of the consequences of retinal vein occlusion. Where an underlying risk factor for arteriosclerosis is clearly present, secondary prevention measures should be commenced, although their effectiveness remains controversial.

Retinal artery occlusion

Retinal artery occlusion is usually embolic. Common predisposing factors are carotid atherosclerosis, valvular heart disease, arrhythmias and infective endocarditis. Remaining cases represent vasculitis, mainly giant cell arteritis (p. 718).

Retinal artery occlusion presents with painless unilateral visual loss, the extent of which depends on whether central or branch occlusion has occurred (peripheral occlusions may be asymptomatic). Transient occlusion of the internal carotid or ophthalmic artery causes transient visual loss, or amaurosis fugax (p. 727). Typical fundoscopic findings in central occlusion are a transiently pale retina with a 'cherry-red' macular spot, developing around 1 hour after occlusion (Fig. 17.6). In branch occlusions, there is no cherry-red spot, and the retinal pallor is regional.

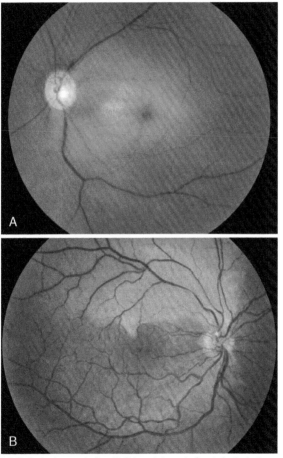

Fig. 17.6 Retinal artery occlusion. (A) Colour photograph of central retinal artery occlusion showing a classic cherry-red spot and a superior optic disc haemorrhage. (B) Superior branch retinal artery occlusion as a result of an embolus, showing a pale segment of retina. (A, From Duker JS, Waheed NK, Goldman DR. Handbook of retinal OCT. Saunders, Elsevier Inc.; 2014. B, From Bowling B. Kanski's Clinical ophthalmology, 8th edn. Elsevier Ltd; 2016.)

17

Age-related macular degeneration

Age-related macular degeneration is the most common cause of visual impairment in the Western world. There are two forms: atrophic (dry) and neovascular (wet). Dysfunction of the retinal pigment epithelium causes overlying photoreceptor death. Choroidal neovascularisation, growing under and into the overlying retina, may occur, distorting the anatomy of the photoreceptors and forming scarring. Both forms are preceded by deposits under the retinal pigment epithelium ('drusen'), often followed by the development of focal areas of macular hypo- and hyperpigmentation, where diseased retinal pigment epithelial cells have precipitated their pigment (age-related maculopathy).

The atrophic form presents with gradual onset of central visual blurring, accompanied, to a lesser degree, by visual distortion. Large (geographic) central patches of atrophy are seen, with areas of adjacent hyperpigmentation. In the neovascular form, sudden onset of central distortion, progressing within weeks, is the predominant symptom. Apart from age, the main risk factor appears to be smoking.

Antivascular endothelial growth factor injections are effective therapy for many cases of the neovascular form. Unfortunately, timely treatment is expensive and labour-intensive, and delayed treatment can lead to irreversible visual loss. In all cases, visual rehabilitation with appropriate magnifiers, improved lighting and adaptation of everyday living objects remains important adjunctive therapy.

Dermatology

Skin disease is common and is important to treat because impaired skin function not only can be life-threatening, but also can severely impair quality of life. People with skin disease can suffer the effects of stigma, stemming from others' belief that skin changes represent contagious disease. Assessment of the skin is valuable in the management of any medical problem and, conversely, assessment of other body systems is important when managing skin disease. This chapter covers common skin diseases and those that are important as components of general medical conditions. Skin infections are also discussed in Chapter 5.

A glossary of dermatological words is shown in Box 18.1.

Presenting problems in skin disease

Lumps and lesions

A new or changing lump is one of the key dermatology presentations. The challenge is distinguishing benign from malignant disease. Detailed history and examination are essential:

Change: Is this new, or has a preexisting lesion changed—in size, colour, shape or surface? Has change been rapid or slow? Is there pain, itch, inflammation, bleeding or ulceration?

Patient: Age? Fair-skinned and freckled? Sun exposure (sunbeds/lived in sunny climates, photoprotection)?

Site: Sun-exposed or covered site? The scalp, face, upper limbs and back in men and face, hands and lower legs in women are the most sun-exposed sites.

Similar lesions: These might include actinic keratoses or basal cell papillomas.

Morphology: Tenderness, size, symmetry, regularity of border, colour, surface characteristics and the presence of crust, scale and ulceration must be assessed. Stretching the skin and using a magnifying lens can be helpful.

Dermatoscopy: This can be used to detect the presence of abnormal vessels, such as in basal cell carcinoma, or the characteristic keratin cysts in basal cell papillomas. It is invaluable for pigmented and vascular lesions.

Clinical examination in skin disease

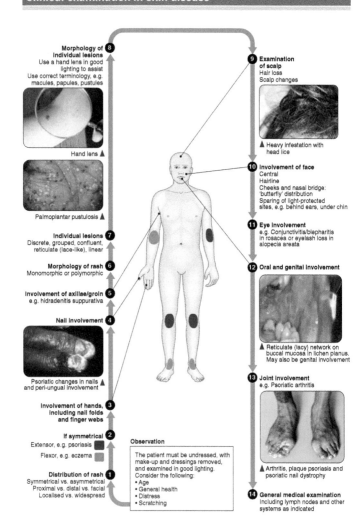

8 Morphology of individual lesions
Use a hand lens in good lighting to assist
Use correct terminology, e.g. macules, papules, pustules

Hand lens ▲

Palmoplantar pustulosis ▲

7 Individual lesions
Discrete, grouped, confluent, reticulate (lace-like), linear

6 Morphology of rash
Monomorphic or polymorphic

5 Involvement of axillae/groin
e.g. hidradenitis suppurativa

4 Nail involvement

Psoriatic changes in nails and peri-ungual involvement ▲

3 Involvement of hands, including nail folds and finger webs

2 If symmetrical
Extensor, e.g. psoriasis ■
Flexor, e.g. eczema ■

1 Distribution of rash
Symmetrical vs. asymmetrical
Proximal vs. distal vs. facial
Localised vs. widespread

9 Examination of scalp
Hair loss
Scalp changes

▲ Heavy infestation with head lice

10 Involvement of face
Central
Hairline
Cheeks and nasal bridge: 'butterfly' distribution
Sparing of light-protected sites, e.g. behind ears, under chin

11 Eye involvement
e.g. Conjunctivitis/blepharitis in rosacea or eyelash loss in alopecia areata

12 Oral and genital involvement

▲ Reticulate (lacy) network on buccal mucosa in lichen planus. May also be genital involvement

13 Joint involvement
e.g. Psoriatic arthritis

▲ Arthritis, plaque psoriasis and psoriatic nail dystrophy

14 General medical examination
including lymph nodes and other systems as indicated

Observation
The patient must be undressed, with make-up and dressings removed, and examined in good lighting. Consider the following:
• Age
• General health
• Distress
• Scratching

Melanocytic naevus or malignant melanoma?

The precise nature of the change should be determined (as described earlier). Does the patient have other pigmented lesions? If the presenting lesion looks different from the others, then suspicion of melanoma is increased; conversely, if the patient has multiple basal cell papillomas, this may be

i	**18.1 Terms used to describe skin lesions**
Macule	A circumscribed flat area of altered colour, ≤1 cm diameter
Patch	As for macule, but larger
Papule	A discrete elevation of skin
Nodule	As for papule, but >1 cm diameter and involving dermis
Plaque	A raised area of skin with a flat top, >1 cm across
Vesicle/bulla	A small (≤1 cm)/larger (>1 cm) blister, respectively
Pustule	A visible accumulation of pus in a blister
Abscess	A localised collection of pus in a cavity
Weal	An evanescent discrete area of dermal oedema
Scale	A flake arising from the stratum corneum
Petechiae, purpura, ecchymosis	Petechiae are flat, pinhead-sized macules of extravascular blood in the dermis; larger ones (purpura) may be palpable; deeper bleeding causes ecchymosis
Burrow	A linear or curvilinear papule, caused by a burrowing scabies mite
Comedone	A plug of keratin and sebum in a dilated pilosebaceous orifice
Telangiectasia	Visible dilatation of small cutaneous blood vessels
Crust	Dried exudate of blood or serous fluid
Ulcer	An area from which the epidermis and the upper dermis have been lost
Excoriation	A linear ulcer or erosion resulting from scratching
Erosion	An area of skin denuded by complete or partial loss of the epidermis
Fissure	A deep, slit-shaped ulcer, e.g. irritant dermatitis of the hands
Sinus	A cavity or channel that permits the escape of pus or fluid
Scar	Permanent fibrous tissue resulting from healing
Atrophy	Loss of substance caused by diminution of the epidermis, dermis or subcutaneous fat
Stria	A linear, atrophic, pink/purple/white lesion in the connective tissue

18

reassuring. Is there a positive family history of melanoma? A suspicious naevus in a patient with a first-degree relative with melanoma probably warrants excision.

The ABCDE 'rule' is a guide to the characteristic features of melanoma: • Asymmetry. • Border irregular. • Colour irregular (moles developing pigment variegation). • Diameter greater than 0.5 cm. • Elevation (+ loss of skin markings).

If there are concerns, biopsy or excision biopsy is indicated.

Rashes

A common presenting complaint in general practice is an eruptive scaly rash, sometimes associated with itching. Causes are summarised in Box 18.2.

i 18.2 Clinical features of common scaly rashes

Type of rash	Distribution	Morphology	Associated clinical signs
Atopic eczema	Face/flexures	Poorly defined erythema and scaling; lichenification	Shiny nails, infra-orbital crease, 'dirty neck'
Psoriasis	Extensor surfaces	Well-defined plaques with a silvery scale	Nail pitting and onycholysis; scalp involvement, axillae and genital areas often affected
Pityriasis rosea	'Fir tree' pattern on torso	Well-defined Small, erythematous plaques Collarette of scale	Herald patch
Pityriasis versicolor	Upper trunk and shoulders	Hypo- and hyperpigmented scaly patches	
Drug eruption	Widespread	Macules and papules Erythema and scale Exfoliation	Mucosal involvement, erythroderma
Lichen planus	Distal limbs Flexor aspect of wrists; lower back	Shiny, flat-topped violaceous papules with Wickham's striae	White lacy network on buccal mucosa; nail changes, alopecia
Tinea corporis	Asymmetrical, often isolated lesions	Scaly plaques that expand with central healing	Nail involvement
Secondary syphilis	Trunk, proximal limbs, palms and soles	Red macules and papules	History of chancre Malaise, fever

History

Age at onset and duration: Atopic eczema often starts in infancy or early childhood, and pityriasis rosea and psoriasis start between the ages of 15 and 40 years. Drug eruptions are acute in onset, with a clear temporal relationship between starting the medicine and the onset of the rash.

Site of onset: Flexural sites are involved in atopic eczema, and extensor surfaces and scalp in psoriasis. Symmetry suggests endogenous disease, such as psoriasis, whereas asymmetry is more common with exogenous causes, such as contact dermatitis or herpes zoster.

Itch: Eczema is extremely itchy, psoriasis less so.

Preceding illness and systemic symptoms: Guttate psoriasis may be preceded by a β-haemolytic streptococcal sore throat. Almost all patients with infectious mononucleosis (p. 120) treated with amoxicillin develop an erythematous maculopapular eruption.

The morphology of the rash and the characteristics of the lesions are important (see Box 18.2).

Management is that of the cause, where possible.

Blisters

There are a limited number of conditions that present with blisters (Box 18.3). Blistering occurs because of loss of cell adhesion within the epidermis or subepidermal region, and the presentation depends on the site or level of blistering within the skin. This in turn reflects the underlying pathogenesis:

Split high in the epidermis (below the stratum corneum): Intact blisters are uncommon, as the blister roof is so fragile that it ruptures easily, leaving erosions (e.g. pemphigus foliaceus, staphylococcal scalded skin syndrome and bullous impetigo).

Split lower in the epidermis: Intact flaccid blisters and erosions may be seen (e.g. pemphigus vulgaris and toxic epidermal necrolysis).

i	**18.3 Causes of acquired blisters**	
	Localised	Generalised
Vesicular	Herpes (simplex or zoster), impetigo, pompholyx	Eczema herpeticum[a], dermatitis herpetiformis, acute eczema
Bullous	Impetigo, cellulitis, stasis oedema, acute eczema, insect bites, fixed drug eruptions	Toxic epidermal necrolysis [a], erythema multiforme/Stevens–Johnson syndrome [a], bullous pemphigoid, pemphigus [a], epidermolysis bullosa acquisita, bullous lupus erythematosus, porphyria cutanea tarda, pseudoporphyria, drug eruptions
aUsually also mucosal involvement.		

18

Subepidermal split: Tense-roofed blisters occur. Examples include bullous pemphigoid (Fig. 18.1), epidermolysis bullosa acquisita and porphyria cutanea tarda.

Foci of separation at different levels of the epidermis: Multilocular bullae (made up of coalescing vesicles) occur, as in dermatitis.

A history of onset, progression, mucosal involvement, drugs and systemic symptoms should be sought. Clinical assessment of the distribution, extent and morphology of the rash should then be made. The Nikolsky sign is useful: sliding lateral pressure from a finger on normal-looking epidermis can dislodge the epidermis in conditions with intra-epidermal defects, such as pemphigus and toxic epidermal necrolysis.

A systematic approach should be taken to diagnosis:

Exclude infection: for example, herpes simplex, varicella zoster, *Staphylococcus aureus.*

Consider common skin disorders in which blistering occurs uncommonly: for example, severe peripheral oedema, cellulitis, allergic contact dermatitis, eczema.

Remember blisters may develop in drug eruptions: for example, fixed drug eruption, erythema multiforme and vasculitis. Toxic epidermal necrolysis (p. 748) is a medical emergency.

Consider immunobullous disease: Bullous pemphigoid, pemphigus, linear IgA disease, bullous lupus.

Investigations and management are guided by the presentation and differential diagnosis, as described below under the specific diseases.

Itch

Itch describes the unpleasant sensation that leads to scratching or rubbing. The terms 'itch' and 'pruritus' are synonymous; however, 'pruritus' is often used when itch is generalised. Itch can arise from primary cutaneous disease or be secondary to systemic disease, which may cause itch by central or peripheral mechanisms. Many common primary skin disorders are associated with itch:

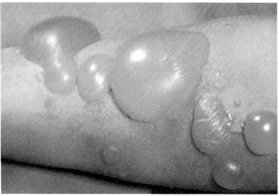

Fig. 18.1 Bullous pemphigoid. Large tense and unilocular blisters.

Generalised pruritus:
• Scabies. • Eczemas. • Prebullous pemphigoid. • Urticarias. • Xeroderma of old age. • Psoriasis.

Localised pruritus:
• Eczemas. • Lichen planus. • Dermatitis herpetiformis. • Pediculosis. • Tinea infections.

If itch is not connected with primary skin disease, many causes should be considered, including:
• Liver diseases—mainly cholestatic diseases, for example, primary biliary cholangitis. • Malignancies—for example, generalised itch in lymphoma. • Haematological conditions—for example, generalised itch in chronic iron deficiency or itch provoked by water (aquagenic pruritis) in polycythaemia. • Endocrine diseases—for example, hypo- and hyperthyroidism. • Chronic kidney disease—severity of itch not clearly associated with plasma creatinine. • Psychogenic causes—for example, 'delusions of infestation'.

Pruritus is common in pregnancy, and may be caused by one of the pregnancy-specific dermatoses. Diagnosis is particularly important in pregnancy, as some disorders can be associated with increased fetal risk.

Management

Management of the underlying primary skin condition or medical condition may alleviate the itch. For those with persisting symptoms despite specific management, symptomatic relief includes sedation (H_1 antagonist antihistamines), emollients and counter-irritants (e.g. topical menthol-containing preparations). UVB phototherapy is useful in itch from a variety of causes, although the only robust evidence of efficacy in generalised itch (not because of skin disease) is in chronic kidney disease. Other treatments include tricyclic antidepressants and opiate antagonists.

Photosensitivity

Photosensitivity is an abnormal response of the skin to UVR or visible radiation, either from sunlight, sunbeds or phototherapy. The UVB band of sunlight (wavelength 300–320 nm) accounts for its 'sunburning' effects. Chronic UVR exposure increases skin cancer risk and photo-ageing. Erythema on acute exposure is a normal response. Abnormal photosensitivity occurs when a patient reacts to lower doses than would normally cause a response. Causes include:

Immunological conditions—for example, polymorphic light eruption, chronic actinic dermatitis, solar urticatria.

Metabolic—porphyrias.

Photo-aggravated skin diseases—for example, lupus erythematosus, erythema multiforme and rosacea. These are exacerbated by sunlight but not caused by it.

Drugs—for example, thiazides, tetracyclines and fluoroquinalones.

Clinical assessment

Key sites are the face, top of ears, neck, bald scalp, back of hands and forearms. Shaded sites, for example, under the chin, are spared. Some conditions (e.g. solar urticaria) develop rapidly after sunlight exposure, whereas others, such as cutaneous lupus, take several days to evolve.

18

Investigations and management

The patient should be referred to a specialist centre for phototesting, provocation, patch or photopatch testing, and screening for lupus and porphyrias.

Management depends on diagnosis. Phototoxic drugs should be stopped, and associated diseases treated. Counselling regarding sun avoidance, protective clothing and sunscreens is essential.

Sunscreens: Modern sunscreens offer protection against UVB and most UVA wavelengths. The SPF describes the ratio of the dose of UVR required to produce erythema with, as opposed to without, the sunscreen. In practice, people use 25% to 33% of the amount of sunscreen required for the stated SPF; thus, an SPF30 sunscreen will usually offer SPF10 in practice. All sunscreens offer only partial protection, at best, and are no substitute for avoiding exposure and covering up.

Leg ulcers

Leg ulcer is not a diagnosis, but a symptom of an underlying disease that has caused complete loss of the epidermis, leaving dermis layers exposed. Ulcers on the lower leg are frequently caused by vascular disease, but there are other causes, as summarised in Box 18.4.

Clinical assessment

A history of the leg ulceration and any predisposing conditions should be elicited. Examination of the site and surrounding skin should include assessment of the venous and arterial vasculature and neurological examination. The site of the ulceration gives clues as to its aetiology (Fig. 18.2).

Leg ulceration as a result of venous disease

Clinical assessment

This is a common clinical problem in middle to old age. Clinical signs include:
• Varicose veins. • Haemosiderin deposition. • Oedema. • Lipodermatosclerosis: firm induration of the skin of the leg, with a shiny appearance,

i 18.4 Causes of leg ulceration	
Venous hypertension	Sometimes following DVT
Arterial disease	Atherosclerosis, vasculitis, Buerger's disease
Small-vessel disease	Diabetes mellitus, vasculitis
Haematological disorders	Sickle-cell disease, cryoglobulinaemia, spherocytosis, immune complex disease, polycythaemia
Neuropathy	Diabetes mellitus, leprosy, syphilis
Tumour	Squamous cell carcinoma, basal cell carcinoma, malignant melanoma, Kaposi's sarcoma
Trauma	Injury, factitious

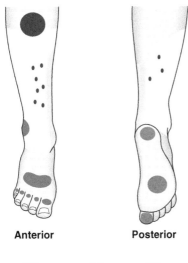

Anterior   **Posterior**

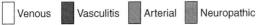

☐ Venous ■ Vasculitis ■ Arterial ■ Neuropathic

Fig. 18.2 Causes of lower leg ulceration.

producing the 'inverted champagne bottle' sign. • Ulcers are typically on the medial lower leg. • Malignant transformation of a chronic ulcer into squamous cell carcinoma: termed 'Marjolin's ulcer'.

Leg ulceration as a result of arterial disease

Deep, painful and punched-out ulcers on the lower leg, especially if they occur on the shin and foot and in the context of intermittent claudication, are likely to be as a result of arterial disease. Risk factors include smoking, hypertension, diabetes mellitus and hyperlipidaemia. The foot is cyanotic and cold, and the surrounding skin is atrophic and hairless. Peripheral pulses are absent or reduced. A vascular surgical assessment should be sought urgently.

Leg ulceration as a result of vasculitis

Vasculitis can cause leg ulceration either directly through epidermal necrosis as a result of damage to the underlying vasculature or indirectly because of neuropathy.

Leg ulceration as a result of neuropathy

The most common causes of neuropathic ulcers are diabetes and leprosy. The ulcers occur over weight-bearing areas such as the heel. Microangiopathy also contributes to ulceration in diabetes. This is discussed in detail on p. 442.

Investigations

• FBC • Urea and electrolytes. • Glucose. • Bacterial swab. • Doppler ultrasound.

Management

Advise weight loss (if obese), smoking cessation and gentle exercise. Oedema should be reduced with the use of compression bandages (once arterial sufficiency is excluded, ratio of ankle:brachial systolic pressure >0.8), elevation of the legs when sitting and the judicious use of diuretics. If purulent, use weak potassium permanganate soaks. Nonadherent absorbent dressings (alginates, hydrogels or hydrocolloids) should be changed daily for highly exudative ulcers. Surrounding venous eczema should be treated with topical glucocorticoid. Skin grafts may hasten healing of clean ulcers.

Abnormal pigmentation

Depigmentation, hypopigmentation and hyperpigmentation are covered on pp. 763–764.

Hair and nail abnormalities

These may be a marker for systemic disease or a feature of skin conditions (e.g. psoriasis). Specific disorders are covered on pp. 764–767.

Acute skin failure

Acute skin failure is a medical emergency, causing failure of thermoregulation, fluid balance and resistance to infection. Commonly, there is widespread dermal vasodilatation that provokes high-output cardiac failure and increased protein loss from the skin and often from the gut. There is often accompanying erythroderma (erythema affecting at least 90% of the body surface), although severe autoimmune blistering diseases and Stevens–Johnson syndrome/TEN can produce acute skin failure without erythroderma.

Causes include:

• Eczema. • Psoriasis. • Pityriasis rubra pilaris (a variant of psoriasis).
• Cutaneous T-cell lymphoma (Sézary's syndrome).

Erythrodermic patients are systemically unwell with shivering and hypothermia, but may also be pyrexial and unable to lose heat because of damage to sweat gland function and sweat duct occlusion. While the cause is treated, rehydration, temperature control and treatment of infection are vital.

Skin tumours

Skin cancer is categorised as non-melanoma skin cancer (NMSC) and melanoma. NMSC comprises basal cell carcinoma (BCC) and squamous cell carcinoma (SCC). The latter has precursor non-invasive states of intra-epithelial carcinoma (Bowen's disease; BD) and dysplasia (actinic keratosis; AK). Melanoma is much rarer than NMSC, but because of metastasis it causes most skin cancer deaths.

UVR is the main risk factor for skin cancer; particularly for SCC and AK, but also for BCC. Melanoma usually arises on intermittently exposed sites, and sunburn is an additional risk factor. Sunbed use is a risk factor for both melanoma and NMSC, and risk is reduced by sunscreens. Other factors include genetic predisposition (e.g. in xeroderma pigmentosum) and immunosuppression; organ transplant recipients have an increased risk of skin cancer, particularly SCC. Chronic inflammation is also a risk factor for SCC (e.g. chronic skin ulcers, lupus), as is scarring skin disease, for example, epidermolysis bullosa.

Malignant tumours

Basal cell carcinoma

This is a common, slow-growing malignant tumour that rarely metastasises but that can invade locally ('rodent ulcer'). Early BCCs usually present as pale, translucent papules or nodules, with overlying superficial telangiectatic vessels (nodular BCC). If untreated, they increase in size and ulcerate, forming a crater with a rolled, pearled edge and ectatic vessels (Fig. 18.3). A superficial multifocal type of BCC presents as a red/brown plaque or patch with a raised, thread-like edge, often on the trunk, and may be up to 10 cm in diameter. Less commonly, a morphoeic, infiltrative BCC presents as a poorly defined, slowly enlarging, sclerotic yellow/grey plaque.

Management

The choice of treatment modality depends on local expertise and interest, and includes surgery, cryotherapy, radiotherapy, photodynamic therapy or the topical immunomodulator imiquimod. All treatments used optimally can produce excellent cure rates.

Squamous cell carcinoma

SCC usually arises on sun-exposed areas with diverse clinical appearances, including keratotic nodules, exophytic erythematous nodules, infiltrating firm tumours and ulcers. Histological grade varies from well differentiated to anaplastic, and lymph node metastasis may occur.

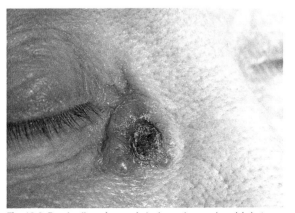

18

Fig. 18.3 Basal cell carcinoma. A slowly growing, pearly nodule just below the inner canthus. The central crust overlies an ulcerated area.

Management

Complete surgical excision is the treatment of choice. Other options include curettage and cautery for small, low-risk lesions, and radiotherapy if surgery is not feasible. Wide excision has a cure rate of around 90% to 95%. In patients who are at high risk for further SCC, systemic retinoids may reduce the rate of occurrence, but rapid appearance of tumours occurs on drug cessation.

Actinic keratosis

Actinic keratoses are hyperkeratotic erythematous lesions arising on chronically sun-exposed sites (Fig. 18.4). Histology shows dysplasia, although the diagnosis is usually clinical. They are treated easily and effectively with liquid nitrogen. If there are a large number of lesions, then the topical cytotoxic 5-fluorouracil may be required; alternatively, topical imiquimod or photodynamic therapy may be used. Progression to SCC is rare, but should be suspected if there is ulceration, bleeding or pain.

Bowen's disease

BD is an intraepidermal carcinoma that usually presents as a slow-growing, erythematous, scaly plaque on the lower legs of fair-skinned elderly women. It can resemble eczema or psoriasis, but is usually asymptomatic and does not respond to topical glucocorticoids. Transformation into SCC occurs in less than 3% of cases. A biopsy is usually required for diagnosis, but non-surgical photodynamic therapy is preferred on the legs, as it spares normal tissue and is associated with good healing.

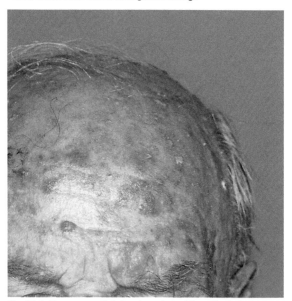

Fig. 18.4 Numerous actinic keratoses in a white patient who had lived for years in the tropics.

Cutaneous lymphoma

Cutaneous T-cell lymphoma (mycosis fungoides, MF) develops slowly over many years from polymorphic patches and plaques. B-cell lymphomas present as nodules or plaques. Both can mimic eczema and psoriasis, so a high index of suspicion is required for diagnosis.

Treatment is symptomatic and does not alter prognosis. In early disease, systemic or local glucocorticoids may be indicated; alternatively, narrow-band UVB phototherapy (for patch stage MF) or PUVA (for plaque stage MF) may be used. In advanced disease, localised radiotherapy, electron beam radiation or antilymphoma chemotherapy may be needed.

Melanoma

Melanoma is a malignant tumour of epidermal melanocytes and has metastatic potential. Incidence has increased over recent decades. Early detection and treatment are essential because of the lack of effective therapies for metastatic disease. The main risk factors for melanoma are:
• Prolonged UVR exposure. • Pale skin. • Large numbers of naevi.
• Positive family history (several associated genes now identified).

Clinical features

Melanoma can occur at any age and site, but it is rare before puberty and typically affects the leg in females and back in males.

Five subtypes occur:

Superficial spreading malignant melanoma (Fig. 18.5): Most common type in Caucasians. A macular pigmented lesion with a superficial radial growth pattern, which over time may become palpable (vertical spread).

Nodular melanoma: A rapidly growing nodule, typically found on the trunk in men. It may bleed, ulcerate and metastasise.

Lentigo maligna melanoma: Occurs most often on exposed skin of the elderly as a pigmented macular area. It is preceded by a prolonged preinvasive phase (lentigo maligna).

Acral lentiginous melanoma: Occurs on the palms and soles, particularly in dark-skinned people.

Subungual melanoma: Rare. It presents with a painless streak of pigmentation under a nail.

Diagnosis

Any new or changed naevi should be assessed using the ABCDE rule (p. 736) and excised if doubt remains.

Management

The lesion should be excised with a wide margin. The Breslow thickness of tumour (the maximal depth from epidermal granular cell layer to deepest tumour cells) is critical for management and prognosis. Clinical staging is essential, to establish whether disease is localised or metastatic. In more advanced disease, treatment often involves wider local excision, sentinel lymph node mapping and biopsy. Prognosis for metastatic disease is poor and treatment is palliative, but improvement can occur with immunotherapy, and tumour-targeted genetic treatments are under development.

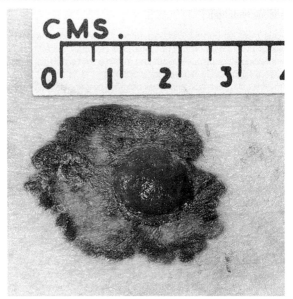

Fig. 18.5 Superficial spreading melanoma. The radial growth phase was present for around 3 years before the invasive amelanotic nodule developed within it. Note the irregular outline, asymmetrical shape and different hues, including depigmented areas signifying spontaneous regression.

Benign skin lesions

Keratoacanthoma

This benign tumour presents as an isolated nodule often 5 cm or more in diameter, with a central keratin plug that grows rapidly over weeks to months, then spontaneously resolves. It is associated with chronic sun exposure and usually occurs on the face. Clinically and histologically, it resembles SCC. Most are treated by curettage or excision to rule out SCC and to avoid the scar resulting from spontaneous resolution.

Freckles

These are most common in sun-exposed sites in fair-skinned individuals and represent focal over-production of melanin with normal melanocyte number. They become darker with sun exposure and are associated with a familial sun-sensitive phenotype.

Lentigines

These are dark brown macules 1 mm to 1 cm across. They are associated with chronic sun exposure and become more common with age. Biopsy may be needed to distinguish them from melanoma.

Basal cell papilloma

These are common benign epidermal tumours (also called seborrhoeic warts) that appear over the age of 35 years. They vary in colour from yellow to dark brown, and have a greasy, 'stuck-on' appearance. They can be left alone or treated by cryotherapy or curettage if they are cosmetically trouble-some. If there is a suspicion of melanoma, biopsy should be undertaken.

Melanocytic naevi

Melanocytic naevi (moles) are localised benign clonal proliferations of mela-nocytes. Moles are a usual feature of most human beings, and it is quite normal to have 20 to 50. Individuals with high sun exposure also show more moles, that is, there is clear evidence for both genetic and environ-mental factors. Most melanocytic naevi appear in early childhood, at ado-lescence and during pregnancy or oestrogen therapy. The appearance of a new mole is less common after the age of 25.

Clinical features

Acquired melanocytic naevi are classified according to the microscopic location of the melanocyte nests:

• Junctional naevi are usually circular and macular, and mid- to dark brown.
• Compound and intradermal naevi are nodules, because of the dermal component, and may be hair-bearing. • Intradermal naevi are usually less pigmented than compound naevi. Their surfaces may be smooth, cerebri-form, hyperkeratotic or papillomatous.

Management

Melanocytic naevi are normal and do not require excision, except when malignancy is suspected (p. 745) or when they repeatedly become inflamed or traumatised. Some individuals wish to have them removed for cosmetic reasons.

Common skin infections and infestations

Bacterial infections

Impetigo

Impetigo is a common, highly contagious, superficial bacterial skin infection. There are two main presentations: bullous impetigo, caused by a staphylo-coccal epidermolytic toxin, and nonbullous impetigo (Fig. 18.6), which can be caused by either *S. aureus* or streptococci, or both. *Staphylococcus* is the most common agent in temperate climates; streptococcal impetigo is seen in hot, humid areas. Nonbullous disease particularly affects young children, often in late summer. Outbreaks can arise with overcrowding or poor hygiene, or in institutions. Coexisting skin conditions, such as abra-sions, infestations or eczema, predispose to impetigo.

In nonbullous impetigo, a thin-walled vesicle develops, ruptures rapidly and is rarely seen intact. Dried exudate, forming golden crusting, arises on an erythematous base. In bullous disease, the toxins cleave the superficial epidermis, causing intact blisters containing clear to cloudy fluid; these last

18

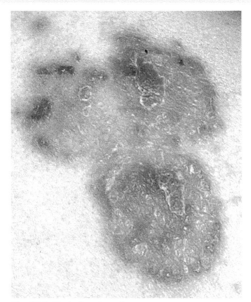

Fig. 18.6 Nonbullous impetigo.

2 to 3 days. The face, scalp and limbs are commonly affected, but sites of eczema can also be involved. Constitutional symptoms are uncommon. A bacterial swab should be taken from blister fluid or active lesions before treatment. Around one-third of the population are nasal carriers of *Staphylococcus*, so nasal swabs should also be obtained.

In mild, localised disease, topical treatment with mupirocin or fusidic acid is usually effective and limits spread. Staphylococcal nasal carriage should be treated with topical mupirocin. In severe cases, oral flucloxacillin or clarithromycin is indicated. If nephritogenic streptococci are isolated, systemic antibiotics should be considered to reduce the risk of streptococcal glomerulonephritis (p. 217).

Staphylococcal scalded skin syndrome

This is a serious exfoliating condition predominantly affecting children, particularly neonates. Systemic circulation of epidermolytic toxins from a *S. aureus* infection cause a split in the superficial epidermis and peeling of the skin.

The child presents with fever, irritability, skin tenderness and erythema, often starting in the groin and axillae and around the mouth. Blisters and superficial erosions develop over 1 to 2 days. Bacterial swabs should be taken from possible sites of primary infection (throat, nose, etc.). Diagnosis is made on the clinical appearance and histological examination of a skin snip taken from the edge of one of the peeling areas, to determine the plane of cleavage and thus exclude the differential diagnosis of toxic epidermal necrolysis, which involves the full thickness of the epidermis. Systemic antibiotics and intensive support-ive measures should be commenced immediately. Family members should be screened and treated for staphylococcal carriage.

Toxic shock syndrome

This condition is covered on p. 127.

Folliculitis, furuncles and carbuncles

Hair follicle inflammation can be superficial, involving just the ostium of the follicle (folliculitis), or deep (furuncles and carbuncles).

Superficial folliculitis: The primary lesions are follicular pustules and erythema. It is often infective, caused by *S. aureus*, but can also be sterile and caused by physical (e.g. traumatic epilation) or chemical (e.g. mineral oil) injury. Staphylococcal folliculitis is most common in children, and often occurs on the scalp or limbs. The pustules usually heal in 7 to 10 days, but can become more chronic, and in older children and adults can progress to a deeper form of folliculitis.

Deep folliculitis (furuncles and carbuncles): A furuncle (boil) is an acute *S. aureus* infection of the hair follicle, which becomes pustular and fluctuant, and is often exquisitely tender. The lesions eventually rupture to discharge pus and, because they are deep, leave a scar. Deep infection of several contiguous hair follicles forms a carbuncle, which is an exquisitely tender nodule, often on the neck, shoulders or hips, and is associated with severe constitutional symptoms. Treat-ment is with an appropriate antistaphylococcal antibiotic or incision and drainage.

Cellulitis and erysipelas

Cellulitis is inflammation of subcutaneous tissue caused by bacterial infec-tion. In contrast, erysipelas is bacterial infection of the dermis and upper subcutaneous tissue, although in practice it may be difficult to distinguish between them. The most common organism causing both conditions is group A streptococci, although swabs are often culture-negative. There is often a predisposing cause, such as a portal of entry for infection, for example, tinea pedis, or an underlying predisposition to infection such as varicose leg ulcer or diabetes.

Diagnosis is based on clinical findings of erythema, heat, swelling, pain and sometimes fever, with a leucocytosis, raised inflammatory markers and positive streptococcal serology. Erysipelas (Fig. 18.7) typically has a well-defined edge, indicating involvement of the dermis. It usually affects the face. Cellulitis most commonly involves the legs. Blistering and regional lymphadenopathy may occur in both conditions. Treatment is usually with IV flucloxacillin, or in cases of penicillin sensitivity, clarithromycin, clindomy-cin or vancomycin. In mild cases, oral antibiotics are indicated.

Mycobacterial infections

Mycobacterium leprae is covered on p. 142.

Scrofuloderma describes the skin changes overlying lymph nodes or joints infected with *M. tuberculosis*. In lupus vulgaris, direct skin inoculation

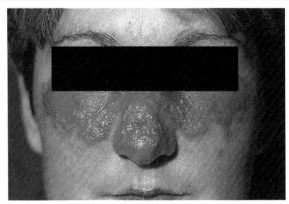

Fig. 18.7 Erysipelas. Note the blistering and crusted rash with raised erythematous edge.

with *M. tuberculosis* causes red–brown scarring inflammatory plaques. Granulomas on skin biopsy are suggestive of mycobacterial infection. Culture of organisms may be tricky, but PCR can assist with diagnosis.

Erythrasma

Erythrasma is a mild localised infection of the skin caused by *Corynebacterium minutissimum*, which often is part of the normal skin flora. It can provoke an asymptomatic or mildly itchy eruption in flexures and toe clefts. Lesions are well defined and red/brown, and scaly. *C. minutissimum* has characteristic coral-pink fluorescence under Wood's light. Treatments include a topical azole cream such as miconazole or a topical antibiotic.

Viral infections

Herpes virus infections

These are described on p. 124.

Papillomaviruses and viral warts

Viral warts are caused by the DNA human papillomavirus (HPV) and are extremely common, being transmitted by direct contact with the virus in either living skin or shed skin fragments. Most people suffer from one or more warts at some point during their life. There are more than 90 different subtypes. HPV subtypes 16 and 18 are spread by sexual contact and are strongly associated with subsequent development of cervical carcinoma. Vaccinations are now available against HPV-16 and -18 and are recommended for adolescent females before they become sexually active. Immunosuppressed patients are at greater risk of infection with HPV.

Clinical features

Common warts are initially smooth, skin-coloured papules that become hyperkeratotic and 'warty'. Warts can be classified on their clinical appearance:

Plantar warts (verrucae): Found on the sole of the foot. These are characterised by a horny collar surrounding a roughened surface. Paring reveals capillary loops that distinguish plantar warts from corns.

Mosaic warts: Mosaic-like sheets of warts.

Plane warts: Smooth, flat-topped papules, usually on the face and the dorsum of the hands.

Facial warts: Often filiform.

Genital warts: Papillomatous and exuberant.

Management

Most viral warts resolve spontaneously but slowly, and do not require treatment. Therapeutic options for problematic warts include:

• Topical salicylic acid (first-line). • Cryotherapy. • Imiquimod or podophyllin for genital warts. • Intralesional bleomycin (for recalcitrant warts).

Molluscum contagiosum

Molluscum contagiosum is caused by a DNA poxvirus infection. It is most common in children over the age of 1 year and the immunosuppressed. The classic lesion is a dome-shaped, 'umbilicated', skin-coloured papule with a central punctum. Lesions tend to be multiple, and are often in sites of apposition, such as the side of the chest and the inner arm. No treatment is required, as these lesions resolve spontaneously, but can take several months to do so. If active resolution is sought, curettage or cryotherapy may be tried, or topical agents such as salicylic acid, podophyllin or imiquimod.

Orf

Orf is a parapoxvirus skin infection and is an occupational risk for those who work with sheep and goats. Inoculation of the virus, usually into the skin of a finger, causes significant inflammation and necrosis, which resolve in 2 to 6 weeks. No specific treatment is available unless there is evidence of secondary infection. Erythema multiforme can be provoked by orf.

Fungal infections

Dermatophytes are fungi capable of causing superficial skin infections known as ringworm or dermatophytosis. The causative fungi (*Microsporum*, *Trichophyton*, *Epidermophyton*) can originate from the soil (geophilic) or animals (zoophilic) or be confined to human skin (anthropophilic).

Clinical forms of cutaneous infection include:

Tinea corporis: This condition should be considered in the differential diagnosis of the red scaly rash on the body. Lesions are erythematous, annular and scaly, with a well-defined edge and central clearing. They may be single or multiple and are usually asymmetrical. *Microsporum canis* (from dogs) and *Trichophyton verrucosum* (from cats) are common culprits. Ill-advised topical glucocorticoid application leads to disguising and worsening of the signs (tinea incognito).

Tinea cruris: This is common worldwide and is usually caused by *T. rubrum*. Itchy erythematous plaques extend from the groin flexures on to the thighs.

18

Tinea pedis (athlete's foot): This is the most common fungal skin infection in the UK and United States and is usually caused by anthropophilic fungi such as *T. rubrum*, *T. interdigitale* and *Epidermophyton floccosum*. Clinical features include an itchy rash between the toes, with peeling, fissuring and maceration.

Tinea capitis: This dermatophyte scalp infection is most common in children. It presents with inflammation and scaling, pustules and partial hair loss. Infection may be within the shaft (endothrix), causing broken hairs at the surface ('black dot'), or outside the hair shaft (ectothrix) with minimal inflammation. Kerion is a boggy, inflammatory area of tinea capitis, usually caused by zoophilic fungi.

Onychomycosis: This causes yellow–brown discoloration and crumbling of the nail plate, which usually starts distally and spreads proximally.

Candidaisis: See p. 172.

Pityriasis versicolor: This persistent superficial skin condition is caused by the commensal yeasts *Malassezia globosa*, *M. sympadialis* or *M. furfur*. It is more frequent in warm, humid climates, and is more severe and persistent in the immunocompromised. It causes scaly, oval macules on the upper trunk, which are usually hypopigmented.

Diagnosis and management

In all cases of suspected dermatophyte infection, the diagnosis should be confirmed by skin scraping or nail clippings. Treatment can be topical (terbinafine or miconazole cream) or systemic (terbinafine, griseofulvin or itraconazole) for stubborn disease and hair or nail involvement.

Infestations

Scabies

Scabies is caused by the mite *Sarcoptes scabiei*. It spreads in households and environments where there is a high frequency of intimate personal contact.

Diagnosis is made by identifying the scabietic burrow, usually found on the edges of the fingers or toes or on the sides of the hands and feet. The clinical features include secondary eczematisation elsewhere on the body; the face and scalp are rarely involved, except in infants. Even after successful treatment, the itch can continue, and occasionally nodular lesions persist.

Treatment involves two applications, 1 week apart, of an aqueous solution of either permethrin or malathion to the whole body, excluding the head. Household contacts should also be treated. In some clinical situations, such as poor adherence, immunocompromised individuals and heavy infestations ('Norwegian' scabies), systemic treatment with a single dose of ivermectin is appropriate.

Head lice

Infestation with the head louse, *Pediculus humanus capitis*, is common and highly contagious. Head lice are spread by direct head-to-head contact.

Scalp itching leads to scratching, secondary infection and cervical lymphadenopathy. The diagnosis is confirmed by identifying the living louse or nymph on the scalp or on a black sheet of paper after careful fine-toothed combing of wet hair following conditioner application. The empty egg cases ('nits') are easily seen adhering strongly to the hair shaft.

Topical dimeticone, permethrin, carbaryl or, less often, malathion in lotion or aqueous form is recommended for the infected individual and any infected contacts. Treatment is applied on two separate occasions at 7 to 10 days' interval. Body lice and pubic (crab) lice are similar, the latter being predominantly sexually transmitted. Treatment is as for head lice.

Acne and rosacea

Acne vulgaris

Acne is a common chronic inflammation of the pilosebaceous units affecting more than 90% of adolescents. The key components are increased sebum production, colonisation of pilosebaceous ducts by *Propionibacterium acnes*, which in turn causes inflammation, and occlusion of pilosebaceous ducts. Family history may be positive, suggesting that genetic factors are important.

Acne usually affects the face and trunk. Greasiness of the skin (seborrhoea) accompanies open comedones (blackheads–dilated keratin-filled follicles) and closed comedones (whiteheads–caused by accumulation of sebum and keratin deeper in the pilosebaceous ducts). Inflammatory papules, nodules and cysts occur and may arise from comedones.

Management

Mild disease is managed with topical antibiotics such as erythromycin, dessicants such as benzoyl peroxide, or topical retinoids.

Moderate inflammatory acne is treated with a 3- to 6-month course of oral tetracyclines (e.g. limecycline). Oestrogen-containing oral contraceptives may help in women.

In severe cases, oral isotretinoin is highly effective. Side effects include drying of the skin and mucous membranes. Isotretinoin may elevate serum triglycerides and derange liver function; both should be checked before commencing the drug. Isotretinoin is highly teratogenic, and a strict pregnancy prevention programme and regular pregnancy testing are required. Depression and suicide are also reported associations, so predrug screening for depressive symptoms and mood monitoring during therapy are important.

Rosacea

Rosacea is a persistent facial eruption of unknown cause, largely occurring in middle age (Fig. 18.8). It is characterised by erythema, telangiectasia, papules and pustules. A bulbous appearance of the nose, known as rhinophyma, may be part of the disease, and is caused by sebaceous gland hypertrophy. The papulo-pustular element of disease usually responds well to tetracyclines, but the erythema and telangiectasia do not; these may require laser therapy.

18

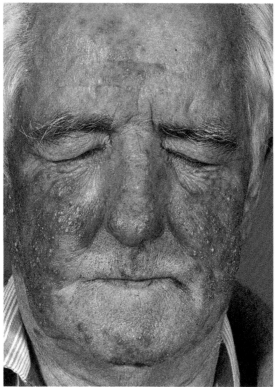

Fig. 18.8 Rosacea. The colour is distinctive, and the typical papulo-pustular rash involves the cheeks, centre of the forehead and chin.

Eczema

The terms 'eczema' and 'dermatitis' are synonymous. There are several clinical variants, all characterised by erythema, ill-defined oedema, papules, vesicles, exudation, fissuring, scaling and dyspigmentation.

Atopic eczema

Generalised, prolonged hypersensitivity to common environmental antigens, including pollen and house dust mites, is the hallmark of atopy, in which there is a genetic predisposition to produce excess IgE. Atopic individuals may develop any combination of asthma, hay fever, food allergies and atopic eczema. Filaggrin gene mutations increase the risk of developing atopic eczema by more than threefold, emphasising the importance of epidermal barrier impairment in this disease. Decreased skin barrier function may permit greater penetration of allergens through the epidermis. Other genes are also implicated.

Acute atopic eczema presents with severe itch, redness and swelling. Papules and vesicles may be evident, along with scaling and cracking of the skin, which is excessively dry. With chronic disease, lichenification may be found (dry, leathery skin thickening with increased markings, secondary to constant rubbing/scratching). The distribution of atopic eczema varies with the age of the patient: in infancy and adulthood, the eczema tends to affect the face and trunk, whereas in childhood, it affects the limb flexures, wrists and the ankles (Fig. 18.9). Management is described below.

Seborrhoeic eczema

This is an erythematous red scaly rash affecting the scalp (dandruff), central face, nasolabial folds, eyebrows and central chest. It may be caused by overgrowth of *Malassezia* yeasts. Management includes the use of ketoconazole or selenium-containing shampoo, in combination with a mild topical glucocorticoid.

Discoid eczema

This is common and characteristically consists of discrete coin-shaped eczematous lesions, which may become infected, most commonly on the limbs of men.

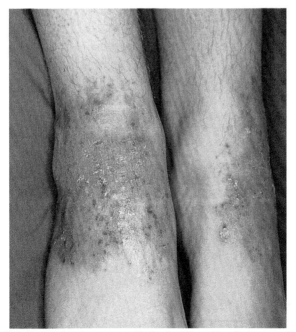

18

Fig. 18.9 Atopic subacute eczema on the fronts of the ankles of a teenager. These are sites of predilection, along with the cubital and popliteal fossae, in atopic eczema.

Irritant eczema and allergic contact eczema

These terms refer to eczematous eruptions of the skin in response to exogenous agents. Detergents, alkalis, acids, solvents and abrasive dusts are common causes of irritant eczema. Allergic contact eczema represents a delayed hypersensitivity reaction to an exogenous antigen. Nickel, parabens (a preservative in cosmetics and creams), colophony (in sticking plasters) and balsam of Peru (in perfumes) are common causes of allergic contact eczema. The distribution of eczema may reveal the cause. Allergen avoidance is the key control measure.

Asteatotic eczema

This occurs in dry skin, most often on the lower legs of the elderly, as a rippled or 'crazy paving' pattern of fine fissuring on an erythematous background. Low humidity caused by central heating, over-washing and diuretics are contributory factors.

Gravitational eczema

This occurs on the lower legs and is often associated with signs of venous insufficiency (oedema, red or bluish discoloration, loss of hair, induration, haemosiderin pigmentation and ulceration).

Lichen simplex

This describes a localised plaque of lichenified eczema caused by repeated rubbing or scratching. Common sites include the neck, lower legs and anogenital area.

Pompholyx

Intensely itchy vesicles and bullae occur on the palms, palmar surface and sides of the fingers and soles. Pompholyx may have several causes, which include atopic eczema, irritant and contact allergic dermatitis and fungal infection.

Investigation and management of eczema: Bacterial and viral swabs should be taken where supra-infection is suspected. HSV may cause a widespread infection, eczema herpeticum; small, punched-out lesions within worsening eczema suggest secondary HSV infection. Skin scrapings to rule out secondary fungal infection should be considered. Total and specific IgE and skin prick tests are not usually helpful. Patch tests should be performed if contact allergic dermatitis is suspected.

Alongside advice, education and support, emollients and topical glucocorticoids are mainstays of treatment for all eczema types.

Emollients (e.g. emulsifying ointments): Applied as bath additives, soap substitutes or directly to the skin. These limit water loss and reduce the amount of topical glucocorticoid required. Sedative antihistamines are useful if sleep is interrupted.

Topical glucocorticoids: Mild (hydrocortisone) and moderately potent (clobetasone butyrate) glucocorticoids are used on the face, whereas potent (betamethasone valerate) and highly potent (clobetasol propionate) forms are restricted to the trunk and limbs. The side effects of topical glucocorticoids (thinning, striae, fragility, purpura and systemic effects) need to be considered with prolonged use, although 'steroid phobia' and under-treatment is often more problematic. The least potent corticosteroid that is effective should be used for the shortest possible time. Topical tacrolimus and pimecrolimus may be useful glucocorticoid-sparing agents, particularly on the face.

Phototherapy: Narrow-band UVB may be useful in atopic eczema resistant to topical treatment.

Psoriasis and other erythematous scaly eruptions

Psoriasis

Psoriasis is a chronic inflammatory hyperproliferative skin disease characterised by demarcated erythematous scaly plaques, particularly on the extensor surfaces and scalp. It follows a relapsing and remitting course. The prevalence is 1.5% to 3% in European populations but less in African and Asian populations. Pathology reveals keratinocyte proliferation and an inflammatory infiltrate. The cause is unknown, but there is a large familial component, and several linked genes have been identified. Precipitating factors include:

• Trauma. • Infection (strep. throat, HIV) • Drugs (β-blockers, antimalarials, lithium). • Stress/anxiety.

Clinical presentations:

Plaque psoriasis: This the most common type, consisting of raised, erythematous plaques with silvery scale arising on the elbows, knees and back (Fig. 18.10). The scalp is involved in around 60% of patients. Nail disease is common, with pitting of the nail plate, onycholysis or subungual hyperkeratosis (Fig. 18.11). Psoriasis of the flexures (e.g. natal cleft, axillae, submammary folds) looks red, shiny and symmetrical, but not scaly.

Guttate psoriasis: This is most common in children and adolescents, and often follows a streptococcal sore throat. The onset is rapid, with small, droplet-shaped, scaly plaques. Guttate psoriasis responds well to phototherapy, but many patients later develop plaque psoriasis.

Erythrodermic psoriasis: Generalised erythrodermic psoriasis is a medical emergency (p. 742).

Pustular psoriasis: This may be generalised or localised. The rare generalised form is an emergency, presenting with large numbers of sterile pustules on an erythematous background. The patient is unwell, with swinging pyrexia, and requires hospital admission. The localised form is less serious, although extremely uncomfortable and affects the palms and the soles (palmoplantar pustulosis). This condition is closely linked to smoking.

Psoriatic arthropathy: See p. 621.

18

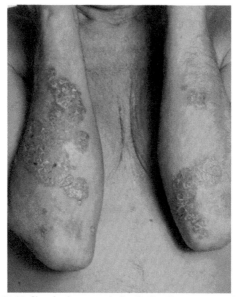

Fig. 18.10 Chronic plaque psoriasis affecting the extensor surfaces.

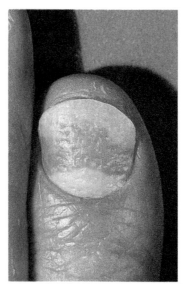

Fig. 18.11 Coarse pitting of the nail and separation of the nail from the nail bed (onycholysis). These are both classic features of psoriasis.

Diagnosis and management

The diagnosis is clinical but should include swabs to exclude infection and rheumatology consultation if joints are affected. Disease impact scores (e.g. Dermatology Life Quality Index, DLQI) are also valuable.

The psychosocial impact of psoriasis is considerable, and reassurance and counselling are vital. Treatment should be individualised according to disease impact, after full discussion of side effects. Limited chronic plaque psoriasis is manageable with topical agents only, whereas more extensive disease may require phototherapy or systemic agents.

Topical agents: Dithranol, tar and vitamin D analogues (calcitriol, calcipotriol) all reduce plaques. Glucocorticoids are used sparingly, mainly for flexures.

Phototherapy: UVB or PUVA is effective in moderate to severe psoriasis, but extensive PUVA carries a long-term risk of skin cancer.

Systemic agents: Retinoids, methotrexate or ciclosporin are effective, but may cause significant side effects. Infliximab, etanercept and adalimumab may be considered when other treatments have failed.

Pityriasis rosea

This is an idiopathic, self-limiting exanthem affecting young adults. A 'herald patch' appears first, a 1 to 2 cm oval lesion with a pink centre, a darker periphery and a collarette of scale; 1 to 2 weeks later a widespread papulosquamous eruption develops in a symmetrical 'fir tree' pattern on the trunk. Treatment is with emollients and mild topical glucocorticoids.

Lichenoid eruptions

Lichen planus

Lichen planus is an idiopathic rash characterised by intensely itchy polygonal papules with a violaceous hue, most commonly involving the flexural aspects of the wrists, and the lower back (Fig. 18.12). Between 30% and 70% of patients have oral mucosal involvement: an asymptomatic fine, white, lacy network of papules known as Wickham's striae.

The diagnosis is clinical, but biopsy for histopathology may be required in atypical cases. Potent topical glucocorticoids may ease the itch; ciclosporin, retinoids or phototherapy may be needed for recalcitrant cases. The condition is usually self-limiting, but rarely may persist for years.

Urticaria

Urticaria ('hives') is caused by localised dermal oedema secondary to a temporary increase in capillary permeability, mediated by mast cell degranulation releasing histamine and other mediators. If oedema involves subcutaneous or submucosal layers, the term angioedema is used.

Clinical features

Acute urticaria may be associated with angioedema of the lips, face, tongue and throat, and even with anaphylaxis. By definition, the lesions last less than 24 hours. Urticarial vasculitis has a similar clinical presentation, but lesions last more than 24 hours. Most cases are idiopathic, but physical, drug-induced, infection-related and autoimmune forms exist (Box 18.5).

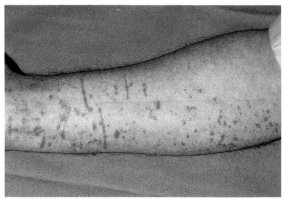

Fig. 18.12 Lichen planus. Glistening discrete papules involving the volar aspects of the forearm and wrist. Note the lesions along scratch marks (Köbner's phenomenon).

 18.5 Causes of urticaria

Acute and chronic urticaria

- Autoimmune because of production of antibodies that cross-link the IgE receptor on mast cells
- Allergens in foods, inhalants and injections
- Drugs (see Box 18.9)
- Physical, e.g. heat, cold, pressure, sun, water
- Contact, e.g. animal saliva, latex
- Infection, e.g. intestinal parasites
- Other conditions, e.g. systemic lupus erythematosus, pregnancy
- Idiopathic

Urticarial vasculitis

- Hepatitis B
- Systemic lupus erythematosus
- Idiopathic

A record of possible allergens, including drugs (see Box 18.9), should be determined. A family history must be sought in angioedema, to determine the likelihood of underlying C1 esterase inhibitor deficiency. Dermographism (urticaria appearing after firm pressure on the skin) may be elicited on examination.

Investigations

These should be guided by the history. Some or all of the following may be appropriate:

• FBC: eosinophils suggest parasitic infection or drug reaction. • ESR: elevated in vasculitis. • U&Es, LFTs and TFTs: to detect underlying disorders. • Total and specific IgE to possible allergens, for example, shellfish and peanuts. • Antinuclear factor: positive in SLE and urticarial vasculitis. • C_3 and C_4 complement levels: if low (complement consumption), check for C1 esterase inhibitor deficiency. • Infection screen: hepatitis and HIV. • Skin biopsy: if urticarial, vasculitis suspected.

Management

Avoid potential triggers, such as NSAIDs and codeine-containing preparations. Nonsedating antihistamines (e.g. loratadine) are the mainstay of management. H_2-blockers (e.g. ranitidine) may be added in cases refractory to H_1-blockers alone. Montelukast, UVB therapy or short-course glucocorticoids may be tried in resistant cases. Those with features of angioedema should carry a kit for self-administration of adrenaline (epinephrine) (p. 363).

Bullous diseases

Toxic epidermal necrolysis

TEN is a severe mucocutaneous blistering disease that is usually caused by a drug reaction (see Box 18.9). Some 1 to 4 weeks after drug commencement, pyrexia, erythema and blistering develop, rapidly involving all skin and mucous membranes. Blisters coalesce and denude, leaving painful erythematous skin. Skin snip allows early diagnosis.

Treatment involves stopping the causative drug. Intensive care is needed, with sterile dressings and emollients, scrupulous fluid balance and monitoring for infection. Sepsis and multi-organ failure are major risks. There is no evidence that immunoglobulins, glucocorticoids or ciclosporin improve outcomes.

Immunobullous diseases

Box 18.6 summarises the clinical features of the immunobullous disorders.

Bullous pemphigoid

Bullous pemphigoid is the most common immunobullous disease, with an average age of onset of 65 years.

Clinical features and diagnosis

After a prodrome of itchy erythematous rash, tense bullae develop (see Fig. 18.1). Mucosal involvement is uncommon. Biopsy reveals subepidermal blistering, an eosinophil-rich infiltrate, and IgG and C3 at the basement membrane on immunofluorescence.

Management

Very potent topical glucocorticoids may be sufficient in frail elderly patients. Tetracyclines have a role; however, most require systemic glucocorticoids, often with steroid-sparing immunosuppressants. The condition often burns out over a few years.

Pemphigus

Pemphigus is less common than bullous pemphigoid and affects patients aged 40 to 60 years. It may occur secondary to drugs or malignancy ('paraneoplastic pemphigus').

18

18.6 Clinical and investigational findings in the immunobullous disorders

Disease	Age	Site of blisters	Nature of blisters	Involves mucous membranes	Treatment
Pemphigus vulgaris	40–60 years	Trunk, head	Flaccid and fragile, many erosions	100%	Systemic steroids, cyclophosphamide
Bullous pemphigoid	≥60 years	Trunk (esp. flexures) and limbs	Tense (see Fig. 18.1)	Occasionally	Systemic steroids, azathioprine
Dermatitis herpetiformis	Young, associated with coeliac disease	Elbows, lower back, buttocks	Excoriated and often ruptured	No	Dapsone, gluten-free diet
Pemphigoid gestationis	Young pregnant female	Periumbilical and limbs	Tense	Rare	
Epidermolysis bullosa acquisita	All ages	Widespread	Tense, scarring	Common (50%)	Immunosuppressants, but poor response
Linear IgA disease	All ages	Widespread	Tense, annular ('string of beads')	Frequent	Dapsone, prednisolone

Clinical features and diagnosis

Skin and mucosae are usually involved, although the skin may be spared. The blisters are flaccid, easily ruptured and often not seen intact. Biopsy shows intra-epidermal blistering, acantholysis and positive direct immunofluorescence for IgG and C3. Circulating epidermal autoantibodies can be used to monitor activity. Investigations should screen for underlying autoimmune disease and malignancy.

Management

High-dose systemic glucocorticoids are usually required. Azathioprine, cyclophosphamide and IV immunoglobulins may be used as glucocorticoid-sparing agents.

Dermatitis herpetiformis

DH is an autoimmune blistering disorder that occurs in up to 10% of individuals with coeliac disease. Almost all patients with DH have evidence of partial villous atrophy, even if asymptomatic.

Intact vesicles or blisters are uncommon, as the condition is so pruritic that excoriations on extensor surfaces of arms, knees, buttocks, shoulders and scalp may be the only signs.

Direct immunofluorescence shows granular IgA in the papillary dermis. A gluten-free diet may suffice, but, if not, the condition is usually highly responsive to dapsone.

Pigmentation disorders

Decreased pigmentation

Vitiligo

Vitiligo is an acquired condition affecting 1% of the population worldwide. It may be familial and is associated with other autoimmune diseases.

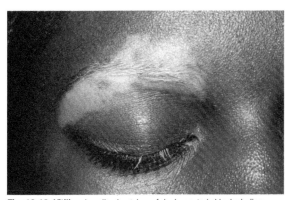

Fig. 18.13 Vitiligo. Localised patches of depigmented skin, including some white hairs. (*From White GM, Cox NH. Diseases of the skin. London: Mosby; 2000; copyright Elsevier.*)

Clinical features

Focal loss of melanocytes causes patches of sharply defined depigmentation. Generalised vitiligo is often symmetrical and frequently involves the hands, wrists, feet, knees, neck and around the body orifices. Associated hair may also depigment (Fig. 18.13). Segmental vitiligo is restricted to one part of the body, but not necessarily a dermatome. Some spotty perifollicular pigment may be seen within the depigmented patches and is often the first sign of repigmentation. Sensation in the depigmented patches is normal (unlike in tuberculoid leprosy). The course is unpredictable, but most patches remain static or enlarge; a few repigment spontaneously.

Management

Protecting the patches from excessive sun exposure with clothing or sunscreen may be helpful to avoid sunburn. Camouflage cosmetics may help those with dark skin. Potent topical glucocorticoids have limited efficacy in repigmentation. Narrowband UVB is the most effective repigmentary treatment available for generalised vitiligo, but even prolonged courses often produce an unsatisfactory outcome. Autologous melanocyte transfer, using split-skin or blister roof grafts, is occasionally employed on dermabraded recipient skin.

Oculocutaneous albinism

Albinism results from genetic reductions in melanin biosynthesis in skin and eyes; however, the number of melanocytes is normal (unlike vitiligo). It is usually inherited as an autosomal recessive trait; several types can be distinguished by genetic analysis. From birth, patients have complete absence of pigment, resulting in pale skin and white hair, and also failure of melanin production in the retina and iris. This causes photophobia, poor vision not correctable with refraction, rotatory nystagmus and alternating strabismus.

These patients are at greatly increased risk of sunburn and skin cancer, and assiduous protection from sun damage is essential.

Increased pigmentation

This is mostly caused by hypermelanosis, but other pigments may occasionally be deposited in the skin, for example, an orange tint in carotenaemia or a bronze hue in haemochromatosis.

Endocrine pigmentation: Chloasma describes discrete patches of facial pigmentation that occur in pregnancy and in some women taking oral contraceptives. Diffuse pigmentation may also occur in Addison's disease, Cushing's syndrome, Nelson's syndrome and chronic renal failure.

Drug-induced pigmentation: See Box 18.7.

Hair disorders

Alopecia

The term means nothing more than loss of hair and is a sign rather than a diagnosis. It is subdivided into localised or diffuse types, and also into scarring or nonscarring alopecia. The causes of alopecia are summarised in Box 18.8.

i	18.7 Drug-induced pigmentation	
Drug	**Appearance**	
Amiodarone	Slate-grey, exposed sites	
Arsenic	Diffuse bronze pigmentation with raindrop depigmentation	
Bleomycin	Often flexural, brown	
Busulfan	Diffuse brown	
Chloroquine	Blue–grey, exposed sites	
Clofazimine	Brown–grey, exposed sites	
Mepacrine	Yellow	
Minocycline	Slate-grey, scars, temples, shins and sclera	
Phenothiazines	Slate-grey, exposed sites	
Psoralens	Brown, exposed sites	

i	18.8 Classification of alopecia	
Localised		**Diffuse**
Nonscarring		
Tinea capitis, alopecia areata, androgenetic alopecia, traumatic (trichotillomania, traction, cosmetic), syphilis		Androgenetic alopecia, telogen effluvium, hypo- or hyperthyroidism, hypopituitarism, diabetes mellitus, HIV disease, nutritional deficiency, liver disease, postpartum, alopecia areata, syphilis, drug-induced (chemotherapy)
Scarring		
Developmental defects, discoid lupus erythematosus, herpes zoster, pseudopelade, tinea capitis/kerion, morphoea, idiopathic		Discoid lupus erythematosus, radiotherapy, folliculitis decalvans, lichen planopilaris

Alopecia areata: This common, nonscarring autoimmune condition appears as well-defined, noninflamed bald patches, usually on the scalp. Pathognomonic 'exclamation mark' hairs are seen (broken hairs, tapering towards the scalp) during active hair loss. Eyebrows, eyelashes, body hair and beard may be affected. The hair usually regrows spontaneously in small bald patches, but the outlook is less good with larger patches and when the alopecia appears early in life or is associated with atopy. Alopecia totalis describes complete loss of scalp hair, and alopecia universalis complete loss of all hair.

Androgenetic alopecia: Male-pattern baldness is physiological in men older than 20 years of age, although it can also occur in teenagers. It also occurs in women, usually after the menopause. The distribution is of bitemporal recession and then crown involvement.

18

Investigations

These should include FBC, U&Es, LFTs, TFTs, iron studies, an autoantibody profile and, in cases where lupus or lichen planus is suspected, a scalp biopsy.

Management

Specific causes, such as iron deficiency, should be treated. Hair may spontaneously regrow in alopecia areata; if not, there may be some response to topical or intralesional glucocorticoids, PUVA or immunotherapy. Some males with androgenetic alopecia are helped by systemic finasteride or topical minoxidil. In females, antiandrogen therapy, such as cyproterone acetate, can be used. Wigs are often appropriate for extensive alopecia.

Hypertrichosis

A generalised increase in hair, hypertrichosis is commonly a side effect of drugs, for example, ciclosporin, minoxidil or diazoxide. Eflornithine inhibits hair growth and may be useful if the cause cannot be removed.

Hirsutism

Hirsutism is the growth of terminal hair in a male pattern in a female. Most cases are idiopathic and, although it may occur in hyperandrogenism, Cushing's syndrome and polycystic ovary syndrome, very few patients have a demonstrable hormonal abnormality. Psychological distress is often significant, and oral contraceptives containing an antiandrogen (e.g. cyproterone acetate), laser therapy or topical eflornithine may be beneficial.

Nail disorders

The nails can be affected by both local and systemic disease. The nail apparatus consists of the nail matrix and the nail plate, which arises from the matrix and lies on the nail bed.

Nail-fold examination may reveal dilated capillaries and ragged cuticles in connective tissue disease (Fig. 18.14) or the boggy inflammation of paronychia, which occurs in individuals undertaking wet work, those with diabetes or poor peripheral circulation, and subsequent to vigorous manicuring.

Normal variants

Longitudinal ridging and beading of the nail plate occur with age. White transverse patches (striate leuconychia) are often caused by airspaces within the plate.

Nail trauma

Nail biting/picking: These are very common. Repetitive proximal nail-fold trauma results in transverse ridging and central furrowing of the nail.

Chronic trauma: Trauma from poorly fitting shoes and sport can cause thickening, disordered nail growth (onychogryphosis) and subsequent ingrowing toenails.

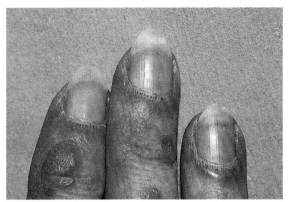

Fig. 18.14 Dermatomyositis. Erythema, dilated and tortuous capillaries in the proximal nail fold and Gottron's papules on the digits are important diagnostic features (p. 627).

Splinter haemorrhages: Fine, linear, dark brown longitudinal streaks in the plate (p. 105) are usually caused by trauma, especially if distal. Uncommonly, they can occur in nail psoriasis and are also characteristic of infective endocarditis (p. 302).

Subungual haematoma: Red, purple or grey–brown discoloration of the nail plate, usually of the big toe, is usually caused by trauma, although a history of trauma may not be clear. The main differential is subungual melanoma, although rapid onset, lack of nail-fold involvement and proximal clearing as the nail grows indicate haematoma. If there is diagnostic doubt, a biopsy may be needed.

Nail involvement in systemic disease

Beau's lines: These transverse grooves appear at the same time on all nails, a few weeks after an acute illness, moving out to the free margins as the nails grow.

Koilonychia: This concave or spoon-shaped deformity of the plate is a sign of iron deficiency.

Clubbing: In the early stages, the angle between the proximal nail and nail fold is lost. In its more established form, there may be swelling of the distal digits or toes. Causes include: • Respiratory: bronchogenic carcinoma, asbestosis, suppurative lung disease (empyema, bronchiectasis, cystic fibrosis), idiopathic pulmonary fibrosis. • Cardiac: cyanotic congenital heart disease, subacute bacterial endocarditis. • Other: inflammatory bowel disease, biliary cirrhosis, thyrotoxicosis, familial causes.

Discoloration of the nails: Whitening is a rare sign of hypoalbuminaemia. 'Half and half' nails (white proximally and red-brown distally) may be found in renal failure. Antimalarials and some other drugs may discolour nails.

18

Skin disease in general medicine

Conditions involving cutaneous vasculature

Vasculitis

Vasculitis usually presents as palpable purpura. The diagnosis is confirmed by biopsy. The causes and treatments are covered on p. 628.

Pyoderma gangrenosum

PG presents initially as a painful, tender, inflamed nodule or pustule that breaks down centrally and rapidly progresses to an ulcer with an indurated, undermined purplish or pustular edge (Fig. 18.15). Lesions may be single or multiple and may be ulcerative, pustular, bullous or vegetative. PG usually occurs in adults in association with underlying inflammatory bowel disease, inflammatory arthritis, blood dyscrasias, immunodeficiencies or HIV. The diagnosis is largely clinical, as histology is not specific. Analgesia, treatment of secondary bacterial infection and supportive dressings are important. Systemic treatment with tetracyclines, systemic glucocorticoids, dapsone, ciclosporin or other immunosuppressants is often required.

Pressure sores

Localised, prolonged, pressure-induced ischaemia can cause pressure sores, which occur in up to 30% of the hospitalised elderly, with considerable morbidity, mortality and expense. The main risk factors are immobility, poor nutrition and tissue hypoxia—for example, with anaemia, peripheral vascular disease, diabetes, sepsis and skin atrophy.

Prevention is key and involves identification of at-risk patients and regular repositioning and use of pressure-relieving mattresses.

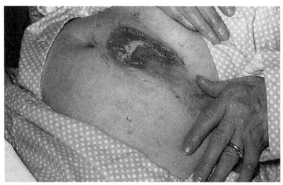

Fig. 18.15 Pyoderma gangrenosum. A large indolent ulcer in a patient with rheumatoid arthritis. Note healing in one part.

Connective tissue disease

Lupus erythematosus

The autoimmune disorder lupus erythematosus can be subdivided into systemic lupus erythematosus (SLE) (p. 622) and cutaneous lupus, which includes discoid lupus (DLE) and subacute cutaneous lupus erythematosus (SCLE).

DLE: This presents as scaly red plaques, with follicular plugging, on photo-exposed areas of the face, head and neck, which resolve with scarring and pigmentary change. Scalp involvement causes scarring alopecia. Most patients with DLE do not develop SLE.

SCLE: Patients may have extensive cutaneous involvement, usually aggravated by sun exposure, with an annular, polycyclic or papulosquamous eruption. Systemic involvement is uncommon and the prognosis usually good.

A diagnosis of cutaneous lupus is confirmed by histopathology and immunofluorescence. The diagnosis of SLE is described on p. 624. Drug-induced lupus should always be considered (Box 18.9).

i	18.9 Clinical patterns of drug eruptions	
Reaction pattern	**Appearance**	**Examples of causative drugs**
Exanthematous	Erythema, maculo-papular	Antibiotics, anticonvulsants, gold, penicillamine, NSAIDs, carbimazole, biological therapies
Urticaria and angioedema	Itchy weals, sometimes with angioedema	Salicylates, opiates, NSAIDs, antibiotics, dextran, ACE inhibitors
Lichenoid	See Fig. 18.12	Gold, penicillamine, antimalarials, anti-TB drugs, thiazides, NSAIDs, β-blockers, ACE inhibitors, PPIs, quinine, sulphonamides, lithium, sulphonylureas, dyes
Purpura and vasculitis	Palpable purpura/necrosis	Allopurinol, antibiotics, ACE inhibitors, NSAIDs, aspirin, anticonvulsants, diuretics, OCP
Erythema multiforme	See Fig. 18.17	See p. 773
Erythema nodosum	Red/purple raised tender swellings	See p. 774
Exfoliative dermatitis	May be erythroderma	Allopurinol, carbamazepine, penicillins, isoniazid, gold, lithium, penicillamine, ACE inhibitors
Toxic epidermal necrolysis	See p. 761	Anticonvulsants, sulphonamides, sulphonylureas, NSAIDs, terbinafine, antiretrovirals, allopurinol

18

i	**18.9 Clinical patterns of drug eruptions—cont'd**	
Reaction pattern	**Appearance**	**Examples of causative drugs**
Photosensitivity	See p. 739	Thiazides, amiodarone, quinine, fluoroquinolones, sulphonamides, phenothiazines, tetracyclines, NSAIDs, retinoids, psoralens
Drug-induced lupus	Discoid or urticarial	Allopurinol, thiazides, ACE inhibitors, hydralazine anticonvulsants, β-blockers, gold, minocycline, penicillamine, lithium
Psoriasiform rash	See Fig. 18.10	Antimalarials, β-blockers, NSAIDs, lithium, anti-TNF
Acneiform eruptions	Rash resembles acne	Lithium, anticonvulsants, OCP, anti-TB drugs, androgenic/glucocorticoid steroids, EGFR antagonists, e.g. cetuximab
Pigmentation	–	See Box 18.7 (p. 765)
Pseudoporphyria	Blisters, hypertrichosis on hands	NSAIDs, tetracyclines, retinoids, furosemide, nalidixic acid
Drug-induced immunobullous disease	See Fig. 18.1	Penicillamine, ACE inhibitors, vancomycin
Fixed drug eruptions	Round erythema, oedema ± bullae	Tetracyclines, sulphonamides, penicillins, quinine, NSAIDs, barbiturates, anticonvulsants
Hair loss	Diffuse	Cytotoxics, retinoids, anticoagulants, lithium, anticonvulsants, antithyroid drugs, OCP, infliximab
Hypertrichosis	See p. 766	Diazoxide, minoxidil, ciclosporin

Cutaneous lupus may respond to topical glucocorticoids or immunosuppressants. Antimalarials and photoprotection are also important, and systemic immunosuppression or low-dose UVA1 phototherapy may be required for resistant disease.

Systemic sclerosis

This autoimmune multisystem disease is described on p. 625. Skin features start with Raynauld's syndrome, digital ulcers and fibrosis. Dilated nail-fold capillaries and ragged cuticles are common.

Morphoea

Morphoea is a localised cutaneous form of scleroderma that can affect any site at any age. It presents as a thickened violaceous plaque, which may become hyper- or hypopigmented. Topical glucocorticoids, immunosuppressants or phototherapy can be effective.

Dermatomyositis

This rare multisystem disease is described on p. 627. Cutaneous features include a violaceous 'heliotrope' rash periorbitally, involving the upper eyelids. A more extensive, photoaggravated rash may involve the trunk, limbs and hands, with papules over the knuckles (Gottron's papules, see Fig. 18.14).

Granulomatous disease

Granuloma annulare

This is common, and may be reactive, although a trigger is usually not apparent. It is generally asymptomatic, and may present as an isolated dermal granulomatous lesion with a raised papular annular edge, or may be more generalised. An association with diabetes has been proposed but not confirmed. Lesions often resolve spontaneously. Intralesional glucocorticoids or cryotherapy can be used for localised disease, and UVB or UVA1 phototherapy or PUVA for generalised disease.

Necrobiosis lipoidica

This condition is important to recognise because of its association with diabetes mellitus. Typically, the lesions appear as shiny, atrophic and slightly yellow plaques on the shins (Fig. 18.16). Underlying telangiectasia is easily seen. Minor knocks may precipitate slow-healing ulcers. Less than 1% of people with diabetes have necrobiosis, but more than 85% of patients with necrobiosis will have or will develop diabetes.

No treatment is very effective. Potent topical or intralesional glucocorticoids are used, as is PUVA.

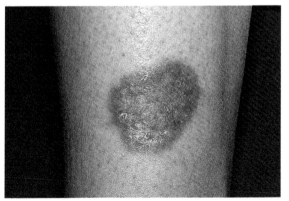

Fig. 18.16 Necrobiosis lipoidica. An atrophic yellowish plaque on the skin of a person with diabetes.

Sarcoidosis

Cutaneous manifestations of sarcoid are seen in about one-third of patients with systemic disease. Variants include:
• Erythema nodosum. • Dusky infiltrated plaques on the nose and fingers (lupus pernio). • Scattered brownish-red, violaceous or hypopigmented papules or nodules that vary in number, size and distribution.

Porphyria

The porphyrias are a group of rare disorders of the haem biosynthesis pathway (p. 205). Some have cutaneous manifestations.

Cutaneous porphyrias: fragility and blisters

Acquired porphyria cutanea tarda (PCT) is the most common porphyria to cause these symptoms. PCT is caused by a chronic liver disease (e.g. alcohol, hepatitis C), in combination with hepatic iron overload. The underlying liver disease is usually only diagnosed on investigation of the skin presentation. Typical features are increased skin fragility, blistering erosions, hypertrichosis, scarring and milia occurring on light-exposed areas, particularly the backs of the hands. Other porphyrias that can cause similar skin features include variegate porphyria and hereditary coproporphyria.

Cutaneous porphyria: pain on sun exposure

Erythropoietic protoporphyria is a rare but important inherited porphyria. The presentation is usually in early childhood, although the diagnosis is often delayed, because physical signs are often minimal despite the child crying from pain on sunlight exposure.

Abnormal deposition disorders

Xanthomas

Deposits of fatty material in the skin, subcutaneous fat and tendons (see p. 250) may be the first clue to primary or secondary hyperlipidaemia.

Amyloidosis

Cutaneous amyloid may present as periocular plaques in primary systemic amyloidosis (p. 204 and amyloid associated with multiple myeloma, but is uncommon in amyloidosis secondary to chronic inflammatory diseases. Amyloid infiltration of blood vessels may manifest as 'pinch purpura' following skin trauma. Macular amyloid, pruritic grey–brown macules or patches, usually on the back, is more common in darker skin types.

Genetic disorders

Neurofibromatosis

This is described on p. 697.

Tuberous sclerosis

This is an autosomal dominant condition with hamartomas affecting many systems. Diagnosis is made on the basis of the classical triad of mental retardation, epilepsy and skin lesions:

• Pale oval patches on the skin (ash leaf macules). • Yellowish-pink papules on the face (adenoma sebaceum). • Peri-/subungual fibromas. • Connective tissue naevi (shagreen patches, often on the lower back).

Gum hyperplasia, retinal phakomas (fibrous overgrowth), renal, lung and heart tumours, cerebral gliomas and calcification of the basal ganglia may also occur.

Reactive disorders

Erythema multiforme

Erythema multiforme has characteristic clinical and histological features, and is thought to be an immunological reaction triggered by infections (e.g. herpes simplex, orf, *Mycoplasma*), drugs (especially sulphonamides, penicillins and barbiturates) and occasionally sarcoidosis, malignancy or SLE. A cause is not always identified. Lesions are multiple, erythematous, annular, targetoid 'bull's eyes' and may blister (Fig. 18.17). Stevens–Johnson syndrome is a severe variant with marked blistering, mucosal involvement (mouth, eyes and genitals) and systemic upset.

Identification and removal/treatment of triggers are essential. Analgesia and topical glucocorticoids may provide symptomatic relief. Supportive care is required in Stevens–Johnson syndrome, including ophthalmology input.

Erythema nodosum

This septal panniculitis of subcutaneous fat causes painful, indurated violaceous nodules on the shins and lower legs. Malaise, fever and joint pains are common. The lesions resolve slowly over a month, leaving bruise-like marks.

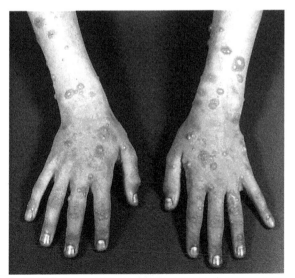

18

Fig. 18.17 Erythema multiforme with blistering lesions in a young woman.

Causes include:

• Infections: bacteria (streptococcus, mycobacteria, *Brucella*, *Rickettsia*, *Chlamydia*, *Mycoplasma*), viruses (hepatitis B, infectious mononucleosis) and fungi. • Drugs: for example, sulphonamides, sulphonylureas, oral contraceptives. • Systemic diseases: sarcoidosis, inflammatory bowel disease, malignancy. • Pregnancy.

The underlying cause should be determined and treated. Bed rest and oral NSAIDs may hasten resolution. Tapering systemic glucocorticoids may be required in stubborn cases.

Acanthosis nigricans

This is a velvety hyperkeratosis and pigmentation of the major flexures, particularly the axillae. Causes include obesity, insulin resistance syndromes and malignancy, usually adenocarcinoma, particularly gastric. Pruritus is a feature of malignancy-associated acanthosis, and the mucous membranes may be involved.

Drug eruptions

Cutaneous drug reactions are common, and almost any drug can cause them. Drug reactions may reasonably be included in the differential diagnosis of most skin diseases. Presentations are summarised in Box 18.9. Common to most drug eruption is symmetry, and a temporal relationship to the commencement of the suspected drug. Eosinophilia or abnormal LFTs may occur, but there are no specific investigations that help.

Management

• Withdrawal of the offending drug. • Oral antihistamines for itch. • Short course of oral prednisolone or potent topical glucocorticoid for symptomatic relief.

19

Ageing and disease

In the developed world, improvements in life expectancy have increased the proportion of older people in the population. For example, the UK population has grown by 11% in the past 30 years, but the number of those aged over 65 years has grown by 24%. Although the proportion of the population aged over 65 years is greater in developed countries, most older people live in the developing world. Two-thirds of the world population aged over 65 years live in developing countries at present, and this is projected to rise to 75% in 2025.

Geriatric medicine is concerned particularly with frail older people, in whom reductions in physiological capacity increase susceptibility to disease and mortality. These patients frequently suffer from multiple comorbidities, and illness often presents in atypical ways with delirium, falls or loss of mobility and day-to-day functioning. Frail older people are also prone to adverse drug reactions, partly because of polypharmacy and partly because of age-related changes in responses to drugs and their elimination. Disability is common in old age, but patients' function can often be improved by the interventions of a multidisciplinary team (Box 19.1).

Comprehensive geriatric assessment

Comprehensive geriatric assessment (p. 776), performed by a multidisciplinary team, is a powerful means of identifying and managing the factors affecting the health and well-being of older people. Evidence shows that it reduces death or deterioration, increases the chances of living independently at home and may also improve cognitive function.

Frailty makes investigation more taxing for patients, and a judgement must be made, often together with the family, about how much investigation is safe and appropriate in each case. The approach should be guided by:
• The views of the patient and family. • The patient's general health. • Will the investigation alter management? • Will management benefit the patient? • Advance directives.

Comprehensive geriatric assessment

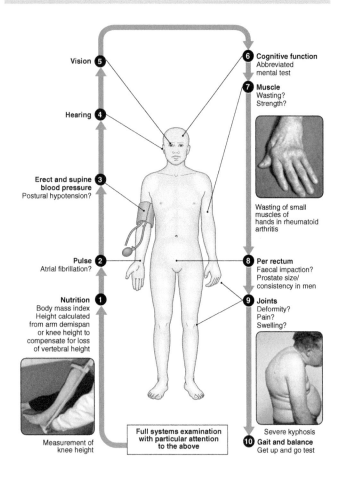

Vision **5**

Hearing **4**

Erect and supine **3**
blood pressure
Postural hypotension?

Pulse **2**
Atrial fibrillation?

Nutrition **1**
Body mass index
Height calculated
from arm demispan
or knee height to
compensate for loss
of vertebral height

Measurement of
knee height

6 Cognitive function
Abbreviated
mental test

7 Muscle
Wasting?
Strength?

Wasting of small
muscles of
hands in rheumatoid
arthritis

8 Per rectum
Faecal impaction?
Prostate size/
consistency in men

9 Joints
Deformity?
Pain?
Swelling?

Severe kyphosis

10 Gait and balance
Get up and go test

Full systems examination
with particular attention
to the above

19.1 Multidisciplinary team and functional assessment	
Team member	**Activity assessed and promoted**
Physiotherapist	Mobility, balance and upper limb function
Occupational therapist	Activities of daily living, e.g. dressing, cooking, home environment and care needs
Dietitian	Nutrition
Speech and language therapist	Communication and swallowing
Social worker	Care needs, discharge planning, organising institutional care
Nurse	Motivation, initiation of activities, promotion of self-care, education, feeding, continence, skin care, communication with family and team
Doctor	Diagnosis and management of illness, team coordinator

19.2 Investigations to identify acute illness

- Full blood count
- U&Es, LFT, calcium, glucose
- CXR
- ECG
- CRP: useful marker for occult infection or inflammation
- Blood and urine cultures if pyrexial

Presenting problems in geriatric medicine

Although the common presenting problems are described individually here, in reality older patients often present with several at the same time, particularly confusion, incontinence and falls. These share some underlying causes and may precipitate each other.

The approach to most presenting problems in old age can be summarised as follows:

Obtain a collateral history: Find out the patient's usual status (e.g. mobility, cognitive state) from a relative or carer.

Check medication: Have there been any recent changes?

Search for and treat any acute illness: See Box 19.2.

Identify and reverse predisposing risk factors: These depend on the presenting problem.

Falls

Falls are very common in older people, with 40% of those over 80 falling each year. Although only 10% to 15% of falls result in serious injury, virtually all fragility fractures in the elderly result from falls. Falls also lead to loss of

> ### 19.3 Risk factors for falls
>
> - Muscle weakness
> - History of falls
> - Gait or balance abnormality
> - Use of a walking aid
> - Visual impairment
> - Arthritis
> - Impaired activities of daily living
> - Depression
> - Cognitive impairment
> - Age >80 years
> - Psychotropic medication

confidence and fear and are frequently the 'final straw' that makes an older person decide to move to institutional care. Management will vary according to the underlying cause.

Acute illness

Falling is one of the classical atypical presentations of acute illness in the frail. The reduced reserves in older people's integrative neurological function mean that they are less able to maintain their balance when challenged by acute illness. Suspicion should be high when falls have occurred suddenly over a few days. Common underlying illnesses include infection, stroke, metabolic disturbance and heart failure. Thorough examination and investigation are required to identify these (Box 19.2). Recently started psychotropic or hypotensive drugs may also cause falls. Once the underlying acute illness has been treated, falls may stop.

Blackouts

A proportion of older people who 'fall' have, in fact, had a syncopal episode. A witness history is useful, as patients may not remember loss of consciousness. If syncope is a possibility, perform appropriate investigations (p. 63).

Mechanical and recurrent falls

Among patients who have tripped or are uncertain how they fell, those with repeated episodes in the past year or unsteadiness during a 'get up and go' test require further assessment. This test involves asking the seated patient to stand up, walk 3 m, turn and go back to the chair. A normal performance takes under 12 seconds. Many such patients are frail, with multiple medical problems and chronic disabilities. Falls are associated with well-established risk factors (Box 19.3). Common pathologies identified include cerebrovascular disease, Parkinson's disease and osteoarthritis of weight-bearing joints. Calculation of fracture risk using tools such as FRAX should be performed, and DEXA bone density scanning should be considered in patients with a 10-year risk of major fracture of more than 10%.

Falls can be prevented by multiple risk factor intervention (Box 19.4), which requires a multidisciplinary approach. The most effective is balance

19.4 Multifactorial interventions to prevent falls

- Balance and exercise training
- Rationalisation of medication (hypnotic, anticholinergic, hypotensive and psychotropic)
- Correction of visual impairment (e.g. cataracts)
- Home environmental hazard assessment and safety education
- Calcium and vitamin D supplementation in institutional care

and exercise training by physiotherapists. Rationalising medication may help to reduce sedation, although many older patients are reluctant to stop their hypnotic. It will also help reduce postural hypotension, defined as a drop in BP of more than 20 mmHg systolic or more than 10 mmHg diastolic pressure on standing from supine. Observation of gait may reveal other treatable underlying disease (e.g. Parkinson's disease) contributing to falls.

If osteoporosis is diagnosed, specific drug therapy should be considered (p. 631).

Dizziness

Dizziness is very common, affecting at least 30% of those aged over 65 years, according to community surveys. Acute dizziness is relatively straightforward, and common causes include:
• Hypotension caused by arrhythmia, acute myocardial infarction, gastro-intestinal bleed or pulmonary embolism. • Acute posterior fossa stroke. • Vestibular neuronitis.

Older people, however, more commonly present with recurrent dizzy spells. They often find it difficult to describe the sensation they experience. The most effective way of establishing the cause(s) of the problem is to determine which of the following is predominant, even if more than one is present: • Lightheadedness, suggestive of reduced cerebral perfusion. • Vertigo, suggestive of labyrinthine or brainstem disease. • Unsteadiness/poor balance, suggestive of joint or neurological disease.

In lightheaded patients, aortic stenosis, postural hypotension and arrhythmias should be considered and excluded, but vasovagal syndrome and postural hypotension are the commonest causes. Vertigo is most often caused by benign positional vertigo (p. 649), but with other neurological signs merits further brain imaging (e.g. MRI).

Delirium

Delirium is transient reversible cognitive dysfunction. The differential diagnosis and management are covered on p. 66).

Urinary incontinence

Urinary incontinence is defined as the involuntary loss of urine, sufficiently severe to cause a social or hygiene problem. It occurs in all age groups but

> **i** 19.5 Causes of transient incontinence
>
> - Restricted mobility
> - Acute confusional state
> - Urinary tract infection
> - Severe constipation
> - Drugs, e.g. diuretics, sedatives
> - Hyperglycaemia
> - Hypercalcaemia

becomes more prevalent in old age. Although age-dependent changes in the lower urinary tract predispose older people to incontinence, it is not an inevitable consequence of ageing, and always requires investigation. Urinary incontinence is frequently precipitated by acute illness in old age and is commonly multifactorial (Box 19.5). Different types of incontinence are covered on p. 245.

Prescribing and deprescribing

The large number of comorbidities that accompany ageing often leads to polypharmacy (defined as the use of four or more drugs). Adverse drug reactions cause up to 20% of admissions in people over 65 years of age. The risk of polypharmacy is compounded by age-related changes in pharmacodynamic and pharmacokinetic factors (p. 11), and by impaired homeostatic mechanisms, such as baroreceptor responses, plasma volume and electrolyte control. Older people are especially sensitive to drugs that can cause postural hypotension or volume depletion. Nonadherence to drug therapy also rises with the number of drugs prescribed.

The clinical presentations of polypharmacy are extremely diverse, so for any presenting problem in old age, the possibility that the patient's medication is a contributory factor should always be considered. Common adverse drug reactions in old age are shown in Box 19.6.

Deprescribing is as important as prescribing in older people. Regular review of medications is vital to ensure that medications are still required, are still working and are not causing side-effects, and to ascertain whether the patient is actually taking them.

Hypothermia

Hypothermia occurs when the body's core temperature falls below 35°C. The very young are susceptible because they have poor thermoregulation and a high body surface area-to-weight ratio, but the elderly are at highest risk.

Clinical assessment

Diagnosis is dependent on recognition of the environmental circumstances and measurement of core (rectal) body temperature. Clinical features depend on the degree of hypothermia:

	19.6 Common adverse drug reactions in old age
Drug class	**Adverse reaction**
NSAIDs	Gastrointestinal bleeding and peptic ulceration Renal impairment
Diuretics	Renal impairment, electrolyte disturbance Gout Hypotension, postural hypotension
Warfarin	Bleeding
ACE inhibitors	Renal impairment, electrolyte disturbance Hypotension, postural hypotension
β-Blockers	Bradycardia, heart block Hypotension, postural hypotension
Opiates	Constipation, vomiting Delirium Urinary retention
Antidepressants	Delirium Hyponatraemia (SSRIs) Hypotension, postural hypotension Falls
Benzodiazepines	Delirium Falls
Anticholinergics	Delirium Urinary retention Constipation

Mild hypothermia (32°C–35°C): Shivering, lethargy, dehydration, tachypnoea.

Moderate hypothermia (28°C–32°C): Violent shivering, slurred speech, slow movement, ataxia.

Severe hypothermia (<28°C): Depressed conscious level, muscle stiffness, not shivering, bradycardia, hypotension, ECG J waves, dysrhythmias.

Critical (<23°C): Coma, dilated, unreactive pupils, cardiac standstill.

It is very difficult to diagnose death reliably by clinical means in a cold patient. Resuscitative measures should continue until the core temperature is normal, and only then should a diagnosis of brain death be considered.

Investigations

Haemoconcentration and metabolic acidosis are common. J waves, which occur at the junction of the QRS complex and the ST segment, may be seen on the ECG (Fig. 19.1). Cardiac dysrhythmias, including ventricular

19

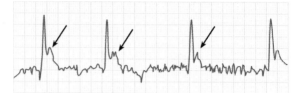

Fig. 19.1 ECG showing J waves (arrows) in a hypothermic patient.

fibrillation, may occur. Serum aspartate aminotransferase and CK may be elevated secondary to muscle damage; serum amylase is often high because of subclinical pancreatitis. If the cause of hypothermia is not obvious, additional tests should identify thyroid and pituitary dysfunction, hypoglycaemia and the possibility of drug intoxication.

Management

Mild hypothermia: Patients should be maintained in a warm room, with additional thermal insulation (blankets and/or space film blanket) and heat packs placed on the abdomen and groin. They should be given warm fluids to drink and an adequate calorie intake. Rewarming at 1° to 2°C/hour is ideal, and underlying conditions should be treated.

Severe hypothermia (<28°C): This is associated with metabolic disturbance and cardiac dysrhythmias. In the presence of cardiopulmonary arrest, rapid rewarming (>2°C/hour) is needed to restore perfusion and is best achieved by cardiopulmonary bypass or extracorporeal membrane oxygenation. Pleural, peritoneal or bladder lavage with warmed fluids is an alternative if the former methods are not available. In addition to supplementary oxygen, warm IV fluids should be given and acidosis corrected. Monitoring of cardiac rhythm and ABGs is essential.

Rehabilitation

Rehabilitation aims to improve the ability of people of all ages to perform day-to-day activities and to restore their physical, mental and social capabilities as far as possible.

The process

Rehabilitation is a problem-solving process focused on improving a patient's physical, psychological and social function. It entails:

Assessment: The nature and extent of the patient's problems can be identified using the International Classification of Functioning, Disability and Health framework, which focuses on health conditions (e.g. stroke), associated physical impairments (e.g. arm weakness), effect on activity (e.g. inability to dress as a result of arm weakness) and restriction of participation in activities (e.g. inability to go out as unable to dress oneself). Such an assessment ensures a whole-person functional approach, rather than a focus merely on disease.

Goal-setting: Goals are specific to the patient's problems, realistic and agreed between the patient and the rehabilitation team.

Intervention: This includes active treatments, individualised to the patient's circumstances, to achieve the set goals and to maintain the patient's health and quality of life.

Reassessment: There is ongoing re-evaluation of the patient's function and progress towards the set goals, with modification of the interventions if necessary. This requires regular review by all members of the rehabilitation team, the patient and the carer.

Oncology

Cancer is now the third leading cause of death worldwide. By 2030, it is projected that there will be 26 million new cancer cases and 17 million cancer deaths per year. In 2008, developing nations with low per capita expenditure on health care accounted for 56% of new cancer cases and 75% of cancer deaths.

The most common solid organ malignancies arise in the lung, breast and gastrointestinal tract, but the most common form worldwide is skin cancer. Cigarette smoking accounts for more than 20% of all global cancer deaths, 80% of lung cancer cases in men and 50% of lung cancer cases in women worldwide, which could be prevented by smoking cessation. Diet and alcohol contribute to a further 30% of cancers, including those of the stomach, colon, oesophagus, breast and liver. Lifestyle modification could reduce these if steps were taken to avoid animal fat and red meat, reduce alcohol, increase fibre, increase fresh fruit and vegetable intake and avoid obesity. Infections account for a further 15% of cancers, including those of the cervix, stomach, liver, nasopharynx and bladder, and some of these could be prevented by infection control and vaccination.

The 10 hallmarks of cancer

The formation and growth of cancer constitute a multistep process, during which sequentially occurring gene mutations result in the formation of a cancerous cell. The key characteristics of carcinogenesis, referred to as the hallmarks of cancer, are:

1. Genome instability and mutation

Normally, cellular DNA repair mechanisms are so effective that spontaneous mutations are corrected, but in cancer cells mutations accumulate despite these mechanisms.

Clinical examination of the cancer patient

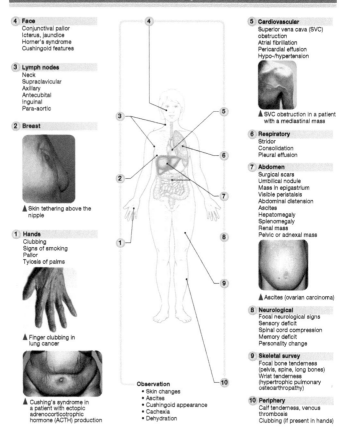

4 Face
Conjunctival pallor
Icterus, jaundice
Horner's syndrome
Cushingoid features

3 Lymph nodes
Neck
Supraclavicular
Axillary
Antecubital
Inguinal
Para-aortic

2 Breast

▲ Skin tethering above the nipple

1 Hands
Clubbing
Signs of smoking
Pallor
Tylosis of palms

▲ Finger clubbing in lung cancer

▲ Cushing's syndrome in a patient with ectopic adrenocorticotrophic hormone (ACTH) production

5 Cardiovascular
Superior vena cava (SVC) obstruction
Atrial fibrillation
Pericardial effusion
Hypo-/hypertension

▲ SVC obstruction in a patient with a mediastinal mass

6 Respiratory
Stridor
Consolidation
Pleural effusion

7 Abdomen
Surgical scars
Umbilical nodule
Mass in epigastrium
Visible peristalsis
Abdominal distension
Ascites
Hepatomegaly
Splenomegaly
Renal mass
Pelvic or adnexal mass

▲ Ascites (ovarian carcinoma)

8 Neurological
Focal neurological signs
Sensory deficit
Spinal cord compression
Memory deficit
Personality change

9 Skeletal survey
Focal bone tenderness (pelvis, spine, long bones)
Wrist tenderness (hypertrophic pulmonary osteoarthropathy)

Observation
• Skin changes
• Ascites
• Cushingoid appearance
• Cachexia
• Dehydration

10 Periphery
Calf tenderness, venous thrombosis
Clubbing (if present in hands)

2. Resistance to cell death

Healthy cells die by apoptosis, autophagy and necrosis. Apoptosis, or programmed cell death, is markedly reduced in many cancers. In autophagy, cellular constituents are degraded by lysosomal activity. Radiotherapy and chemotherapy can increase autophagy, causing cancer cells to enter a state of reversible dormancy. Necrosis is premature cell death with release of cellular contents into the tissues. This induces inflammation, angiogenesis and release of factors that increase cellular proliferation and tissue invasion, enhancing carcinogenesis.

3. Sustained proliferative signalling

Cancer cells can sustain proliferation beyond what would be expected for normal cells; this is typically attributed to growth factors, which bind to receptors that activate a tyrosine kinase signalling cascade, changing gene expression and promoting cellular proliferation and growth. Cancer cells can also stimulate proliferation by producing excess receptors or abnormal receptors, which signal without ligand binding.

4. Evasion of growth suppressors

In healthy tissues, cell-to-cell contact in dense cell populations acts as an inhibitory factor on proliferation. This contact inhibition is typically absent in many cancer cell populations.

5. Replicative immortality

During normal cell replication, telomeres shorten progressively as fragments of telomeric DNA are lost. This shortening acts a mitotic clock, eventually preventing further division. The telomerase enzyme adds nucleotides to telomeres, allowing continued cell division. It is almost absent in normal cells but is expressed at significant levels by many human cancers.

6. Induction of angiogenesis

Cancers require a functional vascular network to ensure continued growth and cannot grow beyond 1 mm^3 without stimulating angiogenesis. Angiogenic growth factors, such as vascular endothelial growth factor and platelet-derived growth factor, cause normally quiescent vasculature to sprout new vessels that help sustain tumour growth.

7. Activation of invasion and metastasis

Local tissue invasion is followed by infiltration of nearby blood and lymphatic vessels by cancer cells. Malignant cells are eventually transported through haematogenous and lymphatic spread to distant sites within the body, where they form micrometastases that will eventually grow into macroscopic metastatic lesions.

8. Reprogramming of energy metabolism

Cancer cells can reprogram their glucose metabolism to limit energy production to glycolysis, even in the presence of oxygen. Although this 'aerobic glycolysis' is much less efficient at energy production than oxidative phosphorylation, it yields glycolytic intermediates that can generate the nucleosides and amino acids necessary for the production of new cells.

9. Tumour-promoting inflammation

Tumour-associated inflammatory responses are now known to promote cancer progression. Cytokines alter blood vessels to permit migration of neutrophils from the blood vessels into the tissues. Other intrinsic cascade systems that contribute to inflammation include the complement system activated by bacteria and the coagulation and fibrinolytic systems activated by necrosis. Growth factors and pro-angiogenic factors may be released by immune cells into the surrounding tumour microenvironment. In particular, reactive oxygen species, which are actively mutagenic, will accelerate the genetic evolution of surrounding cancer cells, enhancing growth and cancer progression.

10. Evasion of immune destruction

Cancer cells continuously shed surface antigens into the circulation, prompting an immune response from cytotoxic T cells, natural killer cells and macrophages. The immune system provides continuous surveillance, eliminating cells that undergo malignant transformation.

Cancers develop and progress when there is loss of recognition by the immune system, lack of susceptibility because of escape from immune cell action and induction of immune dysfunction, often via inflammatory mediators.

Environmental and genetic determinants of cancer

Most cancers are the result of a complex interaction between genetic factors and exposure to environmental carcinogens.

Environmental factors

Environmental triggers for cancer have mainly been identified through epidemiological studies. The principal known environmental causes are summarised in Box 20.1.

Smoking is established beyond doubt as a major cause of lung cancer. Similarly, most carcinomas of the cervix are related to infection with human papillomavirus (HPV subtypes 16 and 18). For carcinomas of the bowel and breast, epidemiology indicates an environmental component. For example, breast cancer incidence in women of Far Eastern origin remains low upon migration to a country with a Western lifestyle but rises in subsequent generations to levels similar to those observed in the host country residents. Possible environmental causes include diet (higher saturated fat and/or dairy intake), reproductive patterns (later first pregnancy) and lifestyle (increased use of artificial light and shift in diurnal rhythm).

Genetic factors

A number of inherited cancer syndromes are recognized, accounting for 5% to 10% of all cancers. They result from inherited mutations in genes regulating cell growth, cell death and apoptosis. Examples include the *BRCA1*, *BRCA2* and *AT* (ataxia telangiectasia) genes that cause breast and some other cancers, the *FAP* gene that causes bowel cancer and the *RB* gene that causes retinoblastoma. Although carriers of these mutations have a greatly elevated risk of cancer, none has 100% penetrance, and additional genetic and environmental factors also operate.

20.1 Environmental factors that predispose to cancer

Environmental aetiology	Processes	Diseases
Occupational exposure (see 'Radiation')	Dye and rubber manufacturing (aromatic amines)	Bladder cancer
	Plumbing, demolition, shipbuilding (asbestos)	Lung cancer, mesothelioma
	Vinyl chloride (PVC) manufacturing	Liver angiosarcoma
	Petroleum industry (benzene)	Acute leukaemia
Chemicals	Chemotherapy (e.g. melphalan)	AML
Cigarette smoking	Carcinogens in inhaled smoke	Lung and bladder cancer
Viral infection	EBV	Burkitt's lymphoma and nasopharyngeal cancer
	HPV	Cervical cancer
	HBV and HCV viruses	Hepatocellular carcinoma
Bacterial infection	*Helicobacter pylori*	Gastric MALT lymphomas, gastric cancer
Parasitic infection	Liver fluke (*Opisthorchis sinensis*)	Cholangiocarcinoma
	Schistosoma haematobium	Squamous bladder cancer
Dietary factors	Low-roughage/high-fat diet	Colonic cancer
	High nitrosamine intake	Gastric cancer
	Aflatoxin from *Aspergillus flavus*	Hepatocellular cancer
Radiation	UV exposure	Basal cell carcinoma
		Melanoma
		Nonmelanocytic skin cancer
	Nuclear fallout	Leukaemia, solid tumours
	Diagnostic exposure	Cholangiocarcinoma following Thorotrast usage
	Therapeutic radiotherapy	Medullary thyroid cancer
		Sarcoma
Inflammatory bowel disease	Ulcerative colitis	Colon cancer
Hormonal	Diethylstilbestrol	Vaginal cancer
	Oestrogens	Endometrial/breast cancer

20

20.2 ECOG performance status scale

0	Fully active, able to carry on all usual activities without restriction and without the aid of analgesics
1	Restricted in strenuous activity, but ambulatory and able to carry out light work or pursue a sedentary occupation. This group also contains patients who are fully active, as in grade 0, but only with the aid of analgesics
2	Ambulatory and capable of all self-care, but unable to work. Up and about more than 50% of waking hours
3	Capable of only limited self-care, confined to bed or chair more than 50% of waking hours
4	Completely disabled, unable to carry out any self-care and confined totally to bed or chair

Assessing and investigating a cancer patient

Clinical assessment

A full history should include questions about potential risk factors such as smoking and occupational exposures. A thorough clinical examination is essential to identify metastases, to discover any coexisting conditions that may affect the management plan and to determine the extent of disease, as assessed by staging investigations.

The overall fitness of a patient is assessed using the ECOG performance status scale (Box 20.2). The outcome for patients with a performance status of 3 or 4 is worse in almost all malignancies than for those with a status of 0 to 2, and this should inform the approach to treatment in individual patients.

Staging means determining the extent of the tumour by clinical examination, imaging and, in some cases, surgery. The outcome is recorded using a standard classification (Box 20.3) that guides treatment decisions, indicates prognosis and allows comparisons to be made between different groups of patients.

Immunohistochemistry of biopsies

IHC staining for tumour markers can provide useful diagnostic information and guide treatment decisions. Common examples include:

- **Oestrogen and progesterone receptors:** Indicate that the tumour may be sensitive to hormonal manipulation.
- **Alpha-fetoprotein (AFP) and human chorionic gonadotrophin (hCG);** Favour germ-cell tumours.
- **Prostatic specific antigen (PSA):** Favours prostate cancer.
- **Carcinoembryonic antigen, cytokeratin** and **epithelial membrane antigen (EMA):** These favour epithelial carcinomas.
- **HER2 receptor:** In breast cancer, high HER2 levels predict response to trastuzumab (Herceptin), an antibody to the HER2 receptor.
- **IHC of lymphoma biopsies:** Helpful in the diagnosis and classification of lymphomas.

i 20.3 TNM classification	
Extent of primary tumour*	
TX	Not assessed
T0	No tumour
T1, T2, T3, T4	Increases in primary tumour size or depth of invasion
Increased involvement of nodes*	
NX	Not assessed
N0	No nodal involvement
N1, N2, N3	Increases in involvement
Presence of metastases	
MX	Not assessed
M0	Not present
M1	Present

Exact criteria for size and region of nodal involvement have been defined for each anatomical site.

Imaging

Imaging is critical for locating the primary tumour, staging the disease and determining the response to treatment. The various modalities are complementary:

- *Ultrasound* is useful for lesions in the liver, kidney, pancreas and reproductive organs. It is also used for guiding biopsies in breast and liver. Endoscopic ultrasound is helpful in staging upper gastrointestinal and pancreatic cancers.
- *CT* is particularly useful in imaging the thorax and abdomen. With modern scanners it is possible to detect colorectal cancers and adenomas ≥ 10 mm diameter.
- *MRI* is the preferred technique for brain and pelvic imaging, and is widely employed to stage rectal, cervical and prostate cancers.
- *Positron emission tomography (PET)* visualises metabolic activity of tumour cells and is widely used, often in combination with CT (PET–CT), to evaluate the extent of the disease, particularly potential distant metastasis.

Biochemical markers

20

Many cancers produce circulating substances called tumour markers. Unfortunately, most are neither sufficiently sensitive nor sufficiently specific to be used in isolation for diagnosis. Some are useful in population screening, diagnosis, determining prognosis, response evaluation, detection of relapse and imaging of metastasis. Tumour markers in routine use are outlined in Box 20.4.

20.4 Commonly used serum tumour markers

Name	Natural occurrence	Tumours
Alpha-fetoprotein	Found in yolk sac and fetal liver tissue. Transient elevation in liver diseases	Ovarian nonseminomatous germ cell tumour (80%), testicular teratoma (80%), hepatocellular cancer (50%)
Beta-2-microglobulin	On surface of lymphocytes, macrophages, some epithelial cells	Non-Hodgkin's lymphoma, myeloma
Calcitonin	Peptide from C cells of thyroid. Used to screen for MEN 2	Medullary cell carcinoma of thyroid
CA-125	Raised in any cause of ascites, pleural effusion or heart failure. Can be raised in inflammatory conditions	Ovarian epithelial cancer (75%), GI cancer (10%), lung cancer (5%) breast cancer (5%)
CA-19.9	Found in epithelium of fetal stomach, intestine and pancreas. Eliminated only via bile; any cholestasis can cause rise	Pancreatic cancer (80%), mucinous tumour of ovary (65%), gastric cancer (30%), colon cancer (30%)
Carcinoembryonic antigen	Found in intestinal mucosa during embryonic and fetal life. Elevated in smokers, cirrhosis, chronic hepatitis, ulcerative colitis, pneumonia	Colorectal cancer, especially with liver metastasis, gastric, breast and lung cancer, mucinous cancer of ovary
Human chorionic gonadotrophin	Hormone from placental syncytiotrophoblasts. Used for disease monitoring in hydatidiform mole and as a pregnancy test	Choriocarcinoma (100%), hydatidiform mole (97%), ovarian nonseminomatous germ cell tumour (50%–80%), seminoma (15%)
Placental alkaline phosphatase	Isoenzyme of alkaline phosphatase	Seminoma (40%), ovarian dysgerminoma (50%)
Prostate-specific antigen	A serine protease that liquefies semen in the prostate. Can be raised in benign prostatic hypertrophy and prostatitis	Prostate cancer (95%)
Thyroglobulin	Matrix protein for thyroid hormone synthesis in normal thyroid follicles	Papillary and follicular thyroid cancer

20.5 Nonmetastatic manifestations of malignant disease

Feature	Common cancer site associations
Weight loss and anorexia	Lung, gastrointestinal tract
Fatigue	Any
Hypercalcaemia	Myeloma, breast, kidney
Prothrombotic tendency	Ovary, pancreas, gastrointestinal tract
Syndrome of inappropriate antidiuretic hormone secretion (SIADH) Ectopic ACTH	Small cell lung cancer (SCLC)
Lambert-Eaton myasthenic syndrome	SCLC
Subacute cerebellar degeneration	SCLC, ovarian cancer
Acanthosis nigricans	Stomach, oesophagus
Dermatomyositis/polymyositis	Stomach, lung

Presenting problems in oncology

In the early stages of cancer, the tumour is small, and the patient is usually asymptomatic. With progression, localised signs or symptoms develop because of mass effects and/or invasion of local tissues. Later, symptoms may occur at distant sites as a result of metastatic disease or from non-metastatic manifestations because of production of biologically active hormones by the tumour (Box 20.5) or as the result of an immune response to the tumour.

Palpable mass

A palpable mass detected by the patient or physician may be the first sign of cancer. Primary tumours of the thyroid, breast, testis and skin are often detected in this way, whereas palpable lymph nodes in the neck, groin or axilla may indicate secondary spread. Hepatomegaly may be the first sign of primary liver cancer or tumour metastasis, whereas skin cancer may present as an enlarging or changing pigmented lesion.

Weight loss and fever

20

Unintentional weight loss is a characteristic feature of advanced cancer, but can have other causes such as thyrotoxicosis, chronic inflammatory disease and chronic infection. Fever can occur in any cancer secondary to infection, but may be a primary feature in lymphoma, leukaemia, renal and liver cancers. The presence of unexplained weight loss or fever warrants investigation to exclude occult malignancy.

Thromboembolism

Thrombosis and disseminated intravascular coagulation are common complications of cancer. Cancer cells activate the coagulation system via factors such as tissue factor, cancer procoagulant and inflammatory cytokines. Thrombus formation may occur as part of a host response to the cancer (i.e., acute phase, inflammation, angiogenesis) or via a reduction in the levels of inhibitors of coagulation or impairment of fibrinolysis. This prothrombotic tendency can be enhanced by therapy such as surgery, chemotherapy, hormone therapy and radiotherapy, and by in-dwelling venous catheters. In some patients, the thromboembolism is the first presenting feature of the underlying cancer.

Ectopic hormone production

Cancer may sometimes present with a metabolic abnormality as a result of ectopic production of hormones by tumour cells, including insulin, ACTH, vasopressin (ADH), fibroblast growth factor (FGF)-23, erythropoietin and parathyroid hormone-related protein (PTHrP) This can result in a wide variety of presentations (Box 20.6).

Neurological paraneoplastic syndromes

These syndromes are thought to be caused by an immunological response to the tumour that damages nerves or muscles. The most common underlying cancers are lung, pancreas, breast, prostate, ovary and lymphoma.

- **Peripheral neuropathy** results from axonal degeneration or demyelination.
- **Encephalomyelitis** presents with diverse symptoms, depending on the location of lesions. Lumbar puncture shows raised CSF protein and lymphocytic pleocytosis. MRI shows meningeal enhancement, and serum anti-Hu antibodies may be present. Small cell lung cancer is the usual cause (75%).

i	**20.6 Ectopic hormone production by tumours**	
Hormone	**Consequence**	**Tumours**
ACTH	Cushing's syndrome	SCLC
Erythropoietin	Polycythaemia	Kidney, hepatoma, cerebellar haemangioblastoma, uterine fibroids
FGF-23	Hypophosphataemic osteomalacia	Mesenchymal tumours
PTHrP	Hypercalcaemia	Squamous cell lung cancer, breast, kidney
Vasopressin (ADH)	Hyponatraemia	SCLC

- *Cerebellar degeneration:* The rapid onset of cerebellar ataxia may be the presenting feature of underlying malignancy. MRI or CT show cerebellar atrophy. Patients may have circulating anti-Yo, Tr and Hu antibodies, but these are nonspecific and may be negative.
- *Retinopathy* rarely complicates cancer, causing blurred vision, episodic visual loss, impaired colour vision and ultimately blindness. The electroretinogram is abnormal, and antiretinal antibodies are present.
- *Lambert-Eaton myasthenic syndrome* causes proximal muscle weakness that improves on exercise. Underlying cancer is present in about 60% of cases. Diagnosis is by EMG.
- *Dermatomyositis* or *polymyositis* (p. 627) may be the presenting feature of some cancers.

Cutaneous manifestations of cancer

Nonmetastatic skin manifestations of cancer include:

- *Pruritus:* lymphoma, leukaemia, CNS tumours.
- *Acanthosis nigricans:* may precede gastric cancers by years.
- *Vitiligo:* malignant melanoma.
- *Pemphigus:* lymphoma, Kaposi's sarcoma, thymoma.
- *Dermatitis herpetiformis:* gastrointestinal lymphoma.

Chapter 18 describes the clinical features and management of these skin conditions.

Emergency complications of cancer

Spinal cord compression

This complicates 5% of cancers, most commonly myeloma, prostate, breast and lung cancers with bony metastases. It often results from posterior extension of a vertebral body mass, but intrathecal metastases also occur.

Clinical features

Symptoms start with back pain, particularly on coughing and lying flat. Cord compression then causes sensory loss in distal dermatomes and weakness distal to the block. Finally, urinary retention and bowel incontinence develop. The thoracic region is most commonly affected, causing upper motor neuron signs, but lumbar spine involvement may cause nerve root compression with predominant lower motor neuron signs.

Management

Cord compression is an emergency. Management involves:

• Confirming the diagnosis with an urgent MRI scan. • Administering high-dose glucocorticoids: dexamethasone 16 mg IV stat then 8 mg twice daily orally. • Providing adequate analgesia. • Referring the patient for surgical decompression or urgent radiotherapy.

Neurosurgery produces superior outcome and survival compared with radiotherapy alone, and should be considered first for all patients. Radiotherapy is used for the remaining patients in cancer types likely to be radiosensitive. Prognosis depends on tumour type, but the neurological deficit at presentation is the strongest predictor of outcome.

20

▋ Superior vena cava obstruction

SVCO is a common complication of cancer that can occur through extrinsic compression or intravascular blockage. Extrinsic compression is usually caused by lung cancer, lymphoma or metastatic tumours. Intrinsic obstruction occurs with thrombus around a central catheter or thromboembolism secondary to cancer.

Clinical features

The patient develops oedema of the arms, face and neck, distended neck and arm veins and dusky skin over the face, arms and neck. Collateral vessels develop on the chest wall over a few weeks. Headache caused by cerebral oedema may occur and is aggravated by bending or lying down.

Investigations and management

CT thorax confirms the diagnosis and distinguishes between extra- and intravascular causes. A tumour biopsy is important to guide treatment. Very chemosensitive tumours (e.g. germ cell tumours and lymphoma) are treated with chemotherapy alone, but for other tumours radiotherapy is required. This relieves symptoms within 2 weeks in 50% to 90% of patients. Stenting is a useful alternative, as it works rapidly even with chemo- or radio-resistant tumours. Initial treatment should be followed by treatment of the primary tumour, as long-term outcome depends strongly on the prognosis of the underlying cancer.

▋ Hypercalcaemia

Hypercalcaemia is the commonest cancer-related metabolic disorder, with a prevalence of up to 20% in cancer patients. The incidence is highest in myeloma and breast cancer (approximately 40%), intermediate in non-small cell lung cancer and low in colon, prostate and small cell lung carcinomas. It is most commonly caused by PTHrP (80%), which stimulates osteoclastic bone resorption and increases renal calcium reabsorption. Bone metastases account for around 20% of cases. Mechanisms such as ectopic PTH secretion are rare.

Clinical features

The symptoms of hypercalcaemia are nonspecific, including drowsiness, delirium, nausea and vomiting, constipation, polyuria, polydipsia and dehydration.

Investigations and management

Measure the serum total calcium, adjusting for albumin (which is often low in cancer). Management requires:

• IV 0.9% saline 2 to 4 L/day • Zoledronic acid 4 mg IV *or* pamidronate 60 to 90 mg IV • In severe symptomatic hypercalcaemia refractory to zoledronic acid, denosumab (initially 60 mg subcutaneous, repeat dosing based on response) is an alternative

Bisphosphonates will usually normalise serum calcium within 5 days, but if not, treatment can be repeated, with maintenance infusions given 3 to 4 times weekly to outpatients.

Neutropenic fever

Neutropenia is common in malignancy, resulting from chemotherapy, radiotherapy if bone marrow is irradiated or malignant infiltration of the bone marrow. Neutropenic fever is defined as a pyrexia of 38°C for more than 1 hour in a patient with neutrophils of less than 0.5×10^9/L or less than 1.0×10^9/L if the nadir is expected to be less than 0.5×10^9/L in the next 24 hours. The risk of sepsis is related to the severity and duration of neutropenia and the presence of risk factors such as IV cannulae or bladder catheters. Neutropenic fever is an emergency that, if untreated, carries a high mortality.

Clinical features

Presentation is with high fever and nonspecific malaise. Examination is usually unhelpful, although hypotension signifies poor prognosis and may progress to shock and organ failure.

Investigations and management

An infection screen should be requested, including peripheral and central line blood cultures, urine culture, CXR and throat, central line and wound swabs. Empirical IV antibiotics are given pending culture results. Antibiotic choice is based on local guidelines and resistance patterns. Piperacillin–tazobactam or meropenem are used commonly, either alone or with gentamicin. Metronidazole is added for suspected anaerobic infection, and teicoplanin for suspected Gram-positive infection (e.g. patients with central lines). Antibiotics should be reviewed after culture results or if there is no response within 36 to 48 hours. Liposomal amphotericin B should be considered for antifungal cover. Granulocyte–colony-stimulating factor (G–CSF) is not used routinely in neutropenia. Supportive therapy with IV fluids, inotropes, ventilation or haemofiltration, may be required.

Tumour lysis syndrome

This refers to the metabolic sequelae following the acute destruction of a large number of cells during cancer treatment. It is usually seen with bulky, chemosensitive disease, including lymphoma, leukaemia and germ cell tumours.

Clinical features

Release of cellular contents causes transient hypocalcaemia, hyperphosphataemia, hyperuricaemia and hyperkalaemia. Acute renal impairment may occur with precipitation of uric acid crystals in the renal tubular system. Symptoms associated with the multiple electrolyte abnormalities include fatigue, nausea, vomiting, arrhythmias, heart failure, syncope, tetany, seizures and sudden death.

Investigations and management

Monitor serum biochemistry regularly for 48 to 72 hours after treatment in patients at risk. Pretreatment serum LDH correlates with tumour bulk and indicates increased risk. Elevated potassium is an early feature. Risk can be reduced by maintaining generous hydration and urine output and by using prophylactic allopurinol or recombinant urate oxidase (rasburicase) to reduce uric acid levels. If normal treatment fails, haemodialysis may be required.

20

Metastatic disease

Metastatic disease is the major cause of mortality and morbidity in cancer patients. In most cases treatment is palliative; however, treatment of a solitary metastasis is occasionally curative.

Brain metastases

Brain metastases occur in 10% to 30% of adults and 6% to 10% of children with cancer, causing significant morbidity. Lung and breast are the tumours which metastasise most commonly to the brain.

Clinical features

Presentation is with headaches (40%–50%), focal neurological dysfunction (20%–40%), cognitive dysfunction (35%), seizures (10%–20%) and papill-oedema (<10%).

Investigations and management

Diagnosis is by CT or contrast-enhanced MRI. In solitary brain metastasis, surgery and adjuvant radiotherapy can increase survival. In patients with multiple brain metastases, median survival untreated is approximately 1 month. Uncontrolled trials suggest glucocorticoids (dexamethasone 4 mg four times daily) can increase survival to 2 to 3 months, and whole-brain radiotherapy improves survival to 3 to 6 months. Anticonvulsants may be required to control seizures. Prognosis is better in those with brain metastases from breast cancer or from an undetected primary tumour.

Lung metastases

These are common in breast, colon and renal cancer and tumours of the head and neck. Diagnosis is usually by CXR or CT. Solitary lesions require investigation p. 311 to exclude a primary lung tumour. Patients with two or more pulmonary nodules are assumed to have metastases. Treatment depends on the extent and type of disease; for solitary lesions, surgery may be considered.

Liver metastases

Liver metastases can be the life-limiting component of disease in colorectal cancer, ocular melanoma, neuro-endocrine tumours and other tumours. Presentations include right upper quadrant pain, jaundice, deranged liver function or abnormal imaging. In selected cases, resection, chemoembolisation or radiofrequency ablation of metastases improve survival. If these are not feasible, symptoms may respond to systemic chemotherapy.

Bone metastases

Bone is the third most common metastatic site, after lung and liver. Bone metastases are a major problem in patients with myeloma, breast or prostate cancers, but are also seen with kidney, thyroid and other cancers.

Clinical features

The main presentations are pain, pathological fracture and spinal cord compression (see earlier). The pain is often progressive and worst at night and is initially reduced by activity but later becomes constant and exacerbated by movement. Pathological fractures are most common with breast cancer.

Investigations and management

The most sensitive test for bone metastases is isotope bone scanning; however, this can be falsely positive in healing bone and falsely negative in multiple myeloma. Plain X-rays should be taken for bone pain, as some lytic lesions may not be detected on bone scan. In patients with a single lesion, a biopsy is required, as primary bone tumours may resemble metastases on X-ray.

The goals of management are:

• Pain relief. • Preservation and restoration of function. • Skeletal stabilisation. • Local tumour control.

Surgery may be needed for skeletal instability (e.g. spinal fracture or a large lytic lesion in a weight-bearing bone). Intravenous bisphosphonates (e.g. pamidronate) are effective at improving pain and hypercalcaemia and reducing fractures. In breast and prostate cancer, hormonal therapy may be effective. Radiotherapy can also be useful. In breast carcinoma, chemotherapy may be used in the management of bony metastases.

Malignant pleural effusion and ascites

Management of these important complications of cancer is described elsewhere (p. 316 and 503).

Therapeutics in oncology

The approach to anticancer therapy depends on the specific goal:

- **Palliative chemotherapy** is used to treat patients with metastatic disease. The goal is an improvement in symptoms and quality of life, so treatment should be well tolerated with minimum adverse effects.
- **Adjuvant chemotherapy** is given after an initial intervention designed to remove all macroscopic disease. Chemotherapy is then given to attempt eradication of any remaining micrometastatic disease. The goal is an improvement in survival.
- **Neoadjuvant chemotherapy** is where chemotherapy is given before a planned major treatment. This may reduce the scale of surgery required, shorten hospitalisation and improve the fitness of the patient before interval debulking. The goal is increased survival.
- **Chemoprevention** is the use of medication to prevent cancer developing in patients identified as being at particular risk.

Surgery in cancer

Biopsy

For accurate diagnosis of cancer, a biopsy is necessary. Although cytology can be obtained with fine needle aspiration, a solid biopsy is usually preferred. This can be a core biopsy, an image-guided biopsy or an excision biopsy.

Excision

Surgical excision offers the best chance of cure in early, localised colorectal, breast and lung cancer. The appropriate selection of cases should be guided

20

by multidisciplinary teams involving surgeons who are expert in the particular cancer. This is especially true for prostate and transitional cell carcinoma of the bladder, in which radiotherapy and surgery may be equally effective.

Palliation

Surgery may be effective in palliating symptoms, for example, the treatment of faecal incontinence with a defunctioning colostomy, fixation of pathological fractures, decompression of spinal cord compression and the treatment of fungating skin lesions.

Systemic chemotherapy

Chemotherapeutic drugs have their greatest activity in proliferating cells, but are not specific for cancer cells, and their side effects result from their antiproliferative actions in normal tissues such as the bone marrow, skin and gut.

Combination therapy

The dosing schedule and interval are determined by the choice of drugs and recovery of the cancer and normal tissues. Commonly, chemotherapy is administered in cycles every 21 or 28 days, repeated for up to six cycles. Changing treatments can increase the effectiveness, but may increase toxicity too, and such developments are evaluated in clinical trials.

- **Low-dose therapy** is usual for palliative chemotherapy. Cycles are repeated after marrow recovery (neutrophils $>1.0 \times 10^9$/L and platelets $>100 \times 10^9$/L).
- **High-dose therapy** is used to achieve a higher cell kill but results in more marrow toxicity. This can be minimised using G–CSF. This approach allows more drug to be delivered, at the cost of greater toxicity.
- **Dose-dense therapy** involves fractionating the intended dose and administering each fraction more frequently (e.g. weekly). Each dose produces less toxicity, but the anticancer effect is related to the accumulative dose over time.
- **Alternating therapy** involves alternating different drugs. Most commonly used with haematological malignancies, it is designed to treat different subpopulations of cancer cells.

Adverse effects

Most cytotoxics have a narrow therapeutic window with significant adverse effects (Fig. 20.1). Nausea and vomiting are common, but with modern antiemetic regimens, such as the combination of dexamethasone and ondansetron, most patients now tolerate chemotherapy well. Myelosuppression is common to all cytotoxics, and this limits doses and can cause life-threatening complications. Neutropenia can be limited by growth factors such as G–CSF that accelerate the repopulation of myeloid precursor cells. More recently, G–CSF has been used successfully to 'accelerate' chemotherapy where the rate-limiting factor was previously the peripheral neutrophil recovery time.

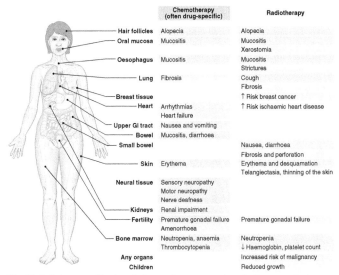

	Chemotherapy (often drug-specific)	Radiotherapy
Hair follicles	Alopecia	Alopecia
Oral mucosa	Mucositis	Mucositis Xerostomia
Oesophagus	Mucositis	Mucositis Strictures
Lung	Fibrosis	Cough Fibrosis
Breast tissue		↑ Risk breast cancer
Heart	Arrhythmias Heart failure	↑ Risk ischaemic heart disease
Upper GI tract	Nausea and vomiting	
Bowel	Mucositis, diarrhoea	
Small bowel		Nausea, diarrhoea Fibrosis and perforation
Skin	Erythema	Erythema and desquamation Telangiectasia, thinning of the skin
Neural tissue	Sensory neuropathy Motor neuropathy Nerve deafness	
Kidneys	Renal impairment	
Fertility	Premature gonadal failure Amenorrhoea	Premature gonadal failure
Bone marrow	Neutropenia, anaemia Thrombocytopenia	Neutropenia ↓ Haemoglobin, platelet count
Any organs		Increased risk of malignancy
Children		Reduced growth

Fig. 20.1 Adverse effects of chemotherapy and radiotherapy. Acute effects are shown in pink and late effects in blue.

Radiation therapy

Radiotherapy involves treating the cancer with ionising radiation; for certain localised cancers, it may be curative. Ionising radiation can be delivered using radioactive isotopes or by high-energy radiation beams, usually X-rays. Three methods are usually employed:

- **Teletherapy:** application from a distance by a linear accelerator.
- **Brachytherapy:** direct application of a radioactive source to a tumour, delivering very high, localised radiation doses. Used for localised cancers of the head and neck, cervix and endometrium.
- **Intravenous radioisotope:** for example, [131]iodine for cancer of the thyroid and [89]strontium for the treatment of bone metastases from prostate cancer.

Most treatments are delivered by linear accelerators, which produce high energy electron or X-ray beams. These cause lethal and sublethal damage to DNA. Treatment is targeted using CT and MRI images to maximise exposure of the tumour and minimise exposure of normal tissues. In addition, conformal radiotherapy uses shaped beams to allow more precise targeting of the tumour and reduce normal tissue exposure.

Fractionation (delivering the radiation in small daily doses) allows normal cells to recover from radiation damage whereas lesser recovery occurs in malignant cells. Radical treatments may entail doses given 5 days a week for 4-6 weeks, totalling 20-30 fractions. whereas for palliative treatments a smaller number of fractions (1–5) is usually adequate.

20

Both normal and malignant tissues vary widely in their sensitivity to radio-therapy. Germ cell tumours and lymphomas are extremely radiosensitive, but most cancers require doses close to or beyond that which can be tolerated by adjacent normal structures. Normal tissue also varies in its radio-sensitivity, with the central nervous system, small bowel and lung being among the most sensitive.

Adverse effects

The side effects of radiotherapy (Fig. 20.1) depend on the normal tissues affected, their radiosensitivity and the dose delivered. A localised acute inflammatory reaction commonly occurs towards the end of most radical treatments. For example, skin reactions are common with breast or chest wall radiotherapy, and proctitis and cystitis with treatment to the bladder or prostate. Late effects developing 6 weeks or more after radiotherapy occur in 5% to 10% of patients. Examples include brachial nerve damage and subcutaneous or pulmonary fibrosis after breast cancer treatment, and shrinkage and fibrosis of the bladder after treatment for bladder cancer. There is a risk of inducing cancer after radiotherapy.

Hormone therapy

This is most commonly used in the treatment of breast and prostate cancer. Breast tumours that are positive for oestrogen receptors respond to anti-oestrogen therapy. Drugs that reduce oestrogen levels or block the effects of oestrogen on the receptor reduce relapse rates and death at least as much as chemotherapy, and in advanced cases can induce stability and remissions lasting months to years.

In prostate cancer, the luteinising hormone-releasing hormone (LHRH) analogue goserelin and/or the antiandrogen bicalutamide reduce androgen levels and provide good long-term control of advanced disease, but are unproven following potentially curative surgery.

Progestogen treatment is associated with response rates of 20% to 40% in metastatic endometrial cancer. In breast cancer, progestogens are used in patients whose disease has progressed despite antioestrogen therapy.

Immunotherapy

Stimulating the patient's immune system with interferons can sometimes alter the natural history of a malignancy. Although solid tumours show little benefit, interferons are active in melanoma and lymphoma, and may be beneficial as adjuvants (after surgery and chemotherapy, respectively) to delay recurrence.

Rituximab is strikingly effective immunotherapy, increasing complete response rates and improving survival in diffuse large cell non-Hodgkin's lymphoma when combined with chemotherapy. It is also effective in palliating advanced follicular non-Hodgkin's lymphoma (p. 579).

Biological therapies

Novel treatments designed to block the signalling pathways responsible for the growth of specific tumours are emerging.

Gefitinib/Erlotinib

These agents inhibit the activity of the EGFR, which is over-expressed in many solid tumours.

Imatinib

Imatinib was developed to inhibit the *BCR-ABL* gene product, tyrosine kinase, that is responsible for chronic myeloid leukaemia (p. 576), which it does extremely effectively.

Bevacizumab

This antibody inhibits VEGF-A, a key stimulant of angiogenesis in tumours. It has activity in colorectal, lung, breast, renal and ovarian cancers.

Trastuzumab

Trastuzumab (Herceptin) targets *HER2*, an oncogene that is over-expressed in some breast and gastric cancers. It is effective as a single-agent therapy, and is also used in conjunction with chemotherapy. Cardiac failure is an important side effect.

Evaluation of treatment

The evaluation of treatment involves the assessment of overall survival duration, response to treatment, remission rate, disease-free survival and response duration, quality of life and treatment toxicity. Criteria have been established to categorise response (e.g. RECIST, Box 20.7).

Late toxicity of therapy

Late toxicities are particularly important for young patients who are living longer after intense multimodality therapy. For example, radiotherapy can retard bone and cartilage growth; impair intellect and cognitive function;

i 20.7 Response evaluation criteria in solid tumours (RECIST)	
Response	**Criteria**
Complete response	Disappearance of all target lesions
Partial response	At least a 30% decrease in the sum of the longest diameter of target lesions, taking as reference the baseline sum longest diameter
Progressive disease	At least a 20% increase in the sum of the longest diameter of target lesions, taking as reference the smallest sum longest diameter recorded since the treatment started and at least a 5 mm increase or the appearance of one or more new lesions
Stable disease	Neither sufficient shrinkage to qualify for partial response nor sufficient increase to qualify for progressive disease, taking as reference the smallest sum longest diameter since the treatment started

20

and cause dysfunction of the hypothalamus, pituitary and thyroid. Late consequences of chemotherapy include heart failure as a result of cardiotoxicity, pulmonary fibrosis, nephrotoxicity and neurotoxicity.

Premature gonadal failure can result from chemotherapy or radiotherapy and leave a patient subfertile. Patients should be made aware of this before treatment is initiated, and sperm or egg storage should be offered before treatment starts. Erectile dysfunction is seen in patients receiving high radiotherapy doses to the pelvis, as in prostate cancer. Infertility and pubertal delay are potential late effects of therapy in children, especially boys. Additional social or psychological support may be required.

Second malignancies may be induced by cancer treatment and occur at greatest frequency following chemoradiation. Secondary acute leukaemia (mostly AML) can occur 1 to 2 years after chemotherapy, and osteosarcoma, soft tissue sarcoma and leukaemia after radiotherapy.

Specific cancers

The diagnosis and management of many organ-specific cancers are covered in the relevant chapters. Here we discuss the approach to common tumours not covered elsewhere.

Breast cancer

Globally, the incidence of breast cancer is second only to lung cancer, and it is the leading cause of cancer deaths in women. Invasive ductal carcinoma with or without ductal carcinoma in situ (DCIS) accounts for 70% of cases, whereas invasive lobular carcinoma accounts for most other cases. DCIS constitutes 20% of breast cancers detected by mammography screening. One third are multifocal and it carries a high risk of becoming invasive. Pure DCIS does not cause lymph node metastases. Lobular carcinoma *in situ* predisposes towards developing cancer in either breast (7% at 10 years). The staging and survival of breast cancer are shown in Box 20.8.

Pathogenesis

Both genetic and hormonal factors are important: 5% to 10% of breast cancers are associated with inherited mutations in *BRCA1*, *BRCA2*, *AT* or *TP53*. Prolonged oestrogen exposure associated with early menarche, late

i	**20.8 5-year survival rates for breast cancer by stage**	
Tumour stage	Stage definition	5-year survival (%)
I	Tumour <2 cm, no lymph nodes	96
II	Tumour 2–5 cm and/or mobile axillary lymph nodes	81
III	Chest wall or skin fixation and/or fixed axillary lymph nodes	52
IV	Metastasis	18

menopause and use of HRT is associated with increased risk. Other risk factors include obesity, alcohol, nulliparity and late first pregnancy. There is no definite evidence linking the contraceptive pill to breast cancer.

Clinical features

Breast cancer usually presents following mammographic screening or as a palpable mass with nipple discharge in 10% and pain in 7% of patients. Presentation with diffuse skin induration is less common and carries an adverse prognosis. Some 40% of patients (mainly larger primary tumours) have axillary nodal disease. Distant metastases occur to bone (70%), lung (60%), liver (55%), pleura (40%), adrenals (35%), skin (30%) and brain (10%–20%).

Investigations

Following clinical examination, patients should have mammography or ultrasound, and an aspiration biopsy for cytology or core biopsy for histology. Biopsies are examined for tumour type, ER and progesterone receptor status and HER2 status. If metastasis is suspected, CT thorax and abdomen and an isotope bone scan are required.

Management

Surgery (lumpectomy or mastectomy) is the principal treatment for most patients. Local excision is as effective as mastectomy if negative resection margins can be achieved. Lymph nodes are also sampled during surgery. Adjuvant radiotherapy is given to reduce the risk of local recurrence to 4% to 6%. Adjuvant hormonal therapy improves disease-free and overall survival in patients with ER-positive tumours. Patients at low risk with small ER-positive tumours should receive tamoxifen. If they are premenopausal they should receive an LHRH analogue.

Adjuvant chemotherapy is offered to patients at higher risk of recurrence (tumour >1 cm, ER-positive or involved axillary nodes). Adjuvant trastuzumab (monoclonal antibody to HER2) should be given in addition to chemotherapy for women with early HER2-positive breast cancer.

Metastatic disease management includes radiotherapy for painful bone metastases and aromatase inhibitors, which inhibit adrenal and adipose oestrogen production. Advanced ER-negative disease may be treated with combination chemotherapy.

Ovarian cancer

Ovarian cancer is the most common gynaecological tumour in Western countries. Some 90% are epithelial in origin, and up to 7% have a positive family history. Patients often present late with vague abdominal discomfort, low back pain, bloating, altered bowel habit and weight loss. Occasionally, peritoneal deposits are palpable as an omental 'cake' and nodules in the umbilicus.

Pathogenesis

The risk of ovarian cancer is increased with *BRCA1* or *BRCA2* mutations, and Lynch type II families have ovarian, endometrial, colorectal and gastric tumours. Advanced age, nulliparity, ovarian stimulation and Caucasian descent all increase risk, whereas suppressed ovulation (pregnancy, prolonged breastfeeding, contraceptive pill) appears to protect.

20

Investigations

USS and CT imaging are fundamental. Serum CA-125 is elevated. Surgery is important in the diagnosis, staging and treatment of ovarian cancer, and in early cases, palpation of viscera, peritoneal washings and biopsies are performed to define disease extent.

Management

In early disease, surgery (tumour excision, total abdominal hysterectomy, bilateral salpingo-oophorectomy and omentectomy) followed by adjuvant chemotherapy with carboplatin with or without paclitaxel is standard treatment. In advanced disease, debulking surgery is undertaken, followed by adjuvant chemotherapy with carboplatin and paclitaxel. Bevacizumab is indicated for patients with high-grade tumours. Monitoring for relapse includes CA-125, clinical examination and CT imaging as required. Second-line chemotherapy is aimed at improving symptoms.

Endometrial cancer

Endometrial cancer accounts for 4% of all female malignancies and presents with postmenopausal bleeding.

Pathogenesis

The duration of oestrogen exposure is important, so nulliparity, early menarche, late menopause and unopposed HRT increase the risk. Obesity is also a risk factor.

Investigations

The diagnosis is by endometrial biopsy.

Management

Surgery (hysterectomy and bilateral salpingo-oophorectomy, peritoneal cytology and lymph node sampling) is used for staging and treatment. For more invasive tumours, adjuvant pelvic radiotherapy is recommended. Adjuvant chemotherapy and hormonal therapy are also used in advanced disease.

Cervical cancer

This is the second most common gynaecological tumour worldwide and the leading cause of death from gynaecological cancer. The usual presentation is an abnormal smear test, but locally advanced disease can present with vaginal bleeding, discomfort or discharge or with bladder, rectal or pelvic wall symptoms. Occasionally, patients present with bone and lung metastases.

Pathogenesis

Cervical cancer is strongly associated with sex at a young age, multiple sexual partners and infection with HPV. Teenagers in the UK are now routinely immunized against HPV.

Investigations

Diagnosis is by smear or cone biopsy. Cystoscopy and sigmoidoscopy are indicated if there are symptoms of bladder, colon or rectal involvement. MRI is often used to characterise the primary tumour. A CXR is performed to detect pulmonary metastasis. CT abdomen and pelvis is performed to look for liver metastasis and lymph nodes, hydronephrosis and hydroureter.

Management

This depends on stage:

- **Premalignant disease:** laser ablation or diathermy.
- **Microinvasive disease:** loop excision of the transformation zone or simple hysterectomy.
- **Invasive but localised disease:** radical surgery.

Chemotherapy and radiotherapy, including brachytherapy, may be given as primary treatment, especially in patients with bulky or locally advanced disease, or lymph node or parametrium invasion. In metastatic disease, cisplatin-based chemotherapy may improve symptoms, but does not increase survival significantly.

Head and neck tumours

Head and neck cancers are typically squamous tumours arising in the nasopharynx, hypopharynx and larynx. They are most common in elderly males, but oropharyngeal cancers are increasing in younger ages, including women. Presentation depends on the site and extent of the primary tumour (Box 20.9).

20.9 Common presenting features by location in head and neck cancer

Hypopharynx

- Dysphagia
- Odynophagia
- Referred otalgia
- Enlarged lymph nodes

Mouth

- Nonhealing ulcers
- Ipsilateral otalgia

Nasal cavity and sinuses

- Discharge (bloody) or obstruction

Nasopharynx

- Nasal discharge or obstruction
- Conduction deafness
- Atypical facial pain
- Diplopia
- Hoarse voice
- Horner's syndrome

Oropharynx

- Dysphagia
- Pain
- Otalgia

Salivary gland

- Painless swelling
- Facial nerve palsy

20

Pathogenesis

The tumours are strongly associated with excessive use of alcohol and tobacco, but other risk factors include EBV for nasopharyngeal cancer and HPV infection for oropharyngeal tumours.

Investigations

This involves direct inspection and biopsy of the primary site, usually by endoscopy and examination under anaesthesia. CT of the primary site and the thorax is required to complete staging.

Management

In the absence of lymph node involvement, long-term remission can be achieved in 90% of patients with surgery or radiotherapy. The choice of treatment often depends on patient preference, as surgery can be cosmetically mutilating. Patients with lymph node involvement or metastasis receive combined surgery and radiotherapy (often with radiosensitising chemotherapy), resulting in long-term remission in around 60% to 70%. Palliative surgery, radiotherapy or chemotherapy are used for palliation in recurrent or metastatic tumour.

Carcinoma of unknown origin

Some patients are found to have metastatic disease at their initial presentation, before diagnosis of a primary site. Biopsy often reveals adenocarcinoma, but the primary site is not always clear.

Investigations

It is necessary to find a compromise between exhaustive investigation to find the primary tumour and obtaining sufficient information to plan appropriate management. Biopsy of an accessible metastasis is usually appropriate. Histology and immunohistochemistry may assist the pathologist in determining the primary site, therefore a biopsy is preferred over fine needle aspiration. A careful history (including familial) and examination should guide additional tests, including renal and liver function, tumour markers and CT of chest and abdomen. Endoscopy may be required for GI symptoms, and a myeloma screen if there are lytic bone lesions.

Management

Always ensure that a curable diagnosis has been excluded. For example, lung metastases in testicular teratoma do not preclude cure; nor do one to two liver metastases in colorectal cancer. A multidisciplinary oncology team may help to avoid unnecessary investigations; for example, an hCG-based pregnancy test in a young man with lung metastases might reveal a potentially curable teratoma. Palliative treatment with analgesia, surgery, radiotherapy or chemotherapy may help symptoms, and need not wait for a definitive diagnosis. Selected patients remain cancer-free for some years after resection of a single adenocarcinoma metastasis.

Multidisciplinary teams

Meeting regularly, multidisciplinary teams provide a valuable forum for patient-centred, interdisciplinary communication to coordinate care and decision making. They allow individual clinicians to discuss complex cases and draw on the collective experience of the team.

Specific roles of the multidisciplinary team include:

- planning diagnostic and staging procedures
- deciding the appropriate primary treatment
- arranging assessment of the patient by the oncology team before chemotherapy or radiotherapy
- identifying the additional needs of the patient, for example, physiotherapy, psychological support, symptom control, nutritional care or postoperative rehabilitation
- ensuring patient access to accurate information on treatment, prognosis, side effects, and so on
- coordinating follow-up
- when appropriate, guiding transition from curative to palliative treatment
- facilitating recruitment into clinical trials
- agreeing protocols to deliver high-quality care
- collecting and reviewing audit data to ensure quality care

Laboratory reference ranges

Units

SI units are a subset of the metre–kilogram–second system of units and were agreed on for everyday commercial and scientific work in 1960 by the International Bureau of Weights and Measures. SI units have been adopted widely in clinical laboratories, but non-SI units are still used in many countries. Therefore values in both SI and non-SI units are given for common measurements in this book. The SI unit system is, however, recommended.

Exceptions to the use of SI units

Blood pressure: By convention, BP is excluded from the SI unit system and is measured in mmHg (millimetres of mercury).

Mass concentrations: Mass concentrations (such as g/L and μg/L) are used instead of molar concentrations for all protein measurements and for substances with insufficiently defined composition.

Bioassay: Some enzymes and hormones are measured by 'bioassay', in which the activity in the sample is compared with the activity (rather than the mass) of a standard sample from a central source. Bioassay results are given in standardised 'units' (U/L), or 'international units' (IU/L), which are derived from the activity in the standard sample.

Laboratory reference ranges in adults

The reference ranges quoted later (Boxes 21.1–21.7) are largely from the Departments of Clinical Biochemistry and Haematology, Lothian Health University Hospitals Division, Edinburgh, United Kingdom. Reference ranges vary between laboratories, depending on the assays used (especially enzyme assays). The origin of reference ranges and the interpretation of 'abnormal' results are discussed on p. 3. Collection requirements, which may be critical to obtaining a meaningful result, are specified by local laboratories according to assay requirements. Unless otherwise stated, reference ranges shown apply to adults; values in children may be different.

Many analytes can be measured in either serum (the supernatant of clotted blood) or plasma (the supernatant of anticoagulated blood); specific assay kits may require one or the other. Sometimes the distinction is critical (e.g. plasma is required to measure fibrinogen because it is largely absent from serum; serum is required for electrophoresis to detect paraproteins because fibrinogen migrates as a discrete band in the zone of interest).

21.1 Normal values for haematological blood tests

Analysis	Reference range	
	SI units	Non-SI units
Bleeding time (Ivy)	<8 mins	–
Blood volume		
Male	65–85 mL/kg	–
Female	60–80 mL/kg	–
Coagulation screen		
PT	10.5–13.5 secs	–
APTT	26–36 secs	–
D-dimers		
Interpret in relation to clinical presentation	<200 ng/mL	–
ESR[a]		
Adult male	0–10 mm/hour	–
Adult female	3–15 mm/hour	–
Ferritin		
Male (and postmenopausal female)	20–300 µg/L	20–300 ng/mL
Female (premenopausal)	15–200 µg/L	15–200 ng/mL
Fibrinogen	1.5–4.0 g/L	0.15–0.4 g/dL
Folate		
Serum	2.8–20 µg/L	2.8–20 ng/mL
Red cell	120–500 µg/L	120–500 ng/mL
Haemoglobin		
Male	130–180 g/L	13–18 g/dL
Female	115–165 g/L	11.5–16.5 g/dL
Haptoglobin	0.4–2.4 g/L	0.04–0.24 g/dL
Iron		
Male	14–32 µmol/L	78–178 µg/dL
Female	10–28 µmol/L	56–157 µg/dL
Leucocytes (adults)	$4.0–11.0 \times 10^9$/L	$4.0–11.0 \times 10^3$/mm^3

21.1 Normal values for haematological blood tests—cont'd

Analysis	Reference range SI units	Non-SI units
Differential white cell count		
Neutrophils	$2.0–7.5 \times 10^9$/L	$2.0–7.5 \times 10^3$/mm^3
Lymphocytes	$1.5–4.0 \times 10^9$/L	$1.5–4.0 \times 10^3$/mm^3
Monocytes	$0.2–0.8 \times 10^9$/L	$0.2–0.8 \times 10^3$/mm^3
Eosinophils	$0.04–0.4 \times 10^9$/L	$0.04–0.4 \times 10^3$/mm^3
Basophils	$0.01–0.1 \times 10^9$/L	$0.01–0.1 \times 10^3$/mm^3
Mean cell haemoglobin	27–32 pg	–
Mean cell volume	78–98 fl	–
Packed cell volume or haematocrit		
Male	0.40–0.54	–
Female	0.37–0.47	–
Platelets	$150–350 \times 10^9$/L	$150–350 \times 10^3$/mm^3
Red cell count		
Male	$4.5–6.5 \times 10^{12}$/L	$4.5–6.5 \times 10^6$/mm^3
Female	$3.8–5.8 \times 10^{12}$/L	$3.8–5.8 \times 10^6$/mm^3
Red cell lifespan		
Mean	120 days	–
Half-life (^{51}Cr)	25–35 days	–
Reticulocytes	$25–85 \times 10^9$/L	$25–85 \times 10^3$/mm^3
Transferrin	2.0–4.0 g/L	0.2–0.4 g/dL
Transferrin saturation		
Male	25%–50%	–
Female	14%–50%	–
Vitamin B$_{12}$		
Normal	>210 ng/L	–
Intermediate	180–200 ng/L	–
Low	<180 ng/L	–

[a]Higher values in older patients are not necessarily abnormal.

21

i	**21.2 Normal values for biochemical tests in venous blood**	
	Reference range	
Analyte	**SI units**	**Non-SI units**
α_1-antitrypsin	1.1–2.1 g/L	110–210 mg/dL
ALT	10–50 U/L	–
Albumin	35–50 g/L	3.5–5.0 g/dL
Alkaline phosphatase	40–125 U/L	–
Amylase	<100 U/L	–
AST	10–45 U/L	–
Bile acids (fasting)	<14 μmol/L	–
Bilirubin (total)	3–16 μmol/L	0.18–0.94 mg/dL
Caeruloplasmin	0.16–0.47 g/L	16–47 mg/dL
Calcium (total)	2.1–2.6 mmol/L	4.2–5.2 mEq/L or 8.5–10.5 mg/dL
Carboxyhaemoglobin[a]	0.1%–3.0%	–
Chloride	95–107 mmol/L	95–107 mEq/L
Cholesterol (total)	Ideal level varies according to cardiovascular risk (see cardiovascular risk chart, p. 294)	
HDL-cholesterol	Ideal level varies according to cardiovascular risk, so reference ranges can be misleading. The National Cholesterol Education Programme Adult Treatment Panel III defines low HDL-cholesterol as <1.0 mmol/L (<40 mg/dL)	
Complement		
C3	0.81–1.57 g/L	–
C4	0.13–1.39 g/L	–
Total haemolytic complement	0.086–0.410 g/L	–
Copper	10–22 μmol/L	64–140 μg/dL
C-reactive protein	<5 mg/L	
Creatine kinase; total		
Male	55–170 U/L	–
Female	30–135 U/L	–
CK MB isoenzyme	<6% of total CK	–
Creatinine		
Male	64–111 μmol/L	0.72–1.26 mg/dL
Female	50–98 μmol/L	0.57–1.11 mg/dL

21.2 Normal values for biochemical tests in venous blood—cont'd		
	Reference range	
Analyte	SI units	Non-SI units
GGT		
Male	10–55 U/L	–
Female	5–35 U/L	
Glucose (fasting)	3.6–5.8 mmol/L	65–104 mg/dL
HbA₁c	4.0%–6.0% 20–42 mmol/mol Hb	–
Immunoglobulins		
IgA	0.8–4.5 g/L	–
IgE	0–250 kU/L	–
IgG	6.0–15.0 g/L	–
IgM	0.35–2.90 g/L	–
Lactate	0.6–2.4 mmol/L	5.4–21.6 mg/dL
LDH; total	125–220 U/L	–
Lead	<0.5 µmol/L	<10 µg/dL
Magnesium	0.75–1.0 mmol/L	1.5–2.0 mEq/L or 1.82–2.43 mg/dL
Osmolality	280–296 mOsmol/kg	–
Osmolarity	280–296 mOsmol/L	–
Phosphate (fasting)	0.8–1.4 mmol/L	2.48–4.34 mg/dL
Potassium[b]	3.6–5.0 mmol/L	3.6–5.0 mEq/L
Protein (total)	60–80 g/L	6–8 g/dL
Sodium	135–145 mmol/L	135–145 mEq/L
Triglycerides (fasting)	0.6–1.7 mmol/L	53–150 mg/dL
Troponins	Interpretation of troponins I and T is covered on p. 282	
Tryptase	0–135 mg/L	–
Urate		
Male	0.12–0.42 mmol/L	2.0–7.0 mg/dL
Female	0.12–0.36 mmol/L	2.0–6.0 mg/dL
Urea	2.5–6.6 mmol/L	15–40 mg/dL
Vitamin D, 25(OH)D		
Normal	>50 nmol/L	>20 ng/mL
Insufficiency	25–50 nmol/L	10–20 ng/ml

continued

21

21.2 Normal values for biochemical tests in venous blood—cont'd

	Reference range	
Analyte	SI units	Non-SI units
Deficiency	<25 nmol/L	<10 ng/mL
Zinc	10–18 µmol/L	65–118 µg/dL

CO up to 8% may be found in heavy smokers.
Serum values are, on average, 0.3 mmol/L higher than plasma values.

21.3 Normal values in arterial blood

	Reference range	
Analysis	SI units	Non-SI units
PaO_2	12–15 kPa	90–113 mmHg
$PaCO_2$	4.5–6.0 kPa	34–45 mmHg
Hydrogen ion	37–45 nmol/L	pH 7.35–7.43
Bicarbonate	21–29 mmol/L	21–29 mEq/L
Oxygen saturation	>97%	

21.4 Normal values for hormones in venous blood

	Reference range	
Hormone	SI units	Non-SI units
ACTH, plasma	1.5–13.9 pmol/L (0700–1000 hours)	7–63 ng/L
Aldosterone		
Supine (at least 30 mins)	30–440 pmol/L	1.09–15.9 ng/dL
Erect (at least 1 hour)	110–860 pmol/L	3.97–31.0 ng/dL
Cortisol	Dynamic tests required–see Ch. 10	
FSH		
Male	1.0–10.0 IU/L	–
Female: *early follicular*	3.0–10.0 IU/L	–
postmenopausal	>30 IU/L	–
Gastrin (plasma, fasting)	<40 pmol/L	<83 pg/mL

i	**21.4 Normal values for hormones in venous blood—cont'd**	
	Reference range	
Hormone	SI units	Non-SI units
GH Dynamic tests usually required—see Ch. 10	<0.5 µg/L excludes acromegaly (if IGF-1 in reference range). >6 µg/L excludes GH deficiency	<2 mIU/L >18 mIU/L
Insulin	Highly variable with plasma glucose and body habitus	
LH		
Male	1.0–9.0 IU/L	
Female: *early follicular*	2.0–9.0 IU/L	
postmenopausal	>20 IU/L	
17β-Oestradiol		
Male	<160 pmol/L	<43 pg/mL
Female: *early follicular*	75–140 pmol/L	20–38 pg/mL
postmenopausal	<150 pmol/L	<41 pg/mL
PTH	1.6–6.9 pmol/L	16–69 pg/mL
Progesterone (luteal phase in women)		
Consistent with ovulation	>30 nmol/L	>9.3 ng/mL
Probable ovulatory cycle	15–30 nmol/L	4.7–9.3 ng/mL
Anovulatory cycle	<10 nmol/L	<3 ng/mL
PRL	60–500 mIU/L	2.8–23.5ng/mL
Renin concentration		
Supine (at least 30 mins)	5–40 mIU/L	–
Sitting (at least 15 mins)	5–45 mIU/L	–
Erect (at least 1 hour)	16–63 mIU/L	–
Testosterone		
Male	10–38 nmol/L	290–1090 ng/dL
Female	0.3–1.9 nmol/L	10–90 ng/dL
TSH	0.2–4.5 mIU/L	–
Thyroxine (free), (free T$_4$)	9–21 pmol/L	0.7–1.63 ng/dL

continued **21**

Hormone	Reference range	
	SI units	Non-SI units
Triiodothyronine (free), (free T$_3$)	2.6–6.2 pmol/L	0.16–0.4 ng/dL

Notes
1. Many hormones are unstable, and collection details are critical; refer to local guidance.
2. Interpretation depends on factors such as sex (e.g. testosterone), age (e.g. FSH in women), pregnancy (e.g. thyroid function tests, prolactin), time of day (e.g. cortisol) or regulatory factors (e.g. insulin/glucose, PTH/[Ca^{2+}]).
3. Reference ranges may be method-dependent.

21.5 Normal values in urine

Analyte	Reference range	
	SI units	Non-SI units
Albumin	See p. 211	
Calcium (normal diet)	Up to 7.5 mmol/24 hours	Up to 15 mEq/24 hours or 300 mg/24 hours
Copper	<0.6 µmol/24 hours	<38 µg/24 hours
Cortisol	20–180 nmol/24 hours	7.2–65 µg/24 hours
Creatinine		
Male	6.3–23 mmol/24 hours	712–2600 mg/24 hours
Female	4.1–15 mmol/24 hours	463–1695 mg/24 hours
5-HIAA	10–42 µmol/24 hours	1.9–8.1 mg/24 hours
Metadrenalines		
Normetadrenaline	0.4–3.4 µmol/24 hours	73–620 µg/24 hours
Metadrenaline	0.3–1.7 µmol/24 hours	59–335 µg/24 hours
Oxalate	0.04–0.49 mmol/24 hours	3.6–44 mg/24 hours
Phosphate	15–50 mmol/24 hours	465–1548 mg/24 hours
Potassium[a]	25–100 mmol/24 hours	25–100 mEq/24 hours
Protein	<0.3 g/L	<0.03 g/dL
Sodium[a]	100–200 mmol/24 hours	100–200 mEq/24 hours
Urate	1.2–3.0 mmol/24 hours	202–504 mg/24 hours
Urea	170–600 mmol/24 hours	10.2–36.0 g/24 hours
Zinc	3–21 µmol/24 hours	195–1365 µg/24 hours

[a]The urinary output of sodium and potassium reflects dietary intake and varies widely. The values quoted are for a 'Western' diet.

21.6 Normal values in CSF

Analysis	SI units	Non-SI units
	Reference range	
Cells	<5 × 10^6 cells/L (all mononuclear)	<5 cells/mm^3
Glucose[a]	2.3–4.5 mmol/L	41–81 mg/dL
IgG index[b]	<0.65	–
Total protein	0.14–0.4 g/L	0.014–0.045 g/dL

[a]Interpret in relation to plasma glucose. Values in CSF are approximately two-thirds of plasma levels.
[b]A crude index of increase in IgG attributable to intrathecal synthesis.

21.7 Normal values in faeces

Analyte	SI units	Non-SI units
	Reference range	
Calprotectin	<50 µg/g	–
Elastase	>200 µg/g	–

Index

Note: Page numbers followed by "f" indicate figures, "t" indicate tables, and "b" indicate boxes.